TEXTBOOK OF PULMONARY MEDICINE
VOLUME 2

ADVANCED RESPIRATORY PATHOLOGIES AND CRITICAL CARE PERSPECTIVES

Edited by:
Dr. Marie Hyacinth Chiong Tumara

ALLIED
HEALTH
PRESS

Textbook of Pulmonary Medicine Volume 2

Advanced Respiratory Pathologies and Critical Care Perspectives

Editor: **Dr. Marie Hyacinth Chiong Tumara**

Allied Health Press
4164 Lakeshore Road
Burlington ON L7L 1A4
Canada
www.alliedhealthpress.com
Email: orders@arclereducation.com

ISBN: 978-1-77956-813-7

ABOUT THE EDITOR

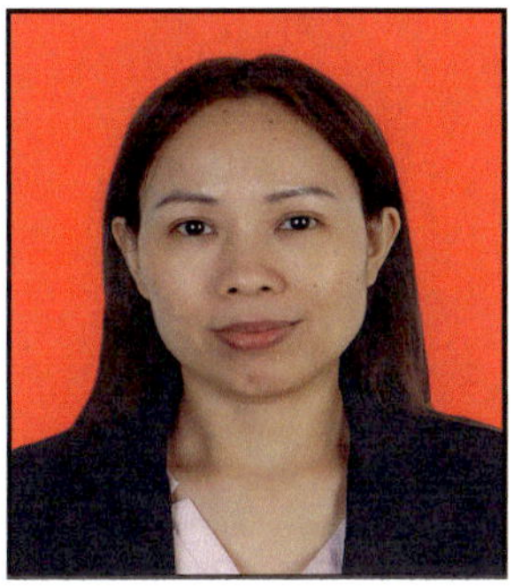

Dr. Marie Hyacinth Chiong Tumara, MD, FPCP, is an Internist with over 16 years of clinical practice and 11 years of government health service. She currently serves as Medical Director and OFW PEME Physician, with expertise in occupational and maritime medicine. A Fellow of the Philippine College of Physicians, she has authored research and medical reports and actively contributes to policy development in hospital and clinical settings. She is presently pursuing her Master's in Health and Hospital Management at Xavier University–Ateneo de Cagayan.

Brief Table of Contents

Getting Started with This Book

Chapter Openers

A list of Chapter Outline is presented providing a brief Introduction to what will be covered in the chapter.

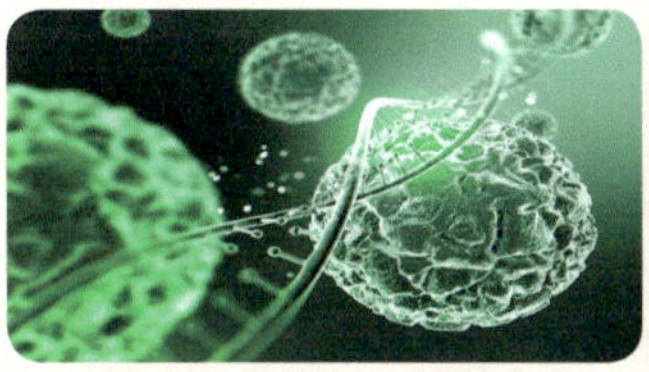

Introduction

Often referred to as the science of life, biology is a broad field of study aimed at comprehending the several kinds of life on Earth, from tiny creatures to sophisticated multicellular entities. Comprising several subfields, including molecular biology, ecology, and evolutionary biology, each of which advances our knowledge of living systems, this field clarifies the mechanisms controlling life events, including development, reproduction, and interaction with the surroundings, which is the central goal of biology. Moreover, biology fills in the void between the natural sciences and medicine by offering a necessary understanding of health, illness, and the interactions between organisms and their environments. Dealing with urgent global issues such as climate change, biodiversity loss, and new diseases depends on an awareness of these complex biological interactions, therefore highlighting the critical part biology plays in modern civilization. Fundamentally, biology explores and tests ideas about the living world using the scientific method. Through methodical observation and experimentation,

LEARNING OBJECTIVES

After studying this chapter, you will be able to:

1. Discuss the scientific method in biology;
2. Explain the cell theory;
3. Discuss the genetics and heredity;
4. Evolution and natural selection;
5. Focus on ecology and ecosystems;
6. Learn about human biology;
7. Evaluate the plant biology;
8. Explain the microbiology;
9. Focus on current trends in biology.

1.1. The Scientific Method in Biology

Learning Outcome

1. Describe the steps of the scientific method;
2. Focus on hypothesis formation;
3. Learn about experimental design.

Learning Outcomes

The beginning of each section of every chapter contains a set of Learning Outcomes that inform students of concepts they should understand. These outcomes help students understand what they should be able to do if they have mastered the material in that section.

Test Your Knowledge

Throughout each chapter, Test Your Knowledge cues you to note which topics have been covered and to self-test your understanding of the material presented.

Test Your Knowledge

1. Explain why correlation does not imply causation in scientific experiments.
2. How does the scientific method help reduce the influence of personal opinions in research?

Chapter Summary

The Summary Section appear at the end of each chapter and summarize main concepts covered throughout the chapter. These points provide key concepts in an engaging and meaningful way.

Summary

The investigation of biological principles highlights the importance of a comprehensive view of life by reflecting the intricate interactions that occur within living systems. The complexity of biology goes beyond individual species or systems, as this essay highlights; it also includes the interactions that mold ecosystems and affect biodiversity. Researchers can conduct in-depth analyses of metabolomic data using sophisticated technologies like MetaboAnalyst, which offer insights into the molecular mechanisms underlying these interactions. As demonstrated by the developments in MetaboAnalyst, for example, the integration of diverse omics data promotes a thorough understanding of metabolic pathways and helps identify important biological markers necessary for research on development and disease (Chong et al., 2018). Additionally, the phenomenon of ecological invasions is a key component of biological research and a vital field of study. The introduction of non-native species into unfamiliar habitats has significant ramifications and calls for multidisciplinary management strategies. Examining the origins and effects of these biological incursions, invasion science has become a crucial field that highlights the need to comprehend ecological dynamics and community interactions. As interest in biological invasions increases, new findings are emerging that put conventional ecological theories and practices to the test. The importance of incorporating various scientific viewpoints is shown by this developing discipline, which also highlights how invasive species shape ecosystems and advances our knowledge of ecological resilience (David et al., 2013). When taken as a whole, these discoveries from invasion science and metabolomics highlight the value of multidisciplinary biology research. Fostering cross-disciplinary collaboration and utilizing technological breakthroughs to improve our comprehension of intricate biological interactions are crucial as we look to the future of biological research. In addition to deepening our understanding of the complexities of life, this method lays the groundwork for tackling urgent environmental issues. Future studies can ensure the continued relevance of biology in a world that is constantly changing by acknowledging the interconnection of biological systems and opening the door to creative solutions that support sustainability and biodiversity conservation. We might imagine a thorough comprehension of life that serves both academia and society at large through ongoing investigation and integration of scientific knowledge.

Knowledge Assessment

The chapter includes material designed to review and reinforce each content. It includes Critical Thinking Questions to help test of your understanding of information presented in the chapter and Short answer Questions to review your understanding of the key concepts presented in the chapter.

Critical Thinking Questions

1. **Who is known as the "Father of Modern Biology"?**
   a. Aristotle
   b. Charles Darwin
   c. Gregor Mendel
   d. Louis Pasteur
2. **What is the basic unit of life?**
   a. Atom
   b. Molecule
   c. Cell
   d. Organism
3. **Which branch of biology studies the interaction of organisms with their environment?**
   a. Genetics
   b. Ecology
   c. Physiology
   d. Botany
4. **Which macromolecule is the main source of energy for living organisms?**
   a. Proteins
   b. Lipids
   c. Carbohydrates
   d. Nucleic acids
5. **DNA is primarily responsible for which function in living organisms?**
   a. Energy production
   b. Protein synthesis
   c. Storing genetic information
   d. Regulating body temperature

Short Answer Questions

1. What is biology, and why is it important to study biology?
2. What are the three main domains of life, and how are they different from one another?
3. Define homeostasis and give an example of how it works in living organisms.
4. What is the cell theory, and why is it fundamental to biology?
5. How do autotrophs and heterotrophs differ in the way they obtain energy?
6. What is the scientific method, and how is it applied in biological research?
7. Discuss how biology helps address global challenges such as climate change, disease, and food security.
8. Explain the levels of biological organization from the smallest unit to the largest. Provide examples at each level.
9. Describe the relationship between structure and function in biology, giving specific examples from cells or organs.
10. How has the discovery of genetics shaped our understanding of inheritance and variation among organisms?

Supplementary Materials

Key Terms: A list of key terms is given for quick reference

KEY TERMS FROM THIS CHAPTER

Annotation enrichment analysis	Biological structure	Cell
Cell theory	Cellular structure	Ecology
Ecosystems	Genetics	Human biology
Microbiology	Natural selection	Organism
Plant biology		

Further Resources: Recommendations for additional readings, websites, and multimedia resources.

References

1. Argelaguet, R., Velten, B., Arnol, D., Dietrich, S., Zenz, T., Marioni, J. C., Buettner, F., et al. (2018). Multi-omics factor analysis—A framework for unsupervised integration of multi-omics data sets. *Molecular Systems Biology, 14*. https://doi.org/10.15252/msb.20178124.
2. Bacher, S., Blackburn, T. M., Essl, F., & Genovesi, P. (2017). *Socio-Economic Impact Classification of Alien Taxa (SEICAT).* https://core.ac.uk/download/286567949.pdf (accessed on 8th March 2025).
3. Barnett, R., Brace, S., Cucchi, T., & Dobney, K. (2013). *Divergent Evolutionary Processes Associated with Colonization of Offshore Islands.* https://core.ac.uk/download/20664364.pdf (accessed on 8th March 2025).

Detailed Table of Contents

CHAPTER 5

Sarcoidosis and Pulmonary Vasculitides 143

CHAPTER 6

Lungs in Systemic Diseases 181

CHAPTER 7

Occupational and Environmental Lung Diseases 221

CHAPTER 8

Disorders of Pleura and MediastinalDiseases 259

CHAPTER 9

Disorders of the Diaphragm and Chest Wall 295

CHAPTER 10

Congenital Anomalies of the Respiratory System 331

CHAPTER 11

Lung Transplantation 365

LIST OF FIGURES

PREFACE

The respiratory system performs essential processes that sustain life by facilitating the exchange of gases, maintaining acid-base balance, and protecting the body from extrinsic insults. Over time, the complexity of pulmonary physiology and pathology has been uncovered through scientific observation and clinical experience. Understanding the mechanisms by which various factors cause lung dysfunction enables health workers to diagnose, treat, and manage a wide range of lung ailments. Respiratory diseases can affect not only lung anatomy but also produce a systemic effect, thus proving the coordination of pulmonary health and overall health.

Advances in diagnostic imaging, molecular biology, and treatments have expanded the range of clinical options for patients with respiratory system diseases. Even with this breadth, the specialty remains challenging due to disease heterogeneity, synergistic overlap of clinical presentations, and the necessity of individualized care approaches. Increasing awareness of occupational exposures, environmental factors, and genetic predisposition further underscores the necessity of comprehensive expertise in this area. In addition, transplantation medicine and critical care are rapidly developing specialties necessitating the most up-to-date expertise.

Textbook of Pulmonary Medicine – Volume 2 is a comprehensive handbook covering a broad spectrum of pulmonary diseases and their treatment. Volume 2 aims to add depth to core information with more advanced specialist fields relevant to high-level clinical practice and research. The book provides insight into disease mechanisms, diagnostic methods, and therapeutic options, all designed to help practitioners offer effective and informed treatment to patients.

Chapter 1 deals with cor pulmonale and pulmonary embolism, two conditions with significant cardiovascular and respiratory interactions. The chapter provides pathophysiology, clinical features, diagnostic approaches, and treatment for these serious conditions.

Chapter 2 focuses on acute respiratory distress syndrome (ARDS), a critical illness with an abrupt onset of respiratory failure and a multifaceted inflammatory reaction. The chapter deals with diagnostic criteria, supportive care, and new therapeutic interventions.

Chapter 3 addresses interstitial lung disease (ILD) and lung cancer, their pathogenesis, clinical presentation, diagnostic problems, and current management. It includes an introduction to fibrotic and inflammatory interstitial disease and bronchogenic carcinoma.

Chapter 4 broadens the ambit to pulmonary neoplasia other than bronchogenic carcinoma, describing less common tumors, their pathology, and clinical features.

Chapter 5 discusses sarcoidosis and pulmonary vasculitides, focusing on their systemic nature and lung involvement. The discussion points include diagnostic criteria, differential diagnosis, and immunomodulatory treatment.

Chapter 6 addresses lung involvement in systemic illnesses and illustrates how multisystem disease interferes with pulmonary function and requires integrated care.

Chapter 7 addresses occupational and environmental lung diseases, highlighting the significance of exposures in disease etiology. Chapter 7 reports on common agents, clinical presentation, preventive interventions, and therapeutic interventions.

Chapter 8 covers pleural and mediastinal diseases, including pleural effusions, pneumothorax, and mediastinal masses, and explains how to diagnose and treat them.

Chapter 9 addresses chest wall and diaphragm disorders with structural and functional defects affecting breathing.

Chapter 10 addresses congenital respiratory anomalies and discusses developmental defects, clinical presentation, and management options at different ages.

Chapter 11 is devoted to lung transplantation, covering indications, operative techniques, immunosuppression, and post-transplant care.

Chapter 12 addresses critical care in pulmonary medicine and briefly covers ventilatory support modalities, management of respiratory failure, and complications of critical illness.

This textbook is intended for pulmonologists, critical care clinicians, respiratory therapists, and residents seeking extensive information in pulmonary medicine beyond the basics. It is also beneficial for general practitioners and other health care professionals who manage patients with complex respiratory diseases. The chapters provide a synthesis of scientific evidence and clinical application to support decision-making across the many health care settings.

This book is an extensive resource that aims to increase knowledge, sharpen clinical expertise, and ultimately lead to improved patient outcomes within the area of respiratory medicine.

COR PULMONALE AND PULMONARY EMBOLISM

1

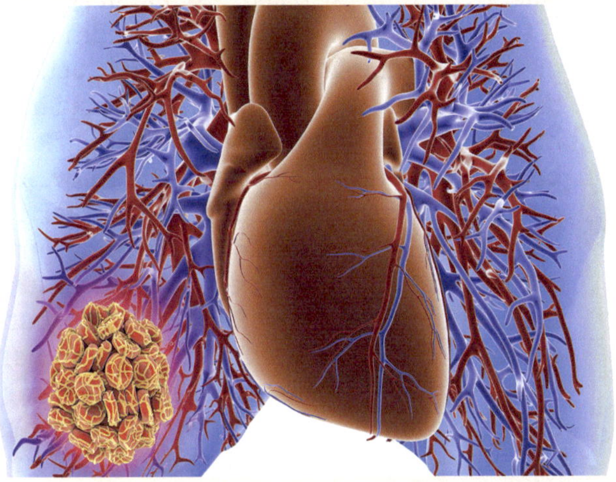

Introduction

The conditions of cor pulmonale and pulmonary embolism are severe pulmonary and cardiovascular disorders that are frequently accompanied by complex diagnostic and therapeutic issues. Cor pulmonale, or right ventricular hypertrophy secondary to pulmonary hypertension, typically develops as a result of lung parenchymal or vascular disease. Pulmonary embolism, however—a pulmonary arterial obstruction typically due to dislodged blood clots from peripheral veins—can result rapidly and produce abrupt respiratory failure or sudden death. The interplay between the two requires an intimate understanding of their pathophysiology, symptomatology, and the implications of delayed diagnosis and treatment. The diagnostic setting of pulmonary embolism is evolving as earlier methods of assessment, such as clinical history and imaging, are also being streamlined. New investigations have highlighted the diagnostic significance of electrocardiographic (ECG) changes, illustrating how some of them can uniformly signal pulmonary embolism. For instance, right ventricular

LEARNING OBJECTIVES

After studying this chapter, you will be able to:

1. Explain the pathophysiology of cor pulmonale.
2. Describe the pathophysiology of pulmonary embolism.
3. List the symptoms and clinical presentation.
4. Discuss the diagnostic approaches.
5. Explore the treatment options for cor pulmonale.
6. Understand the treatment options for pulmonary embolism.

strain patterns are strongly associated with pulmonary embolism and provide valuable clinical input in emergency settings. Accurate diagnosis, particularly in emergency cases, is crucial as it influences the management and outcome of the patient. Therefore, awareness of the subtle presentation of both pulmonary embolism and Cor pulmonale is essential to clinicians who aim to optimize patient care and improve overall survival.

Besides, advanced medical technology and diagnostic tools can enhance the detection of lung illnesses, thereby overcoming the limitation of the paucity of specialized medical experts. For example, sophisticated rule-based expert systems are being developed to assist primary care doctors in diagnosing complex pulmonary conditions, such as Cor pulmonale and pulmonary embolism. The systems utilize extensive patient data—including medical history, clinical findings, and imaging scan results—to facilitate timely decision-making. If properly integrated into clinical practice, these technologies have the potential to drastically reduce the burden of undiagnosed lung diseases, ultimately leading to better health outcomes for at-risk patients and those already suffering from Cor pulmonale or pulmonary embolism (Figure 1.1).

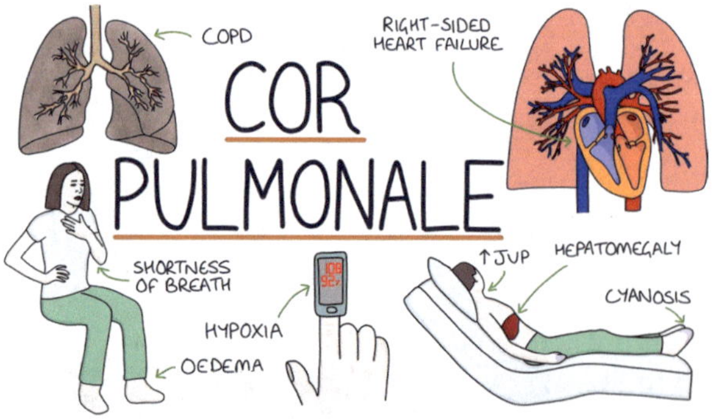

Figure 1.1. Understanding Cor pulmonale.

Source: https://i.ytimg.com/vi/GGkajjvMEAQ/maxresdefault.jpg.

Definition of Cor Pulmonale

Cor pulmonale is the alteration of the right side of the heart secondary to chronic pulmonary diseases, optimally defined by sustained pulmonary hypertension. Cor pulmonale is significant because it not only implies pathologic changes in the lung parenchyma but also involves the heart's compensatory response to increased vascular resistance. Pulmonary hypertension can be due to several causes, such as chronic obstructive pulmonary disease (COPD), pulmonary fibrosis, or conditions like pulmonary embolism that cause obstructions in the blood flow. The prevalence of Cor pulmonale highlights the complexity of the interplay between respiratory function and cardiovascular status, emphasizing the urgent need for early diagnosis and intervention to mitigate further occurrences. This interdependence illustrates the profound impact of chronic respiratory disease on cardiovascular mechanisms, necessitating treatment strategies that target both lung and cardiac health simultaneously. Chronic Cor pulmonale is one specific type of this disorder, which oftentimes arises insidiously from longstanding pulmonary disease, most commonly found in middle-aged and older adults. There is a strong association with smoking, which is a major risk factor in promoting primary pulmonary diseases, further leading to Cor pulmonale. In chronic Cor pulmonale patients, common underlying conditions are bronchiectasis, chronic bronchitis, and pulmonary tuberculosis sequelae. Systematic monitoring of patients often denotes current symptoms as a history of shortness of breath and long-standing coughing, supplemented by physical signs that are indicative of right heart overstrain. With new diagnostic imaging techniques, including chest X-ray and echocardiography, it is important to establish a diagnosis and assess the degree of right ventricular hypertrophy, thus the importance of an integrated process of patient assessment and management (Devi et al., 2009).

In addition, the clinical importance of Cor pulmonale extends far beyond the pulmonary system and has a substantial impact on the patient's overall morbidity and mortality. Due to the heart's compensatory mechanisms in response to increased pulmonary artery pressures, patients may initially be asymptomatic or exhibit non-specific signs and symptoms. However, as the disease advances, right heart failure symptoms become more pronounced and lead to complications such as edema and a reduction in respiratory function. Treatment of Cor pulmonale requires a greater understanding of its etiologic underpinnings and a multidisciplinary approach to halt the progression of worsening quality of life and prevent acute decompensation. Effective treatment would likely include pharmacologic intervention through the reduction of pulmonary pressures in addition to modifications in lifestyle, evidence of an integrated response to this intricate dance between lung and cardiac function (Bogun et al., 2017).

Definition of Pulmonary Embolism

It is important to study pulmonary embolism (PE) critically and thoroughly, discussing its definition, pathophysiology, and clinical significance. Pulmonary embolism, by definition, involves occlusion of pulmonary arteries mainly by thrombi, which are generally secondary to deep vein thrombosis (DVT). The consequence of such occlusions creates increased pulmonary vascular resistance and decreased blood flow, which eventually leads to serious cardiovascular malfunction. The clinical presentation of PE can be highly variable, from asymptomatic to significant ones, including chest pain, dyspnea, and syncope. Remarkably, symptom severity can be associated with embolus size and patients' underlying cardiopulmonary illnesses. The complexity of PE necessitates prompt identification and treatment to prevent the development of life-threatening situations, particularly where it coincides with developing Cor pulmonale, a state of right heart failure secondary to pulmonary disease. Pulmonary embolism is diagnosed using clinical assessment, imaging methods, and laboratory tests.

Clinical practice guidelines recommend using risk stratification techniques to estimate the likelihood of PE, so it is important for health care practitioners to thoroughly evaluate patients with risk factors such as recent surgery, immobilization, or malignancy. Confirmatory tests like computed tomography pulmonary angiogram (CTPA) and ventilation-perfusion scans are used to directly visualize the blockage and estimate the extent of vascular compromise. Additionally, there is a need to identify shock potential in PE patients, as circulatory collapse can occur quite rapidly. This association of PE with Cor pulmonale illustrates the pathophysiological mechanism of events initiated by right ventricle strain and progressing to heart failure, where the right heart becomes unable to cope with increased pulmonary artery pressure, ultimately impairing systemic circulation (Cecconi et al., 2014). Appreciation of the interaction between Cor pulmonale and pulmonary embolism necessitates an understanding of the wide-ranging implications for treatment outcomes and patient management. New therapies, including anticoagulation, thrombolysis, and surgery, are central to the management of PE. These therapies aim to lyse the clot and promote normal circulation, thereby avoiding the risk of ensuing right heart failure. As has been written about in recent publications, concerns with the management of PE do not stop with short-term treatment; long-term strategies must be utilized to prevent recurrence and ensure patient health. Also, concern regarding cardiovascular health, as set forth in initiatives from organizations such as the World Heart Federation and its demands for priority on preventive care and education within groups at risk for both PE and Cor pulmonale, underscores an equally important emphasis on prevention and education (Thygesen et al., 2012). This interprofessional approach to PE thus further emphasizes the necessity of dedicated clinical recommendations and patient-centered care in seeking improved outcomes (Figure 1.2).

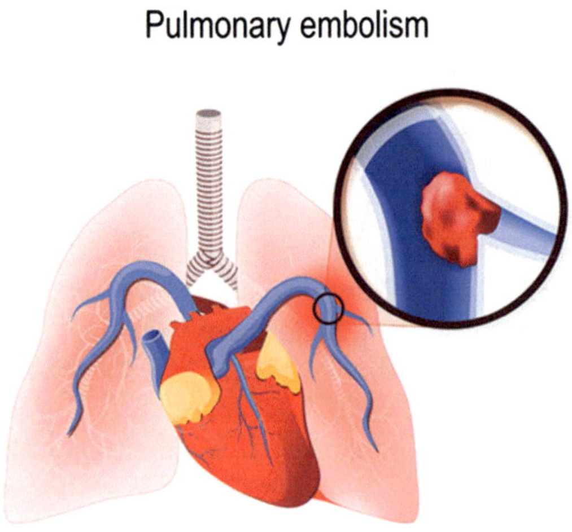

Figure 1.2. Pulmonary embolism.

Source: https://www.aapc.com/codes/webroot/upload/articles_pdf/2022/cca/2022-11-28_17-20-33.webp.

Importance of Understanding Both Conditions

Identification of pulmonary embolism and Cor pulmonale is necessary for an understanding of cardiopulmonary disorders to treat a patient appropriately. Cor pulmonale, or right heart failure resulting from lung disease, is generally a complication of conditions like COPD. Pulmonary embolism, typically caused by venous thromboembolism, tends to be acute and perilous as it is sudden in onset. Appreciation of the unique yet interrelated pathophysiologic processes of such diseases enables medical practitioners to establish treatment approaches tailored to the individual needs of the patient. Failure to comprehend these differences will lead to ineffective or inappropriate interventions, thus jeopardizing patient outcomes and further increasing the cost of care (Halvorsen et al., 2022). Furthermore, the interdependence of cardiopulmonary physiology necessitates a great deal of education and orientation for health professionals as well as health science students. One such example of the heart and lung interdependence is the way one system's pathology can adversely affect the other.

For instance, in patients with pulmonary embolism, abrupt interruption of pulmonary circulatory flow not only leads to increased right ventricular pressure but can also aggravate any pre-existing Cor pulmonale. Therefore, an intimate understanding of the system's dynamics reinforces the importance of evaluating symptoms and treatment modalities holistically. A schooling in this area plays a pivotal function in allowing clinicians to monitor change maximally, manage complications, and individualize patient care (Verhoeff et al., 2017).

Furthermore, through understanding of both Cor pulmonale and pulmonary embolism, health care providers are able to enhance their diagnostic capabilities and therapeutic interventions. Because their clinical presentations overlap, detecting signs and symptoms can expedite timely diagnoses, which are essential for successful interventions.

Delayed diagnosis of pulmonary embolism, for instance, can lead to catastrophic complications like sudden death, while undetected Cor pulmonale can manifest as progressing right heart failure. Hence, understanding the conditions is applicable beyond theoretical knowledge; it encompasses swift decision-making, patient education, and effective multidisciplinary collaboration in assisting patients diagnosed with life-threatening conditions. Hence, encouraging equitable understanding of both conditions is key to enhancing the care level in the healthcare system (Verhoeff et al., 2017).

1.1. Pathophysiology of Cor Pulmonale

Learning Outcome

1. Mechanisms leading to right heart failure;
2. Role of chronic lung diseases;
3. Impact of pulmonary hypertension.

Cor pulmonale pathophysiology is generally controlled by right ventricular (RV) dysfunction secondary to pulmonary hypertension, typically resulting from chronic respiratory illnesses, such as chronic obstructive pulmonary disease (COPD) and interstitial lung disease (ILD). Increased pulmonary vascular resistance due to these underlying diseases causes the right ventricle to sustain higher pressure overload, leading to hypertrophic responses to accommodate the augmented workload. Finally, this adaptation can lead to heart failure if the underlying respiratory condition is not well controlled. Worth noting is that acute exacerbation of these chronic diseases can accelerate the worsening of pulmonary hypertension to acute Cor pulmonale that will require urgent measures to decrease pressure in the RV and maintain appropriate hemodynamic stability (Comfere et al., 2008). In addition to the chronic presentation of Cor pulmonale, acute pulmonary hypertension worsens the course of patients with acute pulmonary embolism who have a sudden presentation. In these situations, an obstructing thrombus within a pulmonary artery can lead to a sudden increase in RV pressure, which can ultimately result in acute Cor pulmonale if the right ventricle cannot manage this acute overload. Acute right heart failure, caused by the inability of the right ventricle to accommodate, is characterized by systemic hypotension and shock. The mechanisms of acute pulmonary hypertension should therefore be well understood in the management of patients with pulmonary embolism. Treatment of these situations aims to reduce right ventricular overload and restore pulmonary perfusion. Overshoots in treatment could include using vasodilators for the lungs and providing inotropic support specifically tailored to the patient's hemodynamic pattern (Comfere et al., 2008). Furthermore, the pathophysiologic relationships between pulmonary embolism and Cor pulmonale are emphasized by the fact that both conditions significantly impact the heart's electrical characteristics.

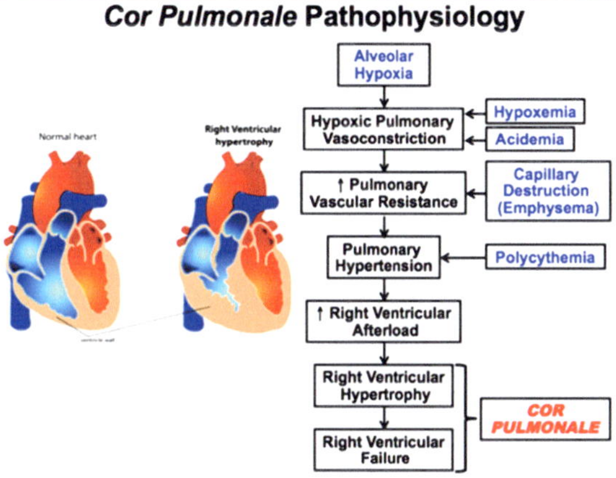

Figure 1.3. Pathophysiology of Cor pulmonale.

Source: https://external-content.duckduckgo.com/iu/?u=https%3A%2F%2Fo.quizlet.com%2FjeCdBLblnZzpItR8odM4hA.png&f=1&nofb=1&ipt=f14d8c555539c33242acde642adc0070a1b64c59733202a929b2ed4446a86089.

ECG changes in relation to Cor pulmonale, such as the presence of right-axis deviation and peaked P-waves (also known as P pulmonale), can be an index of the pathophysiologic processes involved. Electrocardiograms of patients with acute pulmonary illnesses, including COVID-19, have also shown profound arrhythmias and other changes in proportion to poor outcomes. Findings of such ECG abnormalities provide valuable prognostic information, making the incorporation of cardiovascular assessment in Cor pulmonale management, especially in the context of pulmonary embolism and other acute pulmonary syndromes, essential. An appreciation and understanding of these complex interrelationships are necessary to optimize patient outcomes in those with Cor pulmonale and complications (Figure 1.3).

1.1.1. Mechanisms Leading to Right Heart Failure

The intricate mechanisms leading to right heart failure, particularly in the case of Cor pulmonale and pulmonary embolism, are predominantly due to the increased workload on the right ventricle due to increased pulmonary artery pressure. COPD and pulmonary embolism cause pulmonary hypertension, with the right ventricle needing to create greater pressures to overcome vascular resistance. In COPD patients, the presence of pulmonary artery hypertension is a key factor in right ventricular dysfunction. It is linked with increased mortality and is hence of extreme significance to gain insight into these mechanisms (Mokhatar et al., 2018). The more sensitive right ventricle can then undergo remodeling and dilation, with the subsequent impairment of cardiac output and heart failure if not corrected. To the inherent complexity of the situation is added the sudden impact of pulmonary embolism, which is capable of suddenly increasing right ventricular afterload. This sudden pulmonary artery obstruction results in a sudden increase in pressure and puts the right ventricle to extreme strain. In acute cases, this will manifest as severe right heart strain, and echocardiographic examinations would reveal acute dilation and dysfunction of the right ventricle. High D-dimer and C-reactive protein levels can be used as biomarkers to quantify injury to the right ventricle in such patients (Mokhatar et al., 2018). Patients with pre-existing pulmonary disease, such as those presenting with acute respiratory distress syndrome (ARDS), may have added stress to the right heart. Thus, the interaction between acute pulmonary embolism and chronic disease is a dismal reminder of the importance of sustained cardiovascular function monitoring. Systemic inflammatory processes, such as those in COVID-19 and ARDS, only serve to add to the mechanisms of right heart failure. In COVID-19, pulmonary involvement is usual and is accompanied by serious impairment of the right ventricle, which might be linked with poor outcomes in these patients (Almarawi et al., 2020). The rise in inflammatory mediators can lead to myocardial stress and injury through various mechanisms, including direct viral injury, vasoconstriction induced by hypoxia, and thrombosis. These interactions increase pulmonary vascular resistance, simultaneously altering hemodynamic stability, creating a cycle that increases the chance of developing Cor pulmonale. Awareness of these intricate mechanisms will be required for planning strategies for treating and preventing right heart failure in patients with chronic and acute pulmonary disease (Figure 1.4).

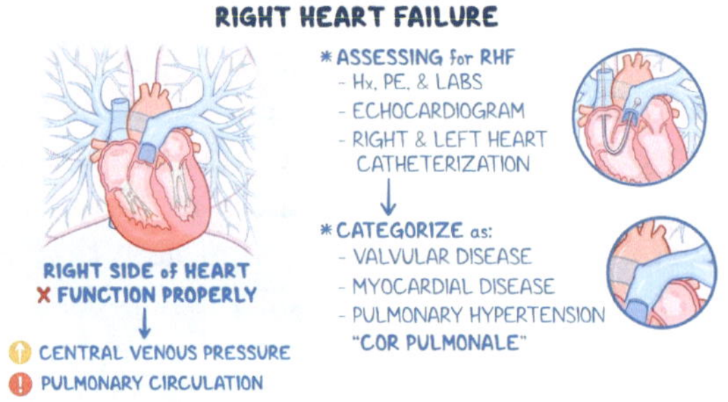

Figure 1.4. Mechanisms leading to right heart failure.

Source: https://www.osmosis.org/_next/image?url=https%3A%2F%2Fd16qt3wv6xm098.cloudfront.net%2FG-99sbibS5WWXNWvwDbNA2ohS0qymxqs%2F_.jpg&w=3840&q=75.

1.1.2. Role of Chronic Lung Diseases

Chronic pulmonary diseases, namely COPD and ILD, are significant culprits of the pathophysiology of Cor pulmonale. These conditions account for the long-term changes in pulmonary architecture and function, leading to chronically elevated pulmonary artery pressure. This elevated resistance to the pulmonary vessels progressively overloads the right ventricle, as it attempts to push blood through the non-compliant pulmonary vascular bed. For instance, in COPD patients, pulmonary hypertension develops as a consequence of the interaction among parenchymal lung damage, vascular remodeling, and hypoxia, which classifies these patients into increased mortality risk groups. Because COPD prevalence is generally underestimated, one should understand its impact on right ventricular function. The association between chronic lung diseases and Cor pulmonale development emphasizes the need for pulmonary condition control and early treatment to avoid cardiovascular complications (Mandoli et al., 2020). The significance of pulmonary hypertension (PH) in chronic lung diseases emphasizes the necessity for better diagnostic and therapeutic strategies. The interactive character of chronic lung disease and PH is a challenge to health professionals, most notably with PH occurring in various degrees of severity. Studies have indicated that mean pulmonary artery pressure (mPAP) in such patients typically does not exceed 30 mmHg; nonetheless, it acts as a final determinant of chronic lung disease morbidity and mortality. Etiologic factors to PH include parenchymal loss as a consequence of lung injury and consequent hypoxia, further entangling the disease picture. Therefore, chronic lung disease plays a role that transcends pulmonary symptoms, in association with systemic consequences such as right heart strain and failure, and ultimately Cor pulmonale (Opitz et al., 2018). Management of chronic lung disease is essential in the prevention of Cor pulmonale, and this involves an integrative approach addressing both pulmonary and cardiovascular health. While pharmacotherapy of PH in chronic lung disease remains scarce now, treatment of the underlying pulmonary disease can be beneficial. PH patients with severe disease might require referral to specialized facilities, which means these patients should be evaluated in pulmonary specialty centers. Also considering the potential benefits of lung volume reduction surgery can illuminate treatment complexity, since balance between improving lung mechanics and increasing pulmonary vascular resistance must be carefully measured. In conclusion, the treatment of the multifaceted implications of chronic lung disease not only aims to improve respiratory function but also strives to ensure right ventricular function is preserved, describing an integrated healthcare model (Mandoli et al., 2020).

1.1.3. Impact of Pulmonary Hypertension

The impact of pulmonary hypertension (PH) on Cor pulmonale is significant because it actually alters the hemodynamics in the pulmonary circuit. Increased pressure within the pulmonary arteries places a tremendous burden on the right ventricle to pump blood against this elevated resistance. This could lead to hypertrophy of the right ventricle and eventually right heart failure, clinically manifested as Cor pulmonale. The progression from pulmonary hypertension to Cor pulmonale is often insidious with few symptoms early on that are non-specific in character, such as exertional dyspnea and fatigue. Therefore, an equanimous understanding of the pathophysiological alterations propelling these changes is required in order to make an early diagnosis and act appropriately. Secondarily, identification of the relationship of pulmonary hypertension and Cor pulmonale assists in planning specific therapies to maximize patient outcomes and prevent irreversible heart failure. The interactive relationships between pulmonary embolisms and pulmonary hypertension add further complexity to the clinical presentation. Acute pulmonary embolism can cause right ventricular failure, acute Cor pulmonale, to arise when there is a sudden rise in the right ventricular afterload. This is particularly serious in situations of extreme acute respiratory distress or massive severe embolism when the acute cardiovascular dynamic effects are immediately lethal. Acute Cor pulmonale secondary to pulmonary embolism typically requires urgent, multidisciplinary care, including cardiology and pneumology, especially in intensive care units (ICUs).

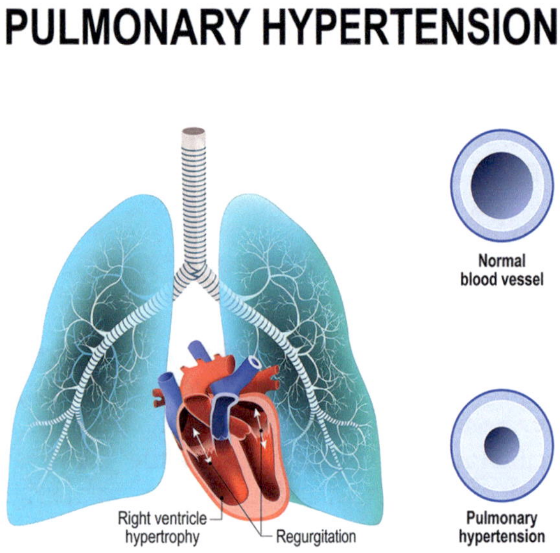

Figure 1.5. Right heart failure impact of pulmonary hypertension.

Source: https://external-content.duckduckgo.com/iu/?u=https%3A%2F%2Fdrraghu.com%2Fwp-content%2Fuploads%2F2021%2F02%2FPulmonary-Hypertension.jpg&f=1&nofb=1&ipt=a559323234d651a49a7755ddd2cbf9c3f22da71fe266a197d8dc6a549628bc92.

The COVID-19 pandemic made these concerns evident, demonstrating how the incorporation of integral care from various specialties impacts overall prognosis. Proper management regimens must be instituted to treat both acute and chronic presentations of pulmonary hypertension and its impact on the right heart. In addition, the diagnostic challenges caused by pulmonary hypertension necessitate careful evaluation methods. Because symptoms are similar between numerous other respiratory disorders, diagnosis is reliant on the use of more than one type of diagnostic approach. These include pulmonary function tests and imaging studies. Right heart catheterization remains the only gold standard for making an absolute diagnosis and assessing disease severity. As pointed out in cases of ILDs, the multisystemic nature of these diseases makes diagnosis challenging due to the convergence of clinical presentations of ILDs and pulmonary hypertension (Sijina et al., 2023). Therefore, a sense of urgency arises for developing maximally optimized diagnostic algorithms and management protocols that best counter the complexities introduced by pulmonary hypertension and its consequences, leading to improved patient care and therapeutic results (Figure 1.5).

Test Your Knowledge

1. What are the mechanisms leading to right heart failure?
2. What is the impact of pulmonary hypertension?

1.2. Pathophysiology of Pulmonary Embolism

Learning Outcome

1. Causes and risk factors;
2. Mechanisms of obstruction in pulmonary circulation;
3. Consequences of embolism on lung function.

Pathophysiologic mechanisms of pulmonary embolism (PE) represent a multi-factorial interaction of events leading to severe hemodynamic changes. On dislodgement of thrombus in deep veins and its migration into venous circulation to ultimately gain access to the pulmonary circuit, pulmonary artery occlusion is caused. This obstruction can cause a sudden increase in pulmonary vascular resistance, which in turn loads the right ventricle as it must deal with this increased pressure to achieve optimal circulation. The consequent right ventricular dysfunction can manifest clinically as Cor pulmonale, a clinical syndrome of secondary right heart failure resulting from pulmonary hypertension. This reveals the importance of understanding the evolution from venous thromboembolism to its impactful role in the cardiovascular system, emphasizing that treatment must account for both the embolic process and the acute right ventricular reaction (Klein, 2022). One of the most essential components of the pathophysiologic impact of PE is the resultant hypoxemia and hypercapnia due to impaired gas exchange. The occluded pulmonary arteries reduce blood flow to sections of the lung, preventing adequate oxygenation, thus leading to ventilation-perfusion mismatching. Mismatching exacerbates underlying pulmonary diseases, particularly COPD. For COPD patients, added stress from pulmonary embolism further compromises general respiratory function and increases the risk of deteriorating cardiac performance, particularly through progressive pulmonary arterial hypertension and Cor pulmonale. These experiences show that PE is not only an isolated incident but part of the continuum of cardiopulmonary pathophysiologic events and, therefore, highlights the importance of careful evaluation and management of such patients (Mokhatar et al., 2018). Furthermore, hemodynamic effects of PE may induce a cascade of systemic effect, which enhances the urgency of conditions. It has been demonstrated in investigations that acute PE is capable of producing various levels of right ventricular overload, which can progress to right heart failure if not treated. Elevated right ventricular pressure also jeopardizes left ventricular filling secondary to interventricular septal bowing, further threatening systemic circulation and oxygenation. This multi-organ manifestation indicates that the pathophysiology of pulmonary embolism exceeds immediate cardiovascular effects and presents in different forms such as syncope, hypotension, and respiratory distress. It is important for clinicians to realize these intricacies in identifying, diagnosing, and treating PE effectively and thereby reducing morbidity and mortality from this potentially lethal disorder (Klein, 2022) (Figure 1.6).

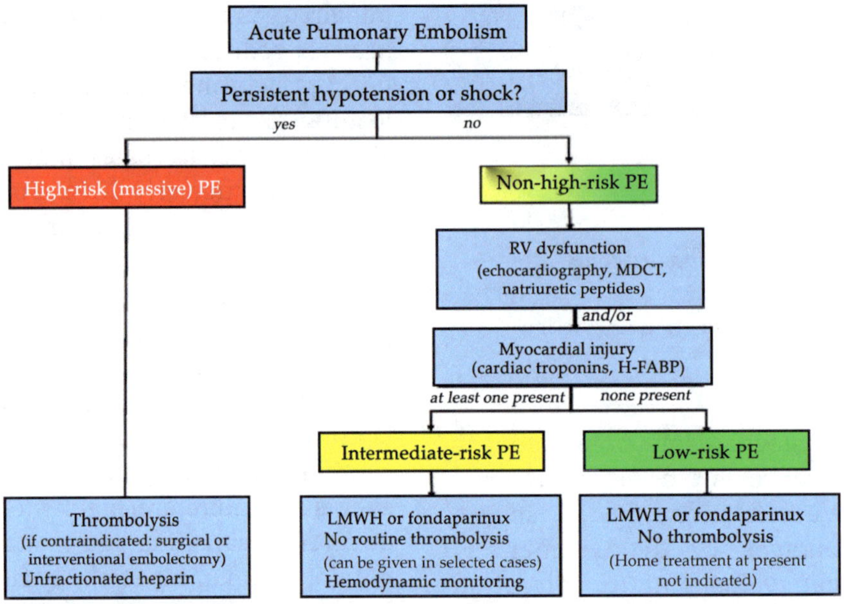

Figure 1.6. Pathophysiology of pulmonary embolism.

Source: https://external-content.duckduckgo.com/iu/?u=https%3A%2F%2Fimage.slidesharecdn.com%2Fptepptx-111013131310-phpapp01%2F95%2Fslide-36-1024.jpg&f=1&nofb=1&ipt=d456ff418f53545e6e7f1da49cc81415560558446709e607f4d1957b5ab2c0a6.

1.2.1. Causes and Risk Factors

Its onset, which is the alteration in right ventricular function due to pulmonary hypertension, is often precipitated by a variety of situations involving chronic lung disease. Among the significant causes is COPD, in which chronic inflammation and bronchial obstruction lead to elevated pulmonary artery pressure. This workload on the right ventricle results in cardiac muscle hypertrophy and remodeling. Other illnesses like ILD and sleep apnea also lead to elevated pressure in the right ventricle. Chronic hypoxia in these conditions worsens pathophysiologic changes, highlighting the need for prompt diagnosis and treatment of underlying pulmonary diseases for the prevention of Cor pulmonale. It is necessary to determine these risk factors because they directly relate to the onset of right heart failure and its complications in Cor pulmonale. Pulmonary embolism, an acute and severe manifestation of pulmonary hypertension, is due to the plugging of pulmonary arteries by thromboembolic material, most commonly due to deep vein thrombosis (DVT). Risk conditions for pulmonary embolism include immobilization of an extended duration, recent surgery, and conditions for underlying disease such as cancer or coagulopathies. All of these risk factors result in an increased tendency for thrombus formation that may continue to cause blockage of blood flow in the pulmonary vasculature. The sudden rise in pressure from the blocked arteries can result in sudden acute Cor pulmonale because the right ventricle cannot compensate for the increased resistance. The interaction between the above risk factors stresses the significance of preventive measures and active management interventions, particularly in high-risk individuals where such an event can be followed by life-threatening complications such as right ventricular failure and systemic hypotension. Apart from the above causes, other acute and chronic conditions may further predispose to the formation of Cor pulmonale and pulmonary embolism. Conditions such as pulmonary artery hypertension and left heart failure also increase stress on the right ventricle and facilitate a right ventricular dysfunction environment. Sudden elevations in pulmonary artery pressure often complicate ICU clinical courses and necessitate therapy to decrease these pressures prior to resulting catastrophic cardiac complications. For instance, treatments that reduce right ventricular afterload, such as using pulmonary vasodilators, play a key role in treating acute circumstances that could otherwise lead to right ventricular failure. Thus, identification of the overall scenario of causes and risk factors is crucial in the creation of effective management plans to avoid the harmful effects of these pulmonary complications as noted by recent literature (Cecconi et al., 2006; Comfere et al., 2008).

1.2.2. Mechanisms of Obstruction in Pulmonary Circulation

Obstructive mechanisms in pulmonary circulation are significant for an understanding of the pathophysiology of Cor pulmonale and pulmonary embolism. Obstructive events can lead to high pulmonary artery pressure, which is detrimental to right ventricular (RV) function. The RV is also designed to be capable of pumping blood into the pulmonary circulation, and any increase in outflow resistance, such as because of a pulmonary embolism, can lead to acute RV dilation. This dilation, along with reduced left ventricular filling, can cause a drastic reduction in cardiac output. With diminishing pulmonary vascular reserve, even subtle rises in pulmonary arterial pressure induce marked hemodynamic changes, ultimately resulting in right atrial hypertension and extremely limited exercise tolerance. Awareness of these dynamics emphasizes the importance of early recognition and therapy of pulmonary obstructions to prevent irreversible RV failure and adverse consequences, such as in Cor pulmonale. Moreover, COPD habitually causes progressive remodeling of the pulmonary vasculature, followed by resultant chronic obstruction. Over time, the heightened pulmonary artery pressure results in right ventricular hypertrophy as the heart attempts to compensate for the increased load due to higher pulmonary artery resistance. The RV adaptations include augmented contractility and vascular elastance modifications, which are transient solutions to a worsening problem. But when pulmonary arterial elastance becomes considerably greater than the capacity of the hearts to compensate, RV performance declines, leading to end-stage Cor pulmonale with marked increases in right atrial pressure. The interaction between chronic obstruction and the structural changes in the RV highlights that long-standing pulmonary disease must be treated with long-term treatment regimens that will abate pulmonary hypertension and enhance cardiac function. Inciting evidence also sets the position of systemic factors in pulmonary vascular occlusion. For instance, certain anticancer treatments are discovered to induce vascular toxicity, with the effect of harmful impacts on both arterial and venous systems, aggravating pulmonary challenges. Some targeted medications, despite being useful against cancer, act inadvertently on vascular pathways, leading to accumulating vascular remodeling and more occurrences of pulmonary embolism. Medications with increased cardiovascular risk may compromise both coronary and pulmonary circulation, with a delicate balance between malignancy treatment and cardiovascular deterioration. Extinction of the vascular side effects of such treatments is essential, as they significantly impact the incidence and severity of pulmonary obstruction, ultimately leading to the onset of Cor pulmonale in susceptible patients (Herrmann et al., 2016; Pinsky, 2016) (Figure 1.7).

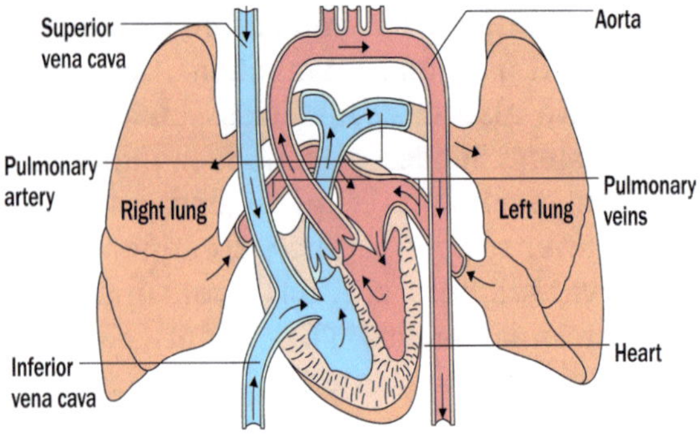

Figure 1.7. Pulmonary and systemic circulation pathway.

Source: https://external-content.duckduckgo.com/iu/?u=https%3A%2F%2Ft3.ftcdn.net%2Fjpg%2F01%2F13%2F31%2F56%2F360_F_113315637_pZU19H00IvvPqJidIZyNLFWvXq5LN2j2.jpg&f=1&nofb=1&ipt=3407bd198c00b86513f6be575d013f2c145a21fbdd02c10ee5c1083ff16b221b.

1.2.3. Consequences of Embolism on Lung Function

The consequences of embolism to lung function are serious, particularly when it is pulmonary embolism (PE) or obstruction in the pulmonary artery. The lack of blood flow to the lungs causes severe respiratory and cardiovascular conditions.

As the embolic zone of the lung becomes ischemic, capacity for adequate gas exchange decreases. Hypoxemia is often found in patients, with secondary shortness of breath and compromise of general pulmonary function. In addition, embolism may be complicated by acute inflammation leading to further exacerbation of lung injury and respiratory mechanics impairment, further enhancing respiratory distress. In severe instances, the resulting lung dysfunction can go on to acute Cor pulmonale, a right ventricular failure secondary to increased pulmonary vascular resistance. Moreover, the abrupt elevation of right ventricular afterload created due to embolic blockage is of critical significance to the function of the heart. The right ventricle of the heart will be required to compensate for increased pressure from the blocked pulmonary circuit, often leading to right ventricular failure. Right ventricular failure is not a solitary cardiac ailment; it illustrates the relationship between lung and heart. The right ventricular strain can lead to ventricular dilation and decreased cardiac output. Without prompt action, the process can proceed towards acute right heart failure, contributing to challenges in both lung function and systemic perfusion. As described, acute Cor pulmonale can occur with conditions like pulmonary embolism due to this sudden cardiac overload, necessitating careful monitoring of hemodynamics to guide proper measures to reduce the resulting pressure overload and prevent further complications (Cecconi et al., 2006). Furthermore, managing the augmented pulmonary artery pressure, a consequential effect of PE, presents significant clinical challenges.

Pressure increases can lead not only to compromised lung function but also to systemic events, including hypotension and decreased organ perfusion. Specifically, the approach to management must address the acute nature of the disorder; typical expectations of management in chronic pulmonary hypertension are not applicable. Instead, clinicians need to immediately employ measures for the reduction of right ventricular afterload and restoration of normal pressures. This can involve the use of pulmonary vasodilators and inotropic agents that are specifically tailored based on the patient's response. Monitoring is essential since acute pulmonary hypertension, if not treated, can lead to severe complications like right ventricular failure. Thus, prompt and accurate intervention must be made to prevent long-term impact on lung function and outcome of the patient (Comfere et al., 2008) (Figure 1.8).

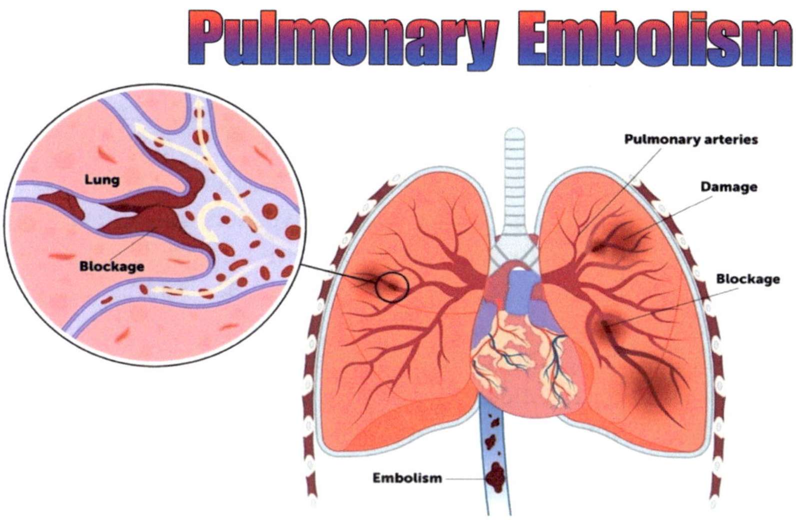

Figure 1.8. Consequences of embolism on lung function.

Source: https://external-content.duckduckgo.com/iu/?u=https%3A%2F%2Fdrsubhakarnadella.com%2Fwp-content%2Fuploads%2F2024%2F08%2FAdobeStock_558730161_copy-7783d25d7de04446ea5685b73e7d1755.webp&f=1&nofb=1&ipt=f4a72373a5b5aafeb25d5dd9b91b35011cf39c103349d2bf8747cf0eb69b9b34.

Test Your Knowledge

1. What are the causes and risk factors?
2. What are the mechanisms of obstruction in pulmonary circulation?

1.3. Symptoms and Clinical Presentation

Learning Outcome

1. Common symptoms of Cor Pulmonale;
2. Common symptoms of Pulmonary Embolism;
3. Differences in clinical presentation between the two conditions.

The presentation of pulmonary embolism (PE) and Cor pulmonale is typically with superimposable signs, and it is challenging to diagnose and therefore treat the patient. Cor pulmonale, characterized by right ventricular hypertrophy due to chronic lung disease, typically presents with dyspnea on exertion, chronic cough, and overall fatigue. In contrast, PE presents acutely with an acute type of dyspnea, pleuritic chest pain, and hemoptysis in a few cases. As both conditions have the potential to lead to right heart failure, discrimination is crucial to establish appropriate therapeutic intervention. Physical examination and clinical history are of the most importance, but diagnostic validity can be compromised by variations in the degree and pattern of symptoms between patients. Early diagnosis of pulmonary embolism is vital because it can have severe morbidity and mortality. Usually, patients with PE may present with tachycardia, dyspnea, or anxiety, all easily mistaken for more innocuous causes. The clinical diagnosis would generally involve the use of a variety of diagnostic agents, such as D-Dimer tests and imaging techniques such as computed tomography pulmonary angiography (CTPA). Surprisingly, it is learned that CTPA is the diagnostic gold standard for PE, yet it is not standardized everywhere, especially in underdeveloped regions. When this is so, other forms of diagnosis like the point-of-care ultrasound (POCUS) have been established, with sensitivity and specificity for the detection of PE, thus indicating the necessity for clinical flexibility (Melo et al., 2025). The presentation of Cor pulmonale, typically chronic and insidious, can overshadow the acute form of pulmonary embolism, thus indicating the necessity for risk stratification. Cor pulmonale patients can present with peripheral edema, ascites, and cyanosis, demonstrating worsening cardiac output. In contrast, the acute deterioration in PE can result in abrupt collapse or syncope. A diagnostic compliance audit for PE shows that while D-Dimer testing is widely utilized, there is an evident need for greater guideline concordance, particularly in complex presentations where Cor pulmonale and PE may present together (Daud et al., 2025). These results are crucial not only for improving patient diagnostic processes but also for maximizing the understanding of the interrelated clinical manifestations of these severe pulmonary ailments.

1.3.1. Common Symptoms of Cor Pulmonale

The clinical presentation of Cor pulmonale is usually characterized by the onset of worsening dyspnea. If the right ventricle is subjected to increased pressure due to pulmonary hypertension, the patient will experience shortness of breath with exertion. This dyspnea, over time, can progress to become severe at rest, limiting activity severely. Some patients may even acquire orthopnea, exacerbation of pain on recumbency, which is more likely to lead to sleep disturbances. These symptoms are often mistakenly attributed to other chronic respiratory or cardiac diseases, so they are difficult to diagnose early. Therefore, being aware of these patterns is important for health care workers because early recognition improves patient outcomes. Moreover, the progressive nature of such symptoms necessitates a proper investigation of contributing underlying pulmonary conditions resulting in Cor pulmonale, as evident from several case reports emphasizing the significance of proper diagnosis and management protocols for effective treatment (Aínguez-López et al., 2024). Apart from dyspnea, peripheral edema is another salient symptom of Cor pulmonale that occurs primarily due to right-sided heart failure. Because the right ventricle cannot hold the increased load from pulmonary circulation, pressure rises in the venous system, and fluid leaks into the surrounding tissue. Water retention in the lower extremities, particularly ankles and feet, leads to pain in patients and further compromises mobility. The amount of edema correlates with the progression of Cor pulmonale, which typically manifests as an overt sign of worsening heart function. The physician should be attentive to this symptom, particularly in patients at risk such as those with COPD. Awareness of how respiratory disease may lead to Cor pulmonale will be incredibly valuable in the formulation of targeted treatments to reverse such unsettling symptoms (Osakwe et al., 2022). Aside from dyspnea and peripheral edema, exertional symptoms and fatigue are common among Cor pulmonale patients. With progression of the disease, the patients complain of fatigue and diminished exercise tolerance, a reflection of the impaired ability of the heart to pump effectively. This is not only due to reduced oxygenation resulting from defective pulmonary function but also due to the body's compensatory responses to cardiac inefficiency. Patients may experience mundane everyday tasks becoming challenging, potentially leading to psychosocial consequences such as anxiety and depression. Fatigue is thus treated as a significant symptom by appropriate evaluation of patient history, exercise levels, and overall impact on quality of life. Thus, a holistic approach taking into consideration both physiological symptoms as well as psychological status is essential in optimally managing patients with Cor pulmonale (Aínguez-López et al., 2024) (Figure 1.9).

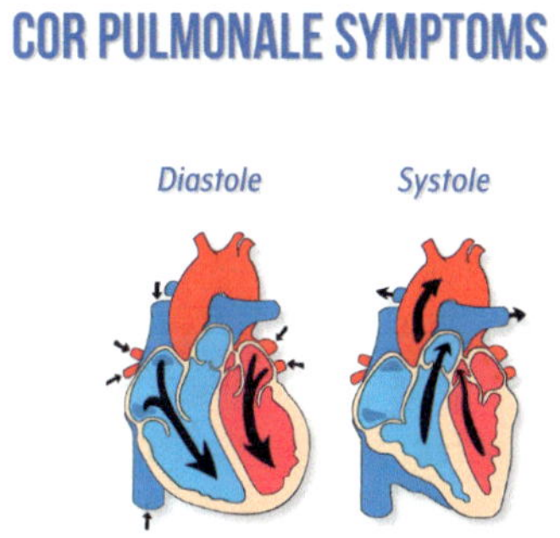

Figure 1.9. Symptoms of Cor pulmonale.

Source: https://external-content.duckduckgo.com/iu/?u=https%3A%2F%2Fi.ytimg.com%2Fvi%2Fi9cq-m39cbc%2Fmaxresdefault.jpg&f=1&nofb=1&ipt=6dfef2a15d82cabaecfc3c8313e880f38ab0d015926d7eaca9a356fce9a2553c.

1.3.2. Common Symptoms of Pulmonary Embolism

Pulmonary embolism (PE) is defined by a variety of symptoms that may have a significant impact on prognosis. Breathlessness is usually the initial presentation with a sudden onset, either at exertion or at rest. The symptom arises as a result of pulmonary artery obstruction, leading to deficient blood flow and attendant hypoxia. Sharp and pleuritic chest pain is yet another common presentation of PE since it can occur due to secondary pleural irritation due to impaired blood supply. The patient will also have symptoms such as cough, which may be productive and, in some cases, cause hemoptysis, further complicating the clinical picture. It is necessary to recognize these symptoms for early diagnosis, especially considering that overlapping signs in patients with other pulmonary illnesses, such as COPD, can hinder PE diagnosis (Liu et al., 2023). Clinical presentation of pulmonary embolism in the majority of instances is nonspecific and can mimic other illnesses, which results in potential underdiagnosis. For instance, patients may have manifestations of extreme anxiety or distress due to hypoxic episodes, which also makes certain diagnoses complicated. Edema of lower limbs is also a feature of PE, particularly if PE is secondary to DVT, and hence correct patient assessment through physical examination for potential thrombotic complications is most essential. Elevated biomarkers, such as D-dimer, are also useful in confirming a diagnosis, given that raised levels may indicate the existence of a thromboembolic episode. Familiarity with these interrelated symptoms is valuable, especially among medical practitioners working with groups with high risk factors for PE, such as patients with past COPD or long-term immobilization (Liu et al., 2023). The urgency of early detection of pulmonary embolism symptoms cannot be overemphasized, given the nature of the condition's potential for rapid deterioration and consequent complications. Common symptoms such as pallor, tachycardia, or hypotension can manifest in more severe cases, indicating a severe condition that requires immediate medical intervention. These hemodynamic instabilities may serve to foster a vicious cycle, exacerbating underlying conditions like Cor pulmonale, in which right ventricular strain worsens the clinical presentation. The association of PE and Cor pulmonale underscores vigorous management strategies in at-risk patients. Clinicians should remain vigilant when diagnosing such symptoms, as timely intervention may significantly improve prognosis, and, therefore, teaching healthcare professionals how to recognize PE signs is a crucial part of healthcare education and patient treatment (Figure 1.10).

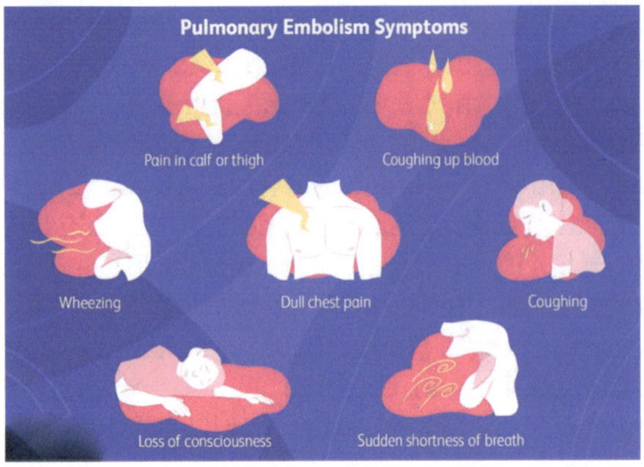

Figure 1.10. Symptoms of pulmonary embolism.

Source: https://external-content.duckduckgo.com/iu/?u=https%3A%2F%2Fwww.verywellhealth.com%2Fthmb%2FGGB5yku1HpVLODD3q2xcpj0u614%3D%2F1100x0%2Ffilters%3Ano_upscale()%3Amax_bytes(150000)%3Astrip_icc()%2Fsymptoms-of-pulmonary-embolus-4163779_final-3a9c69d8313f48ccb5bd880da18ca168.jpg&f=1&nofb=1&ipt=9a94a9319fd29e542a7baa52503edecabbf3c037087d80e0bff3fc1d6057a7c1.

1.3.3. Differences in Clinical Presentation Between the Two Conditions

The clinical presentations of Cor pulmonale and pulmonary embolism (PE) are diametrically opposite, reflecting the pathophysiologic processes responsible for these two conditions. Cor pulmonale, defined as right ventricular hypertrophy and failure secondary to chronic pulmonary hypertension, is characterized by the gradual development of symptoms. Patients have worsening dyspnea, fatigue, and signs of right heart failure such as peripheral edema and jugular venous distension. This devious progression allows the patient to adapt to declining health, and symptoms may be attributed to other chronic pulmonary illnesses. Sudden and dramatic presentation, on the other hand, is the hallmark of pulmonary embolism. Patients typically arrive with abrupt onset of dyspnea, pain, or syncope resulting from abrupt halt in pulmonary blood flow. These striking differences in onset and clinical course of symptoms suggest the need for individualized management and diagnostic approaches to the two disorders. Proceeding to analyze the clinical presentation further, the most frequent symptoms of pulmonary embolism strikingly contrast with those of Cor pulmonale. Most PE patients reported sudden onset dyspnea (81% and 78% in two different studies), then chest pain (56% and 39%), followed by syncope (26% and 22%) (Cenci et al., 2012).

The above symptoms are typically acute and need emergency medical care. However, Cor pulmonale patients may have chronic respiratory symptoms, which may be misattributed to other underlying illnesses, such as COPD. While patients with chronic pulmonary disease can have evidence of Cor pulmonale, both systemic complications and no acute dramatic clinical changes as with pulmonary embolism, this inconsistency must be evaluated entirely because misdiagnosis can significantly impact patient treatment. In addition, the clinical presentations of the disease vary in their potential predictive factors and complications.

For instance, in Cor pulmonale, the chronicity of the disease typically results in secondary complications such as exercise intolerance and effects of right heart failure on the systemic level, which are not always easy to identify. The patients progressively evolve into an increasingly symptomatic state, predisposing them to more complex medical problems later on. On the other hand, pulmonary embolism is an acute hazard with a potential for acute worsening from right ventricular overloading, especially in cases of massive or multiple embolism. Symptoms of systemic hypotension and even shock may follow in severe situations, and intervention should be instantaneous (Comfere et al., 2008). Recognition of such differences in clinical presentation is valuable to medical professionals to ensure the optimal early detection, intervention, and treatment designs tailored to the individualized features of each disorder.

Test Your Knowledge

1. What are the common symptoms of Cor pulmonale?
2. What are the common symptoms of pulmonary embolism?

1.4. Diagnostic Approaches

Learning Outcome

1. Diagnostic tests for Cor Pulmonale;
2. Diagnostic tests for Pulmonary Embolism;
3. Importance of differential diagnosis.

Effective diagnostic tools for Cor pulmonale and pulmonary embolism (PE) are crucial due to the severity of these conditions. Cor pulmonale, as right ventricular failure due to pulmonary hypertension, necessitates expert testing methods. Physical examination and clinical history provide initial assessment in most instances, which may be followed by symptoms such as peripheral edema or jugular venous distension. However, imaging modalities, particularly echocardiography, play a significant role in making the diagnosis by assessing right ventricular size and function. Chest X-rays can also uncover underlying lung disease or abnormalities, whereas computed tomography (CT) pulmonary angiography is still the gold standard for PE diagnosis. Accurate diagnosis is crucial as it dictates therapy choices and results. To this end, an understanding of the entire spectrum of diagnostic workup is essential, particularly since early therapy can significantly reduce mortality due to these conditions. The workup in pulmonary embolism often involves a multidirectional diagnostic approach to properly stratify risk and select therapies. While clinical evaluation is extremely relevant, the inclusion of laboratory work, such as the D-dimer assay, contributes to diagnostic workup. Elevated D-dimer levels are suggestive of thrombosis but must be interpreted alongside clinical findings and imaging. Imaging in high-risk patients is important; CT pulmonary angiography is fast and accurate in imaging vascular obstruction. Bedside ultrasound may also be a helpful adjunct, particularly in urgent cases where routine imaging may be limited. The ability of ultrasound to diagnose tension pneumothorax or right ventricular strain further highlights its use in acute situations. Thus, early and correct diagnosis not only affects management but also enhances the scope for better clinical outcomes in involved patients with such life-threatening conditions (Ahmad et al., 2017). In keeping with the intricate relationship between Cor pulmonale and pulmonary embolism, the importance of diagnostic methods cannot be overemphasized. The double jeopardy of such pulmonary and cardiac complications requires a clear understanding of their pathophysiology for proper diagnosis. Right ventricular strain, typically precipitated by a significant pulmonary embolism, can arise through many clinical parameters that need to be carefully evaluated. Echocardiography remains the prime diagnostic modality for evaluating right ventricular enlargement and dysfunction, thus directing further therapeutic interventions. Also, there is a need for new imaging technologies and diagnostic parameters in the rapidly evolving world of pulmonary medicine. Using the most up-to-date evidence-based practices can optimize risk stratification and timely interventions, thereby decreasing morbidity and mortality rates resulting from these diseases. The critical review of current diagnosis tools available to medical professionals continually redefines treatment models, eventually leading to better patient care (Bellis et al., 2018) (Figure 1.11).

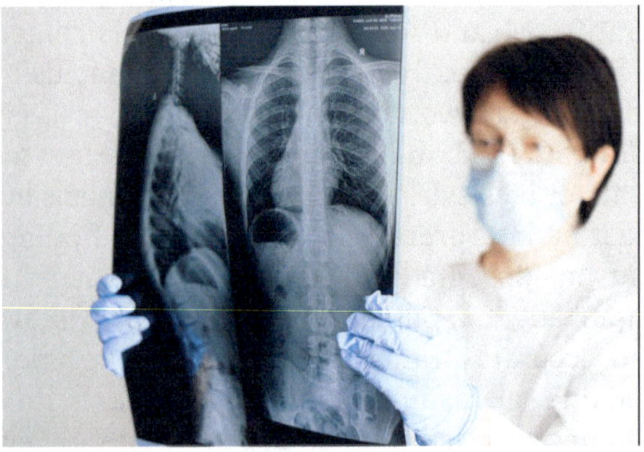

Figure 1.11. Diagnostic approaches of Cor pulmonale.

Source: https://external-content.duckduckgo.com/iu/?u=https%3A%2F%2Fcdn.idntimes.com%2Fcontent-images%2Fcommunity%2F2023%2F07%2Fpexels-anna-shvets-4225923-d4489bb130503f3025efedb692274be1-b36128e13b41ed05fb47228f4257b6b4.jpg&f=1&nofb=1&ipt=846579b4e2d860f51d19673562785efed29413741a2247640bd27f7fab6e9753.

1.4.1. Diagnostic Tests for Cor Pulmonale

Assessment of Cor pulmonale, particularly in cases of pulmonary embolism (PE), requires an extensive diagnostic approach. Pulmonary function tests like spirometry typically constitute the first part of the evaluation of patients with suspected Cor pulmonale. They can detect COPD or other underlying pulmonary diseases that lead to Cor pulmonale. Along with pulmonary function tests, arterial blood gas analysis is equally crucial as it provides information about arterial oxygen and carbon dioxide levels, which can indicate hypoxia or respiratory acidosis in patients with compromised pulmonary function. Combined, these tests provide an underlying understanding of the patient's respiratory status that becomes paramount for subsequent diagnostic steps aimed at establishing Cor pulmonale. Electrocardiography (ECG) is both a primary and a valuable diagnostic tool for the diagnosis of Cor pulmonale. PE patients particularly present with typical ECG results, though most will be normal on ECG at the time of diagnosis. The most frequent abnormality in PE patients is sinus tachycardia, as identified in Hrobar et al. (2019), but this alone is nonspecific. The diagnosis of right ventricular (RV) strain is more specific and occurs more frequently among those with a positive CTPA for PE. The sensitivity and specificity of an ECG in the presence of RV strain in patients presenting with dyspnea further confirm its diagnostic utility in this context. Its utility in the diagnosis of Cor pulmonale secondary to PE should hence be used cautiously and with clinical presentation. Imaging tests such as echocardiography and CTPA play a critical role in diagnosing Cor pulmonale and assessing the underlying conditions, such as PE. Echocardiography allows for assessment of right ventricular size and function, providing vital feedback on the stress placed on the heart by pulmonary hypertension. Furthermore, CTPA plays a critical role in monitoring occlusions of pulmonary arteries and correlating observations directly with the diagnosis of PE. The ability to image alterations in the right heart dynamics, coupled with angio-CT imaging features of PE, constitutes an entire diagnostic process. This combination of modalities verifies suspicion of Cor pulmonale and allows targeted management of the underlying pulmonary pathology, ultimately resulting in better patient outcomes in Cor pulmonale due to PE (Figure 1.12).

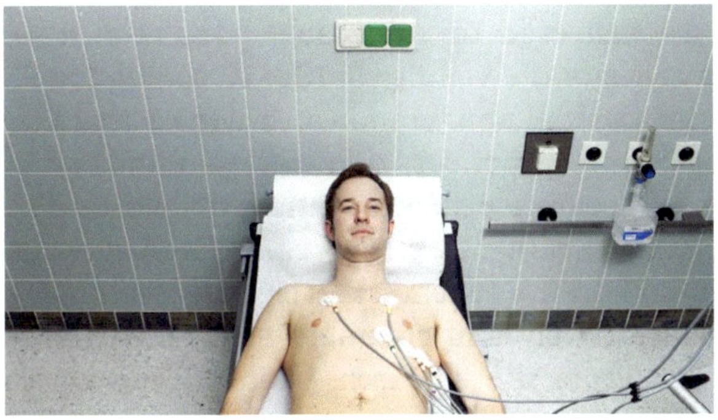

Figure 1.12. Diagnostic tests for Cor pulmonale.

Source: https://i0.wp.com/post.medicalnewstoday.com/wp-content/uploads/sites/3/2021/04/EKG-Male-Doctor-1296x728-Header-1024x575.jpg?w=1155&h=1528.

1.4.2. Diagnostic tests for Pulmonary Embolism

Diagnosing pulmonary embolism (PE) is crucial in managing underlying conditions for Cor pulmonale and involves using various tests to determine the presence and size of the embolism. The D-dimer test is a critical in PE diagnosis, a fibrin degradation biomarker that is usually present in high concentrations in patients with thromboembolism. It is highly sensitive and thus can be applied to rule out PE in low-risk patients. But its specificity is not clearly established; thus, its increase in other conditions too is feasible. Thus, imaging modalities such as CT pulmonary angiography (CTPA) have become a gold standard for diagnosing PE. CTPA not only provides a direct visualization of clots still within the pulmonary arteries but also assists with assessing the overall pulmonary vascular status, which is relevant in managing sequelae of both PE and Cor pulmonale (Halvorsen et al., 2022). Another important diagnostic tool for PE is the use of ultrasound to assess DVT, which typically functions as a precursor to pulmonary embolisms. Compression ultrasonography is the clinician's go-to for detecting DVT in the lower extremities, allowing clinicians to link clots in peripheral veins and potential pulmonary complications. Those results that are positive for DVT mandate further study for PE, usually by CTPA or ventilation-perfusion (V/Q) scans; the latter particularly useful in situations where contrast material is not feasible. V/Q scans also assess airflow and blood flow distribution in the lungs and offer information about regional ventilation and perfusion abnormalities associated with embolic disorders. Identification of V/Q mismatch patterns has the potential to revolutionize treatment and influence the management of patients with Cor pulmonale (Cecconi et al., 2014).

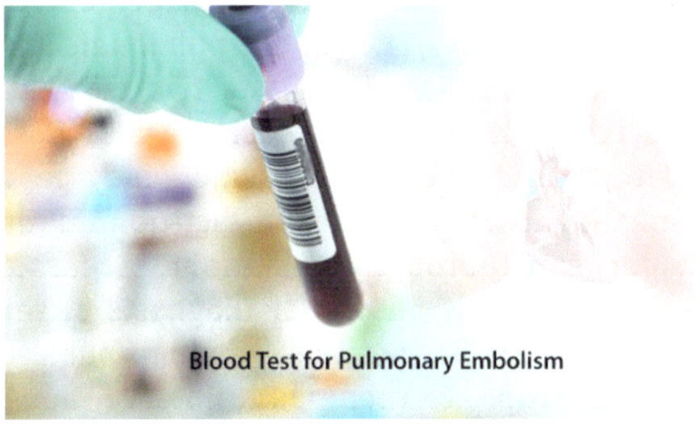

Figure 1.13. Blood test for pulmonary embolism.

Source: https://external-content.duckduckgo.com/iu/?u=https%3A%2F%2Fwww.healthcheckup.com%2Fwp-content%2Fuploads%2F2019%2F10%2FBlood-Test-for-Pulmonary-Embolism1.jpg&f=1&nofb=1&ipt=2db5a99e42a818542b58addd6b82bacc1a3893309e338c0ae459d6f7faa34c0f.

In addition to the previously mentioned tests, ECG changes can provide ancillary data regarding the effect of PE on cardiac function, particularly in those who progress to Cor pulmonale. For instance, yours can have evidence of right ventricular strain on the ECG, for instance, right axis deviation or other alterations that are in keeping with right heart overload. ECG does not diagnose PE, but these alterations may be employed as pointers to avert further evaluation. Moreover, the inclusion of clinical probability models, such as the Wells score, can be useful to stratify the likelihood of PE in patients with respiratory distress or other PE-suggestive symptoms. This combined process of biochemical, imaging, and clinical assessment facilitates a comprehensive diagnostic process, hence enabling early and effective treatment of pulmonary embolism and its implications on Cor pulmonale (Halvorsen et al., 2022) (Figure 1.13).

1.4.3. Importance of Differential Diagnosis

The practice of differential diagnosis plays a crucial role in the clinical management of pulmonary diseases, such as Cor pulmonale and pulmonary embolism (PE). The two diseases share common symptoms such as shortness of breath and chest pain, which may lead to misdiagnosis if medical practitioners do not perform thorough evaluations. Accurate diagnosis not only allows for diagnosis of the primary cause of the patient's symptoms but also directs appropriate therapeutic interventions. For instance, incorrect diagnosis of PE as acute coronary syndrome may result in inappropriate treatment, which could interfere with patient safety and outcome. Thus, professionals are required to be competent in differentiating such serious conditions from one another so that respective proper and timely interventions can be provided, emphasizing the importance of an accurate differential diagnosis in clinical practice, and ongoing education for professionals about the nuances of such complex cases. A differential diagnosis has implications that extend beyond individual patient care and affect healthcare systems at large. Strategic diagnosis of conditions like PE and Cor pulmonale can inform and guide resource allocation, maximizing the quality of care delivered to vulnerable populations. An analysis of the validity of ICD-10 coding for PE with Cor pulmonale indicates wide variability in coding practices, and only a minority of cases accurately identify patient diagnoses. The findings highlight a critical connection between administrative function and clinical assessment, where timely and complete documentation is vital. From the research, while ICD-10 codes for PE with Cor pulmonale are highly specific, they exhibit low sensitivity and positive predictive value, which impacts studies and quality improvement projects to know more about such conditions in a wider scope (Bejjani et al., 2023). In clinical diagnosis, differential diagnosis is a critical instrument that enables the differentiation of underlying conditions and adjustment of treatment protocols accordingly. For instance, a case illustrating the diagnostic challenge of differential diagnosis between PE and acute coronary syndrome underscores the necessity for complete workups involving cardiac biomarker testing and imaging studies (Rao et al., 2025). The use of a multidisciplinary team not only enhances the likelihood of a correct diagnosis but also provides improved patient outcomes. The ability to make a correct diagnosis might lead to the application of certain treatments aimed at the precise etiology of an individual's condition, emphasizing the point that effective management hinges on correct medical identification. Lastly, the importance of differential diagnosis in both Cor pulmonale and pulmonary embolism cannot be overstressed, as it is central to delivering quality healthcare and ensuring maximum patient safety.

Test Your Knowledge

1. What are the diagnostic tests for pulmonary embolism?
2. What is the importance of differential diagnosis?

1.5. Treatment Options for Cor Pulmonale

Learning Outcome

1. Pharmacological interventions;
2. Lifestyle modifications and management;
3. Surgical options and their indications.

Management of Cor pulmonale demands a two-pronged approach: correcting both the intrinsic pulmonary disease and the secondary right ventricular failure. Initial treatment may involve optimization of oxygen therapy, particularly for COPD or other respiratory conditions that compromise pulmonary function. Supplemental oxygen is useful in correcting hypoxemia, thereby reducing the workload on the right ventricle. Secondly, bronchodilators are typically advocated to enhance airflow and reduce airway resistance, ultimately enhancing oxygen delivery. The interdependence between lung function and ventricular performance suggests that by addressing respiratory complications, clinicians can indirectly improve the hemodynamic loads associated with Cor pulmonale, thereby enhancing functional capacity and quality of life in patients. Because right ventricular failure is a potential consequence of acute increases in afterload, as would occur in the context of pulmonary embolism, immediate and appropriate intervention is paramount. Thrombolytic therapy is an essential treatment during the acute presentation of lytic blood clots that occlude pulmonary arteries, thereby decreasing elevated pulmonary vascular resistance. Surgical interventions, such as open pulmonary embolectomy, are also significant in severe cases of thrombolysis failure or contraindication. Surgical indication includes a clear presentation of hemodynamic instability with right ventricular failure, emphasizing the significance of prompt diagnosis and intervention to attain appropriate hemodynamic stability. Application of these measures not only alleviates the acute crisis but also provides a mechanism for long-term management of Cor pulmonale within the framework of an overall care plan. The application of drugs to reduce right ventricular afterload, such as pulmonary vasodilators, plays a major role in the management of chronic Cor pulmonale. These treatments can enhance pulmonary blood flow and thereby improve right ventricular function.

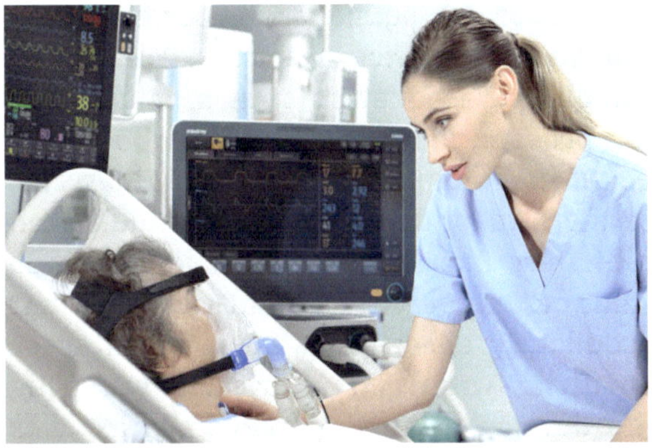

Figure 1.14. Treatment options for Cor pulmonale.

Source: https://external-content.duckduckgo.com/iu/?u=https%3A%2F%2Fwww.10faq.com%2Fassets%2Fimg%2Fwhat-is-cor-pulmonale-08.jpg&f=1&nofb=1&ipt=7fc03dc95247acccfc64ac2bbc6c81ba787d265ec7d3914e531353490cbfe000.

Clinical evidence shows that specific agents, such as phosphodiesterase-5 inhibitors, have been used to increase exercise capacity and quality of life in patients with chronic pulmonary hypertension and Cor pulmonale. Besides, chronic therapy can include the use of diuretics to reverse fluid overload, thus reducing the preload on the heart. It is important to keep a vigilant eye on the balance between treatment efficacy and potential toxic side effects, emphasizing individual treatment protocols to maximize patient benefit. Interactive and adaptive treatment that integrates all therapeutic options is vital for the effective management of Cor pulmonale (Cecconi et al., 2006; Lindem et al., 2006) (Figure 1.14).

1.5.1. Pharmacological Interventions

Pharmacologic treatment forms the core of the treatment of Cor pulmonale and conditions for pulmonary embolism, thereby improving patient outcomes. The treatment arsenal includes numerous classes of drugs that predominantly aim to decrease pulmonary hypertension and improve right ventricular function. For example, pulmonary vasodilators such as nitric oxide and prostacyclin analogs are important in decreasing vascular resistance, hence lessening the afterload for the right ventricle. Additionally, inodilators like milrinone and levosimendan enhance myocardial contractility with vasodilatory effects. It is most advantageous in patients with right ventricular dysfunction who develop acute Cor pulmonale as it can reverse the harmful impact of raised right ventricular pressure (Halvorsen et al., 2022). In summary, a multi-targeted pharmacological approach not only cures the symptoms but also targets the cause of the pathophysiology of Cor pulmonale and pulmonary embolism. Vasoactive medications also play a key therapeutic role in drug treatment of Cor pulmonale, particularly when hemodynamic stabilization is critical. Norepinephrine and sodium nitroprusside are common vasopressors that increase systemic vascular resistance and cardiac output, which can be critical in cases of acute decompensation. In the context of pulmonary embolism patients, anticoagulant therapy such as heparin or low molecular weight heparin plays a critical role in preventing clot enlargement and lowering embolic recurrence risk, thus the workload of the right ventricle (Zochios et al., 2022). The co-administration of anticoagulants and vasopressors aims to treat acute Cor pulmonale from thromboembolic disease and thereby overall cardiovascular stability (Zochios et al., 2022). With careful observation of hemodynamic response, these interventions can be adjusted to enhance patient survival with acute emergencies. In addition, integrating pharmacological interventions into a general treatment plan is necessary to manage patients with Cor pulmonale and pulmonary embolism. Non-pharmacological treatments like oxygen therapy and mechanical ventilation are also used with certain drug therapies to maintain maximal pulmonary function and avoid hypoxemia.

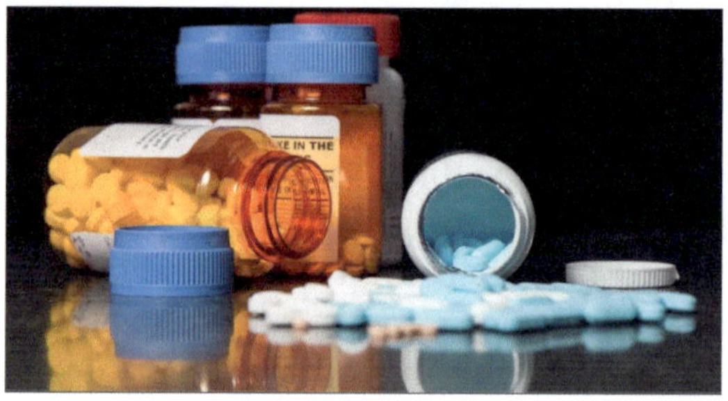

Figure 1.15. Pharmacological interventions treatment for Cor pulmonale.

Source: https://external-content.duckduckgo.com/iu/?u=https%3A%2F%2Fwww.findatopdoc.com%2Fvar%2Ffatd%2Fstorage%2Fimages%2F_aliases%2Ffb_thumb%2Fhealthy-living%2Fmedical-advancements-new-treatments-and-perspectives-on-fibromyalgia%2Fpharmacological-treatments%2F3584078-1-eng-US%2FPharmacological-treatments.jpg&f=1&nofb=1&ipt=01e14df09861f83c7d91ce4409a106299f3efc1540e7c53c75124f89409a1233.

In ARDS patients, Veno-venous extracorporeal membrane oxygenation (VV ECMO) is also considered part of a comprehensive pharmacological package for unloading the right ventricle while ensuring systemic oxygenation. Knowing the mechanisms of right ventricular injury's enables specific pharmacological interventions to enhance RV-PA coupling and reverse stressors like increased pulmonary vascular resistance. This combined strategy highlights the importance of pharmacological therapies within the complex framework of Cor pulmonale and pulmonary embolism management (Zochios et al., 2022) (Figure 1.15).

1.5.2. Lifestyle Modifications and Management

Lifestyle modification is crucial in the management of Cor pulmonale and pulmonary embolism. Smoking cessation forms the most significant component of lifestyle modification because tobacco smoking worsens pulmonary disease and induces thrombosis. It has been found that not only does smoking cause COPD, but it also has an effect on the vascular health at large, making mortality due to pulmonary hypertension and Cor pulmonale greater. The implementation of smoking cessation programs, therefore, has far-reaching effects on the patient's outcome via enhanced lung function and fewer opportunities for subsequent thromboembolic illness.

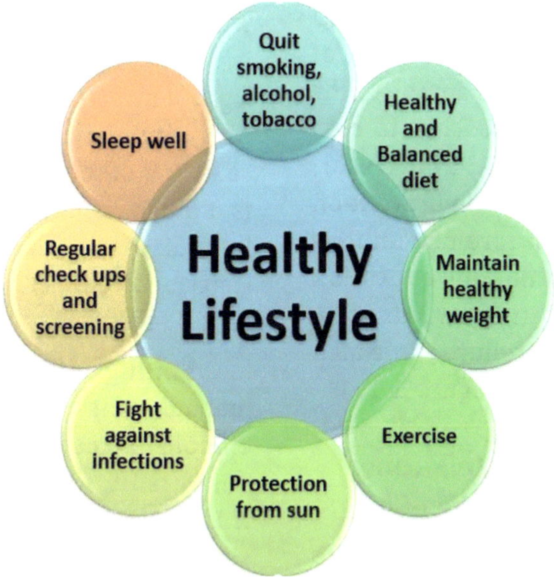

Figure 1.16. Lifestyle modifications.

Source: https://external-content.duckduckgo.com/iu/?u=http%3A%2F%2Fdsresearchcentre.com%2Fstorage%2Fblog%2Fmodification-to-prevent-cancer.jpg&f=1&nofb=1&ipt=915ccfaeb07deafdc917d021ccc49b0adeb562ed6fc28af6fa45f99c84a8abe8.

Lifestyle modification education through regular exercise and appropriate nutritional intake further enhances these services for a comprehensive care approach, improving pulmonary as well as cardiovascular status. Additionally, weight management is an essential aspect of averting the dangers of Cor pulmonale and pulmonary embolism. Obesity can even aggravate respiratory disease by limiting the expansion of the lungs and adding additional burden to the heart, thus causing Cor pulmonale. Thus, physicians must emphasize including a balanced diet and physical activity as key components of a thorough management plan. This practice is also in line with clinical guidelines for practice aimed at the improvement of general health and prevention of thromboembolic disorders, particularly among high-risk populations. In addition, nutrition education can raise patient knowledge on determinants of weight and facilitate long-term lifestyle changes for long-term health improvement and prevention of the progression of respiratory conditions. Moreover, control and management of comorbid diseases, primarily cardiovascular, are also very essential in reducing hospital risk factors of Cor pulmonale and pulmonary embolism. Chronic lung patients most likely have other disease conditions, including cardiovascular disease and hypertension, complicating the disease course. The addition of patient education for such underlying chronic disease conditions, as well as specific lifestyle modifications, can make active management achievable. The GOLD guidelines offer frameworks for the care of COPD, with a focus on coordination among COPD and cardiovascular disease approaches to best optimize patient outcomes (García-Navarro et al., 2025). Moreover, formal education in prevention and accessible treatment for thromboembolic disease, as quoted in current nursing education initiatives, refers to the potential rewards of an educated patient population to reduce associated morbidity (Miller et al., 2014) (Figure 1.16).

1.5.3. Surgical Options and Their Indications

The treatment of pulmonary embolism and Cor pulmonale is often a surgical one when medical management does not relieve symptoms or in high-risk mortality situations. Pulmonary embolectomy and lung transplant are the available surgical options that must be weighed under some clinical circumstances. Pulmonary embolectomy is particularly indicated for cases of massive pulmonary embolism in patients who are hemodynamically unstable or in shock, since timely intervention will be able to restore perfusion and improve oxygenation. It may also be lifesaving in patients who do not respond to anticoagulation therapy, as recent advancements in the interventional therapies for pulmonary embolism (Donovan, 2024) show. Early surgical decision-making also has a profound influence on patient outcomes and is typically guided by a multidisciplinary team. In chronic Cor pulmonale and associated lung disease, surgical procedures such as LVRS or lung transplant are undertaken to consider if conservative measures are unsuccessful. LVRS can be applied to advanced emphysema patients through the reduction of hyperinflation and improvement in respiratory mechanics.

It is particularly indicated in those with a severe drop in quality of life despite optimal medical care. On the other hand, lung transplantation is reserved for patients with end-stage lung disease in whom there is irreversible pulmonary hypertension leading to right ventricular failure and other complications of Cor pulmonale. Both of these require optimal selection of the patient since surgical candidacy is determined by balancing the severity of lung disease with the probability of improved functional capacity with surgery (Thakur et al., 2024).

Timing of surgery is central to the management of Cor pulmonale and pulmonary embolism. Postponement of surgical treatment will result in deteriorating symptoms and irreversible changes in the cardiovascular system, ultimately compromising morbidity and mortality. Clinicians should therefore conduct thorough assessments to determine the extent of right ventricular dysfunction and pulmonary hypertension. Risk stratification, particularly in pulmonary embolism cases, assists in recognizing patients who will most likely respond to surgical treatment. It must be noted that although surgical interventions might offer significant benefits, they carry inherent risks such as anesthesia complications, infection, and postoperative recovery. Continuous monitoring and coordination among experts allow for personalized surgical approaches that optimize patient results in Cor pulmonale and pulmonary embolism management (Donovan, 2024; Thakur et al., 2024) (Figure 1.17).

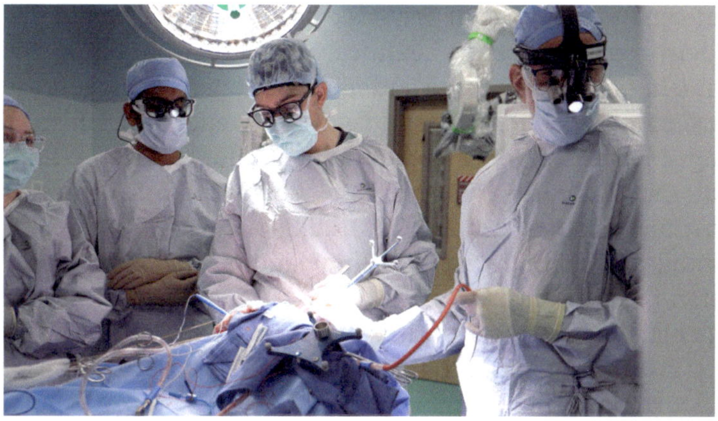

Figure 1.17. Surgical options for Cor pulmonale.

Source: https://external-content.duckduckgo.com/iu/?u=https%3A%2F%2Fnewsnetwork.mayoclinic.org%2Fn7-mcnn%2F7bcc9724adf7b803%2Fuploads%2F2023%2F02%2FResection-of-an-epileptic-focus-Team-16x9-1.jpg&f=1&nofb=1&ipt=d45d228a9acb246b16deafb137dcfd0e454bc26dfd4debb762dcaf63f3ccdec2.

Test Your Knowledge

1. What are the pharmacological interventions?
2. What are the surgical options and their indications?

1.6. Treatment Options for Pulmonary Embolism

Learning Outcome

1. Anticoagulation therapy;
2. Thrombolytic therapy;
3. Surgical interventions and catheter-based treatments.

The management of pulmonary embolism (PE) encompasses a spectrum of approaches based on severity and the patients' health. In acute, high-risk PE, prompt measures are imperative to reversing hemodynamic instability. The first line of treatment is anticoagulation therapy, which typically begins with unfractionated heparin or low molecular weight heparin, which effectively halts clot extension. In the case of massive PE or in PE presenting with hemodynamic collapse, stronger modalities such as thrombolysis may be used to lyse the embolus rapidly. Additionally, surgery such as embolectomy is a viable option for specific patients for whom thrombolytic therapy cannot be initiated. Each of these treatment regimens attempts to reverse the acute effects of PE without inducing complications such as Cor pulmonale that may arise in the setting of prolonged hypoxia and right ventricular overload. More recent advancements in models of treatment have also highlighted the possibility of outpatient treatment for selected patients with low-risk PE. Current guidelines support ambulatory care or early discharge practices for this group, particularly after verifying their clinical stability through a thorough assessment. Analysis using the national database has indicated that a significant percentage of low-risk patients are suitable for treatment at home, which not only helps deliver more effective healthcare resources but also promotes satisfaction and comfort among patients. In this regard, more and more patients have favorable outcomes with early discharge regimens, which have similar rates of recurrent venous thromboembolism and bleeding as inpatients with longer lengths of stay. These findings underscore the importance of accurately selecting low-risk patients and using appropriate treatment modalities to optimize care and minimize in-hospitalizations (Farmakis et al., 2024). Long-term management of pulmonary embolism needs careful observation to control potential complications, particularly chronic thromboembolic pulmonary hypertension (CTEPH) and Cor pulmonale. Patients with PE are also in danger of these severe sequelae, particularly if they are treated poorly or experience recurrent attacks. Follow-up is a continuation of anticoagulation therapy for a defined period, often between three and six months, to prevent recurrences of thromboembolic events. In those who have CTEPH develop, surgery with pulmonary endarterectomy may be considered in addition to other therapies such as pulmonary vasodilators. The combined efforts of physicians like pulmonologists and cardiologists are responsible for the follow-up of such patients, referring them to their treatment plan promptly, and giving the optimal outcomes (Thakur et al., 2024) (Figure 1.18).

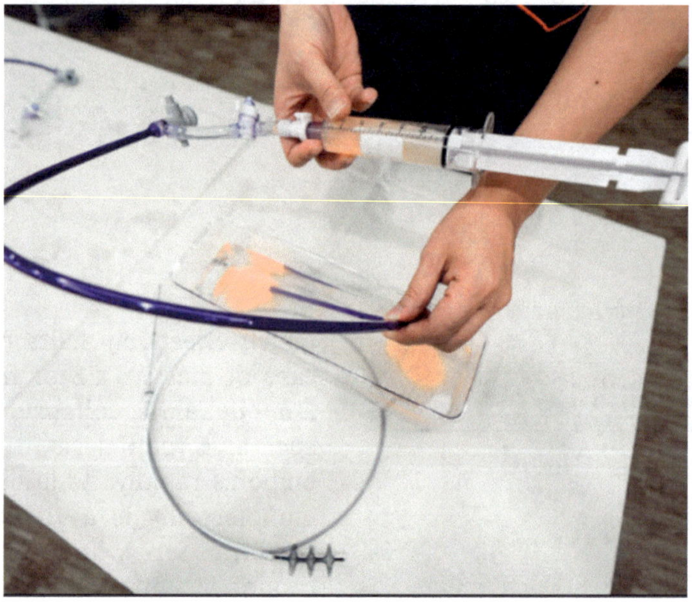

Figure 1.18. Pulmonary embolism treatment.

Source: https://external-content.duckduckgo.com/iu/?u=https%3A%2F%2Fnuhsplus.edu.sg%2Fimages%2Fdefault-source%2Fdefault-album%2Fpulmonary-embolism---image.png%3Fsfvrsn%3D95e6bcc2_1&f=1&nofb=1&ipt=9b68658b4d3a5ad39a45ec3d9aafe629b67809f544a3728b8225e161757e88aa.

1.6.1. Anticoagulation Therapy

Anticoagulant therapy is a cornerstone to the management of pulmonary embolism (PE), a leading cause of Cor pulmonale. By preventing further clot formation and lysis of clots that already form, anticoagulants play a crucial role in preventing the acute right ventricular overload that could lead to Cor pulmonale. Large numbers of PE patients require therapeutic interventions soon after diagnosis and, therefore, rapid anticoagulation is essential. Pre-existing conditions, such as venous thromboembolism, place the patient at risk for recurrent occurrence and thus make the function of anticoagulant therapy not merely therapeutic but also preventive. This is particularly relevant in the acute and critical care setting, where prompt intervention can profoundly impact the patient's outcome and prognosis. Multidisciplinary collaborative care enhances the efficacy of treatment regimens, while addressing the complexity of both conditions, and has a considerable impact on the health of patients who are at risk of evolving acute Cor pulmonale (Arrigo et al., 2023). Therapeutic use of anticoagulants includes multiple agents, like unfractionated heparin, low molecular weight heparins, and direct oral anticoagulants. Anticoagulant choice is often determined by the renal function of the patients, bleeding risk, and need for rapid reversal in emergent situations. Unfractionated heparin is used most universally in the critical care setting due to ease of monitoring and reversibility, which is paramount in the acute setting of Cor pulmonale secondary to PE. Accordingly, the application of direct oral anticoagulants provides a viable option for outpatient therapy, with ease in dosing and less monitoring. However, the balance between efficacy and safety remains the hallmark of anticoagulation therapy; the physician must balance risks versus benefits to attain maximum patient outcome in this high-risk patient population (Halvorsen et al., 2022). Moreover, with accumulating data on the long-term effects of anticoagulation, particularly among the at-risk recurrent pulmonary embolism population, therapy for prolonged duration has become a key part of clinical guidelines. The interrelationship between anticoagulant treatment and prevention or worsening of Cor pulmonale underscores the importance of ongoing clinical observation and inter-disciplinary team efforts. Personalization of anticoagulation treatment to not just decrease acute hazard but also to alter longer-term models of well-being is of paramount importance to improve quality of life and prevent morbidity. Such a need becomes even more apparent in the context of sudden setbacks during the COVID-19 pandemic, where the incidence of PE escalated exponentially alongside acute respiratory illnesses, thereby increasing the risk of Cor pulmonale. As is highlighted, the coming together of a number of specialties encourages a multidisciplinary style of treatment critical in patients combating these complex health conditions (Arrigo et al., 2023) (Figure 1.19).

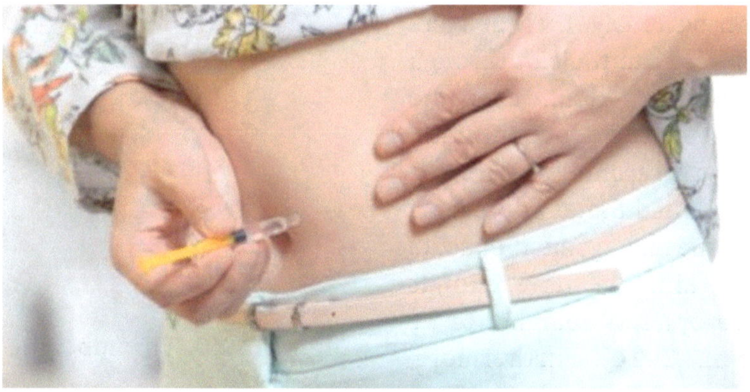

Figure 1.19. Anticoagulant selection is cornerstone of pulmonary embolism treatment.

Source: https://external-content.duckduckgo.com/iu/?u=https%3A%2F%2Fwww.acepnow.com%2Fwp-content%2Fuploads%2F2025%2F03%2FAdobeStock_214753653-500x261.jpg&f=1&nofb=1&ipt=55c87e90bf2c23603868b418ae5acb1e017f62be8f0400ec099ac51271f6dba1.

1.6.2. Thrombolytic Therapy

Thrombolysis therapy has emerged as an important treatment in the management of pulmonary embolism (PE), particularly in severe or high-risk cases. The therapy enables very rapid dissolution of thrombi that cause pulmonary artery occlusion and hence very significantly corrects hemodynamic instability as well as reduces complications, such as Cor pulmonale. This therapeutic option is of very high importance because delay in the management of acute PE is associated with high mortality and morbidity.

Even if anticoagulation remains the treatment of choice in first-line therapy, thrombolysis can be a crucial addition in the most serious cases of large clots, effectively eliminating the immediate risks. It is thus essential to balance the benefits of thrombolytic therapy against its inevitable risks, particularly complications of bleeding. It hence necessitates careful patient selection based on their clinical presentation and comorbid conditions. Enhanced technology has fortified the application of catheter-directed thrombolytic therapy (CDT) for expanding therapeutic interventions for severely affected PE. Unlike traditional systemic thrombolysis, where medications are administered intravenously, CDT delivers thrombolytic drugs directly to the clot through a catheter, resulting in lower systemic exposure and possibly a reduced incidence of fatal bleeding. As quoted by the recent literature, the growth of CDT in the United States represents an evolving pattern in the management of acute pulmonary embolism, although its economic impact on healthcare systems remains to be achieved (Abele et al., 2024). Furthermore, ongoing clinical trials and research continue to monitor the efficacy and safety profile of various thrombolytic agents, highlighting the need for more evidence to establish the most effective application of this therapeutic approach. However, despite the positive outcomes associated with thrombolytic therapy, caution and judicious patient selection are still necessary clinically. The management strategy for PE must consider not only the clinical presentation of the thromboembolic process but also the overall implications of treatment on the patients' health, especially concerning predisposing diseases such as Cor pulmonale. Non-thrombotic causes of acute pulmonary disease must also be managed differently, as reflected in the variety of clinical presentations across various patients (N/A, 2018). Lastly, inclusion of thrombolytic therapy within the total therapy for pulmonary embolism requires consideration of carefully evaluated risks against benefits. It is thus an important ingredient in the formulation of therapeutic modalities for this lethal disorder (Figure 1.20).

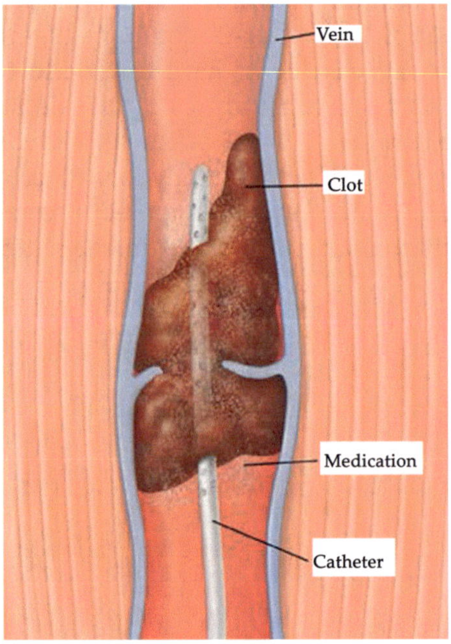

Figure 1.20. Thrombolytic therapy.

Source: https://api.kramesstaywell.com/Content/6066ca30-310a-4170-b001-a4ab013d61fd/ucr-images-v1/Images/cross-section-of-vein-with-blood-clot-showing-catheter-releasing-medication-into-clot-277284.

1.6.3. Surgical Interventions and Catheter-Based Treatments

The treatment of pulmonary embolism (PE) has evolved dramatically, with catheter-based procedures and surgery becoming central to minimizing its complications. Among these, surgical thrombectomy remains a foremost surgical intervention, while it is typically reserved for those with large PE who are unresponsive to anticoagulation or thrombolysis. This is a direct extraction of the thrombus from the pulmonary arteries, thus normalizing hemodynamics and significantly improving hemodynamic stability. According to a recent study, thrombectomy by surgery is very effective with a mortality rate of around 23.2% in patients undergoing this procedure, which proves it to be a life-saving procedure for those with a high chance of death due to PE complications, e.g., development of Cor pulmonale (Maqsood et al., 2024). In addition to surgical thrombectomy, catheter therapies have also gained popularity as minimally invasive interventions for PE treatment. Therapies include varied procedures like catheter-directed thrombolysis and mechanical thrombectomy, which are a safe approach for selective embolic treatment with minimal systemic anticoagulation risks. Of note is the rising trend of increased catheter-directed therapy use, particularly among patients who need urgent treatment without the associative risks of major surgery. The potential of reduced major bleeding complications, noted in some 4.9% in recent analyses of data, highlights their favorable profile as compared to conventional anticoagulation strategies with greater mortality (Oettinger et al., 2024). The practice is indicative of the requirement for dynamic adjustment of treatment strategies in line with patient-specific risk factor and clinical presentation. The inclusion of catheter-based and operative interventions into the practice of clinical medicine for treatment of PE not only provides short-term relief from thrombotic obstruction but also significantly contributes to long-term outcome, particularly with respect to preventing Cor pulmonale. Facilitation of collaboration between interventional radiologists and surgical staff is crucial in optimizing the treatment algorithm for patients, especially those with acute right heart strain or hemodynamic instability. Recent data indicate that although surgical procedures carry a reduced mortality risk compared to anticoagulation therapy, they also require wise patient selection for maximum benefit. Treatment in PE is evolving, with more studies needed to enhance these interventions further and evaluate their impact on all-cause mortality and quality of life in patients with this serious condition (Maqsood et al., 2024) (Figure 1.21).

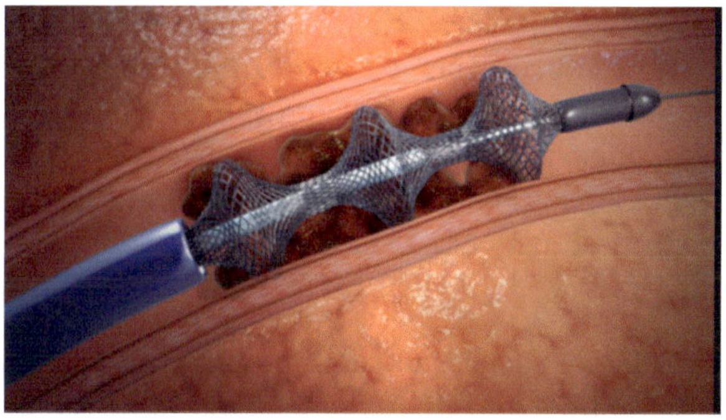

Figure 1.21. Surgical interventions and catheter-based treatments of pulmonary embolism.

Source: https://external-content.duckduckgo.com/iu/?u=https%3A%2F%2Fwww.huntingtonhealth.org%2Fwp-content%2Fuploads%2F2021%2F07%2FHH_072121-News-Post_FlowTriever_Hero-600x337.jpg&f=1&nofb=1&ipt=10b3aff208762b72f16d3c32b641517 02fd0bbf495319f1e6708a9d3ad1f47ed.

Test Your Knowledge

1. What is anticoagulation therapy?
2. What is thrombolytic therapy?

Summary

The intricate relationship between Cor pulmonale and pulmonary embolism emphasizes the importance of thorough knowledge of these serious conditions, particularly within the context of early diagnosis and treatment. As discussed in this essay, Cor pulmonale with right ventricular hypertrophy due to pulmonary hypertension often arises from acute and chronic pulmonary pathology. Perhaps the most common acute complication of respiratory disease, pulmonary embolism has the capability of inducing staggering morbidity and mortality if not promptly diagnosed and managed. Recent studies emphasize the importance of emerging diagnostic technology, such as shear wave elastography, which may assist clinicians in determining venous thrombus stiffness and, consequently, embolic potential in affected individuals (Akramova et al., 2024). Moreover, some patient groups, i.e., intracranial hemorrhage, present special difficulties in the management of pulmonary embolism. For example, anticoagulation therapy timing in the case presented in patients with pulmonary embolism, as well as nontraumatic intracranial hemorrhage, is an important factor, since early treatment raises the risk of adverse consequences like death and neurological impairment (Chang et al., 2024). These findings are important for clinicians to balance the benefits of anticoagulation with complications, particularly in high-risk groups for both conditions. The more nuanced findings based on existing research emphasize that one strategy may not be sufficient; rather, a case-by-case approach is necessary for varied clinical presentations. In short, effective management of pulmonary embolism and Cor pulmonale is a multidisciplinary approach involving proper assessment, early intervention, and a thorough understanding of the interrelated pathophysiologic mechanisms underlying such processes. Evolving the diagnostic approach and treatment protocols is important to enhance patient outcomes and avoid the development of fatal complications. With the addition of newer diagnostic techniques and individualized treatment protocols, physicians are more capable of managing the nuances of patients with pulmonary embolism and its potential evolution into Cor pulmonale. Additional research in this field is needed to continuously enhance our understanding and treatment protocols, ultimately improving patient outcomes and survival rates in this recalcitrant area of medicine.

In any discussion of Cor pulmonale and pulmonary embolism, it is crucial to highlight the integral relationship between pulmonary hypertension and right ventricular failure. Cor pulmonale, or right ventricular enlargement and failure due to elevation in pulmonary vascular resistance, is caused most frequently by chronic respiratory illness in the form of COPD and ILD. In addition, acute pulmonary embolism can initiate sudden hemodynamic alterations, leading to acute right heart strain or failure. These two conditions emphasize the intricate interaction between the lung and the heart, with a focus on comprehensive assessment in patients with symptoms of respiratory distress or heart failure. Lastly, understanding the etiologic pathophysiologic mechanisms is necessary for clinicians to effectively intervene and optimize patient outcomes, as these conditions have significant morbidity and mortality implications. The clinical presentation of Cor pulmonale and pulmonary embolism may range from a few signs to a full-blown presentation, thus making diagnosis and management more complex. Cor pulmonale patients may present with peripheral edema, fatigue, and dyspnea that are masked as pulmonary disease exacerbations. Pulmonary embolism, on the other hand, presents acutely with hemoptysis, pleuritic chest pain, and tachypnea, eliciting an urgent response. Risk factors for recent surgery, immobility for a long duration, and hypercoagulability significantly enhance pulmonary embolism risk, which highlights the recognition of high-risk populations. Continuous monitoring and early diagnostic imaging, such as CT pulmonary angiography, remain crucial in the differentiation of these entities. Such alertness in the clinical environment can lead to early intervention, thereby reducing the morbidity and mortality of Cor pulmonale and pulmonary embolism. Current studies have begun to shed light on the complicated interactions between COVID-19 and its potential impact upon the cardiovascular system, which are particularly relevant to Cor pulmonale as well as pulmonary embolism. Siripanthong et al. (2022) describes how COVID-19 patients may experience myocardial damage as a result of direct viral infection in addition to indirect hypercoagulability, and this has implications regarding long-term cardiovascular sequelae. The association of viral infection with increased risk of venous thromboembolism only serves to heighten the vital need to keep a vigilant watch for symptoms of pulmonary embolism in infected patients. Furthermore, (Halvorsen et al., 2022) also brings to attention that emerging evidence indicates the importance of continued research into interactions of respiratory and cardiovascular systems during and following COVID-19. Thus, practitioners need to keep these changing dynamics in mind to manage patients with pre-existing cardiovascular ailments or complications arising from viral illnesses.

KEY TERMS FROM THIS CHAPTER

- Anticoagulation therapy
- Chest pain
- Chronic lung disease
- Cor pulmonale
- D-dimer test
- Deep vein thrombosis (DVT)
- Dyspnea
- Hemoptysis
- Jugular venous distension (JVD)
- Peripheral edema
- Pulmonary embolism (PE)
- Pulmonary hypertension
- Pulmonary infarction
- Right heart failure
- Right ventricular hypertrophy
- Saddle embolus
- Tachypnea
- Thrombolysis

Critical Thinking Questions

1. **Cor pulmonale is defined as:**
   a. Left ventricular failure due to lung disease
   b. Right ventricular enlargement and failure secondary to pulmonary hypertension
   c. Acute myocardial infarction
   d. Systemic hypertension causing heart failure
2. **The most common cause of pulmonary embolism is:**
   a. Air embolism
   b. Fat embolism
   c. Deep vein thrombosis (DVT)
   d. Septic emboli
3. **Which of the following is a classic clinical sign of acute pulmonary embolism?**
   a. Sudden onset of pleuritic chest pain and dyspnea
   b. Gradual weight loss
   c. Productive cough with green sputum
   d. Bilateral leg edema
4. **What is the typical chest X-ray finding in Cor pulmonale?**
   a. Cardiomegaly with prominent right atrium and right ventricle
   b. Bilateral alveolar infiltrates
   c. Large pleural effusion only
   d. Normal chest X-ray
5. **Which diagnostic test is considered the gold standard for confirming pulmonary embolism?**
   a. Chest X-ray
   b. D-dimer test
   c. Ventilation-perfusion (V/Q) scan
   d. CT pulmonary angiography

Short answer Questions

1. Define Cor pulmonale.
2. What is the most common cause of Cor pulmonale?
3. Name three clinical features of Cor pulmonale.
4. What is the primary pathophysiological mechanism leading to Cor pulmonale?
5. Which diagnostic test is most helpful in confirming pulmonary embolism?

Answer to Critical Thinking Questions

1. (b); 2. (c); 3. (a); 4. (a); 5. (d).

References

1. Mohr, K., Keeling, B., Kaier, K., Neusius, T., Rosovsky, R. P., Moriarty, J. M., Rosenfield, K., Abele, C., Farmakis, I. T., Keller, K., Barco, S., Channick, R. N., Giri, J. S., Lookstein, R. A., Todoran, T. M., Christodoulou, K. C., Hobohm, L., Lanno, M., Reed, J., . . . Secemsky, E. A. (2024). Modelling costs of interventional pulmonary embolism treatment: implications of US trends for a European healthcare system. *European Heart Journal Acute Cardiovascular Care, 13*(6), 501–505. https://doi.org/10.1093/ehjacc/zuae019Agustí García-Navarro, À., Anzueto, A., Barnes, P. J., Bourbeau, J., et al. (2025). *Global Initiative for Chronic Obstructive Lung Disease 2023 Report: GOLD Executive Summary*. https://core.ac.uk/download/647990828.pdf (accessed on 30th June 2025).
2. Ahmad, S., Delaney, M., & Flora, B. (2017). Focused sonography in cardiac arrest. https://core.ac.uk/download/322433236.pdf (accessed on 30th June 2025).
3. Akramova, E. G., & Kapustina, E. P. (2024). Shear wave elastography values of thrombus in patients with lower extremity deep vein thrombosis for pulmonary embolism detection: The ROC analysis. *Almanac of Clinical Medicine*. https://www.semanticscholar.org/paper/7a72011e7a34c36151663bab96bf1cc94a072541 (accessed on 30th June 2025).
4. Almarawi, H., Alwani, M., & Arabi, A. (2020). Right ventricular involvement in COVID-19 patients: A rapid review. *Heart Views: The Official Journal of the Gulf Heart Association, 21*, 193–194. https://www.semanticscholar.org/paper/d4f34b8b4dee663bf7d2319770abb316c665ee4a (accessed on 30th June 2025).
5. Amin, S., Shahab, A., Qazi, A. R., Yunus, H., Saeed, L., Khan, A., Rehman, M. E. U., et al. (2023). A rare incidence of hepatocellular carcinoma with tumor thrombus extending to the right heart. *Cureus, 15*. https://www.semanticscholar.org/paper/7a21c4e4b4de42fffb86b13c596f10018c58477f (accessed on 30th June 2025).
6. Arrigo, M., Price, S., Harjola, V., Huber, L. C., Schaubroeck, H., Vieillard-Baron, A., Masip, J., et al. (2023). Diagnosis and treatment of right ventricular failure secondary to acutely increased right ventricular afterload (acute Cor pulmonale): A clinical consensus statement of the Association for Acute Cardiovascular Care of the European Society of Cardiology. *European Heart Journal. Acute Cardiovascular Care, 13*, 304–312. https://www.semanticscholar.org/paper/8acf5a61d862e140b87507fa874e4de5306f7fa1 (accessed on 30th June 2025).
7. Bejjani, A., Khairani, C., Lo, Y., Jiménez, D., Barco, S., Mahajan, S., Caraballo, C., et al. (2023). Abstract 17709: ICD-10 codes have low sensitivity and suboptimal positive predictive value for identifying cases of pulmonary embolism with Cor pulmonale in electronic healthcare records. *Circulation*. https://www.semanticscholar.org/paper/51222234054a8b21b1750d5460882d7df57d476a (accessed on 30th June 2025).
8. Bogun, L., Brynza, M., Bychkova, O., Lysenko, A., et al. (2017). Respiratory failure & Cor pulmonale. https://core.ac.uk/download/144471261.pdf (accessed on 30th June 2025).
9. Cecconi, M., De Backer, D., Antonelli, M., Beale, R., Bakker, J., Hofer, C. K., Jaeschke, R., et al. (2014). Consensus on circulatory shock and hemodynamic monitoring. Task force of the European Society of Intensive Care Medicine. *Intensive Care Medicine, 40*, 1795–1815. https://doi.org/10.1007/s00134-014-3525-z (accessed on 30th June 2025).
10. Cecconi, M., Johnston, E., & Rhodes, A. (2006). What role does the right side of the heart play

in circulation? https://core.ac.uk/download/29469393.pdf (accessed on 30th June 2025).

11. Cenci, C., Miniati, M., Monti, S., Poli, D., et al. (2012). Clinical presentation of acute pulmonary embolism: Survey of 800 cases. https://core.ac.uk/download/pdf/8687670.pdf (accessed on 30th June 2025).
12. Chang, K., Hambach, B., Nareddy, S., Prucnal, C., Hernandez, E., & Sovory, L. (2024). Abstract 4139732: Timing of anticoagulation in pulmonary embolism with nontraumatic intracranial hemorrhage: A multi-national database study. *Circulation*. https://www.semanticscholar.org/paper/0ce24587dcc805c6f83b194d9bcfdb43ae94694d (accessed on 30th June 2025).
13. Comfere, T. B. O., Gajic, O., Mankad, S. V., Mour, G., et al. (2008). Arterial pulmonary hypertension in noncardiac intensive care unit. https://core.ac.uk/download/pdf/8230925.pdf (accessed on 30th June 2025).
14. Daud, M., Anees, M., Wazir, H. U., Ahmad, Z., Umar, Z., Arif, W., Ahmad, S., et al. (2025). Comprehensive evaluation of the diagnostic approach to pulmonary embolism: Analysis of D-dimer utilization, imaging modalities (CTPA and V/Q scan), and clinical risk stratification tools. *Indus Journal of Bioscience Research*. https://www.semanticscholar.org/paper/c67a40796bcec10e35b98727c17518a3a7f6ded9 (accessed on 30th June 2025).
15. De Bellis, A., D'Abramo, M., Frati, G., Greco, E., et al. (2018). Surgical embolectomy for acute massive pulmonary embolism: State of the art. https://core.ac.uk/download/188822613.pdf (accessed on 30th June 2025).
16. Devan, K. S. (2006). *Expert System with An Embedded Imaging Module for Diagnosing Lung Diseases*. https://core.ac.uk/download/301113939.pdf (accessed on 30th June 2025).
17. Devi, P. L. (2009). A study on etiology and clinical profile of chronic Cor pulmonale. https://core.ac.uk/download/235665579.pdf (accessed on 30th June 2025).
18. Domínguez-López, J. A., & Mendoza-Razo, L. E. (2024). Cor triatriatum sinister in a young adult: An unusual cause of syncope. *Cureus, 16*. https://www.semanticscholar.org/paper/815c727526acf1592e1a3e46c37cbbcd35c6e763 (accessed on 30th June 2025).
19. Donovan, K. M. (2024). Pulmonary embolism triage: When to do what. *Methodist DeBakey Cardiovascular Journal, 20*, 65–67. https://www.semanticscholar.org/paper/9eb896834abfb2e028b7cec4f6fb89b618fc52d7 (accessed on 30th June 2025).
20. Farmakis, I., Valerio, L., Christodoulou, K., Giannakoulas, G., Hobohm, L., Keller, K., Lurz, P., et al. (2024). Trends in home treatment and early discharge of patients with low-risk pulmonary embolism. *European Heart Journal*. https://www.semanticscholar.org/paper/ba12e9ede130ac87e434303deafc1d40ccb11153 (accessed on 30th June 2025).
21. Ghorbanpouryami, F., Pishgahi, M., Safari, S., Yousefifard, M., et al. (2020). Electrocardiographic findings of COVID-19 patients and their correlation with outcome: A prospective cohort study. https://core.ac.uk/download/327264299.pdf (accessed on 30th June 2025).
22. Halvorsen, S., Mehilli, J., Cassese, S., Hall, T. S., Abdelhamid, M., Barbato, E., De Hert, S., et al. (2022). 2022 ESC guidelines on cardiovascular assessment and management of patients undergoing non-cardiac surgery. *European Heart Journal, 43*, 3826–3924. https://doi.org/10.1093/eurheartj/ehac270 (accessed on 30th June 2025).
23. Herrmann, J., Yang, E. H., Iliescu, C., Çilingiroğlu, M., Charitakis, K., Hakeem, A., Toutouzas, K., et al. (2016). Vascular toxicities of cancer therapies. *Circulation, 133*, 1272–1289. https://doi.org/10.1161/circulationaha.115.018347 (accessed on 30th June 2025).

24. Hrobar, P., Isles, C., Kourounis, G., Mackay, J., et al. (2019). ECG in suspected pulmonary embolism. https://core.ac.uk/download/186328202.pdf (accessed on 30th June 2025).

25. Klein, J. (2022). Another study shows electronic cigarettes harm lungs: It is time for researchers to move from the tobacco playbook to a tobacco endgame. *American Journal of Respiratory and Critical Care Medicine, 205*, 1265–1266. https://www.semanticscholar.org/paper/daa7bdb5971e1fdd5653a1e3672823ba5f3083e5 (accessed on 30th June 2025).

26. Ks, S., Seru, N. K., Mohan, M. S., Basnet, S., & Amit, K. (2023). Case study: Interstitial lung disease with pulmonary arterial hypertension and *Cor pulmonale. Asian Journal of Hospital Pharmacy*. https://www.semanticscholar.org/paper/b6d1fe62346d2a925dd3e5dfe41c9639ea9cfb59 (accessed on 30th June 2025).

27. Lindem, T., & Randen, H. P. (2006). Bør akutt massiv lungeemboli opereres? Pasientkasus og litteraturstudie. https://core.ac.uk/download/30899918.pdf (accessed on 30th June 2025).

28. Liu, X., Jiao, X., Gong, X., Nie, Q., Li, Y., Zhen, G., Cheng, M., et al. (2023). Prevalence, risk factor and clinical characteristics of venous thrombus embolism in patients with acute exacerbation of COPD: A prospective multicenter study. *International Journal of Chronic Obstructive Pulmonary Disease, 18*, 907–917. https://www.semanticscholar.org/paper/1d80ed40c4ec20970914006f1d7356c7b02ea86c (accessed on 30th June 2025).

29. Mandoli, G., Sciaccaluga, C., Bandera, F., Cameli, P., Esposito, R., D'Andrea, A., Evola, V., et al. (2020). Cor pulmonale: The role of traditional and advanced echocardiography in the acute and chronic settings. *Heart Failure Reviews, 26*, 263–275. https://www.semanticscholar.org/paper/72495bda003989708e51d91fdc59a00858f7ad60 (accessed on 30th June 2025).

30. Maqsood, M., Zhang, R. S., Zlotnick, D. M., Parikh, S., & Bangalore, S. (2024). Outcomes with treatment interventions for clot-in-transit in patients with pulmonary embolism: A meta-analysis. *The Journal of Invasive Cardiology*. https://www.semanticscholar.org/paper/43615f3605ee199863031ab979298e4f47ddb238 (accessed on 30th June 2025).

31. Melo, R. H., Gioli-Pereira, L., Lourenço, I. D., Passos, R. H., Bernardo, A. T., & Volpicelli, G. (2025). Diagnostic accuracy of multi-organ point-of-care ultrasound for pulmonary embolism in critically ill patients: A systematic review and meta-analysis. *Critical Care, 29*. https://www.semanticscholar.org/paper/98a195aff601a5756d05893a9fdd04d49f60f1ca (accessed on 30th June 2025).

32. Miller, A. (2014). Clinical practice guideline for venous thromboembolism. https://core.ac.uk/download/230485911.pdf (accessed on 30th June 2025).

33. Mokhatar, S. (2018). Evaluation of cardiac function by echocardiography in chronic obstructive pulmonary disease patients and its correlation with disease severity. *Journal of Medical Science and Clinical Research*. https://www.semanticscholar.org/paper/57055298a2daaee5afcc669c5de44ac25609037d (accessed on 30th June 2025).

34. N/A. (2018). Guidelines on the diagnosis and management of acute pulmonary embolism: The Task Force for the Diagnosis and Management of Acute Pulmonary Embolism of the European Society of Cardiology (ESC). https://core.ac.uk/download/226186779.pdf (accessed on 30th June 2025).

35. Oettinger, V., Von Zur Muehlen, C., Hilgendorf, I., Wolf, D., Rilinger, J., Gauchel, N., Maier, A., et al. (2024). Recent secular trends of catheter-directed therapy for treatment of pulmonary embolism: A retrospective cohort study based on German national data. *European Heart*

Journal. https://www.semanticscholar.org/paper/547e8b43fcd156ad0d504e9ed096ea726c6d9f2f (accessed on 30th June 2025).

36. Opitz, I., & Ulrich, S. (2018). Pulmonary hypertension in chronic obstructive pulmonary disease and emphysema patients: Prevalence, therapeutic options and pulmonary circulatory effects of lung volume reduction surgery. *Journal of Thoracic Disease, 10*(Suppl 23), S2763–S2774. https://www.semanticscholar.org/paper/e3d45ed70a16105699d8b24f55cd120bfd9839a4 (accessed on 30th June 2025).
37. Osakwe, O., & Das, B. B. (2022). Successful pulmonary endarterectomy after acute pulmonary embolism and reversal of acute Cor pulmonale in an 11-year-old boy with nephrotic syndrome. *Children, 9*. https://www.semanticscholar.org/paper/177f497d242040b14f9746a79834064c462948a3 (accessed on 30th June 2025).
38. Pinsky, M. R. (2016). The right ventricle: Interaction with the pulmonary circulation. *Critical Care, 20*. https://doi.org/10.1186/s13054-016-1440-0 (accessed on 30th June 2025).
39. Rao, J., Wang, Z., & Chen, H. (2025). Effective management of pulmonary embolism after initial diagnosis of acute coronary syndrome: A case report highlighting differential diagnosis challenges. *Frontiers in Medicine, 12*. https://www.semanticscholar.org/paper/a094e749f3097c1f89d81a55736f02041a9c85b2 (accessed on 30th June 2025).
40. Siripanthong, B., Asatryan, B., Hanff, T. C., Chatha, S., Khanji, M. Y., Ricci, F., Muser, D., et al. (2022). The pathogenesis and long-term consequences of COVID-19 cardiac injury. *JACC: Basic to Translational Science, 7*, 294–308. https://doi.org/10.1016/j.jacbts.2021.10.011 (accessed on 30th June 2025).
41. Thakur, Y., Meshram, R., & Taksande, A. (2024). Navigating pediatric Cor pulmonale: A comprehensive review of diagnosis and management. *Cureus, 16*. https://www.semanticscholar.org/paper/0c55d708784169569baf14219459599de5d6815e (accessed on 30th June 2025).
42. Thygesen, K., Alpert, J. S., Jaffe, A. S., Simoons, M. L., Chaitman, B. R., White, H. D., & Writing Group Joint ESC for the Universal Definition of MI. (2012). Third universal definition of myocardial infarction. *Global Heart, 7*, 275–275. https://doi.org/10.1016/j.gheart.2012.08.001 (accessed on 30th June 2025).
43. Verhoeff, K., & Mitchell, J. R. (2017). Cardiopulmonary physiology: Why the heart and lungs are inextricably linked. *AJP Advances in Physiology Education, 41*, 348–353. https://doi.org/10.1152/advan.00190.2016 (accessed on 30th June 2025).
44. Zochios, V., Yusuff, H., Conway, H., Lau, G., & Schmidt, M. (2022). The right ventricle during veno-venous extracorporeal membrane oxygenation in acute respiratory distress syndrome: Can we protect the injured ventricle? *ASAIO Journal, 68*, 456–460. https://doi.org/10.1097/mat.0000000000001655 (accessed on 30th June 2025).

ACUTE RESPIRATORY DISTRESS SYNDROME

2

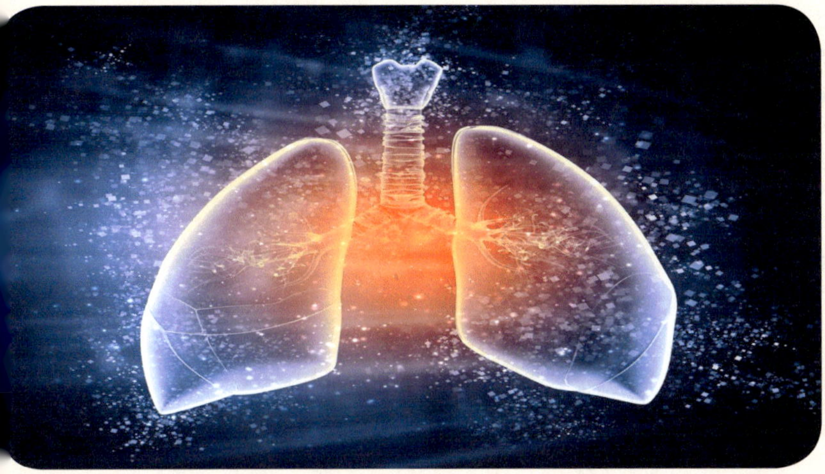

LEARNING OBJECTIVES

After studying this chapter, you will be able to:

1. Explain the pathophysiology of ARDS.
2. Understand the causes and risk factors.
3. Describe clinical presentation.
4. List the treatment options.
5. Explore the prognosis and outcomes.
6. Discuss the prevention strategies.

Introduction

Acute Respiratory Distress Syndrome (ARDS) is a severe and often life-threatening syndrome with a sudden onset of severe respiratory insufficiency. ARDS has refractory bilateral pulmonary infiltrates and hypoxemia that necessitate vigorous medical therapies such as mechanical ventilation. The pathophysiology of ARDS is multifaceted, involving an inflammatory cascade with increased pulmonary vascular permeability and non-cardiogenic pulmonary edema. Therefore, ARDS is frequently a cause of intensive care unit (ICU) admission, indicating its manifestation as a significant source of morbidity and mortality in critically ill patients. Due to its severity and urgency, early detection and treatment are essential to improve patient outcomes and minimize late morbidity, highlighting the need for ongoing investigation into successful treatments and the underlying pathophysiology of the syndrome (Alessandri et al., 2018). Despite a half-century of advances in our understanding of ARDS, treatments remain woefully limited. Researchers have attempted to clarify risk factors and pathogenic contributors to

ARDS, with subsequent gains in the area of understanding biomarkers and physiological processes in the syndrome. The absence of pharmacologic treatments, though, reflects the heterogeneity of ARDS, which renders it intractable to one-size-fits-all solutions. Some of the most promising treatments have been hindered by heterogeneity of patient response and lack of knowledge of the primary targets for treatment. While clinicians and researchers navigate this difficult terrain, one potential solution is to adopt precision medicine strategies that utilize individual patient profiles to inform treatment, delivering interventions that are maximally effective while ensuring optimized clinical outcomes (Calfee et al., 2017). The intensity of ARDS necessitates an interdisciplinary approach that goes beyond medical therapy to even exploring newer biotechnologies. As applied biomolecular technology progresses in its field, there are opportunities for a breakthrough in the management of ARDS, using models similar to those for other complex conditions such as cardiovascular ailments and asthma. The application of advanced bioinformatics and the trend towards precision medicine can enable more personalized treatment by identifying specific biomarkers or gene expression patterns that predict patient responses to treatments. Thus, research on these new therapeutic milieus is imperative, as they may lead to more effective management interventions and improved outcomes for ARDS patients, thus closing a valuable gap in current clinical practice (Calfee et al., 2017) (Figure 2.1).

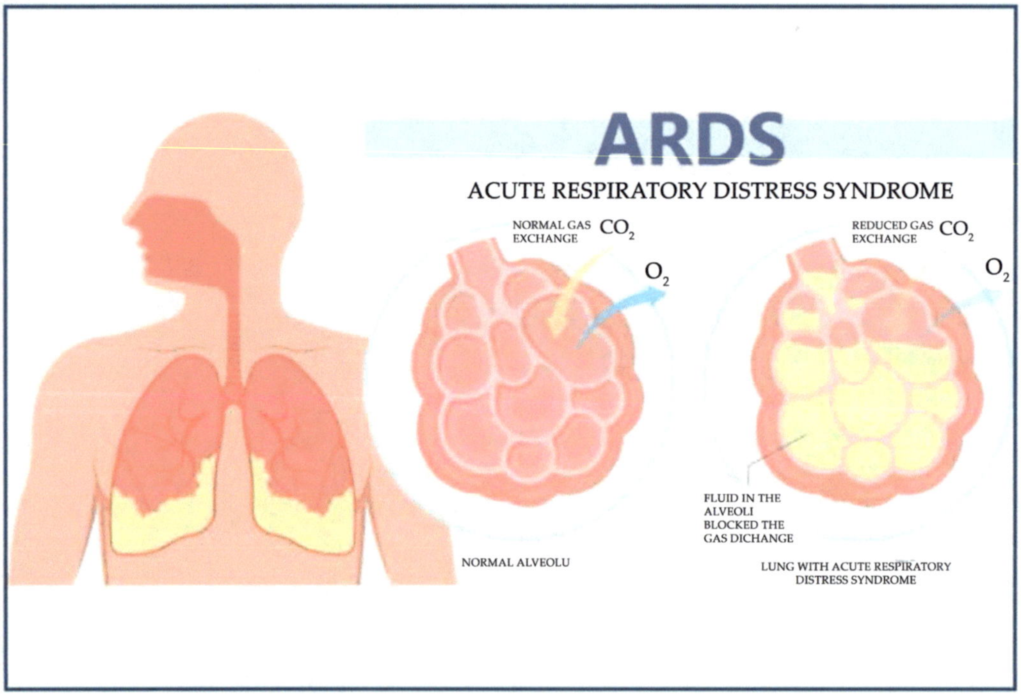

Figure 2.1. Acute respiratory distress syndrome.

Source: https://external-content.duckduckgo.com/iu/?u=https%3A%2F%2Fwww.medicoverhospitals.in%2Fimages%2Farticles%2Facute-respiratory-distress-syndrome-overview.jpg&f=1&nofb=1&ipt=959adc18158779e7a8cadad3457f99038fff430b14924ed548ea4d3b5d6eb15c.

Definition of Acute Respiratory Distress Syndrome (ARDS)

ARDS is a complex, life-threatening illness that encompasses widespread inflammation in the lung and leads to acute respiratory distress. Categorized by clinical presentation and by criteria for diagnosis, ARDS is traditionally characterized by extreme hypoxemia that greatly compromises gas exchange. Modern definitions include the importance of measuring the PaO2/FIO2 ratio and PEEP levels, which are now essential to the diagnosis of this syndrome. Interestingly, newer classification schemes attempt to distinguish ARDS not only from other etiologies of respiratory distress but also from illnesses like heart failure that can have a similar clinical presentation. Such precision in definition is important because incorrect diagnosis can lead to inappropriate management strategies and worsen patient outcome, emphasizing the need for clearly defined, evidence-supported criteria in the clinical setting. The pathophysiologic process of ARDS emphasizes the intricate interplay of direct lung injury and systemic processes that lead to respiratory failure. Sepsis, pulmonary, and aspiration are frequent causes, each having multiple mechanisms to diffuse alveolar damage—cellular damage to the alveolar-capillary membrane results in pulmonary edema and impaired gas exchange. Importantly, indirect systemic damage from extrapulmonary conditions is capable of triggering ARDS, rendering the condition challenging to categorize as an entirely pulmonary process. Furthermore, mechanical ventilation, as essential to patient survival, paradoxically can lead to increased lung injury if not treated carefully. This sort of pathophysiological mechanism knowledge is essential in the development of end-targeted therapies that minimize ventilator-induced lung injury with a view of improving overall outcome (Bai et al., 2013). Aside from knowledge of the pathophysiological basis of ARDS, effective management options are also essential in order to enhance clinical outcomes. Current evidence points towards the benefits of lung-protective ventilation strategies, including low tidal volume and ideal PEEP, which have been shown to enhance survival significantly. Supportive interventions in the form of prone position and use of extracorporeal membrane oxygenation (ECMO) have also been found to be effective adjuncts in treating severe cases. More work has led to more interventions in the pipeline to handle the many variables in ARDS. The dynamic care environment of ARDS reflects an enhanced understanding of the disorder, serving as a stepping stone to an integrated strategy that combines pathophysiological insights with novel therapies within intensive care units (ICUs).

Importance of Understanding ARDS

It is critical that ARDS be understood by many stakeholders involved in the practice of medicine, as proper management of this potentially life-threatening condition could profoundly influence patient outcomes. ARDS is characterized by acute onset of respiratory failure secondary to alveolar-capillary membrane damage and leads to significant morbidity and mortality among critically ill patients. Knowledge of the ARDS pathology and clinical picture enables clinicians to take timely intervention and minimize complications. As highlighted in more recent literature, increased awareness of environmental insults, such as exposure to cigarette smoke, underscores the need for broad-based education on ARDS, leading to more effective prevention and targeted individualized treatment (Bai et al., 2013). Hence, a clear concept of ARDS is crucial for maximizing survival and quality of care. In addition, the understanding of ARDS extends to clinical diagnosis and steps into the field of multidisciplinary care where the role of every member of the healthcare team is essential. Specifically, nursing personnel play a key role in ARDS patient management through rigorous monitoring and individualized care interventions. Literature is available that proves that expert nursing can enhance the clinical outcome for ARDS through fulfilling the physical and psychological needs of patients along with their families (Morais et al., 2024). A nurse's work is to conduct a detailed clinical evaluation and collaborate with the medical team to formulate an all-encompassing recovery plan. This holistic orientation not only answers the patient's actual medical issues but also formulates an environment that minimizes anxiety and fear, which is very common with critical care conditions. Finally, the importance of ARDS knowledge also extends to the formulation of novel treatment protocols with the aim of enhancing patient care. With ongoing research focused on pharmacological and non-pharmacological treatments, increased knowledge of ARDS will support the integration of evidence-based practice in clinical settings. Bai et al. (2013) highlight that advancements in lung-protective ventilation strategies and fluid therapy have improved patient outcomes to a great extent. As studies emerge, clinicians must remain current with these new practices in order to be equipped with the ability to utilize the most effective treatment modalities. This adaptive nature of ARDS care underscores the importance of regular learning practice among health professionals, ultimately yielding better care plans and quality of life for patients suffering from this severe illness (Figure 2.2).

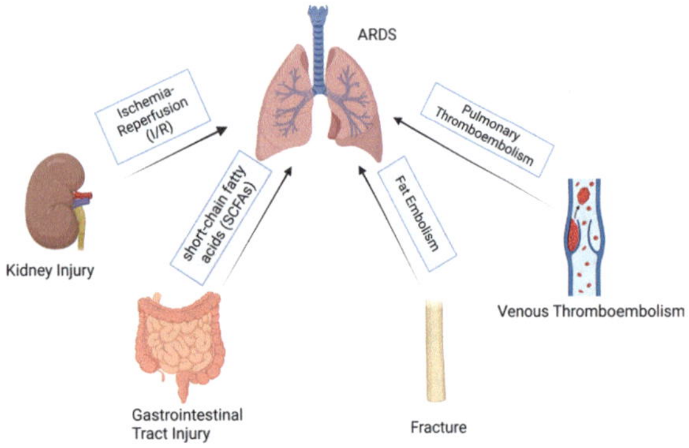

Figure 2.2. Importance of understanding ARDS.

Source: https://onlinelibrary.wiley.com/cms/asset/acaa0bdd-c153-47f8-a377-622b9f72df60/mco270074-fig-0004-m.jpg.

2.1. Pathophysiology of ARDS

Learning Outcome

1. Mechanisms of lung injury;
2. Role of inflammation in ARDS;
3. Impact on gas exchange and lung function.

The pathophysiology of acute respiratory distress syndrome (ARDS) is a complex interplay of inflammatory processes that impair gas exchange and normal pulmonary function. After alveolar-capillary membrane injury, there is a cascade release of inflammatory mediators, leading to increased permeability. This causes proteinaceous pulmonary edema to fill the alveoli, greatly reducing compliance and impairing effective ventilation. Early presentations include hypoxemia, most commonly with associated diffuse bilateral infiltrates on radiography, further deranging respiratory mechanics and oxygenation. It is worth noting that this underlying mechanism should be understood, as it forms the basis for therapeutic interventions aimed at minimizing lung injury and restoring homeostasis, thereby improving outcomes for patients with ARDS. Therapeutic management of ARDS aims at reversing the deleterious consequences of inflammation without impairing the ventilation adequacy. Research has shown that glucocorticoid therapy is very important in reversing this by inhibiting the excessive inflammatory process and promoting resolution of lung injury. Long-term low-to-moderate dose glucocorticoid treatment has been associated with augmented pulmonary physiology and reduced morbidity, as evident by a significant increase in mechanical ventilation-free days among the patients. The treatment is crucial in that it can also result in augmented hospital survival rates, changing the nature of care for ARDS management. All therapeutic decisions taken regarding glucocorticoids involve a careful balancing of potential benefits and risks so that the patient-centric approach is always prioritized while treating this complex syndrome (Meduri et al., 2016). Apart from pharmacotherapy, advances in mechanical ventilation methods have emerged to optimize outcomes in ARDS patients. Inspiratory lung protective ventilation with low tidal volume and augmented positive end-expiratory pressure (PEEP) is applied for minimizing ventilator-induced lung injury while preserving oxygenation. Besides, adjunct treatment such as prone positioning has been identified to maximize ventilation-perfusion matching and increase levels of oxygenation, especially in severe patients who are non-responsive to conventional therapy.

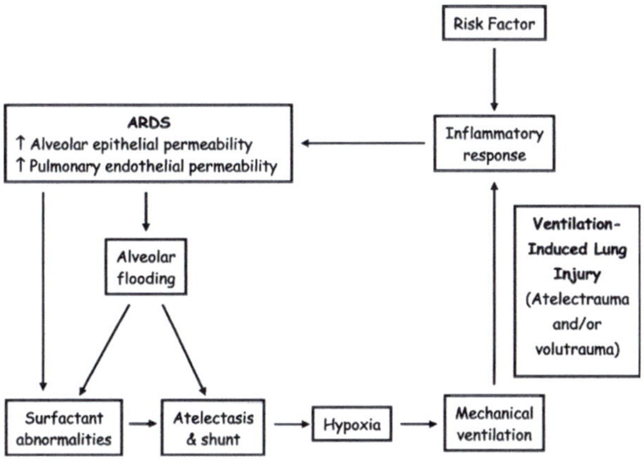

Figure 2.3. Current schematic of the pathophysiology of ARDS.

Source: https://external-content.duckduckgo.com/iu/?u=https%3A%2F%2Fwww.researchgate.net%2Fprofile%2FRuth_Graham7%2Fpublication%2F12416590%2Ffigure%2Ffig1%2FAS%3A784547142717443%401564062023879%2FCurrent-schematic-of-the-pathophysiology-of-ARDS.png&f=1&nofb=1&ipt=824ac6d33205ba017134fa0671c70a1b14733b1a0b86370c8b5e8054eda29de6.

Evidence confirms that these positional therapy maneuvers can yield important clinical advantages, including enhanced respiratory compliance and decreased oxygen requirements. As clinicians continue to refine their approach to the management of ARDS based on new evidence and case series, successful management strategies will continue to focus on reducing mortality and sustaining lung function in severe illness (Azimzadeh et al., 2017) (Figure 2.3).

2.1.1. Mechanisms of Lung Injury

The pathophysiology of lung injury in patients with ARDS includes a complex interaction between inflammatory mechanisms and mechanics. The condition most commonly leads to disruption of the alveolar-capillary membrane with increased permeability and pulmonary edema. Inflammatory mediators, such as cytokines, play a vital role in this process and are responsible for recruiting neutrophils, which augment surface damage to the lung through the elaboration of proteolytic enzymes and reactive oxygen metabolites. During this process, the structure of the normal lung is destroyed, and oxygenation and gas exchange are impaired. An understanding of these mechanisms provides the foundation for creating effective management, particularly because interventions aimed at reducing inflammation hold therapeutic potential. These findings inform clinical practice that not only seeks to enhance respiration but also directly works to safeguard lung tissue from further damage, emphasizing the two-fold focus that is needed in treating ARDS patients. Mechanical ventilation, being a necessary adjunct to the management of respiratory failure, ironically induces further lung injury if poorly managed. Use of high tidal volumes and pressures can lead to volutrauma, where hyperdistention of the alveoli causes cell injury and lung inflammation. The repeated recruitment and decruitment of collapsed lung units can also produce other mechanical stress, referred to as atelectrauma, to contribute to overall lung injury. Present-day research identifies the importance of employing protective ventilation strategies, specifically low tidal volume ventilation, which has been shown significantly to lower mortality in ARDS patients. These strategies are aimed at maintaining decreased airway pressures and judiciously applying positive end-expiratory pressure to prevent repetitive injury to the lung parenchyma. Thus, a comprehensive appreciation of the interaction between mechanisms of lung injury and mechanical ventilation is critical in the planning of therapeutic regimens in ARDS.

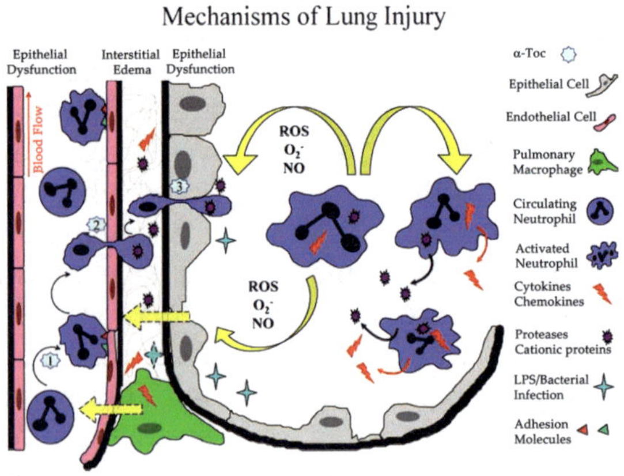

Figure 2.4. Mechanisms of lung injury.

Source: https://www.researchgate.net/profile/Gregory-Downey/publication/9088874/figure/fig1/AS:601589886758923@1520441614244/Mechanisms-of-lung-injury-Step-1-In-response-to-an-inciting-event-such-as-LPS.png.

Recruitment maneuvers are another controversial but potentially useful adjuvant in mechanical ventilation of ARDS. Recruitment maneuvers are applied to re-expand collapsed areas of the lung, enhancing ventilation-perfusion matching and overall oxygenation. However, the application of high airway pressures during the maneuvers is interspersed with worries about potential complications, including bacterial translocation and secondary inflammatory reactions. While benefits have been shown in specific scenarios, the efficacy of recruitment maneuvers in patients with features such as lung fibrosis or stiff chest wall is questionable. Ongoing research is an essential step in establishing the appropriate environments and techniques to facilitate a feasible, individually tailored approach that considers the patient's individual factors and minimizes the risk of further lung injury. In awareness of the nuances involved with these interventions, it will be important to optimize the results for patients with ARDS (Frank et al., 2002; Blanch et al., 2003) (Figure 2.4).

2.1.2. Role of Inflammation in ARDS

ARDS is characterized by massive inflammation, which is the core of its pathogenesis. Injury of lung parenchyma initiates a cascade of inflammatory mediators, leading to neutrophil and other immune cells' infiltration. The inflammatory response aims to limit infection and repair damaged tissue but, when deregulated, exacerbates lung injury. In ARDS, chronic activation of inflammatory processes can produce increased pulmonary vascular permeability and pulmonary edema formation, also causing respiratory failure. Understanding the inflammatory processes in ARDS is critical for focused therapeutic interventions aimed at restoring and offsetting the detrimental effects of inflammation on lung function and patient outcomes. Current research on glucocorticoid therapies has found them effective in modulating these inflammatory processes (Meduri et al., 2016). The inflammatory process in ARDS is further complicated by the interaction between various cytokines and chemokines that coordinate the immune response. Elevated plasma concentrations of pro-inflammatory cytokines such as interleukin-6 and tumor necrosis factor-alpha not only indicate the extent of lung injury but also induce systemic inflammation and result in multiple organ failure. Research has indicated that the responses of individual patients to these inflammatory mediators can be highly variable, making the treatment profile of ARDS complicated. Recent evidence has suggested that personalized therapies aimed at specific areas of inflammation could enhance patient outcomes. For instance, low-dose glucocorticoid treatment has also been described as being associated with increased survival and reduced days of mechanical ventilation in ARDS patients, suggesting the possibility of further research into the inflammatory mechanisms at play (Meduri et al., 2016).

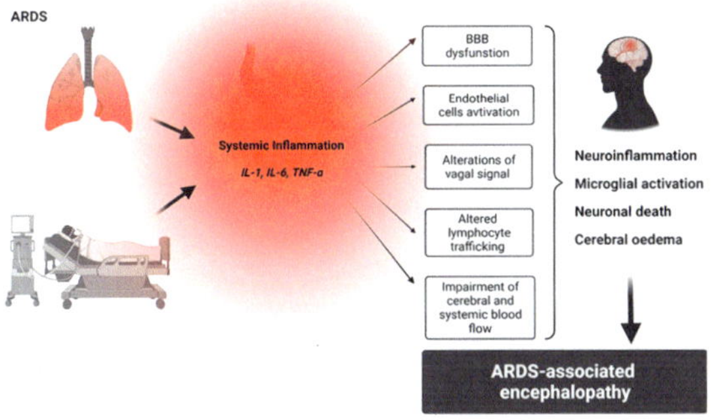

Figure 2.5. Role of inflammation in ARDS.

Source: https://www.researchgate.net/publication/362679774/figure/fig2/AS:11431281098015599@1668743373584/Role-of-inflammation-in-the-development-of-ARDS-associated-secondary-brain-injury.png.

Therapeutic maneuvers designed to modulate inflammation in ARDS have been of particular interest. A single approach is the use of beta-agonists, such as salbutamol, which have been reported to reduce lung water and, remarkably, affect neutrophil activation. Despite *in vitro* findings having established that salbutamol has no significant effect on neutrophil chemotaxis or apoptosis, administration has been associated with increased neutrophil levels in the blood, suggesting an ambivalent association between inflammation and treatment. Much research into modifying the inflammatory response in ARDS is needed to progress effective therapy that minimizes lung injury without abandoning the protective role of inflammation. A thorough understanding and control of such inflammatory processes are the foundation for improved clinical outcome in patients with this acute respiratory syndrome (Figure 2.5).

2.1.3. Impact on Gas Exchange and Lung Function

The complex interaction between the lung and gas exchange is significantly affected in ARDS. The important problem in ARDS is non-cardiogenic pulmonary edema, which results in disturbed gas exchange at the alveolar-capillary interface. This is conveyed by bilateral opacities on chest X-rays and hypoxemia that does not respond to supplemental oxygen. The consequent impairment of lung function can seriously complicate therapy with need for advanced therapeutic maneuvers to reestablish adequate oxygenation and ventilation. Respiratory mechanics also become altered by ARDS in a way that lung compliance is impaired and the work of breathing is increased, which could potentiate the patient's respiratory drive and cause respiratory failure requiring mechanical ventilation (Finney et al., 2014). Gas exchange in patients with ARDS is typically treated with mechanical ventilation strategies aimed at preventing additional lung injury while maximizing oxygen delivery. Lung protective ventilation strategies consist of the use of lower tidal volumes and limiting plateau pressures in a bid to avoid ventilator-induced lung injury. Extracorporeal membrane oxygenation (ECMO) may be an adjunct therapy for ARDS that is particularly severe. Evidence indicates that ECMO can facilitate lung protective ventilation by preventing excessive lung function decline while allowing more limited mechanical support. This method has been discovered to have promise in improving patient outcome for ARDS patients with severe hypoxemia, as indicated by research which shows that ECMO could improve oxygenation while avoiding mechanical loading in diseased lungs (Finney et al., 2014). Despite advances in management strategies, the impact of ARDS on gas exchange and lung function remains a final challenge. Rescue therapy such as recruitment maneuvers, pruning, and inhalation of nitric oxide has been implemented to support oxygenation but with unpredictable impact on long-term mortality. Current data emphasize that a multi-dimensional approach, with careful fluid management, may be required to optimize outcomes. The response heterogeneity to different interventions underlines the need for patient-specific management, taking into account the severity of ARDS and the accompanying comorbidities. Additional research has to further investigate the long-term efficacy of these interventions to lower mortality and enhance functional outcomes in patients with severe ARDS, ensuring therapeutic strategies are optimally adapted and refined (Alessandri et al., 2018) (Figure 2.6).

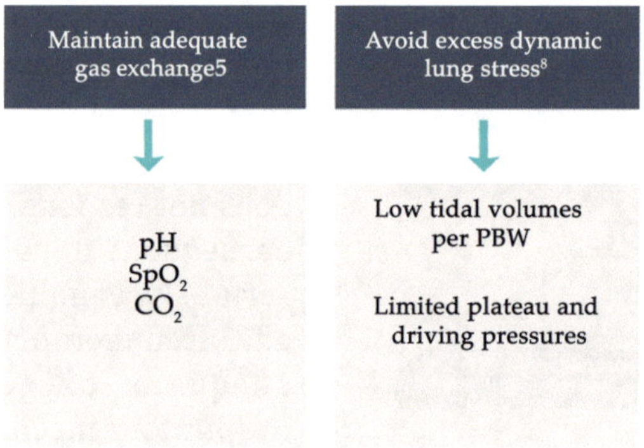

Figure 2.6. ARDS impact on gas exchange and lung function.

Source: https://www.getinge.com/siteassets/start/products-and-solutions/intensive-care/acute-respiratory-distress-syndrome-ards/ards_graphic_04-gas-lung-stress-750x500.jpg/cropbestbetmiddlecenter-640x427-255178229.jpg.

Test Your Knowledge

1. What are the mechanisms of lung injury?
2. What is the role of inflammation in ARDS?

2.2. Causes and Risk Factors

Learning Outcome

1. Common causes of ARDS (e.g., pneumonia, sepsis);
2. Patient demographics and susceptibility;
3. Environmental and genetic risk factors.

ARDS represents a complex clinical syndrome that is caused by a combination of etiologic and risk factors. Among the most recognized pulmonary precipitants, mention should be made of pneumonia, aspiration of gastric contents, and thoracic trauma. All these events can lead to extensive damage and inflammation of the alveolar-capillary membrane, ultimately ending in compromised gas exchange and respiratory failure. Studies show that patients with infections such as pneumonia have a higher risk of developing ARDS due to the inflammation present in the infection. Thoracic trauma also ruins the mechanical stability of the lungs, hence compounding the vulnerability to ARDS. Thus, health care professionals must be familiar with these pulmonary clinical etiologies because they direct prevention efforts and management of patients at risk (Toalongo et al., 2021). However, ARDS etiology does not comprise only pulmonary pathology. Extrapulmonary factors also play an important role in its onset. Pathologies like shock, sepsis, and critical trauma can precipitate ARDS since the systemic inflammatory response in the body can extend to and adversely affect lung tissue. For instance, sepsis not only initiates a generalized inflammatory reaction but also has the potential to produce multiple organ dysfunction, where the risk of respiratory complications is increased. In addition, some of the medical interventions, in particular mechanical ventilation, although required in some cases, can ironically cause lung function to deteriorate in vulnerable patients. It is crucial for medical professionals to identify these extrapulmonary risk factors so that preventive strategies can be begun effectively and therapy can be adjusted for the most vulnerable individuals who are at most significant risk for developing ARDS (Toalongo et al., 2021). Also, genetic susceptibility may influence predisposition to ARDS, providing an additional layer of etiology. Polymorphisms of genes that code for endothelial function and inflammatory cascades have been demonstrated to predispose individuals to ARDS after various insults, according to research. In certain patient populations, such as those undergoing assisted reproductive technologies, the risk factors would manifest in specialty avenues, such as ovarian hyperstimulation syndrome (OHSS), whose occurrence has been proven to induce pulmonary complications like ARDS. The realization of such intricate interplays between biological determinants and clinical conditions can prompt clinicians to more individualized treatment strategies. Thus, knowledge of the intricate etiology and risk factors of ARDS is important not only for improving clinical outcomes but also for enhancing quality of life in patients with this disabling disease.

2.2.1. Common Causes of ARDS (e.g., Pneumonia, Sepsis)

ARDS most commonly presents in critically ill patients and has several common etiologies that contribute to its pathophysiology. These include pneumonia, both community-acquired and hospital-acquired, as well as being the most common etiologies. The causative inflammatory response in the lungs from pathogens leads to alveolar-capillary membrane permeability, ultimately causing pulmonary edema. This is a serious process that seriously impairs gas exchange and may lead to severe respiratory failure if left untreated. Secondly, patients with pneumonia often have mechanical ventilatory demands, and this reflects the strong relationship between ARDS and infectious death. Appropriate management of pneumonia through intensive diagnosis and intervention is critical in avoiding its progression into ARDS, hence promoting survival in the critical care unit. Another frequent etiology of ARDS is sepsis, a systemic inflammatory reaction. The cytokine cascade due to sepsis, particularly the release of inflammatory mediators, will adversely affect lung function directly. As clinical evidence has indicated, sepsis elevates pulmonary vasculature permeability and tends to lead to fluid entry into alveoli, thus obstructing oxygenation. The severity of sepsis as an underlying condition for ARDS is evidenced by the fact that the condition frequently requires intensive care therapy and mechanical ventilation. The knowledge of the interaction between sepsis and ARDS heightens the need for timely identification and treatment of septic patients, which can minimize their susceptibility to the onset of respiratory distress. Extended care plans addressing both the systemic infection and the resulting pulmonary complication are critical to improving patient outcomes. Beyond sepsis and pneumonia, several other causes may also result in ARDS. Environmental stimuli, such as exposure to toxic inhalants or irritants in the lungs, are another key component of lung injury. The deposition of toxic substances could activate biological mechanisms leading to inflammation and injury to alveoli. Additionally, the pathogenic function of fibrinolysis imbalance, including the activity of Plasminogen Activator Inhibitor-1 (PAI-1), has been highlighted in recent research. Increased PAI-1 levels correlate with unfavorable prognosis in acute lung injury (ALI), illustrating the complex pathophysiologic mechanisms of ARDS (Brady et al., 2009). These observations highlight the necessity of having a multi-dimensional approach to learning and managing the various etiologic factors causing ARDS, moving towards improved identification, prevention, and treatment (Bai et al., 2013) (Figure 2.7).

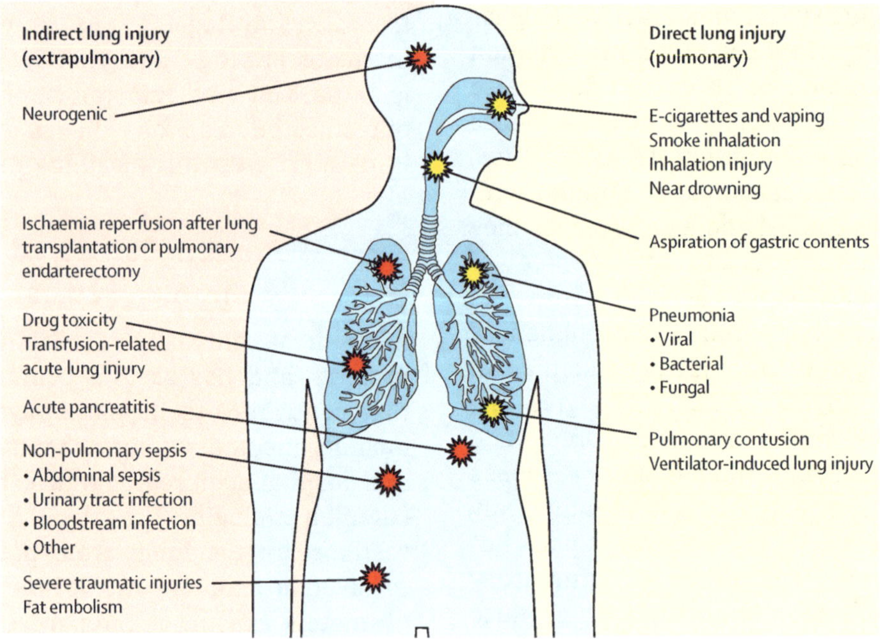

Figure 2.7. Causes of ARDS.

Source: https://www.thelancet.com/cms/10.1016/S0140-6736(22)01485-4/asset/d1d72dd7-db8c-4db9-8198-15b4bc359165/main.assets/gr1_lrg.jpg.

2.2.2. Patient Demographics and Susceptibility

Patient demographics are crucial in determining vulnerability to ARDS. The epidemiological features of populations indicate significant facts about the population groups that are most affected by this syndrome. Research indicates that patient age, gender, and pre-existing medical conditions are significant factors that determine susceptibility. For instance, elderly people, particularly at the age of 50-60 years, are more often hospitalized for ARDS and other respiratory conditions like COVID-19 complications, as indicated through patient sample research conducted in Iran (Abbaszadeh et al., 2020).

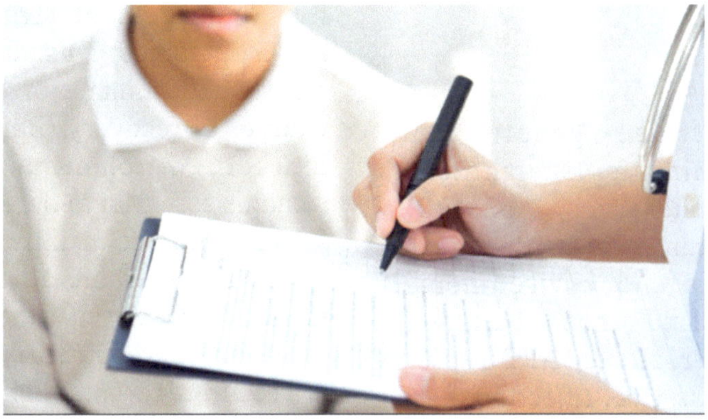

Figure 2.8. Patient demographics and susceptibility.

Source: https://external-content.duckduckgo.com/iu/?u=https%3A%2F%2Fhamid-razavi.com%2Fwp-content%2Fuploads%2F2022%2F02%2FHP-Razavi-Blog-Feb-770x433-1-770x433.jpg&f=1&nofb=1&ipt=b0d3be5116d717d63166eedc54d30b54570c11ac5d869e3b4599d50ae147b784.

Such age susceptibility can be explained by the naturally occurring decline in pulmonary function associated with aging and the increased prevalence of comorbidities characteristic of older individuals, both of which lead to a generally higher risk of complicated respiratory consequences. Gender imbalance plays a significant role in ARDS susceptibility as well. Data reflect an unequal gender representation of males over females, a trend also documented in a broad spectrum of respiratory disorders, including COVID-19. For instance, a study emphasized the sex ratio of COVID-19 patients as approximately 1.93:1 and indicated that male patients had a greater Case Fatality Rate (CFR) (Abbaszadeh et al., 2020). This disparity can be attributed to a range of reasons, including variation in their biological response towards infection and an increased number of underlying medical conditions, such as cardiovascular disease and diabetes, in male patients. Besides, social practices and occupational exposures can also expand such gender-related differences, putting extra emphasis on the need for gender as a demographic variable in ARDS susceptibility. In addition, comorbidities significantly enhance the likelihood of contracting ARDS. Hypertension, chronic respiratory diseases (CRD), and diabetes are frequently documented in those with severe presentations of respiratory distress (Abbaszadeh et al., 2020). These underlying health conditions not only compromise pulmonary function but also enhance the systemic inflammation that is a hallmark of ARDS. It is also fascinating that genetic factors can influence susceptibility to respiratory disease, as has been studied in reports looking at the impact of ACE gene polymorphisms.

Whereas research has provided inconsistent findings regarding the role of genetic factors in SARS progression, male gender and age consistently emerge as independent predictors of ARDS outcome. Understanding these intricate interactions between demographics and health outcomes is crucial to developing targeted prevention and therapy for ARDS (Figure 2.8).

2.2.3. Environmental and Genetic Risk Factors

The interaction between genetic and environmental determinants is significant in the predisposition and severity of ARDS. Genetic predispositions can affect an individual's response to pathogens and environmental stressors. For instance, some genomic variations may predispose a person to ARDS after triggering events such as viral infections, e.g., SARS-CoV-2. However, there remains limited evidence on genetic components, particularly for lung function impairment and how these variants interact with environmental exposures such as occupational hazards and air pollution leading to lung function impairment. The complexity of causation indicates the need for more comprehensive studies on both the genetic susceptibility and the external determinants of ARDS risk across different populations. Environmental risk factors are an essential part of the pathogenesis and course of ARDS, making prevention and care a multifaceted process. Cigarette smoke, outdoor pollution, and occupational dust exposure are implicated in increased incidence and severity of respiratory distress. Notably, pathophysiologic consequences of these environmental stresses may lead to ALI, which is a forerunner of ARDS. Current evidence shows that exposure to such toxins can predispose individuals to more severe clinical courses in the presence of infectious pathogens. Lung-protective ventilation and conservative fluid management strategies have improved ARDS outcomes, yet such environmental factors remain determinants of disease presentation and courses of recovery (Bai et al., 2013). Research into both environmental and genetic risk factors remains essential to the knowledge of how these factors interact in influencing ARDS outcome. While considerable advances have been made in the discovery of candidate genetic variants involved in respiratory disease, more effort is required to establish by what mechanisms such variants may be altered by exposure to the environment. Present research has also come to recognize the complexities of asthma and other respiratory diseases, such as the fact that environmental factors can enhance as well as inhibit the expression of genetic vulnerabilities. An understanding of these closely linked phenomena will enable clinicians to design individualized models of risk assessment and interventions that account for genetic as well as environmental factors, respectively, and thereby improve the management and outcome of ARDS in different populations.

Test Your Knowledge

1. What are the common causes of ARDS?
2. Explore patient demographics and susceptibility?

2.3. Clinical Presentation

Learning Outcome

1. Symptoms and signs of ARDS;
2. Diagnostic criteria and tools;
3. Differentiating ARDS from other respiratory conditions.

Clinical presentation of ARDS includes an acute development of respiratory distress typically within one week of a known insult. The patients have a variety of symptoms, including dyspnea, tachypnea, and hypoxemia. Bilateral pulmonary infiltrates on imaging tests can be observed in initial assessments, complicating the diagnosis as theyoverlap with pneumonia and other lung conditions. Acute cause of this syndrome is perhaps augmented by the existence of underlying disorders, e.g., infection, trauma. Clinical variables such as the urgency and severity of symptoms can play an essential role in modulating management. Of note is the significant contribution of the timing of intervention to managing the sudden deterioration in respiratory function. Early recognition of these symptoms is important in optimizing results and avoiding the progression of the syndrome, making way for immediate treatment. In cases of ARDS caused by infectious etiology, clinical presentation can typically overlap with that of COVID-19, emphasizing the disease's rapid progression. This underscores the value of careful clinical evaluation, possibly with the use of point-of-care ultrasound (POCUS) as an assessment tool. Using POCUS, clinicians can assess lung involvement as the pathologic changes of COVID-19 are peripheral in nature. With such imaging modalities, integration enables clinicians to make instant decisions on patient management and thereby reduce clinical uncertainty. Studies have revealed that the method has a more accurate assessment in the setting of acute dyspnea among patients and is vital in guiding treatment decisions, particularly where it is essential to distinguish between ARDS of various etiologies, including those resulting from viral infections like SARS-CoV-2 (Becherer-Bailey et al., 2020). Moreover, consideration of less common causes of ARDS can shed light on the complex clinical manifestation of the syndrome. For instance, granulomatous diseases like sarcoidosis may present as ARDS only rarely, leading to erroneous diagnosis if the underlying pathology is not ruled out. Patients may be without a previous diagnosis, and thus clinical manifestations become more challenging to manage. Autopsy findings reveal that idiopathic ARDS is potentially caused by underlying sarcoidosis, highlighting the need for more differential diagnoses. This case highlights the importance of an integrated diagnostic process for cases of acute respiratory failure. Understanding the wide range of conditions that can lead to ARDS can significantly enhance therapeutic efforts and outcomes for patient care. This is particularly true in cases of diagnosis after death, highlighting once again how challenging it is to detect atypical presentations (Chan et al., 2018) (Figure 2.9).

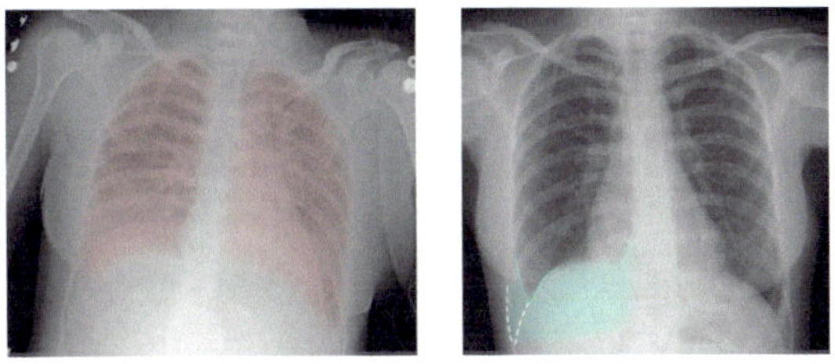

Figure 2.9. Clinical presentation of ARDS.

Source: https://media-us.amboss.com/media/views/60b87936b3d39.jpg.

2.3.1. Symptoms and Signs of ARDS

Early diagnosis of ARDS is crucial for timely treatment and improved outcomes in patients. The significant symptoms of ARDS develop within hours to days following a precipitating event, such as pneumonia, trauma, or sepsis.

Clinically, the patients are typically described by extreme dyspnea, a severe sense of shortness of breath, and abrupt appearance of tachypnea, a pronounced elevation of respiratory rate. The patient's oxygen saturation may fall quite significantly, reflecting gas exchange impairment. The lungs, too, on auscultation may have bilateral rales or crackles because of alveolar fluid. These need to be identified so that early evaluation may occur, hopefully avoiding the serious implications associated with this fatal syndrome. As ARDS progresses, additional clinical findings are more prominent, corresponding with the severity of lung injury and ventilatory dysfunction. Patients will have evidence of increased work of breathing, usually manifesting as accessory muscle recruitment and retractions due to compromised lung compliance. Cyanosis will also be present, reflecting inadequate delivery of oxygen to tissues, and will become evident with or without supplemental oxygen therapy. The evolution into bilateral infiltrates on chest radiograph further confirms the diagnosis of ARDS over other respiratory diseases. Additionally, patients require mechanical ventilation as hypoxemia aggravates, leading healthcare providers to initiate advanced respiratory support strategies. This evolution calls for the critical situation of patients in an integrated fashion to counteract evolving symptoms and signs of the syndrome. It is important to recognize the pathophysiological processes of ARDS to appreciate its clinical presentation. The syndrome results from direct lung injury, such as in pneumonia, and indirect lung injury from systemic disease, such as shock or sepsis. For instance, in some cases of Q fever, ARDS has been noted as a dominant feature, making it imperative for clinicians to be aware of its diverse presentations (Anderson et al., 2007). This intricate interaction of multiple elements leads to intense pulmonary inflammation, increased vascular permeability, and disrupted surfactant function, consequently exacerbating the typical features of ARDS. The overall clinical presentation covers not only respiratory but also systemic symptoms, such as a change in mental status secondary to hypoxemia. With the incorporation of this information, clinicians are better able to navigate the fields of diagnosis and management of ARDS (Dyer et al., 2019) (Figure 2.10).

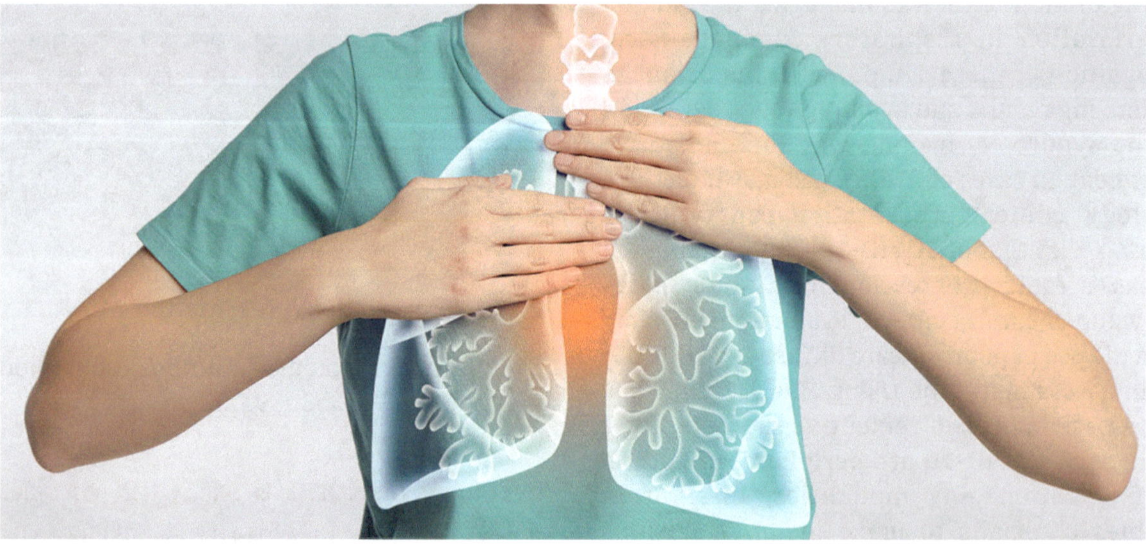

Figure 2.10. Symptoms and signs of ARDS.

Source: https://www.kauveryhospital.com/blog/wp-content/uploads/2024/03/ARDS-Treatment-1200x545_c.jpg.

2.3.2. Diagnostic Criteria and Tools

The diagnosis of ARDS calls for a careful strategy with sensitive diagnostic criteria and tools that guide clinical decision-making. The Berlin definition, first proposed in 2012, places ARDS in three categories of severity—mild, moderate, and severe—based on the severity of hypoxia by the PaO2/FiO2 ratio. Radiographic results, on the other hand, are typically obtained with the help of chest X-rays or computed tomography (CT) scanning for imaging bilateral opacities not entirely explained by effusions, lobar lung collapse, or nodules. Other explanations for respiratory failure, such as cardiogenic pulmonary edema or anatomical disorders, need to be excluded in order to diagnose ARDS and treat accordingly (Azoulay et al., 2016). Diagnostic equipment is part of the effort to establish the etiology of ARDS. Noninvasive diagnostic tests like arterial blood gas analysis and pulse oximetry provide preliminary information about the respiratory condition and oxygenation of the patient. Besides this, advanced techniques like bronchoscopy and bronchoalveolar lavage (BAL) are often employed to gain a better insight into the diagnosis, particularly when infection is a presumed etiology. High mortality rates were seen in a study of critically ill hematological patients for some etiologies of ARDS, pointing to the importance of proper diagnosis. Both invasive pulmonary aspergillosis and unclassified etiology of ARF had high correlation with poor outcomes in this population and emphasized the importance of employing a practical diagnostic approach (Azoulay et al., 2016). While modern diagnostic tools and standards have revolutionized the ARDS process, there are cases when the etiology evades identification. In certain sporadic cases, for example, diseases such as sarcoidosis can show up as ARDS without prior diagnosis, resulting in adverse clinical outcomes. The reality that a 41-year-old female who presented with ARDS was diagnosed with sarcoidosis only postmortem is a testament to the levels of complexity involved in ARDS diagnosis. These occurrences highlight the importance of clinicians not to settle for conventional etiologies of ARDS in their evaluations, as rigidly following typical causatives may result in inappropriate treatment. Therefore, an ongoing study to further define diagnostic strategies is crucial to empower healthcare providers to more accurately identify the myriad subtleties of ARDS and to improve outcomes (Figure 2.11).

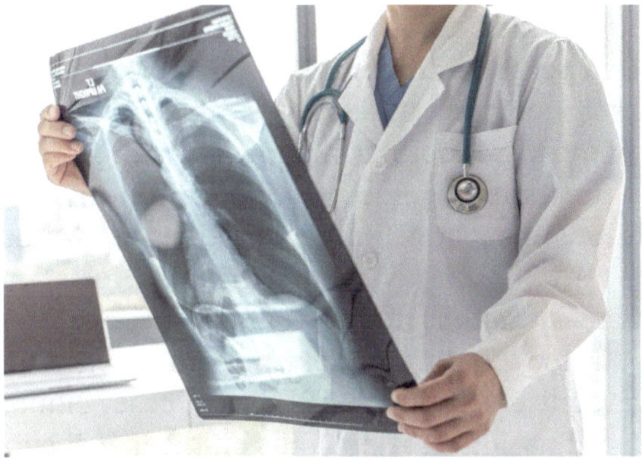

Figure 2.11. The diagnosis of acute respiratory distress syndrome (ARDS).

Source: https://www.apollohospitals.com/sites/default/files/2025-02/Acute-Respiratory-Distress-Syndrome-ARDS-scaled.jpg.

2.3.3. Differentiating ARDS from Other Respiratory Conditions

It is very important to differentiate ARDS from other respiratory conditions in order to treat the patient and obtain an optimal result effectively. ARDS is an acute-onset clinical syndrome with bilateral pulmonary infiltrates and profound hypoxemia, usually in patients with other risk factors such as sepsis, pneumonia, or trauma. In contrast, other conditions like cardiogenic pulmonary edema usually have overlapping symptoms but a different etiology, typically linked with heart failure or overloading of fluid. The differentiation process can significantly impact treatment strategy, which underscores the importance of proper clinical assessment and diagnostic methods for distinguishing between these overlapping presentations. Proper differentiation enables clinicians to effectively manage fluid distribution and oxygenation interventions, reducing complications from delayed therapy and incorrect diagnosis. Diagnostic approaches help differentiate ARDS from other respiratory disorders. Tests such as chest X-ray and lung ultrasonography, for instance, are very helpful in assessing fluid accumulation characteristic of pulmonary edema, which helps differentiate it from ARDS due to permeability increase. These modalities possess certain advantages, including high sensitivity to detect changes in lung water and function to guide treatment. Non-invasive methods, like transpulmonary thermodilution, also give hemodynamic information and enable clinicians to determine the cause of respiratory failure. Therefore, the ability to accurately discriminate ARDS from other similar respiratory illnesses depends on the use of such bedside evaluations, which guide intervention and patient management strategies, particularly within intensive care units (ICUs) (Assaad et al., 2018). The advent of COVID-19 has also complicated discriminating ARDS because the virus can induce respiratory failure that is extremely imitative of classical presentations of ARDS. Critical pneumonia due to SARS-CoV-2 infection often leads to the development of ARDS, primarily due to a cytokine storm involving pro-inflammatory mediators such as interleukin-6 (IL-6) (Kato et al., 2020). This overlap necessitates that clinicians recognize not only clinical symptoms but also be highly sensitive to the potential for viral infections, which can enhance inflammatory processes and result in rapid deterioration. Understanding the pathophysiologic mechanisms involved in ARDS, particularly in the case of COVID-19, enhances clinicians' precision in categorizing respiratory distress and implementing timely interventions. Such precision is vital because managing ARDS in infectious disease can be severely affected by the potential for misclassification, leading to inappropriate treatment measures and adverse patient outcomes.

Test Your Knowledge

1. What are the symptoms and signs of ARDS?
2. What are the diagnostic criteria and tools of ARDS?

2.4. Treatment Options

Learning Outcome

1. Supportive care and mechanical ventilation;
2. Pharmacological interventions;
3. Emerging therapies and clinical trials.

It is crucial to know about the management of ARDS so that patient outcomes can be improved. Traditional management lies heavily in support interventions, with significant emphasis on lung-protective mechanical ventilation and fluid management. The cornerstone of lung-protective ventilation is the application of reduced tidal volumes, which avoid ventilator-induced lung injury and enhance oxygenation. This technique avoids further damage to the alveolar-capillary membrane and avoids aggravating ARDS. While these interventions have proven useful in lowering ARDS-related morbidity, the decrease in mortality is modest, pointing toward a critical need for novel therapeutic drugs. Current pharmacologic interventions have limited application due to the syndrome's heterogeneous nature and the complexity of its pathophysiology, which renders it difficult to identify universally effective treatments (Calfee et al., 2017). Current advances in the understanding of the biological pathways of ARDS have spurred research into more targeted treatments. As one illustration, research into the role of mesenchymal stem cells (MSCs) shows the therapeutic potential of cell-based therapies for the management of ARDS inflammatory and healing processes. MSCs release a myriad of paracrine molecules that can decrease inflammation, regulate endothelial and epithelial permeability, and promote tissue repair, thereby offering a multidimensional approach to treatment. These advances are promising but remain to be translated into successful clinical interventions. The current absence of evidence-based pharmacologic treatments for ARDS challenges researchers to request personalized medicine approaches, applying biomarker discovery in tailoring treatments based on patient profiles (Calfee et al., 2017). The precision medicine model aims to select therapeutic strategies based on a patient's unique biological characteristics, maximizing treatment efficiency. With the progression of treatment modalities, continued research to bridge the gap between experimental data and clinical practice in the management of ARDS is imperative. Various clinical trials are in progress, emphasizing newer agents that act on inflammatory processes and augment alveolar repair. The knowledge acquired through such studies may determine effective therapeutic regimens while complementing the traditional dearth of pharmacologic options. In light of the various challenges in the management of ARDS, collaborative efforts that involve the expertise of researchers, clinicians, and biopharmaceutical companies will be instrumental. As science continues to investigate deeper into the pathophysiology of ARDS, the expansion of the treatment window by intensive research and development may herald a transformative shift in management, ultimately envisioning a world in which the effect of ARDS is significantly mitigated (Aggarwal et al., 2011) (Figure 2.12).

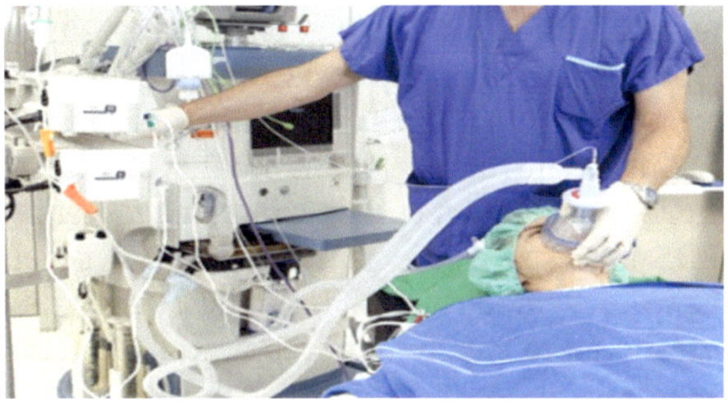

Figure 2.12. Treatment landscape for acute respiratory distress syndrome (ARDS).

Source: https://external-content.duckduckgo.com/iu/?u=https%3A%2F%2Fblogger.googleusercontent.com%2Fimg%2Fb%2FR29vZ2xl%2FAVvXsEho7MZ3dUAE3d2ef0ZXJ4Uzk7X-T0ETcOZCwmjU0GMUTz_bhciThElMxUdhF9ep1A1FeiPKQygwRX9UxO58VIgwCbBuKj7CHFLPP5dQAkvVHyD7ctRuWOmz5sVpQaEhz8_5wseDbJautsk%2Fw1200-h630-p-k-no-nu%2FAcute%2BRespiratory%2BD-istress%2BSyndrome%2BARDS.png&f=1&nofb=1&ipt=99978589348754d440accd4624fa2730b8333f43c7c53d3f6f1b577f644aa4cd.

2.4.1. Supportive Care and Mechanical Ventilation

Supportive care plays a fundamental role in the management of ARDS to stabilize the patient and handle the complex demands of severe respiratory failure. The key objective of supportive care is to achieve sufficient oxygenation and ventilation while preventing lung injury. This is particularly critical because ARDS puts patients at risk of severe complications like hypoxemic respiratory failure and multisystem organ dysfunction. Physicians become responsible for applying interventions in support of respiratory function, including supplemental oxygenation, hemodynamic monitoring, and effective fluid management. Because patients can clinically decline rapidly, frontline clinicians must be proactive and take advantage of evidence-based guidelines and protocols to adapt correspondingly to the dynamically evolving clinical status of ARDS patients to optimize their recovery potential and reduce mortality secondary to this syndrome. Mechanical ventilation emerges as a key factor in the management of ARDS in cases where patients present severe respiratory impairment. Mechanical ventilation is designed to supplement respiratory function and apply lung-protective mechanisms to avoid further injuring the alveoli. Low tidal volume ventilation treatment is commonly applied in managing ARDS and has been shown to improve outcomes compared to traditional modes of mechanical ventilation. In addition to tidal volume problems, the ventilator settings must be closely monitored to avoid such phenomena as ventilator-induced lung injury. Application of specific ventilation strategies can lead to enhanced oxygenation and reduced duration of mechanical support. Customized treatment addresses physiological needs and adheres to the best practices available today, highlighting the importance of modulating mechanical ventilation according to the patient's evolving clinical scenario. With the progress in critical care studies, the role of supportive care and mechanical ventilation is constantly changing, especially in the context of new viral infections such as COVID-19. As noted in the literature, patients with COVID-19 progressively develop hypoxemic respiratory failure that necessitates more sophisticated respiratory support closely mimicking the pathological process found in ARDS (Greenland et al., 2020). This raises the question of how care protocols can be optimized and how the pathogenesis of respiratory failure in such cases can be explained. Moreover, while there are no absolute treatments for ARDS, lung protection strategies in supportive care as well as mechanical ventilation have over time come to the fore in prominent roles (Fanelli et al., 2013). Ongoing research into novel therapeutic options aims to improve outcomes for those suffering from ARDS and its sequelae, ultimately highlighting the synergy between supportive therapy and mechanical ventilation in the successful treatment of this complex syndrome (Figure 2.13).

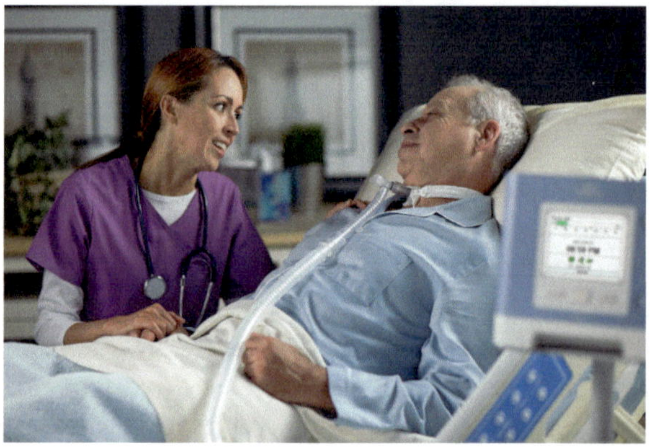

Figure 2.13. Supportive care and mechanical ventilation.

Source: https://external-content.duckduckgo.com/iu/?u=https%3A%2F%2Fwww.brooksidemulticare.com%2Fwp-content%2Fuploads%2F2019%2F12%2F810PhilipsTrilogy18500.jpg&f=1&nofb=1&ipt=6df21a201f5f2142322d8b0365df34f723e0c256244bd3c6a49b574e1df373cc.

2.4.2. Pharmacological Interventions

Pharmacologic treatment is at the heart of therapy for ARDS, a syndrome characterized by fatal pulmonary inflammation and increased alveolar-capillary membrane permeability. Overall, the objectives of such treatment are to counteract the underlying inflammatory process, improve oxygenation, and increase global lung function. Corticosteroids are a foundation of pharmacological treatment, which can suppress inflammation and improve outcomes in patients with ARDS. The implementation of these interventions in the clinical setting is based on evidence that early corticosteroid treatment may lower mortality rates in severe ARDS, as shown by several studies comparing corticosteroid dosing regimens and treatment timing. Thus, the prudent use of these drugs remains a focus in optimizing the therapy of patients with ARDS, highlighted by the evolving body of evidence in critical care. Apart from corticosteroids, the role of neuromuscular blocking agents should not be overlooked in the management of ARDS. These agents are particularly useful in patients with severe hypoxemic respiratory failure because they facilitate lung protective ventilation techniques, reducing respiratory effort and avoiding ventilator-induced lung injury. Administration of neuromuscular blockers can lead to enhanced compliance of the respiratory system and allow for lower tidal volumes, which are required in maintaining lung function and preventing further injury. Clinical practice guidelines typically recommend that the use of these drugs be followed by sedation protocols to facilitate patient comfort and facilitate invasive mechanical ventilation. Careful assessment of potential side effects, such as prolonged muscle weakness, should be done to avoid complications following drug withdrawal support, focusing on the need for individualized treatment regimens and monitoring. To advance further, the pharmacological management of ARDS remains ongoing, especially with the COVID-19 pandemic, where many patients have experienced profound respiratory involvement. Researchers have been looking for a number of new therapeutic agents to act against the intrinsically implicated pathophysiologic mechanisms of ARDS. For example, new evidence suggests that antiviral drugs and other cytokine-targeted drugs, which are a leading cause of ARDS in COVID-19 patients, may be worth the effort. The addition of such new drugs to clinical practice highlights the worth of evidence-based medicine in the intensive care setting, where clinicians strive to use the interventions that will provide the greatest benefits. Later, ongoing research and partnerships among healthcare professionals are central to advancing treatment modalities for this complex syndrome and applying established and emerging pharmacological interventions to their optimal extent, as highlighted in the literature (Greenland et al., 2020; Harris et al., 2016) (Figure 2.14).

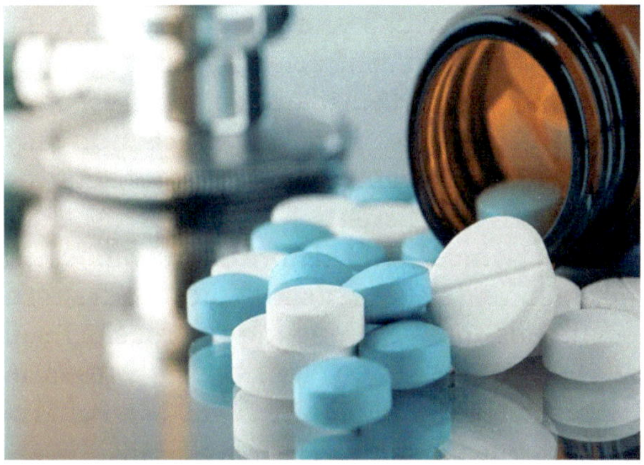

Figure 2.14. Pharmacological interventions.

Source: https://external-content.duckduckgo.com/iu/?u=https%3A%2F%2Fwww.pharmapproach.com%2Fwp-content%2Fuploads%2F2020%2F04%2FPharmacology.jpg&f=1&nofb=1&ipt=da54dc40c1febb341102166148a1e2d304453e950b3ea546d090fe30768f1edc.

2.4.3. Emerging Therapies and Clinical Trials

The emergence of novel treatments and clinical trials for ARDS is a promising avenue for optimizing patient outcomes in this critical illness. Current therapy is often incomplete due to the heterogeneous nature of ARDS with multiple underlying mechanisms and differential sensitivity to therapeutic methods. As highlighted in recent reviews, understanding the biological and analytical approaches necessary for precision medicine is central to identifying successful interventions based on the unique patient profile. This search is critical, especially as there are no widely accepted pharmacologic interventions for ARDS, highlighting the need for new therapies and targeted clinical trials designed with this subtlety (Calfee et al., 2017). Clinical trials in recent years have also witnessed the expansion of nascent treatments to modify the pathophysiologic processes of ARDS directly. For example, the platform of using biomolecular technology in combination with bioinformatics has established novel opportunities for therapy development. With a growing emphasis on the specificity of treatment, scientists are beginning to combine biomarkers to track patient response. This precision medicine approach not only aims to improve efficacy but also offsets the challenges of differential responses in ARDS patients, which have historically complicated therapeutic trials. Utilizing these advanced techniques, new therapeutic approaches can be enabled, potentially resulting in breaks in the care of ARDS (Calfee et al., 2017). Patient-reported outcomes (PROs) are increasingly being noted in the assessment of ARDS therapeutic interventions as well. Traditional methods such as spirometry have not been able to quantify the entire patient experience, including the psychological and functional impact of the disease. Current clinical trials now emphasize the need for holistic PRO measurements to supplement objective measurements. By doing this, researchers can obtain an integrated understanding of treatment outcomes, making it more likely to report significant benefits that directly correspond with patients' daily lives. This focus is a turn toward increased patient-centeredness for ARDS, whereby therapeutic development is directed not merely toward physiological benefit but also toward an enhanced overall quality of life (Figure 2.15).

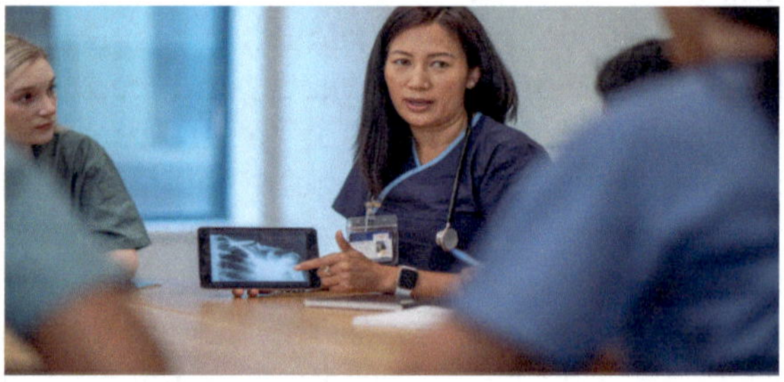

Figure 2.15. Emerging therapies and clinical trials.

Source: https://external-content.duckduckgo.com/iu/?u=https%3A%2F%2Fthemmrf.org%2Fwp-content%2Fuploads%2F2023%2F04%2Ftrials-hero.png&f=1&nofb=1&ipt=c780ea37e5e2d6b61a5d470b64896d0540562a8682f93538d3b9b6b20294ff04.

Test Your Knowledge

1. What is supportive care and mechanical ventilation?
2. What are the emerging therapies and clinical trials?

2.5. Prognosis and Outcomes

Learning Outcome

1. Factors influencing recovery;
2. Long-term effects of ARDS;
3. Statistical outcomes and survival rates.

The prognosis prediction of ARDS remains a complex issue due to various physiological and clinical factors. Studies demonstrate that certain biomarkers can play an important role in outcome prediction among patients with ARDS. For instance, high plasma levels of Plasminogen activator inhibitor-1 (PAI-1) have been linked to greater mortality in children, where findings indicate that for each increase in plasma PAI-1 by one log, the risk of death is almost double after adjusting for age and severity of illness. This finding suggests that PAI-1 may be a valuable prognostic marker, providing clinicians with the means for risk stratification and, by extension, potentially for determining the direction of therapeutic interventions during the initial treatment of ALI and ARDS patients (Brady et al., 2009). The heterogeneity of the syndrome, which increases the variability in the outcome of ARDS, makes it difficult to define uniform treatment protocols. Despite considerable advances over the past half-century in our understanding of its pathogenesis and risk factors, there remains a dearth of effective pharmacologic therapies directed specifically against ARDS. This paucity of target-based treatments can be attributed to the heterogeneity of patient responses to therapies and the limitations in drug trials targeting diverse biological pathways. Thus, researchers emphasize the need for a precision medicine approach comprising an individualized biomarker profile to optimize treatment among ARDS patients (Calfee et al., 2017). This paradigm shift may potentially not only enhance patient population stratification but also clinical outcome in general. Moreover, ARDS has a long-term effect on patient quality of life and outcome, beyond the acute critical care period. Long-term consequences such as pulmonary impairment, psychological impact, and physical health impairment are typically faced by survivors. It is important to understand the determinants of these long-term complications to develop extensive management and rehabilitation strategies. Continued investigation into predictive markers like PAI-1 and integration of new biological and analytical paradigms may uncover the determinants of acute survival and long-term health as well. By addressing the multibody prognosis and outcomes of ARDS, medical professionals can more effectively tailor interventions on an individual basis to enhance the recovery trajectories and quality of life of survivors of such a severe illness (Figure 2.16).

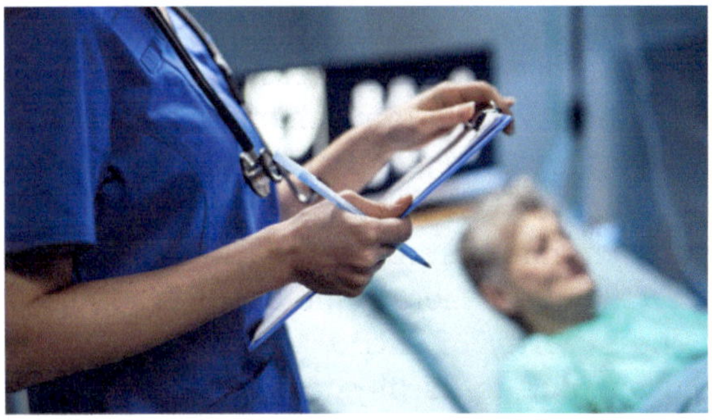

Figure 2.16. Prognosis and outcomes.

Source: https://external-content.duckduckgo.com/iu/?u=https%3A%2F%2Fwww.crossroadshospice.com%2Fmedia%2F5110%2Fprognosis.png&f=1&nofb=1&ipt=615906ddabf1fbd3dd1ba2c78644ea395e5da97aba06fdc3e83fdf0c8924e28e.

2.5.1. Factors Influencing Recovery

The course of recovery from ARDS is governed by a vast array of clinical and non-clinical variables that can significantly impact patient outcomes. Of these, the severity of lung injury at diagnosis takes precedence. More severe levels of ARDS typically have protracted recovery periods due to the extensive damage to the lungs that disrupts gas exchange and subjects them to secondary complications such as infection or organ failure. Comorbid conditions such as cardiovascular disease or diabetes also complicate the recovery process by suppressing overall physiological tolerance. Thus, controlling these factors is essential not only for short-term management strategies but also for long-term recovery planning because understanding the patient's baseline state of recovery can guide therapeutic decisions and improve rehabilitation outcomes. Another very significant aspect of determining recovery from ARDS is the management strategies used, which could be pretty different from facility to facility. Treatment modalities, including the utilization of ventilatory support and pharmacologic therapies, play significant roles in enhancing gas exchange as well as avoiding further injury to the lung. For example, administration of Positive End-Expiratory Pressure (PEEP) using mechanical ventilation enhances oxygenation through the maintenance of alveoli from closing, but must be cautiously managed to avoid hemodynamic instability. In the majority of cases, the ECMO therapy indication is a measure of the severity of ARDS, which also impairs recovery due to its physiological influence on drug pharmacokinetics, sometimes leading to variable therapeutic effects and increased side effects associated with drug use in therapy (Aebi et al., 2017). Thus, treatment modalities must be individually selected and implemented to the distinct clinical picture of each patient in an attempt to optimize outcome. Psychosocial problems also play a role in the recovery following ARDS. Patients who require ICU admissions also develop psychological disturbances in the form of anxiety, depression, and post-traumatic stress disorder (PTSD) that can hamper their recovery course. Social support systems, such as family involvement and availability of rehabilitation facilities, are essential to the development of a healthy recovery environment. Additionally, pain management and prognosis communication can influence the emotional state of a patient and, in turn, ensure they comply with rehabilitation processes. The integration of psychological well-being and physical recovery highlights the need for comprehensive care interventions that target both physiological and psychosocial spheres in recovery. Therefore, intervention against such multi-factorial influences can not only induce physical healing but also be a stimulus for an overall better quality of life among ARDS survivors (Figure 2.17).

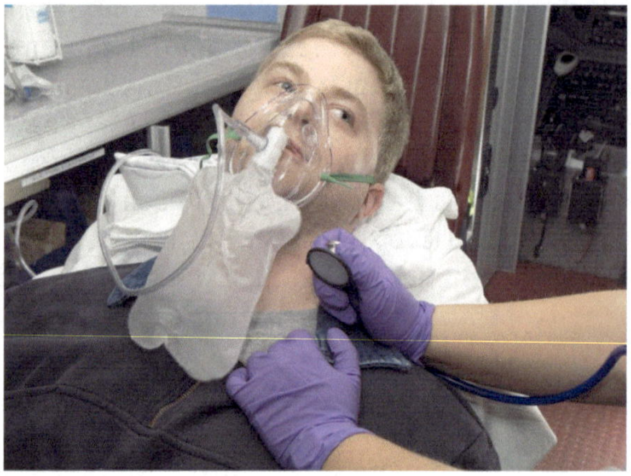

Figure 2.17. Factors influencing recovery from acute respiratory distress syndrome (ARDS).

Source: https://external-content.duckduckgo.com/iu/?u=https%3A%2F%2Fcdn-prod.medicalnewstoday.com%2Fcontent%2Fimages%2Farticles%2F266%2F266682%2Fards-patient.jpg&f=1&nofb=1&ipt=25d51519e5cade642ebb09d74f12dd4781336fa8038f32d53581a6fce8b1cd09.

2.5.2. Long-Term Effects of ARDS

The long-term effects of ARDS significantly affect survivors' physical, psychological, and economic well-being. ARDS survivors are often faced with various chronic pulmonary complications, including impaired lung function and worsening pre-existing illnesses like chronic obstructive pulmonary disease (COPD). The patients also experience exercise intolerance and chronic respiratory symptoms, all of which enhance compromised quality of life. Furthermore, functional disabilities due to ARDS may lead to long-term issues in the return to work, social functioning, and daily activities. This compromising of functional status underscores the necessity for vigorous, comprehensive rehabilitation programs addressing both respiratory function and patient recovery overall. Apart from the physical consequences, psychological impacts are also prominent among ARDS survivors, who usually develop psychological concerns such as PTSD, anxiety, and depression. The near-universal severity of illness, in association with the intensive medical interventions received in their hospital stay, can generate psychological trauma that will impact them long after the acute resolution of the syndrome. Thus, mental health assessment and successful interventions should be integral to post-ARDS care since they can considerably enhance the quality of life for survivors. A few intervention strategies may include cognitive behavioral therapy and other psychological support interventions, which can lead to enhanced mental health results, thereby allowing patients to become better reintegrated within their community. Moreover, advanced treatment techniques in ARDS, such as glucocorticoid therapy and ECMO, are redefining patient outcomes. Empirical evidence suggests that glucocorticoid treatments can induce significant improvements in hospital survival and prevent long-term sequelae of the inflammatory process in ARDS patients (Meduri et al., 2016). ECMO, once viewed as a resuscitation last resort, has now become an inherent component of the treatment regimen in seriously ill ARDS cases and is often used in lung-protective ventilation and potentially to improve long-term outcomes (Finney et al., 2014). Such evolving treatment paradigms highlight the importance of ongoing research and modifications in practice so that care provided not only addresses the problem of short-term survival but also considers long-term consequences of ARDS on patients' health and well-being in general (Figure 2.18).

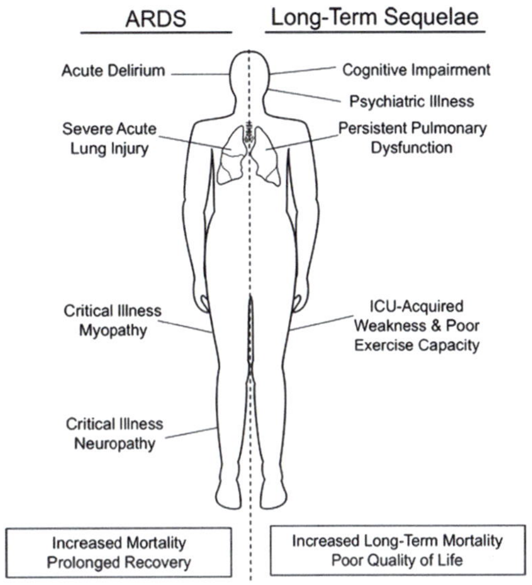

Figure 2.18. The long-lasting effects of the acute respiratory distress syndrome.

Source: https://www.tandfonline.com/cms/asset/805d9be5-ed34-49ab-a501-86d7f38e88ed/ierx_a_1743182_f0001_b.gif.

2.5.3. Statistical Outcomes and Survival Rates

The mortality rates and statistical outcomes of ARDS patients reveal shocking facts about the severe implications of this syndrome. As a guideline, according to the LUNG SAFE study, which followed a representative sample population of ICU patients from across the globe, ARDS accounted for 10.4% of ICU admissions, and a shocking 23.4% of patients required intubation. The incidence of ARDS not only indicates its prevalence but also highlights the significant workload it poses for healthcare systems worldwide. Immediate clinician identification of ARDS was incredibly low within the cohort, reflecting a colossal influence which was potentially detrimental to treatment effectiveness and outcomes overall. These statistics indicate that improved awareness and early detection by physicians enable better treatment of ARDS, thus increasing the chances of survival. Mortality rates from ARDS are a grim indication of its severity. The study revealed that hospital mortality was closely associated with the subtypes of ARDS, with rates rising from 34.9% in mild cases to 46.1% in severe cases — a trend substantiating the classification scheme of the Berlin Definition. The data not only reflect the severity of the prognosis of patients based on the severity classification but also reflect the importance of early and appropriate therapeutic interventions. Also, the data implicates a disturbing association of low clinician recognition rates and poorer mortality results, again necessitating enhanced management guidelines. The adoption of lung protective ventilation strategies may dramatically impact survival rates, as reflected by changes in ICU practices. The debate about optimal ventilatory methods and adjunctive treatments merely serves to add complexity to ARDS management. Use of techniques such as prone positioning and ECMO has found popularity in recent years, which reflects a shift towards more aggressive therapies. The CESAR study, which established the role of ECMOs in managing severe ARDS, showed improved outcomes when these newer techniques were used, particularly in patients with severe influenza infection. Despite this, the contexts and timing under which these modalities would be applied remain controversial among medical practitioners. Considering the ongoing evolution of our knowledge about ARDS, it is important to continue improving treatment approaches to maximize survival rates and enhance overall critical care for patients in ICUs.

Test Your Knowledge

1. What are the factors influencing recovery?
2. What are the long-term effects of ARDS?

2.6. Prevention Strategies

Learning Outcome

1. Identifying at-risk populations;
2. Infection control measures;
3. Strategies for reducing lung injury.

It is vital to integrate appropriate prevention interventions in reducing the incidence of ARDS among critical illness patients. One of the significant measures involves vigilant monitoring of high-risk groups like severe brain injury patients. Since neurological dysfunction comes with respiratory issues, heightened vigilance can aid in early detection and timely intervention for cases of respiratory failure or pneumonia. Therefore, health care workers ought to be equipped with the knowledge and skills of recognizing signs of failing respiratory conditions. Moreover, implementing airway management and mechanical ventilation guidelines can protect patients with compromised airway reflexes, thereby lowering the risk of acquiring ARDS. Emphasis on proactive monitoring and intervention can strongly decrease morbidity associated with pulmonary complications in these vulnerable patients, as indicated by contemporary research (Lee et al., 2012). The second key strategy for preventing ARDS centers on optimizing lung protective ventilation strategies. Adherence to lung-protective ventilation strategies involves application of decreased tidal volumes and avoidance of excessive amounts of positive end-expiratory pressure (PEEP), which has been shown to reduce lung injury. Furthermore, initiation of a fluid-conservative protocol can significantly improve patient outcomes through reduced pulmonary edema and general improvement in respiratory mechanics. The manner in which these strategies are implemented must be approached with careful attention to the specific patient's condition, as under-treatment and overtreatment both pose potential risk. Active clinical trials continue to seek out new ventilation strategies that further reduce the incidence of ARDS and associated complications. This study attests that integrating evidence-based practices into care guidelines is essential for enhancing patient safety and clinical outcomes in critically ill patients (Bai et al., 2013).

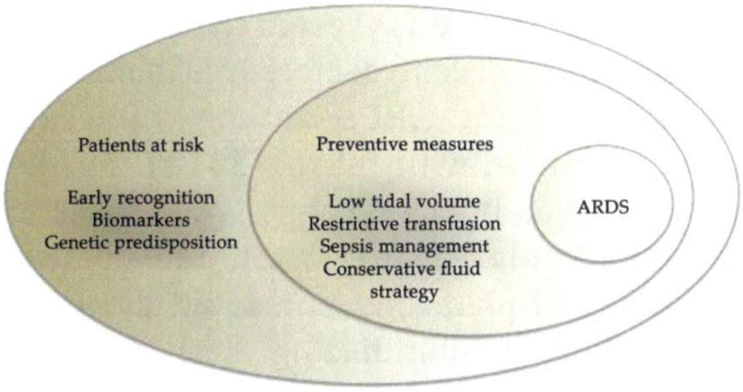

Figure 2.19. Preventive approaches to ARDS.

Source: https://www.researchgate.net/profile/Candelaria-De-Haro/publication/236337150/figure/fig2/AS:202889055215617@1425383928574/Preventive-approaches-to-ARDS.png.

Finally, raising awareness among health staff regarding the complex causality of ARDS and prevention best practices can reinforce institutional programs in addressing this serious condition. Continuing education efforts must reach not only the medical personnel directly involved in caring for patients but also interprofessional teams involved in critical care. This gives an intrinsic understanding of risk factors, such as environmental factors and the effects of tobacco exposure, which enhance clinical consequences among susceptible groups. Increased awareness and knowledge can facilitate more informed decision-making for the prevention and management of ARDS. As the medical community learns more about mechanisms of prevention, the potential for reducing the burden of ARDS becomes increasingly possible. Hence, it becomes essential to create a learning and adaptive culture for practice transformation that aligns with patient care (Lee et al., 2012) (Figure 2.19).

2.6.1. Identifying at Risk Populations

Identifying risk populations for ARDS is crucial in the management and effective intervention of this harmful disorder. Several risk factors identified contribute significantly to the development of ARDS, including predisposing conditions, environmental exposure, and demographics. Critically ill patients, especially those with sepsis, pneumonia, or major trauma, have a greater incidence of ARDS. Current studies have also stressed the adverse impacts of cigarette smoke exposure, which may heighten vulnerability to respiratory distress through exacerbation of lung conditions. It is by understanding such risk factors that medical experts can screen and keep track of vulnerable populations, thereby improving early detection and treatment rates among ARDS patients. Further, advances in biomolecular technology have made it possible to create a more sensitive test to identify vulnerable people. With the analysis of patterns of protein expression in plasma and BAL fluid, it is now possible for researchers to detect biomarkers that have the potential to predict whether a patient will develop ARDS. This precision medicine model is important because current pharmacologic treatments for ARDS are presently constrained by the syndrome's heterogeneous nature and differential response to conventional therapies. As noted in recent literature, combining biologic and analytical approaches can enhance the ability to appropriately target interventions in populations known to be at risk, possibly preventing the development of syndromes and associated morbidity (Calfee et al., 2017). Epidemiologic research further emphasized the importance of understanding environmental determinants in the pathogenesis of ARDS. Exposure to toxicants, allergens, and other pathogenic factors can also significantly raise the likelihood of developing ALI. For instance, adding social determinants of health, for instance, socioeconomic status, ability to access medical treatment, and living conditions, creates a more accurate picture of at-risk populations. As further study continues to shed light on these domains, the field is moving toward recognition of the multi-dimensional character of ARDS risk factors. This broader context is key to creating effective public health interventions and procuring proactive care for at-risk populations, particularly given the high mortality rates inherent to ARDS (Bai et al., 2013).

2.6.2. Infection Control Measures

Infection prevention practices play a significant role in avoiding the hazard of ARDS, particularly in susceptible infections such as COVID-19. The rapid and uncontrolled spread of the SARS-CoV-2 virus has emphasized the significance of robust infection prevention practices in healthcare settings and the community at large. Effective measures include following proper hygiene measures, such as hand hygiene and the use of personal protective equipment (PPE), to reduce the transmission rate. Furthermore, early vaccination drives are essential for developing herd immunity and preventing severe cases resulting in ARDS. As indicated in recent studies, knowledge of the pathways through which these viruses are transmitted can direct targeted interventions and make the argument for a coordinated public health response to emerging public health threats, readying health systems for newly emerging respiratory pathogens as illustrated in global activities concerning COVID-19 (Ansari et al., 2020). In addition, continuous infection control requires continued training and education of healthcare professionals and the general public. Educational campaigns emphasizing symptom recognition, when to seek a doctor, and quarantine's role in reducing spread are all components of an across-the-board approach to preventing ARDS. The ever-present threat posed by emerging viruses, such as the recent outbreaks of MERS-CoV and H7N9, requires infection prevention practices to be regularly reviewed and updated based on new evidence. Coordination of health agencies at a global level is crucial for creating universal protocols that can be applied across various populations. Gaps in knowledge of transmission dynamics emphasize the importance of collaborative action and rigorous research to develop effective infection control measures to minimize the incidence of ARDS among vulnerable individuals (Al-Tawfiq et al., 2014). Further, the role played by new technology in infection prevention cannot be overstated. Telemedicine, mobile health platforms, and rapid diagnostic platforms are revolutionizing the patient care model, particularly in the management of respiratory diseases. These advances make early intervention possible, reducing the risk of disease progression to ARDS by enabling earlier identification of infected individuals. Health systems can leverage analytics to track and predict outbreak patterns, thereby embracing pre-emptive measures to prevent APO. The integration of traditional public health measures with cutting-edge technology presents an interesting avenue through which infection control can be enhanced. By applying a holistic approach consisting of education, technology, and co-operation, the healthcare fraternity can successfully minimize the risks associated with respiratory infections and their potential development into more severe complications such as ARDS (Ansari et al., 2020).

2.6.3. Strategies for Reducing Lung Injury

Effective management strategies for ARDS patients aim to minimize lung damage caused by mechanical ventilation. One of the most important interventions is lung-protective ventilation, where low tidal volumes are used to prevent alveolar stretch damage. The strategy has been shown to reduce mortality rates in comparison to standard high tidal volume ventilator techniques. By avoiding overdistension of the lungs, this strategy follows the overall objective of minimizing ventilator-induced lung injury (VILI). Along with maintaining optimal positive end-expiratory pressure (PEEP), these ventilation strategies improve oxygenation while avoiding repetitive trauma to the lung parenchyma.

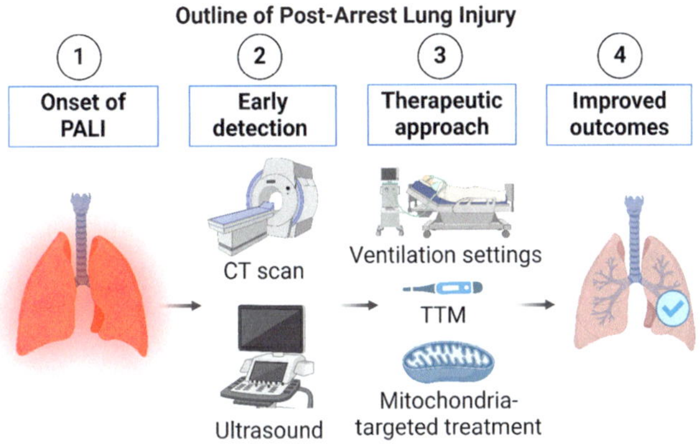

Figure 2.20. Strategies for reducing lung injury.

Source: https://media.springernature.com/lw685/springer-static/image/art%3A10.1186%2Fs40560-024-00745-z/MediaObjects/40560_2024_745_Fig1_HTML.png.

Therefore, the implementation of lung-protective ventilation not only addresses the short-term requirements of oxygenation in patients but also plays a major role in preserving lung integrity in the long term, which is crucial for ARDS recovery. Fluid management also constitutes a critical component of interventions to minimize lung injury in ARDS. Restrictive fluid protocols are increasingly recommended to minimize pulmonary edema and maximize oxygenation outcomes. There is evidence that precise attention to fluid administration leads to better clinical outcomes, including reduced 60-day mortality rates. By avoiding fluid overload, restrictive fluid management not only reduces the occurrence of worsening pulmonary complications but also supports optimal hemodynamics. It also needs to be fine-tuned because under-resuscitation and over-resuscitation both remain potential causes of adverse outcomes. Therefore, employing a strategy of rigorous fluid management can significantly reduce lung injury risk in ARDS patients since it also addresses the underlying pathophysiology of the syndrome and facilitates better recovery patterns. In addition to mechanical ventilation strategies and fluid management, innovative therapies have recently been identified as potential adjuncts in reducing lung injury in ARDS patients. Methods such as prone positioning have been promising in the ways that they increase ventilation-perfusion mismatch, thus improving oxygenation. Rescue therapy in the form of inhaled nitric oxide and ECMO is also another form of oxygenation aid in extreme cases of ARDS. Their overall mortality is, however, inconclusive and remains to be studied. Future studies must focus on personalized medicine approaches, leveraging biomolecules and genetic profiling to predict patient responses to these therapies, as per the literature at hand. Such a shift toward a precision medicine paradigm has the potential to lead to more effective treatment protocols directly aimed at the heterogeneity of ARDS, ultimately reducing lung injury and improving the patient outcome (Calfee et al., 2017) (Figure 2.20).

Test Your Knowledge

1. How to measure infection control?
2. What are the strategies for reducing lung injury?

Summary

ARDS requires a comprehensive understanding of its implications, treatment, and long-term impacts. As a multifaceted disease often initiated by a broad array of etiological factors, including sepsis and trauma, ARDS needs to be treated with prompt and effective interventions to mitigate its impact on patient outcomes. The critical care interventions, notably mechanical ventilation, continue to play a pivotal role in the management of this life-threatening syndrome, impacting both lung function and patient survival (Hillman et al., 2016). Balancing the intervention benefits, such as reduced work of breathing and removal of extravascular lung water, with their risks, including volume trauma and hypoxia, remains the key to optimizing patient care (Adams et al., 2016). The evolving understanding of ARDS forms the foundation for efforts to simplify treatment regimens and ultimately enhance patient recovery course. The complexity of ARDS implies the necessity for multidisciplinary approaches that address not only the pulmonary consequences but also the secondary effects on other organ systems. Research has highlighted the intricate interaction between respiratory failure and overall health, particularly through recent studies on neurological factors in severe cases, with viral infections like COVID-19 as a prime example. This kind of association signals to clinicians the multi-factorial nature of patient presentation, requiring greater caution in monitoring symptoms other than respiratory impairment (Boon et al., 2020). Thus, a treatment paradigm that encompasses both ventilatory support and interdisciplinarity-guided monitoring is imperative to minimize long-term morbidity in patients with ARDS. ARDS management as a whole represents the complexity of critical care medicine, encompassing respiratory, cardiovascular, and even neurologic considerations. Ongoing optimization of therapeutic modalities, in accordance with emerging research and clinical evidence, is fundamentally important to enhancing patient outcomes. An increased awareness of the long-term potential impact of ARDS, including potential neurological manifestations and deterioration in overall health, is crucial for clinicians. As the medical field evolves with new findings and emerging treatment options, a unified effort towards increased interdisciplinary collaboration is needed to avoid the challenges posed by ARDS, thereby fostering wider awareness and improved management of this important syndrome.

ARDS is a severe illness caused by an array of etiologies, producing significant morbidity and mortality in involved patients. Non-cardiogenic pulmonary edema is among the most prevalent manifestations of ARDS, manifesting as bilateral opacities on chest radiograph. Affected patients typically exhibit hypoxemia resistant to standard oxygen therapy, requiring supportive measures such as mechanical ventilation. The syndrome is also a frequent reason for ICU admission, and its successful management is the overriding concern (Alessandri et al., 2018). The last decade has witnessed research aimed at the discovery of definitive therapeutic strategies, though corticosteroids are not typically employed since their efficacy is very restricted in this context. Early detection and supportive care remain the focal points to maximize outcomes for ARDS patients. The treatment of ARDS has also evolved over the years, with new therapeutic modalities promising in the clinical setting. Current rescue therapies include recruitment maneuvers, prone position, inhaled nitric oxide, high-frequency oscillatory ventilation, and ECMO, all of which aim to enhance oxygenation in patients with severe disease (Alessandri et al., 2018). However, while these treatments look promising in reversing hypoxemia, their impact on mortality is unknown and needs investigation of their long-term safety and efficacy. Restrictive fluid management has also been recognized as a potentially useful strategy, since it does not reduce 60-day mortality significantly but can improve patient fluid balance during treatment. These results underscore the importance of patient-specific therapy based on individual patient needs and clinical context in the management of ARDS. More recent studies are also exploring new pharmacologic modalities that have the potential to address the underlying pathophysiologic mechanisms of ARDS. Of the interesting developments is the targeting of tumor necrosis factor-alpha (TNF-α), a cytokine that participates in the inflammatory pathways of ALI. Explorations of selective inhibition of TNFR1, the path through which toxic effects of TNF-α are mediated, have been promising in preclinical models and early human trials. For instance, a trial of the selective TNFR1 blocker GSK1995057 showed significant decreases in pulmonary inflammation and damage in animal and human models of endotoxin exposure. These findings anticipate that customization of the therapies to target specific inflammatory pathways in individuals directly will offer a novel method of preventing or mitigating the development of ARDS. With ongoing research, customization of treatment courses using both conventional and novel therapies will be imperative to optimizing patient outcomes in ARDS.

KEY TERMS FROM THIS CHAPTER

- Acute phase
- Alveolar-capillary membrane
- ARDS berlin
- Bilateral infiltrates
- Cytokine storm
- Exudative phase
- Fibrotic phase
- Hypoxemia
- Lung compliance
- Mechanical ventilation
- Non-cardiogenic pulmonary edema
- Oxygenation index
- PaO_2/FiO_2 ratio
- Positive end-expiratory pressure (PEEP)
- Proliferative phase
- Prone positioning
- Refractory hypoxemia
- Surfactant dysfunction

Critical Thinking Questions

1. **Which of the following is NOT a typical cause of ARDS?**
   a. Sepsis
   b. Aspiration of gastric contents
   c. Pulmonary embolism
   d. Severe trauma
2. **What is the hallmark feature of ARDS on chest imaging?**
   a. Hyperinflated lungs
   b. Bilateral infiltrates
   c. Unilateral lobar consolidation
   d. Cavitary lesions
3. **According to the Berlin definition, which of the following is a requirement for diagnosing ARDS?**
   a. PaO_2/FiO_2 ratio > 300
   b. Symptom onset within 4 weeks of an insult
   c. Evidence of left atrial hypertension
   d. Pulmonary edema from cardiac failure
4. **Which of the following ventilatory strategies is recommended in ARDS?**
   a. High tidal volume (10–12 mL/kg)
   b. Low PEEP
   c. Low tidal volume (4–8 mL/kg)
   d. Rapid respiratory rate (>30/min)
5. **What is a potential benefit of prone positioning in ARDS patients?**
   a. Increases cardiac output
   b. Improves oxygenation
   c. Reduces need for sedation
   d. Decreases tidal volume requirements

Short Answer Questions

1. What is the Berlin definition of Acute Respiratory Distress Syndrome (ARDS), and what are the key criteria?
2. List at least five common direct and indirect causes of ARDS.
3. Describe the pathophysiological changes in the alveolar-capillary membrane in ARDS.
4. What are the typical clinical signs and symptoms of ARDS?
5. What findings are typically seen on a chest X-ray or CT scan in a patient with ARDS?

Answer to Critical Thinking Questions

1. (c); 2. (b); 3. (b); 4. (c); 5. (b).

References

1. Nikpouraghdam, M., Farahani, A. J., Alishiri, G., Heydari, S., Ebrahimnia, M., Samadinia, H., Sepandi, M., Jafari, N. J., Izadi, M., Qazvini, A., Dorostkar, R., Tat, M., Shahriary, A., Farnoosh, G., Zijoud, S. R. H., Taghdir, M., Alimohamadi, Y., Abbaszadeh, S., Ghaleh, H. E. G., & Bagheri, M. (2020). Epidemiological characteristics of coronavirus disease 2019 (COVID-19) patients in IRAN: A single center study. *Journal of Clinical Virology*, *127*, 104378. https://doi.org/10.1016/j.jcv.2020.104378Adams, J. Y., Bradley, L. A., Dempsey, T. M., Kuhn, B., et al. (2016). Management of mechanical ventilation in decompensated heart failure. https://core.ac.uk/download/323070948.pdf (accessed on 30th June 2025).
2. Aebi, A. G. S., Anderson, M., Arlt, S., Barr, H., Barthelemy, O., Beiderlinden, M., et al. (2017). Medication complications in extracorporeal membrane oxygenation. https://core.ac.uk/download/129191716.pdf (accessed on 30th June 2025).
3. Aggarwal, R., Choudhary, S., Hokabaj, S., Mishra, R., et al. (2017). Ovarian hyperstimulation syndrome and pulmonary edema–A rare complication. https://core.ac.uk/download/539902782.pdf (accessed on 30th June 2025).
4. Aggarwal, S., Ajuebor, M. N., Barazzone, C., Beyth, S., Birukova, A., Chan, Y., Corcione, T., et al. (2011). Concise review: Mesenchymal stem cells for acute lung injury: Role of paracrine soluble factor. https://core.ac.uk/download/10082053.pdf (accessed on 30th June 2025).
5. Alessandri, F., Pugliese, F., & Ranieri, M. (2018). The role of rescue therapies in the treatment of severe ARDS. https://core.ac.uk/download/132156803.pdf (accessed on 30th June 2025).
6. Al-Tawfiq, J. A., Charrel, R. N., Gautret, P., Gray, G., et al. (2014). Emerging viral respiratory tract infections—Environmental risk factors and transmission. https://core.ac.uk/download/322846912.pdf (accessed on 30th June 2025).
7. Anderson, A., Aronson, D., Daya, M., Sarmiento, D. M., Collen, J. F., Hartzell, J. D., Kelly, K., et al. (2007). Atypical Q fever in US soldiers. https://core.ac.uk/download/pdf/8382347.pdf (accessed on 30th June 2025).
8. Ansari, A. A., Ceribelli, A., De Santis, M., Gershwin, M. E., et al. (2020). Recommendations for coronavirus infection in rheumatic diseases treated with biologic therapy. https://core.ac.uk/download/323069262.pdf (accessed on 30th June 2025).
9. Assaad, S., Friedman, M. B., Kratzert, W. B., Perrino, A. C., et al. (2018). Assessment of pulmonary edema: Principles and practice. https://core.ac.uk/download/145643671.pdf (accessed on 30th June 2025).
10. Auckburally, A., & Nyman, G. (2017). Review of hypoxemia in the anaesthetized horse: Predisposing factors, consequences and management. https://core.ac.uk/download/46558350.pdf (accessed on 30th June 2025).
11. Azimzadeh, N., Baram, M., Cavarocchi, N. C., Hirose, H., et al. (2017). Prone position: Does it help with acute respiratory distress syndrome (ARDS) requiring extracorporeal membrane oxygenation (ECMO)? https://core.ac.uk/download/83049619.pdf (accessed on 30th June 2025).
12. Azoulay, E., Benoit, D., Bruneel, F., Contejean, A., et al. (2016). Increased mortality in hematological malignancy patients with acute respiratory failure from undetermined etiology: A Groupe de Recherche en Réanimation Respiratoire en Onco-Hématologique (Grrr-OH) study. https://core.ac.uk/download/84044246.pdf (accessed on 30th June 2025).

13. Bai, C., Jones, K. D., Matthay, M. A., Song, Y., et al. (2013). The acute respiratory distress syndrome in 2013. https://core.ac.uk/download/323074044.pdf (accessed on 30th June 2025).
14. Becherer-Bailey, G., Farrow II, R., Mantuani, D., Nagdev, A., et al. (2020). Early multi-organ point-of-care ultrasound evaluation of respiratory distress during SARS-CoV-2 outbreak: Case report. https://core.ac.uk/download/305124175.pdf (accessed on 30th June 2025).
15. Blanch, L., López-Aguilar, J., Piacentini, E., Villagrá, A., et al. (2003). Clinical review: The implications of experimental and clinical studies of recruitment maneuvers in acute lung injury. https://core.ac.uk/download/pdf/3472684.pdf (accessed on 30th June 2025).
16. Boon, P., De Herdt, V., Garrez, I., Hemelsoet, D., et al. (2020). Neurological manifestations and neuro-invasive mechanisms of the severe acute respiratory syndrome coronavirus type 2. https://core.ac.uk/download/323232708.pdf (accessed on 30th June 2025).
17. Brady, S., Curley, M. A. Q., Flori, H., Matthay, M., et al. (2009). Elevated PAI-1 is associated with poor clinical outcomes in pediatric patients with acute lung injury. https://core.ac.uk/download/323078706.pdf (accessed on 30th June 2025).
18. Bustos Toalongo, J. I., Cobos Alvarracín, M. Y., Mesa-Cano, I. C., Ramírez-Coronel, M., et al. (2021). Respiratory distress syndrome: Systematic review. https://core.ac.uk/download/490682694.pdf (accessed on 30th June 2025).
19. Calfee, C. S., & Meyer, N. J. (2017). Novel translational approaches to the search for precision therapies for acute respiratory distress syndrome. https://core.ac.uk/download/323074546.pdf (accessed on 30th June 2025).
20. Chan, V., Lashari, B., Raza, A., Ward, C., et al. (2018). Sarcoidosis presenting as acute respiratory distress syndrome. https://core.ac.uk/download/213444704.pdf (accessed on 30th June 2025).
21. Daly, A. K., Wu, A. K. L., Zhao, B., Hui, D. S. C., Ng, E. K. O., Leung, G. M., Tse, G. M., et al. (2005). Absence of association between angiotensin converting enzyme polymorphism and development of adult respiratory distress syndrome in patients with severe acute respiratory syndrome: A case control study. https://core.ac.uk/download/pdf/3645911.pdf (accessed on 30th June 2025).
22. Dyer, K. (2019). Acute respiratory distress syndrome. https://core.ac.uk/download/226774733.pdf (accessed on 30th June 2025).
23. Fanelli, V., Ghannadian, S., Simonetti, U., Slutsky, A. S., et al. (2013). Acute respiratory distress syndrome: new definition, current and future therapeutic options. https://core.ac.uk/download/301857456.pdf (accessed on 30th June 2025).
24. Finney, S. J. (2014). Extracorporeal support for patients with acute respiratory distress syndrome. https://core.ac.uk/download/77004032.pdf (accessed on 30th June 2025).
25. Frank, J. A., & Matthay, M. A. (2002). Science review: Mechanisms of ventilator-induced injury. https://core.ac.uk/download/pdf/3349195.pdf (accessed on 30th June 2025).
26. Greenland, J. R., London, M. J., Michelow, M. D., Wang, H., et al. (2020). COVID-19 infection: Implications for perioperative and critical care physicians. https://core.ac.uk/download/305124313.pdf (accessed on 30th June 2025).
27. Harris, J., Harris, J., Ista, E., Ista, E., et al. (2016). Clinical recommendations for pain, sedation, withdrawal and delirium assessment in critically ill infants and children: An ESPNIC position

statement for healthcare professionals. https://core.ac.uk/download/46665888.pdf (accessed on 30th June 2025).

28. Jones, P., Kulich, K., Miravitlles, M., van der Molen, T., et al. (2012). Beyond FEV1 in COPD: A review of patient-reported outcomes and their measurement. https://core.ac.uk/download/29469334.pdf (accessed on 30th June 2025).
29. Kato, S., & Kurzrock, R. (2020). Repurposing interleukin-6 inhibitors to combat COVID-19. https://core.ac.uk/download/323310902.pdf (accessed on 30th June 2025).
30. Lee, K., & Rincon, F. (2012). Pulmonary complications in patients with severe brain injury. https://core.ac.uk/download/46972148.pdf (accessed on 30th June 2025).
31. McAuley, D. F., Nathani, N., Perkins, G. D., Smith, R., et al. (2006). *In vitro* and *in vivo* effects of salbutamol on neutrophil function in acute lung injury. https://core.ac.uk/download/12435.pdf (accessed on 30th June 2025).
32. Meduri, G. U., & Schwingshackl, A. (2016). Rationale for prolonged glucocorticoid use in pediatric ARDS: What the adults can teach us. https://core.ac.uk/download/323079960.pdf (accessed on 30th June 2025).
33. Morais, V. S. de, Pinto, A. B. P., & Santos, E. M. de P. dos. (2024). Nurses' role in the treatment of respiratory distress syndrome in newborns. https://core.ac.uk/download/643616467.pdf (accessed on 30th June 2025).
34. Risso, A., Alvarez, J., Bellani, G., Bettini, M., et al. (2016). Epidemiology, patterns of care, and mortality for patients with acute respiratory distress syndrome in intensive care units in 50 countries. https://core.ac.uk/download/54529633.pdf (accessed on 30th June 2025).

INTERSTITIAL LUNG DISEASES AND LUNG CANCER

3

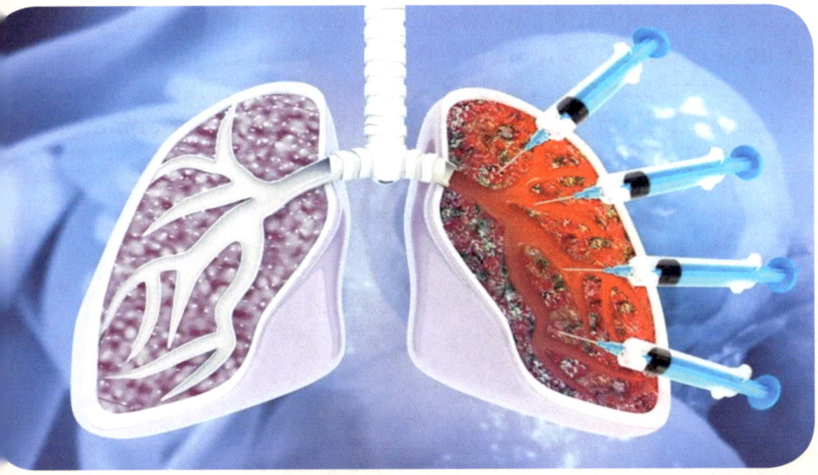

LEARNING OBJECTIVES

After studying this chapter, you will be able to:

1. Understand the types of interstitial lung diseases.
2. Describe the risk factors for interstitial lung diseases.
3. Explain the pathophysiology of interstitial lung diseases.
4. Give an overview of lung cancer.
5. Identify the risk factors for lung cancer.
6. Explore the link between interstitial lung diseases and lung cancer.

Introduction

Interstitial lung diseases (ILDs) are a varied group of interstitial pulmonary diseases with inflammation and fibrosis of the lung interstitium. ILDs seriously impair the function of the lung, leading to disabling symptoms of chronic cough and dyspnea, which eventually lower the quality of life in patients. The increasing prevalence of ILDs is alarming and is contributed to by exposures to environmental toxins, autoimmune disorders, and even idiopathic etiologies. The pathophysiology of these conditions must be known, as they are often overlapping or pose extra risk for lung cancer and hence represent a central area of medical science and public health endeavor. Addressing these interlinked challenges necessitates an integrated understanding of ILDs and their role as precursors to cancer, highlighting the value of enhanced diagnostic and therapeutic interventions in integrated patient management (Dołęga et al., 2024). Lung cancer, a leading cause of cancer death globally, is often complicated by the presence of underlying pulmonary disease, including ILDs. The relationship between fibrosis, inflammation, and malignant transformation remains of continuous interest, as chronic inflammation is a well-documented pathway for causing cellular alterations that lead to cancer formation. Patients with certain types of ILDs, such as idiopathic pulmonary fibrosis, are at increased risk for developing lung cancer due to shared risk factors like exposure and smoking. This ominous correlation necessitates an interdisciplinary intervention by oncologists, pulmonologists, and researchers to further clarify the pathophysiologic links and shared risk factors in ILDs and lung cancer, ensuring that patients are monitored and treated accordingly in both diseases (Assassi et al., 2011). Appropriate management of ILD and lung cancer patients is crucial, with timely diagnosis and treatment potentially having a significant influence on outcomes. Long-term care strategies that incorporate screening for lung cancer among ILD patients are fundamental components of the patient's care. Patient education on potential risks and symptoms of lung cancer can also encourage individuals to come in early for medical care. Therapeutic advancements toward the pathological mechanism of ILDs may, further, hold utility in reducing the incidence of lung cancer among such populations. With increased research into the complex interactions between ILDs and lung cancer, an interdisciplinary preventive, diagnostic, and treatment approach will be essential to enhance patient survival and quality of life (Dołęga et al., 2024) (Figure 3.1).

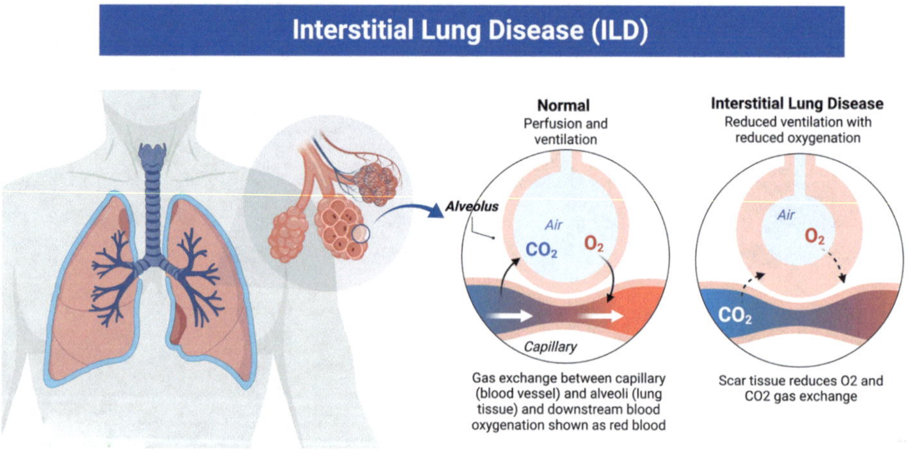

Figure 3.1. Interstitial lung diseases (ILDs).

Source: https://www.chemoexperts.com/images/side-effects/Interstitial%20Lung%20Disease-%20ILD.jpeg.

Definition of Interstitial Lung Diseases (ILDs)

ILDs are a heterogeneous group of pulmonary disorders characterized by inflammation and fibrosis of the interstitial lung tissue. This broad category includes over 200 distinct diseases, which can be classified as idiopathic, autoimmune disease-related, occupational, and drug-induced, among others. The interstitium is the tissue surrounding the alveoli, the minute air spaces where gas exchange occurs. Damage to this region can lead to scarring, compromising lung function, and leading to significant morbidity. The heterogeneity of ILDs makes diagnosis difficult, necessitating a precise classification system that is capable of distinguishing between various conditions and offering recommendations on appropriate therapeutic interventions. Early detection of ILDs is key to successful management as the therapeutic approach varies considerably depending on the etiology and extent of fibrosis. The pathophysiology of ILDs is complex and multifactorial, having both environmental and genetic factors. In the majority of cases, the etiology is unknown, and some ILDs are hence labeled as idiopathic, such as Idiopathic Pulmonary Fibrosis (IPF). Symptoms are a chronic dry cough and progressive dyspnea, and these easily mimic other respiratory diseases. The inflammatory processes associated with ILDs can lead to serious pulmonary complications, with respiratory failure being the most severe among them. Besides, the inherent nature of these diseases predisposes towards secondary complications, such as lung malignancies. The overlap between ILDs and malignancy highlights the importance of constant surveillance and active management protocols to achieve maximum benefit for patients affected by these conditions, bolstering the imperative of multidisciplinary models of care. Advances in the categorization and knowledge of ILDs have established more accurate surveillance and treatment protocols. The term progressive fibrosing interstitial lung diseases (F-ILDs) is especially significant, emphasizing the importance of early identification as part of an effort to improve patient outcomes. Consistent definitions and methodologies for treating F-ILDs are critical since they inform treatments that may modify disease progression. Current consensus among researchers has emphasized antifibrotic therapies in the event that initial management is unable to stop the progression of pulmonary fibrosis (Brown et al., 2023). Furthermore, multidisciplinary care with the inclusion of pulmonary rehabilitation and follow-up monitoring is also able to improve patients' quality of life while serving as important support during their disease. The link between ILDs and cancer of the lung remains an area of active research, necessitating further examination of preventive and therapeutic regimens that may be initiated in response to these interrelated conditions.

Overview of Lung Cancer

Among all the respiratory diseases, lung cancer is a serious health problem with its high mortality and morbidity. Lung cancer is a broad spectrum consisting of two types, which are non-small cell lung cancer (NSCLC) and small cell lung cancer (SCLC), and the latter accounts for approximately 85% of cases. The prognosis in lung cancer patients is generally unfavorable, predominantly due to late diagnosis, when symptoms are more pronounced and therapeutic success is reduced. The etiological factors for lung cancer are primarily tobacco smoking, environmental, and occupational exposures. Recent findings also incriminate genetic predisposition and inflammatory lung diseases in enhancing vulnerability to this malignancy, and hypothesize a multi-factorial etiology for its pathogenesis and advancement. Understanding these risk factors is critical to the early prevention and intervention. With ongoing science in this field of lung cancer, the association between ILDs and lung cancer has been brought to attention. ILDs are a group of heterogeneous disorders of the lungs characterized by inflammation and fibrosis of lung tissue, causing impaired lung function. Patients with certain ILDs, such as idiopathic pulmonary fibrosis, are at heightened risk of lung cancer. This association highlights a significant research area since chronic inflammatory illnesses will drive carcinogenesis through mechanisms involving oxidative damage and cytokine imbalance. Chronic inflammation is actually a known risk factor for most cancers, including lung cancer. Thus, the interaction between ILDs and lung cancer stresses the importance of integrated healthcare strategies in managing patients with chronic lung diseases to avert cancer. Recent findings in lung cancer biology have created new hopes in targeted treatments and immunotherapy, transforming treatment. Molecular analysis of lung cancer has revealed novel genetic alterations, permitting customized treatment regimens to be designed. For instance, those with epidermal growth factor receptor (EGFR) mutations benefit from targeted therapies specifically targeting this pathway. Immunotherapy has also revolutionized treatment planning, with immune checkpoint inhibitors being used to stimulate the patient's immune system against tumor cells. Overall, these advances call for a total rethinking of treatment protocols, with emphasis on the inclusion of genetic screening and personalized therapeutic regimens. Through further research of lung cancer in the context of ILDs, healthcare professionals can optimize patient outcomes and increase long-term survival rates in this challenging disease profile (Figure 3.2).

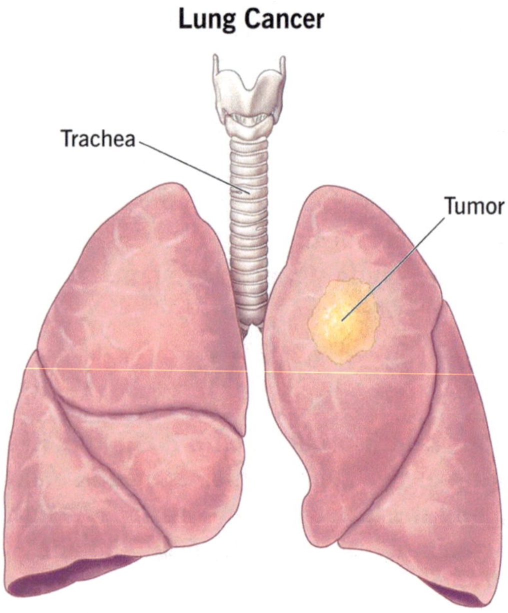

Figure 3.2. Overview of lung cancer.

Source: https://my.clevelandclinic.org/-/scassets/images/org/health/articles/4375-lung-cancer

Importance of Studying the Relationship Between ILDs and Lung Cancer

The relationship between ILDs and lung cancer has also emerged as an important area of research due to the high stakes it presents in patient management and outcomes. ILDs are a group of pulmonary disorders marked by inflammation and fibrosis, which can create a stormy environment within the lungs. The disruption can promote malignant transformation of lung cells, thereby increasing vulnerability to cancer. It is a critical intersection to understand, particularly since ILD patients fare poorly in terms of prognosis as well as their underlying respiratory disease. Overlapping symptomatology can subsequently render proper diagnosis of lung cancer challenging, necessitating vigorous investigations to identify the cancer in already compromised ILD patients, as exemplified by the need for greater awareness in clinical practice. Thus, exploration of this relationship is vital for maximizing diagnosis, treatment planning, and ultimately maximizing survival. Further, research into ILDs and lung cancer provides insights into shared pathobiological mechanisms that may direct the treatment of lung cancer. The inflammation and tissue remodeling of ILDs can lead to alterations within the lung microenvironment, which may yield opportunities for tumor development and growth. By understanding these mechanisms, researchers can potentially identify biomarkers or therapeutic targets that could lead to earlier diagnosis and more personalized therapies for patients at risk of developing lung cancer. The significance of effective management strategies cannot be overstated since current therapies for ILDs, including antifibrotic agents, can decrease some of the cancer-related risks. However, within the realm of rapidly evolving treatment modalities for lung cancer, a complete understanding of the interplay of these diseases is essential to achieve the best patient outcomes and enhance quality of life in affected populations (Geelhoed et al., 2017). In addition, the relationship between ILD and lung cancer must be understood within the realm of public health and resource prioritization. As the prevalence of both ILDs and lung cancer is rising globally, it is increasingly important that medical systems implement specific screening and prevention policies. It is in this understanding that resource diversion can be optimized to enable better early detection programs, which are central to reducing cancer morbidity and mortality rates in individuals who have pre-existing pulmonary disease. In addition, because ILDs and lung cancer have the capability to impair a patient's quality of life significantly, an interdisciplinary model of patient care is paramount. Knowledge of how these disease processes interact can encourage the development of integrated models of care that focus on symptom management, early intervention, and high-quality supportive services, ultimately resulting in a better health-related quality of life for patients with both lung cancer and ILDs at the same time (Assaad et al., 2018).

3.1. Types of Interstitial Lung Diseases

Learning Outcome

1. Idiopathic Pulmonary Fibrosis;
2. Sarcoidosis;
3. Hypersensitivity Pneumonitis.

Interstitial lung diseases (ILDs) are a broad group of interstitial lung disorders, resulting in fibrosis and inflammation of the lung interstitium. Idiopathic Pulmonary Fibrosis (IPF) is a well-known condition, characterized by progressive fibrosis and severely compromised lung function. This particular condition has been shown to have a poor prognosis, with a median survival of almost 21.82 months from diagnosis, indicating the complexity of successful treatment (Creel et al., 2008). Survival differences are also attributed to risk factors by means of variables like gender and age, and higher mortality in men compared to women. An appreciation of the distinctive features of IPF and its impact on lung function is necessary, with special reference to the relationship between ILDs and the development of secondary complications, such as lung cancer. Another large group of ILDs includes those secondary to established causes, such as environmental toxins, autoimmune disease, and medications that were mentioned above. For example, hypersensitivity pneumonitis is caused by immune responses to inhaled organic allergens, leading to varying degrees of lung inflammation and fibrosis.

Scleroderma-associated lung disease also demonstrates how systemic illnesses can manifest as ILD, highlighting the importance of systematic diagnosis and treatment tailored to the underlying etiology. A Maltese study has highlighted that guidelines for managing ILD patients should be standardized and equivalent to international standards, as most patients experience deteriorating lung function over time and require follow-up with repeated evaluations and treatments (Fenech et al., 2012). This sheds light on the extent to which it is important to research the types and the settings of ILDs in relation to lung cancer outcomes.

The clinical relevance of the various ILDs is further exemplified by their potential role in the pathogenesis of lung cancer. Some ILD patients, particularly those with IPF, might be at increased risk of lung cancers due to the chronic inflammation and fibrosis in the lung parenchyma. This risk factor is further augmented by the fact that a majority of those who have IPF are also active or former smokers, further elevating their risk factors. With further research continuing to explore this relationship between ILDs and lung cancer, it is increasingly critical that health care providers incorporate lung cancer screening regimens in the management program of patients diagnosed with ILDs. This allows for increased early detection and intervention, which is essential for better patient outcomes in this at-risk population suffering from concurrent respiratory diseases (Figure 3.3).

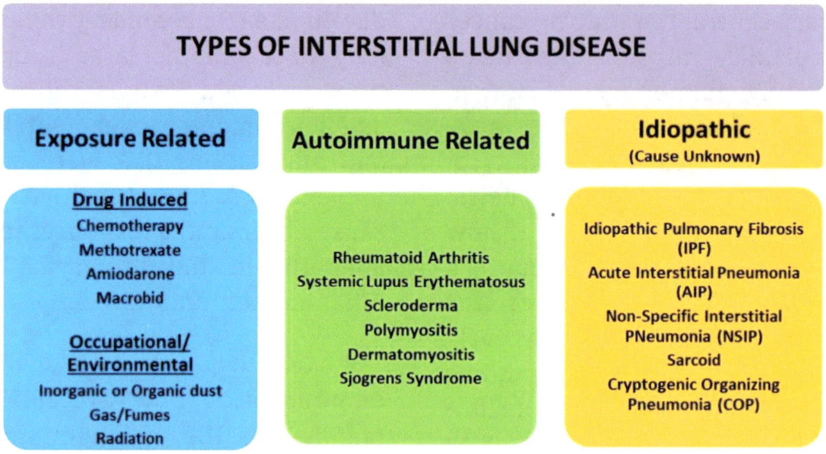

Figure 3.3. Types of interstitial lung diseases.

Source: https://cdn-bejha.nitrocdn.com/kdUuIaPCsuCBPZpAHQVmXEokxbtoxcbd/assets/images/optimized/rev-598d290/respirehab.com/wp-content/uploads/2021/06/ILD-causes-interstitial-lung-disease-classification1.jpg.

3.1.1. Idiopathic Pulmonary Fibrosis

Idiopathic Pulmonary Fibrosis (IPF) is a progressive, chronic ILD with the accumulation of fibrotic tissue in the lungs, leading to severe respiratory impairment. The pathogenesis of IPF is obscure, and this hinders the development of effective therapy. In a cohort-based study involving 331 IPF patients, the median survival after diagnosis was approximately 21.82 months, and a vast gender difference was noted. Male patients exhibited a higher risk of death, with males nearly 2.85 times more at risk of dying from the disease compared to female patients. In addition, patients aged over 69 years demonstrated a higher risk of mortality, highlighting the serious impact of gender and age on survival among IPF patients (Creel et al., 2008). This highlights the need for ongoing research into not only IPF pathophysiology but also its demographic-related survival disparities. One of the main issues with the management of IPF is the often protracted and multicomponent diagnostic process that patients undergo, which can significantly delay intervention. Delay in diagnosis of ILDs, including IPF, has been found to occur relatively commonly, particularly in primary care. A multi-center cohort was analyzed, revealing that appropriate chest CT scans were conducted before consultation with a pulmonologist in 66% of patients. However, most experienced diagnostic delays despite clear imaging evidence of ILD features. Interestingly, patients with documented dyspnea were referred more promptly than those with less acute presentations. Each year of delay not only accelerated fibrotic alterations but resulted in worse outcomes in patients, and this highlights the importance of improved diagnostic testing and greater awareness among primary care physicians (Adegunsoye et al., 2019). Abating these delays in diagnosis potentially could have the ability to improve prognosis and quality of life in IPF patients. Additionally, the link between IPF and lung cancer is a field of growing concern in both the areas of pathology and public health. Individuals with ILD, including IPF, are more likely to develop lung cancer than members of the general population, with rates significantly above the latter. This type of overlap is extremely problematic for doctors who must treat both diseases simultaneously. The endocrine impacts on immunology and fibrotic responses, particularly noted in female IPF patients, could perhaps give some probable directions that link IPF with oncogenic mechanisms (Creel et al., 2008). As the realization of this connection increases, it is well established that IPF patients must be thoroughly screened for lung cancer, including detailed care programs that traverse the range of pulmonary well-being, from fibrotic disorders to cancers. Integration of study results into practice is necessary to improve outcomes in this at-risk population (Figure 3.4).

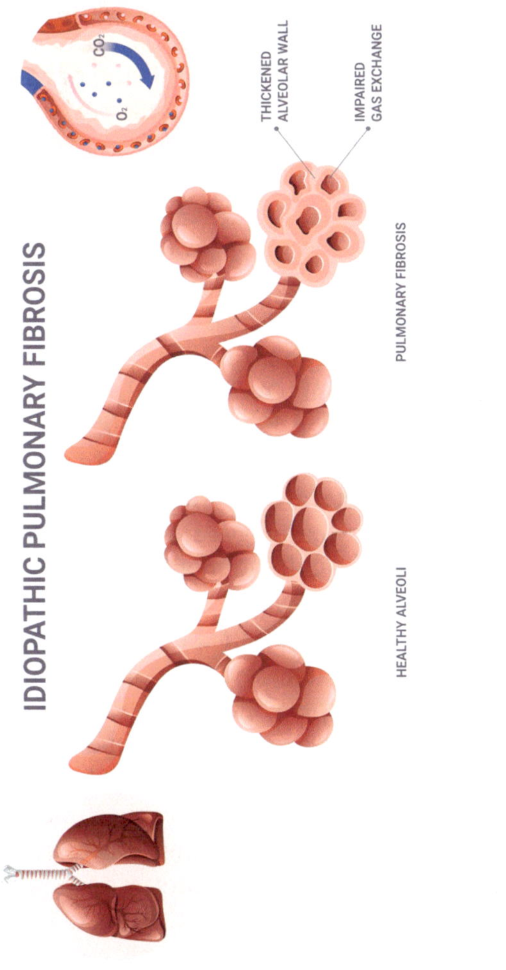

Figure 3.4. Idiopathic pulmonary fibrosis.

Source: https://vumc-reporter.s3.amazonaws.com/uploads/pulmonary-fibrosis-lungs_AdobeStock_688662872.jpg.

3.1.2. Sarcoidosis

Sarcoidosis is a complex inflammatory disease characterized by the occurrence of granulomas in various tissues, initially manifesting in the lungs. As an ILD, sarcoidosis can have far-reaching pulmonary effects and compromise of respiratory function. Sarcoidosis pathophysiology involves an exaggerated immune response, which is thought to be secondary to environmental antigens in the context of genetic predisposition. The disease is typically marked by an enormous variety of respiratory symptoms, including cough, dyspnea, and chest pain, that are similar to other respiratory illnesses. Early and accurate diagnosis is crucial as the disease may heal on its own in some patients, while others present with more complicated forms and necessitate aggressive therapeutic interventions. Recognition of the heterogeneous clinical manifestations is crucial for clinicians to discriminate sarcoidosis from other ILDs to initiate timely treatment and management interventions. The overlapping presentation of sarcoidosis and lung cancer is a tremendous challenge to clinicians. Patients with sarcoidosis have an increased risk of developing malignancies, including lung cancer, due to shared risk factors, including environmental exposures and tobacco use. Chronic inflammation in sarcoidosis is able to play a role in altering cellular microenvironments, thus making carcinogenesis possible. Moreover, the difficulty of differentiating sarcoidosis-associated nodules from lung cancer using imaging examinations provides great difficulty in the management of such patients. It is pertinent that clinicians remain vigilant for malignant alterations among sarcoidosis patients and employ integrative diagnostic approaches to differentiate effectively between such diseases. Consequently, a multi-faceted approach incorporating clinical assessment, imaging, and sometimes biopsy is crucial for effective diagnosis and treatment. In recent years, studies have emerged with emphasis on the importance of addressing the interaction of lung cancer and sarcoidosis in public health initiatives. The realization of the implications of this interaction might encourage cancer prevention through early surveillance and screening behavior among sarcoidosis patients. As cases of sarcoidosis keep on increasing, particularly in the younger population, it is vital to elucidate the underlying factors for the resultant elevated risk of cancer in such patients. Ongoing research is vital in the comprehension of the complex relation between the mechanisms of inflammation and cancer genesis, particularly in ILDs like sarcoidosis. In addition, advances in the therapeutic modalities of sarcoidosis can enhance patient outcomes, not only by suppressing the inflammatory aspect of the disease but also, perhaps, by preventing related cancer risks. Continued research on the epidemiology and the pathogenesis of sarcoidosis will eventually elucidate our understanding of its association with lung cancer and direct proper clinical practices accordingly (Figure 3.5).

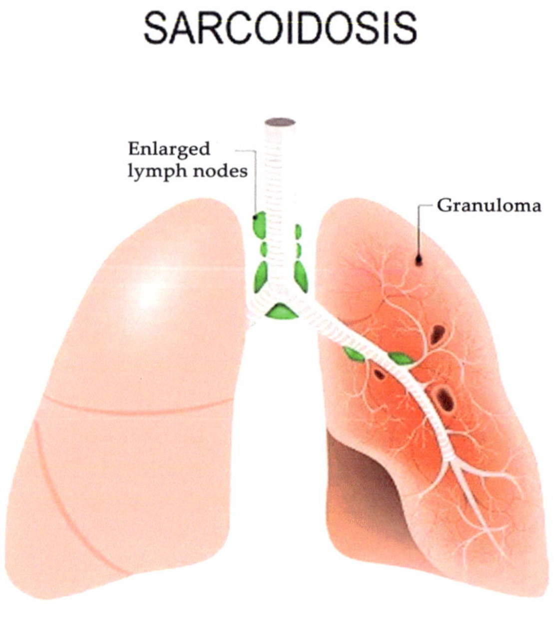

Figure 3.5. Sarcoidosis.

Source: https://drvirendrasingh.com/wp-content/uploads/2023/01/What-is-Sarcoidosis.jpg.

3.1.3. Hypersensitivity Pneumonitis

The study of hypersensitivity pneumonitis (HP) is an essential aspect of the study of ILDs due to its distinct immunological pathophysiology and environmental causes. HP emerges when repeated exposure to organic antigens such as mold spores, dust, and bird droppings causes an exaggerated immune reaction, leading to inflammation and fibrosis of lung tissue. Major features of this condition in its acute and chronic presentation underlie most clinical presentations, tending to encourage a false diagnosis as other pulmonary diseases. Knowledge of clinical implications of HP not only helps in the institution of proper therapeutic regimens but also highlights the need for environmental control to reduce exposure risks. Subsequently, pathogenesis and epidemiological progress in HP over the past few decades highlight its significance in the broader ILD context, bringing to the fore the critical role of environmental health in pulmonary disease treatment as well as intersections (Alfaro et al., 2019). In ILDs and lung cancer, hypersensitivity pneumonitis represents an isolated condition in the context of management and correct diagnosis. The inflammatory pathways associated with HP have been implicated in pulmonary fibrosis, which in turn increases the risk of lung cancer. Although chronic inflammation and fibrogenesis cause a disordered lung architecture, the oncogenic potential of injured lung parenchyma cannot be ruled out. Moreover, HP should be differentiated from other ILDs, such as idiopathic pulmonary fibrosis, given their comparable clinical features but different prognostic implications. The latest information from scientific reports at leading congresses emphasizes the need for greater vigilance in clinical practice concerning the potential link between hypersensitivity reactions, chronic inflammation, and cancer genesis. HP's multifaceted nature warrants further study to better understand its role in ILD pathogenesis as well as lung cancer risk (Alfaro et al., 2020). Treatment of hypersensitivity pneumonitis is both acute and preventive, consisting of long-term measures aimed at restricting exposure to known antigens. It begins with removal of the offending substance and identification and is reinforced by pharmacologic therapy that facilitates reduction in inflammation. Corticosteroids are the traditional drugs used to restrict acute inflammatory responses but are problematic due to their side effects, and continued research is being conducted into other immunomodulatory drugs. Education regarding environmental and occupational exposure is also essential for individuals at risk of HP, with a focus on proactive prevention of exacerbations. As research into hypersensitivity pneumonitis continues to advance, integration of findings from recent studies in ILDs and their systemic impact may offer further insight and directions for maximizing patient outcome in this complex overlap of lung health and environmental exposures (Alfaro et al., 2019) (Figure 3.6).

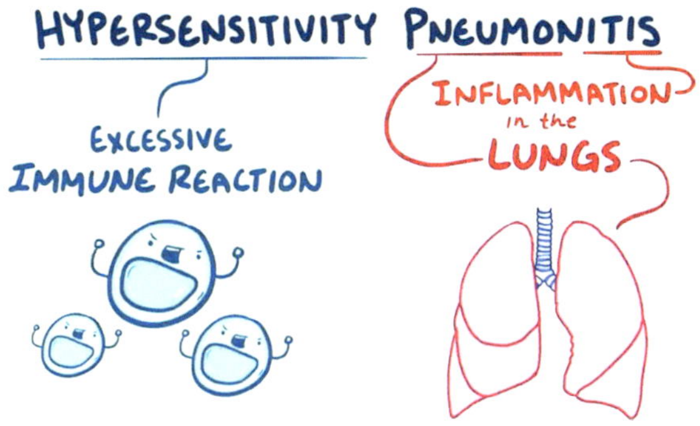

Figure 3.6. Hypersensitivity pneumonitis.

Source: https://external-content.duckduckgo.com/iu/?u=https%3A%2F%2Fosmose-it.s3.amazonaws.com%2FTLDJo7eMQCKYrDWZ55GP07c7RRGSxnr3%2F_.jpg&f=1&nofb=1&ipt=acfefe165d55a87cd8de9e6f72812fa722f89e92e6da0367822d4a319abbca1a.

Test Your Knowledge

1. What is idiopathic pulmonary fibrosis?
2. Explain about hypersensitivity pneumonitis.

3.2. Risk Factors for Interstitial Lung Diseases

Learning Outcome

1. Environmental exposures;
2. Genetic predispositions;
3. Occupational hazards.

It is essential to know the risk factors of ILDs in order to effectively prevent and improve patient outcomes. Age is one of the significant risk factors, and idiopathic pulmonary fibrosis (IPF) is diagnosed at the patient's median age of 69 years. It has been established that patients over the age of 69 have a 1.6 times higher relative risk of death compared to their younger counterparts. Gender is also a significant factor as the mortality rate in men with IPF is approximately 2.85 times higher compared to that of women. The discrepancy suggests a complex interaction between hormonal, immunological, and environmental factors. Understanding the demographic factors influencing ILD risk will enable clinicians to identify high-risk groups and adopt appropriate treatments, with special attention to constant surveillance for early detection. Environmental exposure is most notably involved in the pathogenesis of ILDs, and lifestyle and occupational exposures have been recognized as major causative factors. Workers who are exposed to specific dusts, chemicals, and radiation in the workplace have been reported to be more vulnerable to ILD. Smoking remains a common risk factor that aggravates lung fibrosis and global reduction in lung function. Research indicates the presence of a systemic prothrombotic state in IPF patients, and this implies that derangement of the body's coagulation pathways would further aggravate the illness. Chronic silica or asbestos exposure have been implicated in provoking an accelerated pace of deterioration of lung function and mortality. The interaction of these environmental factors not only increases the risk of ILD occurrence but also highlights the necessity of public health practices to minimize exposure to harmful substances. Finally, genetic susceptibility is a new area in consideration as an ILD risk factor. Specific genetic mutations have also been connected to an increased likelihood of developing conditions like IPF, highlighting that familial histories play an important role in determining individual susceptibility. Additionally, research on the immunological responses of patients in such diseases indicates complex mechanisms wherein genetic markers may influence disease progression and survival in general. For example, the correlation of a systemic prothrombotic state in IPF patients could be a result of intrinsic genetic abnormalities that control coagulation and inflammatory reactions. It necessitates an interdisciplinary research and treatment approach that considers both lifestyle and genetic parameters to delineate the multifactorial etiology of risk factors for ILDs. By embracing an integrative understanding of such factors, healthcare workers can better cope with the needs of patients and minimize the risks of ILDs, finally bridging the knowledge gap among ILDs and lung cancer prevention strategies (Figure 3.7).

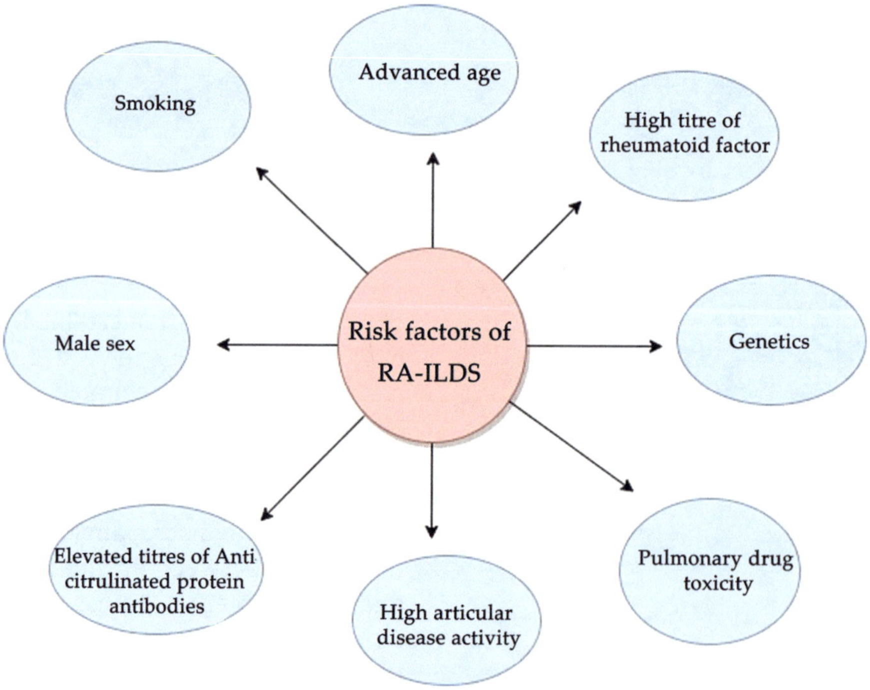

Figure 3.7. Risk factors for interstitial lung diseases.

Source: https://assets.cureus.com/uploads/figure/file/326386/article_river_f4094b60878611ec9c3239a658991556-rheumatoid-arthritis--1-.png.

3.2.1. Environmental Exposures

Environmental exposures also have a very significant contribution to the etiology of ILD and lung cancer with multiple occupational and non-occupational factors playing a role. In contrast, individuals exposed to the agricultural sector are generally at risk of hazardous aerosols like organic and inorganic particles that can compromise respiratory function. Research indicates a link between exposure to pesticides, fungus, and bacteria prevalent in agricultural settings and several pulmonary conditions, highlighting the need for increased monitoring and detection technologies in these environments (N/A). With the evolving agricultural practices, especially with the use of mushroom and greenhouse farming, there are exposure risks that require more vigilance and preventive health measures for the workers to offset such adverse effects on lung health. Additionally, idiopathic pulmonary fibrosis (IPF), which is a severe form of ILD, may be caused by exposures to the environment. Although the ultimate cause of IPF remains unknown, environmental exposures such as air pollution and work exposures can contribute to its pathogenesis. According to statistics, older men are particularly vulnerable to poor outcomes, with survival strongly influenced by their age and sex (Creel et al., 2008). The difficulty of IPF is exacerbated by inadequate treatment, making further research into environmental determinants of the disease more important. These external factors are key not only to treatment but to the creation of preventative measures. The relationship of environmental exposures to lung cancer highlights another important area of public health focus. Epidemiologic studies consistently discover that particulate contaminants and carcinogens found in filthy air can augment cancer risk, particularly among groups of concern whose members are exposed over long times to these toxins. By informing the public and lawmakers of the toxic impact of environmental toxins, there is a chance of inducing stricter controls that limit exposure to undesirable agents in air, soil, and water. Recognizing the crucial role of environmental health in determining lung cancer risk profiles is essential for health professionals to implement more comprehensive preventative programs aimed at reducing the incidence of ILD and environmental factor-induced lung cancer.

3.2.2. Genetic Predispositions

It is important to know genetic predispositions to help explain the complexities of ILDs and how they relate to lung cancer. Research has identified some known genetic markers that influence one's susceptibility to such diseases, which risk pulmonary injury even in the presence of environmental risk factors. As the human genome consists of variations that dictate the response of cells to external stressors, learning about these genetic factors can help explain pathways that result in pathological conditions. For instance, gene variations for inflammation and fibrosis can potentially prescribe the trajectory of ILDs, which in turn can increase lung cancer risk later on. Identification of these genetic predispositions is key to the development of more efficient prevention methods and specific therapeutics for high-risk populations. The role of epigenetics adds another dimension of complexity to the interaction between genetic predispositions and lung disorders. Epigenetic signatures, such as DNA methylation and histone modifications, can alter gene expression without affecting the underlying genetic code. These changes are created by environmental exposures, i.e., toxins and occupational hazards, in combination with genetic susceptibilities to augment lung pathology. An understanding of this interaction can provide a clue as to why individuals develop ILDs or lung cancer and others do not, even when they are exposed equally. When researchers aim to chart the epigenetic map of lung cells, they want to put together a systematic overview of disease-developmental factors. The overlap between genetics and epigenetics is likely to offer useful information in identifying susceptibility to such disabling diseases (Borok et al., 2016). Additionally, the identification of environmental stimuli in addition to genetic susceptibility is essential to a holistic approach to ILDs and lung cancer. Evidence is present to suggest that, although particular variations within the genes may predispose to lung disease, exposure to specific environmental exposures could be a potent trigger. For instance, patients with genetic variations affecting their immune response can become susceptible to the inflammatory pathways that are traditionally seen in ILDs (Althobiani et al., 2024). Moreover, this interaction can also elucidate responses to treatment since treatments can be tailored as per the genetic profile of a person and previous exposure history. Awareness of these dynamic interactions also puts additional spotlight on the need for multidisciplinary strategies, integrating genetics, environmental science, and clinical practice to improve diagnostic and management strategies for patients with these conditions. Thus, the intricate web of genetic vulnerabilities is both risk and promise in addressing ILDs and lung cancer (Figure 3.8).

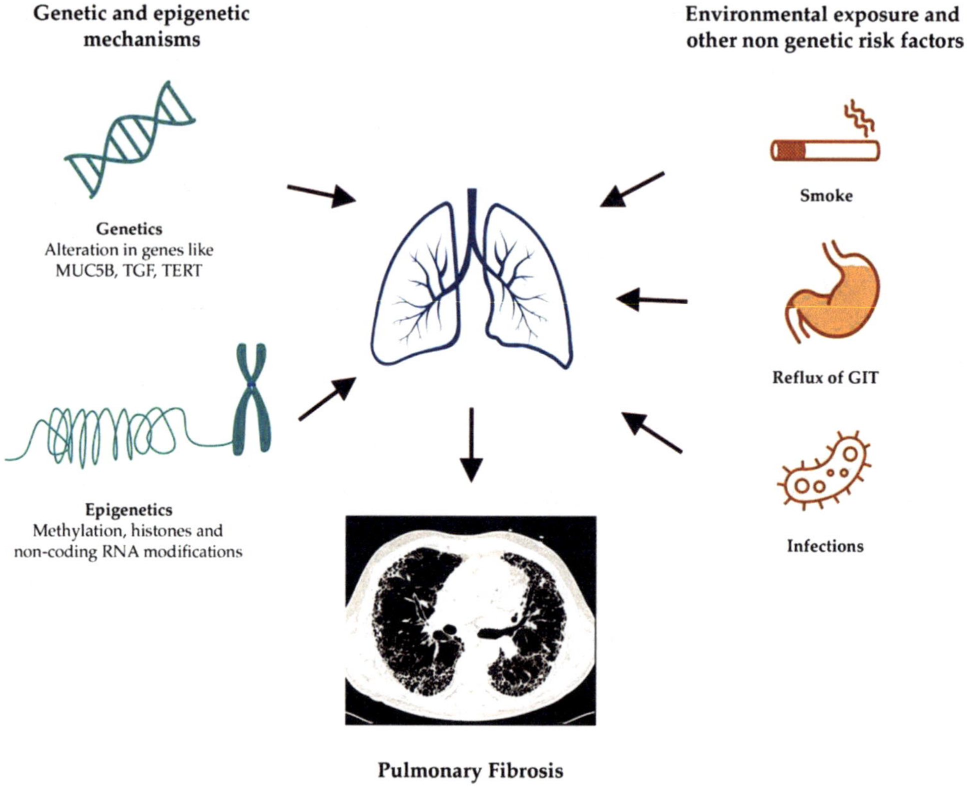

Figure 3.8. Genetic predispositions for interstitial lung diseases.

Source: https://www.mdpi.com/diagnostics/diagnostics-12-03107/article_deploy/html/images/diagnostics-12-03107-g001.png.

3.2.3. Occupational Hazards

Occupational exposures are a significant cause of ILDs and lung cancer, particularly in high-risk activities such as mining and construction. Many toxic substances, including asbestos, silica dust, and coal mine dust, which are known causes of respiratory illness, have exposed workers repeatedly.

For instance, the conditions in underground coal mining are unique; in response, safety standards have been established so that workers don't labor in conditions way below those of the general population. These efforts aim to mitigate the mortality and morbidity due to lung disease that disproportionately affects this industry's workers (Zimmerman et al., 2025). Good supervision and observance of safety guidelines are key to helping limit exposure, but the chronic dangers require additional workplace security measures and instruction. Ineffective compensation practices and long procedures for work-induced health-condition claims further exacerbate the occupational lung disease burden. According to research targeting the South African mining sector, most compensable diseases certified between 2004 and 2012 were for tuberculosis, silicosis, and asbestos disease, indicating a concerning trend in occupational health regulation (Ndaba et al., 2017). The prevailing rates of certification show a systemic breakdown to prevent exposure to toxic substances and to treat employees suffering from such debilitating diseases. Such evidence indicates that there is existing legislation, but the enforcement of protective measures is inadequate. Such a deficiency calls for policy reformulations and employer responsibility to ensure better health outcomes for workers exposed to unsafe work conditions. In addressing the issue of occupational hazards, it is then necessary to examine the interaction between exposure duration and disease expression. Experiments have indicated that exposure to inhaled toxins for as little as a short while can lead to severe health consequences for construction and mining workers, primarily the development of pneumoconiosis and other ILDs. Moreover, identifying the long-term consequences of exposure and determining whether latent periods are required before disease appears remain active research avenues (Ndaba et al., 2017). The complexity of such associations necessitates an integrative approach to occupational health, one that harmonizes risk assessment with early treatment and robust support systems to assist affected workers. The implementation of comprehensive training programs, along with more stringent enforcement of protective protocols, can be those vital steps towards the mitigation of ILDs and lung cancer in exposed occupations (Figure 3.9).

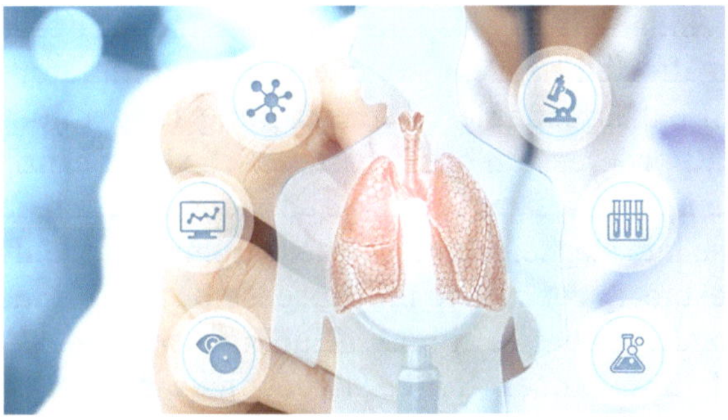

Figure 3.9. Occupational hazards for interstitial lung diseases.

Source: https://www.healio.com/~/media/slack-news/stock-images/pulmonology/l/lungs-digital-3_adobe.jpg.

Test Your Knowledge

1. What are the genetic predispositions?
2. What are the occupational hazards?

3.3. Pathophysiology of Interstitial Lung Diseases

Learning Outcome

1. Mechanisms of lung tissue damage;
2. Inflammatory processes involved;
3. Role of fibrosis in disease progression.

The pathophysiology of ILDs is complex and multifactorial, with nearly entirely interstitial inflammation and fibrosis of the lung interstitium. It is characterized by an abnormal increase in interstitial inflammatory cells and extracellular matrix that results in thickening and hardening of lung tissue. An initial insult, either from environmental or autoimmune factors, triggers an inflammatory response that calls immune cells to affected tissues. The resultant inflammatory milieu is capable of maintaining lung injury and progression of fibrosis, which significantly compromises gas exchange and lung function. In the late stages, scar tissue development not only results in restrictive lung disease but also leads to future complications, including increased risk of lung cancer. Hence, it becomes crucial to understand the mechanism of ILD development and progression in the context of cancer risk. One of the critical parameters behind the pathophysiology of ILD is the balance between injury and repair processes in the alveolar epithelium. The normal repair mechanism is an aggressive one that maintains lung integrity following injury. In ILD, this balance is disturbed, and most abnormal repair processes are preferred to lead to fibrotic change instead of normal healing. Such dysregulation may be due to chronic environmental insult, genetic predisposition, or autoimmune dysregulation to produce an amplification of the inflammatory process and thus remolding of lung architecture. With increasing disease, the dysfunctional biomechanical properties of lung tissue can compromise compliance and improve work of breathing and thus further perpetuate respiratory dysfunction. These pathological changes are important to grasp because not only do they elucidate the pathophysiologic process driving ILD but also the elevated risk for lung cancers associated with this disease. New research indicates that newer imaging modalities may potentially better assess the pathophysiologic characteristics of ILD. For instance, MRI is gaining popularity since it can potentially provide both morphologic and functional data regarding lung pathology without the ill effects of radiation exposure. Although initially applied in limited clinical disorders like cystic fibrosis and acute pulmonary embolism, the contribution of MRI to ILD is under investigation.

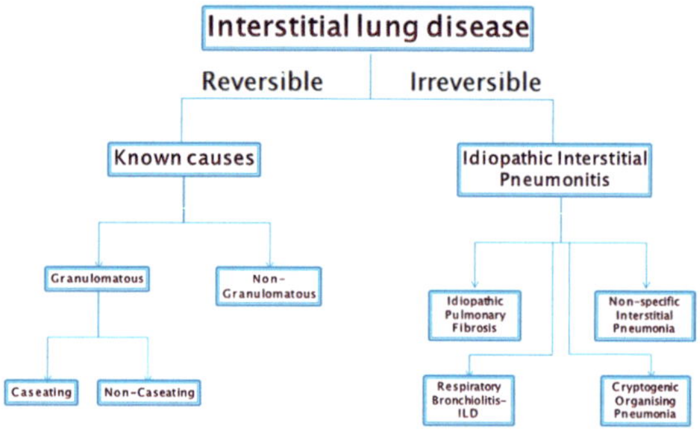

Figure 3.10. Pathophysiology of interstitial lung diseases.

Source: https://external-content.duckduckgo.com/iu/?u=https%3A%2F%2Fpathologia.ed.ac.uk%2Fwp-content%2Fuploads%2F2019%2F02%2FCapture-1.png&f=1&nofb=1&ipt=0c033705aef3161242d9526003d61ec69f660afd017bbdafbe25d1f5c6b0de53.

The newer imaging protocols enhance the ability to comprehensively assess lung perfusion and ventilation, which can prove to be very useful in differentiating disease dynamics and treatment response. With developments in imaging technology, they could aid our capabilities for diagnosing and monitoring ILDs and ultimately make decisions in the management, ultimately furthering patient outcomes in the context of underlying malignancies (Hebestreit et al., 2011; Assaad et al., 2018) (Figure 3.10).

3.3.1. Mechanisms of Lung Tissue Damage

The pathogenesis of lung tissue injury is multifactorial, particularly in the case of ILDs such as idiopathic pulmonary fibrosis (IPF). In IPF, the disease's characteristic aspect is the wound healing response to deranged lung injury, leading to an overwhelming accumulation of collagen and subsequent fibrosis. The disease process is usually driven by a multi-factorial etiology of exposure to environmental agents and genetic predisposition that renders an individual prone to it with increasing age. Research has shown that men are disproportionately affected, with gender- and age-skewed survival rates; males are at greater risk of death compared to females, and individuals aged over 69 years have an increased risk of death from the disease (Creel et al., 2008). It is thus important to understand these population variables controlling lung tissue damage to be able to direct therapeutic interventions and improve prognostic outcomes. Acute pneumonitis and delayed fibrosis following lung irradiation are another source of investigation into the mechanisms of radiation-induced damage to lung tissue. Radiosensitivity may vary considerably between different genetic strains of mice, revealing a complex interaction between inflammation and secondary fibrosis. It has been discovered that strains prone to pneumonitis exhibit distinctive inflammatory patterns of gene expression early following irradiation with considerable activation of pro-inflammatory pathways. On the other hand, fibrosis-susceptible strains show enrichment of genes within the processes of cellular proliferation and repair (Baye et al., 2017). Such an observation explains the heterogeneity of individual responses to lung tissue injury, and the necessity for individualized therapeutic strategies in treating radiation-induced lung disease and its following late sequelae. In addition, the role of systemic influences, such as hormonal effects on the injury of lung tissue, may be a candidate for future research. The fact that survival advantage in females, and more so those with a history of full-term pregnancies, indicates the possibility of an immunomodulatory effect that can protect lung tissue against the stress of challenge or insult (Creel et al., 2008). The physiology behind how hormonal fluctuation results in resistance to injury of lung tissue remains to be conclusively elucidated. There may be a future line of research that investigates the physiological adaptation during pregnancy resulting in this protective mechanism, with potential applications for the creation of novel treatments for not only ILDs but also lung cancer and associated co-morbidities. In conclusion, these findings serve to underscore the intricate interaction between environmental exposures and biological determinants in the regulation of lung health (Figure 3.11).

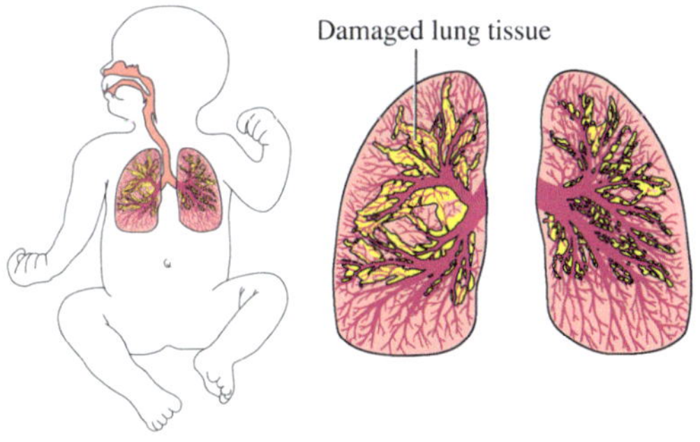

Figure 3.11. Lung tissue damage.

Source: https://www.nhlbi.nih.gov/sites/default/files/inline-images/bronchopulmonary-dysplasia-1.jpg.

3.3.2. Inflammatory Processes Involved

The inflammatory processes lie at the core of ILD pathogenesis and involve an immune response leading to inflammatory cell deposition in the lung interstitium. This disrupts normal lung interstitium architecture and function and, in the majority of cases, leads to fibrosis, which may produce progressive respiratory failure. The inflammatory response is not an uncoordinated event, but rather an intricate interaction between various cytokines, immune cells, and tissue factors. For instance, macrophage and neutrophil activation induce the production of pro-inflammatory cytokines, which can exacerbate lung damage and lead to fibrotic changes. Chronic inflammation, being synonymous with sustained immune cell infiltration, not only contributes to the pathogenesis of ILD but can also create a permissive environment for the genesis of lung cancer, indicating that there is a need for advanced diagnostic and therapeutic methods for both illnesses. Advanced imaging techniques in the investigation of inflammatory phenomena have emerged as valuable tools for understanding ILDs. The application of 99mTc-MIBI scanning in patients provides invaluable information regarding the degree of inflammatory activity of the lungs. This imaging modality can distinguish among various disease states, allowing clinicians to assess disease severity more accurately than other imaging modalities, including high-resolution computed tomography (HRCT). Specifically, studies indicate that the greater accumulation of 99mTc-MIBI correlates with active inflammation and poor clinical prognosis, suggesting it can be employed as a non-invasive biomarker for monitoring disease development and therapeutic response. Therefore, the integration of such new imaging modalities into clinical practice not only broadens the understanding of inflammatory processes in ILDs but also aids in detecting patients at risk for harmful complications, such as lung cancer, early on, thus providing the impetus for early interventions (Assadi et al., 2015). Outside the lungs, ILD inflammation can extend to systemic processes that can potentially foster malignancy. The relationship between tumorigenesis and chronic inflammation is widely documented, with several pathways being identified in the process. It is particularly significant in considering how inflammatory mediators establish a microenvironment for cancer cell survival and proliferation. To this extent, increased research is required to characterize inflammatory patterns using magnetic resonance imaging (MRI) and their association with lung cancer outcomes. Although the clinical utility of lung MRI is yet to be determined in ILDs, it is a non-invasive technology that can provide valuable functional information on lung mechanics and perfusion. With the advancement of diagnostic technologies, their utility in delineating the complex relationships between the inflammatory processes within the lung may offer new data and better management for affected individuals (Heemann et al., 2011).

3.3.3. Role of Fibrosis in Disease Progression

Fibrosis is at the heart of ILDs pathogenesis and intimately linked with lung cancer development. It is pathologically characterized by the deposition of extracellular matrix material, which ravages normal pulmonary architecture and ultimately affects gas exchange and respiratory function. As such diseases as Idiopathic Pulmonary Fibrosis (IPF) advance, cycles of recurrent epithelial damage and aberrant repair increase extensive fibrotic scarring in the lungs. Besides damaging the function of affected lung tissue, it also makes patients susceptible to cancer. Experiments have discovered that fibrotic changes occur years before clinical manifestation of cancer, suggesting latency when structural changes set the stage for neoplastic transformation. Furthermore, the clinical condition of IPF patients reveals a calamitous prognosis, with average survival rates reflecting the severity of this fibrotic condition (Creel et al., 2008). Fibrosis and lung cancer are also revealed in their interaction through the plasticity of lung epithelial cells, which can undergo vast remodeling after injury. Exactly, in pulmonary fibrosis, repeated epithelial damage will lead to dysregulated epithelial cell proliferation as well as disrupted activation of growth factors, permissive for tumorigenesis. Epithelial activation is not a secondary by-product of fibrosis; rather, it represents a significant boundary beyond which the mechanisms favorable for tumorigenesis also contribute to neoplastic development. Evidence exists for the histopathological correlation between extensive pulmonary fibrosis and enhanced lung cancer prevalence, although the precise mechanism has yet to be investigated (Adamson et al., 2011). This knowledge is crucial in order to know how lung cancer may emerge on the basis of well-established fibrotic lung disorders. In conclusion, the role of fibrosis in promoting disease progression, particularly in lung cancer, is one of significant clinical relevance. The evolution from ILDs to malignancy illustrates a complex interplay of pathologic events triggered by chronic inflammation, epithelial damage, and consequent dysregulated repair mechanisms. With the potential to inform patient management and treatment outcomes, further research is needed to dissect the molecular pathways linking fibrosis with cancer. This understanding can ultimately translate to the development of therapies that not only affect the fibrotic process but also minimize the risk for malignancy in the patient. Since survival continues to be a major concern with diseases such as IPF, integrating what is currently understood about fibrosis and tumorigenesis could shape future clinical practice and improve patient outcomes as a whole (Creel et al., 2008) (Figure 3.12).

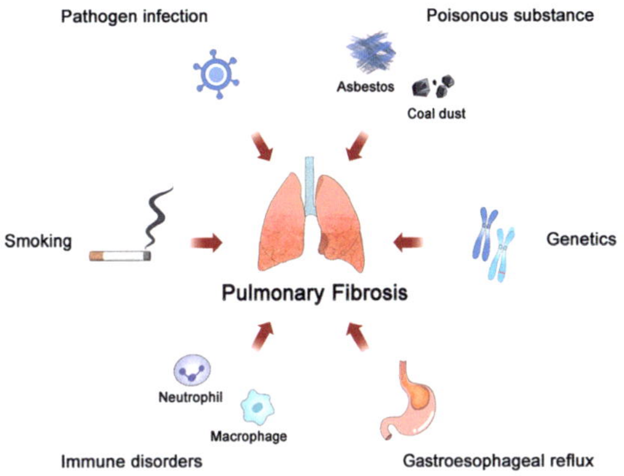

Figure 3.12. Role of fibrosis in disease progression.

Source: https://media.springernature.com/m685/springer-static/image/art%3A10.1038%2Fs41420-024-02078-0/MediaObjects/41420_2024_2078_Fig1_HTML.png.

Test Your Knowledge

1. What are the mechanisms of lung tissue damage?
2. What is the role of fibrosis in disease progression?

3.4. Overview of Lung Cancer

Learning Outcome

1. Types of lung cancer;
2. Common symptoms and diagnosis;
3. Staging and prognosis.

Lung cancer remains to be the most prevalent and deadly form of cancer in the world, characterized by the abnormal overgrowth of cells in lung tissues. Lung cancer may be broadly classified as either NSCLC or SCLC. NSCLC accounts for approximately 85% of all cases, with a number of subtypes such as adenocarcinoma and squamous cell carcinoma, with variations in clinical course and treatment outcomes. Conversely, SCLC is more aggressive and is most commonly linked with smoking and metastasizes extremely rapidly. These subtypes should be recognized to tailor the therapeutic management and predictive results. Advances in molecular biology have also made it possible to identify specific genetic changes that are associated with lung cancer and can direct individualized treatment options and improve patient outcomes. Lung cancer risk factors are multifaceted, both environmental and genetic in nature. The highest risk factor is smoking, and a staggering 85% of all lung cancers are due to tobacco use. Even non-smokers can develop lung cancer due to exposure to secondhand smoke, radon gas, and occupational exposures. Also, certain genetic susceptibilities can predispose one to lung cancer, and understanding the interaction between genetics and environmental damage is essential. ILDs also need to be included in this picture, since certain forms of ILD-induced lung damage confer a risk of cancer. These associations are of paramount importance to know for the sake of possible prevention and early detection. Despite the bleak figures for lung cancer, recent developments in treatment modalities have brought new hope to patients. Traditional modalities like surgery, chemotherapy, and radiation therapy are being increasingly complemented by new approaches like targeted therapy and immunotherapy. These newer approaches target specific molecular targets or utilize the body's immune system to attack cancer cells more selectively. However, recent data show that those patients who have underlying ILDs may respond differently to treatment and experience variable outcomes. For instance, the presence of comorbid ILDs like idiopathic pulmonary fibrosis complicates the therapeutic picture and requires close attention. Additional research into biomarkers and tailored treatment regimens could enhance the effectiveness of lung cancer therapies, ultimately aiming to improve patient outcomes, consistent with evidence for the effectiveness of personalized medicine in treating cancer (Daccord et al., 2016) (Figure 3.13).

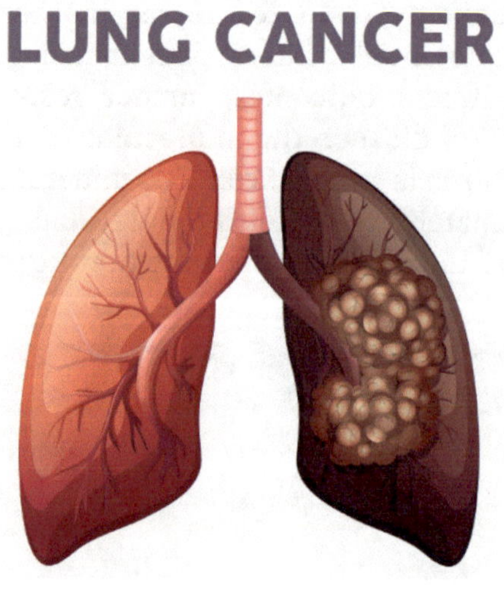

Figure 3.13. Lung cancer.

Source: https://external-content.duckduckgo.com/iu/?u=https%3A%2F%2Fwww.netmeds.com%2Fimages%2Fcms%2Fwysiwyg%2Fblog%2F2019%2F09%2FLung_cancer_big_898.jpg&f=1&nofb=1&ipt=e8129aa7461d9e0ed372b0713ebca9fb80ba6fb8179de9ce4faad5a6a67ba318.

3.4.1. Types of Lung Cancer

The morphology of lung cancer is virtually completely classified into two large groups: non-small cell lung cancer (NSCLC) and small cell lung cancer (SCLC). NSCLC accounts for approximately 85% of all lung cancer and is, in turn, divided into a number of histological subtypes, including adenocarcinoma, squamous cell carcinoma, and large cell carcinoma. All of the subtypes exhibit distinct cellular characteristics and biological behaviors, which dictate prognosis and therapy. Adenocarcinoma that occurs in peripheral lung tissue is the most common subtype among non-smokers. Squamous cell carcinoma, however, has a history of smoking and is found in the central lung zones. It is crucial to note these types because they have different pathophysiology, necessitating targeted therapeutic strategies and clinical decision-making for patient management and follow-up. On the other hand, while it accounts for a minority of lung cancers, small-cell lung cancer is characterized by its early metastatic and aggressive nature. SCLC is significantly linked to smoking and has a high doubling time and growth fraction, characteristics that render it a poor prognosis. This type of lung cancer is more frequently characterized by having limited-stage disease that is treatable with curative intent or extensive-stage disease that more likely requires palliative therapy approaches. The standard treatment for SCLC includes chemotherapy and radiation therapy as foundational components, and immunotherapy presents a hopeful option for certain patient subsets. Given the extreme differences between the clinical behavior and treatment response of SCLC and NSCLC, correct classification of the types of lung cancer is imperative for optimal patient management and future research into targeted therapy. The association between lung cancer and ILDs cannot be overlooked because the presence of certain ILDs may influence the development of different types of cancer. Conditions such as idiopathic pulmonary fibrosis (IPF) are associated with an increased risk of lung cancer, especially NSCLC, since they have the same risk factors, such as smoking and environmental exposure.

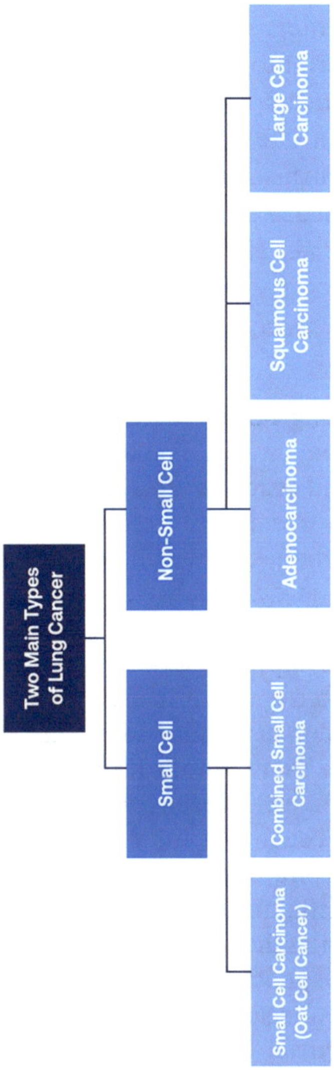

Figure 3.14. Types of lung cancer.

Source: https://www.lung.org/optimize/getmedia/e587a919-8d71-4406-aa11-fa084dc6a3d8/lung-cancer-type-chart.jpg?format=webp.

The literature indicates that the chronic inflammatory environment and fibrotic changes characteristic of ILDs can promote carcinogenesis in lung tissue. Furthermore, biomarkers such as galectin-3 (Gal-3) have been studied to distinguish between benign and malignant processes in patients with coincidental lung cancer and ILDs. These insights emphasize the need for integrated management to address lung cancer and ILDs interactively, prioritizing early diagnosis and individualized treatment regimens in line with advances in recognizing the mechanisms responsible for interconnecting the two disease processes (Bellotti et al., 2018; Daccord et al., 2016) (Figure 3.14).

3.4.2. Common Symptoms and Diagnosis

ILDs and lung cancer share different symptoms in common, which makes their diagnosis difficult and leads to delayed diagnosis, often leading to premature treatment. One of the most common symptoms shared by the two conditions is dyspnea or shortness of breath, which considerably worsens a patient's quality of life. The symptom may also develop slowly and patients often ignore it in early stages. Similarly, chronic cough is another common presentation that can be seen in both ILDs and lung cancer. The patient can present with a chronic non-productive cough that, initially, may be attributed to other respiratory system diseases. In addition, systemic inflammation and tumor burden can start affecting the body, and generalized fatigue as well as spontaneous weight loss can result from these diseases. Early identification of the signs is crucial to enable timey intervention, therefore, it is vital to conduct a thorough clinical assessment to differentiate between these superimposed presentations. ILDs and lung cancer are diagnosed using a combination of the clinical assessment, imaging scans, and, where necessary, tissue biopsy. Diagnostic imaging, such as high-resolution computed tomography (HRCT), is important in identifying the specific patterns evident in ILDs, for example, ground-glass opacities or reticular patterns. Where lung cancer is suspected, the imaging procedures may reveal nodules or masses that require further investigation. Surgical procedures like cryobiopsy have improved diagnostic yield, particularly in obtaining lung tissue samples, and can differentiate between cancer and non-cancerous effectively. Results regarding the diagnostic utility of cryobiopsies indicate that they are superior to traditional methods. They take larger samples of alveolar tissue without creating significant artifacts, thereby allowing easier diagnosis of ILDs and lung cancers (Griff et al., 2019).

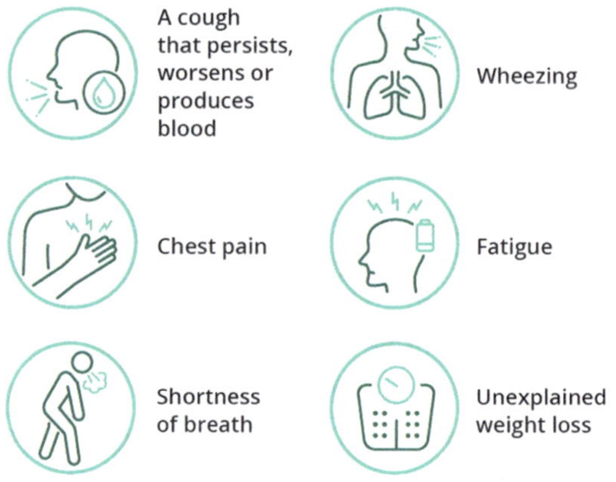

Figure 3.15. Lung cancer symptoms.

Source: https://cdn.cancercenter.com/-/media/ctca/images/others/medical-graphics/old/lung-cancer-symptoms-dt.png.

When developing respiratory symptoms occur, it is essential to consider drug-induced lung adverse events, particularly when patients are undergoing chemotherapy or targeted therapies. For instance, use of imatinib has been associated with the development of pulmonary complications, the specific case being one such scenario where a patient was seen with acute dyspnea and hypoxia after initiating treatment. Interstitial patterns consistent with pulmonary distress were observed on imaging for which drug cessation was necessary. In such situations, awareness about the potential drug-related side effects is crucial because these can emulate or exacerbate symptoms of underlying lung disease. This points to the important overlap between lung health and pharmacologic treatments, where vigilance among cancer-treatment patients is vital because early detection and intervention can prevent huge morbidity (Ciulei et al., 2020) (Figure 3.15).

3.4.3. Staging and Prognosis

The staging and prognosis of ILDs and lung cancer are critical determinants of treatment regimens and predicting patient outcomes. Staging gives one insight into the extent and severity of the disease, and this is fundamental in planning a therapeutic approach. The idiopathic pulmonary fibrosis (IPF) variant of ILDs, for instance, is very heterogeneous in clinical presentation and therefore needs precise stratification. Recent findings have led to the development of diagnostic criteria consisting of clinical, physiological, and radiologic parameters that consistently enhance mortality risk prediction. Nevertheless, even with improvements, about 10% of pulmonary fibrosis remain unclassifiable, exemplifying heterogeneity and complexity associated with such conditions (Daccord et al., 2016). Hence, a robust staging system is vital not only for classifying diseases but also for guiding individualized treatment plans, which is a factor in optimizing clinical benefits. Further, the prognostic factors of lung diseases, particularly of chronic and life-threatening conditions, must be thoroughly considered. Prognosis can also be important in determining the provision of palliative and supportive care, thereby testifying to the importance of personalization. Interestingly, patients with chronic pulmonary diseases, such as chronic obstructive pulmonary disease (COPD), ILD, and lung cancer, share identical physical and psychosocial issues. These diseases tend to create disabling symptoms, such as dyspnea, which enormously impair quality of life. Recognizing the shortcomings of traditional prognostication tools in accurately anticipating the path in ILDs and non-malignant diseases, current research supports the integration of supportive and palliative care interventions based on patient need rather than prognosis alone (Boland et al., 2013). This model of care, thus, calls for greater precision in understanding the patient-specific trajectory. Advancements in staging and prognostication methods have a direct impact on the success of the treatment of ILDs and lung cancer. Identification of molecular disease phenotypes and endotypes may lead to improved comprehension and individualization of therapy.

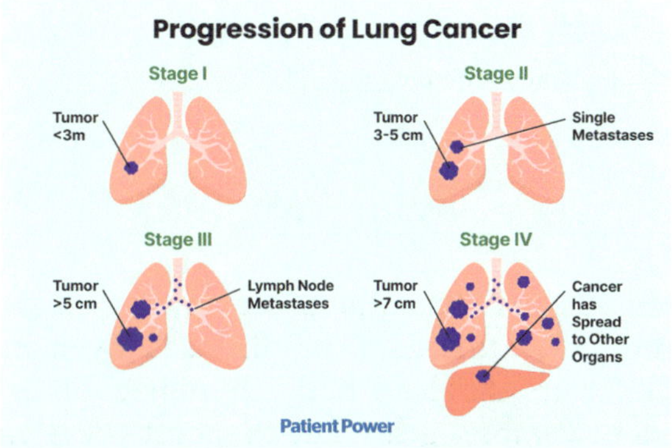

Figure 3.16. Staging and prognosis of lung cancer.

Source: https://images.ctfassets.net/tytuahdkbx9m/5sWVpLtuTWij01vHdv8XiA/dd0e1a37c1d49b951c068f94d1282bdb/PP-GettyImages-1256628174-Lung-Cancer-Stages-3000x2000.png.

For IPF, dividing patients into groups based on their respective disease characteristics may allow clinicians to predict the response to antifibrotic treatment, thus improving treatment accuracy. In addition, future biomarker identification is imperative for earlier diagnosis and tailoring of care strategies. With personalized medicine being targeted to the respiratory domain, healthcare caregivers are better able to predictively anticipate disease progression and improve patient care pathways, with treatments that complement the patient-specific challenges in patients suffering from these complex lung diseases (Boland et al., 2013; Daccord et al., 2016) (Figure 3.16).

Test Your Knowledge

1. What are the types of lung cancer?
2. What is staging and prognosis?

3.5. Risk Factors for Lung Cancer

Learning Outcome

1. Smoking and tobacco use;
2. Environmental pollutants;
3. Genetic factors.

Lung cancer remains a worldwide health problem to this date, predisposed by many risk factors that have both environmental and genetic components. While the most prevalent risk factor is familiar smoking, its impact is amplified among individuals who have experienced respiratory disorders such as ILD. There is evidence that ILD patients are at a high risk of lung cancer due to chronic lung inflammation and tissue remodeling, which can lead to malignant transformation. For instance, individuals who suffer from pulmonary diseases like bronchiectasis and idiopathic pulmonary fibrosis have registered high prevalence of lung cancer. The chronic inflammation associated with these ailments increases the carcinogenicity of environmental toxicants, further emphasizing the need for close surveillance in this group. Furthermore, exposures in certain occupations are outright important to lung cancer hazard, particularly in people with concomitant lung ailments. Workers in the asbestos, silica, and other carcinogen-exposure occupations have increased risks for developing lung cancer, particularly with accompanying respiratory disease. Most noteworthy is the combined effect of occupational risks and combined lung pathology, increasing the risk of cancer. Studies have established that individuals with ILD exposed to asbestos have a high incidence of elevated lung cancer cases (Kobayashi et al., 2024). Such an association necessitates investigation of work history among patients with ILD, emphasizing the need for preventive intervention and surveillance of high-risk individuals.

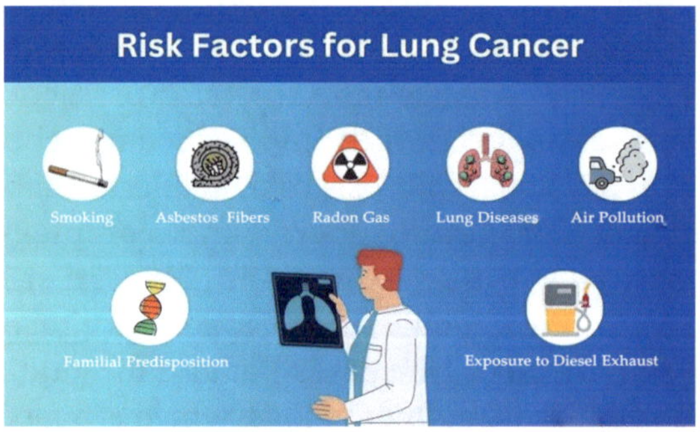

Figure 3.17. Risk factors for lung cancer.

Source: https://www.fitpaa.com/wp-content/uploads/2023/10/Untitled-design-2023-10-02T150518.500-jpg.webp.

Additionally, the correlation between lung cancer and age highlights the necessity of thorough risk evaluation in older populations, particularly those with ILD. As patients grow older, the chances of accompanying conditions, such as COPD and other lung conditions, rise. Older persons' lung cancer depends not only on overall exposure to carcinogens but also on the coexistence of other disabling lung conditions (Yu et al., 2025). These interactions complicate it further to deal with lung cancer clinically. Hence, healthcare professionals should make a point to incorporate age and overall respiratory health into lung cancer risk assessment. It is important to grasp these intricate risk factors while designing effective prevention and intervention programs for high-risk populations, leading to improved health outcomes (Figure 3.17).

3.5.1. Smoking and Tobacco Use

The relationship of smoking and tobacco use to the development of respiratory disease, particularly ILD and lung carcinoma, is evident. Cigarette smoke is an excellent stimulator of inflammation in the lungs, causing structural changes in airways as well as lung parenchyma. These alterations are generally exacerbated in individuals with underlying illnesses such as COPD and rheumatoid arthritis, wherein smoking acts as a significant cofactor for disease progression. The correlation of cumulative smoking history and cellular change in bronchoalveolar lavage (BAL) samples underlines the intrinsic correlation between smoking habit and lung disease, suggesting that even individuals with normal pulmonary status can exhibit extensive inflammatory changes (Karimi et al., 2014). This ominous trend thus underlines the necessity for targeted interventions to decrease smoking-related lung disease. Besides, mounting evidence emphasizes the danger posed by exposure to secondhand smoke, with its adverse impacts on non-smokers, particularly vulnerable populations such as children and pregnant women. The World Health Organization identifies tobacco smoking as the most preventable cause of disease and death worldwide, with an estimated 443,000 deaths in the United States alone each year (DuCasse et al., 2013). Apart from lung cancer, smoking is most linked to many other respiratory conditions, and it is hard to have public health campaigns against its prevalence. With the clinicians' roles, it is largely the case that respiratory therapists take on patients with smoking disease education and intervention therapy. On that note, upcoming healthcare professionals must be equipped with information and expertise to treat tobacco use in the clinic. In spite of the evident hazards, the majority of health curricula, including respiratory therapy curricula, have not provided adequate preparation of students regarding tobacco-related education. A study illustrating how students with very little exposure to respiratory therapy related to tobacco education recognized a disconcerting gap in their education that could leave them unable to effectively educate patients on how to quit smoking and avoid it (DuCasse et al., 2013). The findings reveal that the students are inadequately equipped to combat the public health problem of tobacco smoking, ultimately limiting their ability to combat smoking-induced diseases. As ILD and cancer of the lungs continue to prevail among smokers, improving the educational system in regard to tobacco smoking within healthcare programs is necessary in developing a vigorous reduction of the disease burden.

3.5.2. Environmental Pollutants

The relationship between lung health and air pollutants is known to play a critical role in ILD and the development of lung cancer. Airborne particulate matter, such as fine particulate matter (PM2.5) and nitrogen dioxide (NO2), has been linked to various respiratory diseases and causes chronic inflammation and cellular damage to lung tissues. Particularly, patients with idiopathic pulmonary fibrosis (IPF), the most severe ILD, demonstrate heightened vulnerability to such environmental poisons. It has been found through research that prolonged exposure to toxic chemicals can cause an improper wound-healing response, which in turn causes scarring and fibrosis of lung tissue, significantly increasing the chances of lung cancer in such a patient. Identification of this mechanistic link emphasizes the importance of addressing environmental pollution as a public health issue. In addition, the strong association between exposure to nitrogen dioxide and the incidence of lung cancer in patients with IPF demonstrates the toxic effect of environmental contaminants. A current cohort study depicted that high levels of NO_2 were correlated with a high incidence of lung cancer, which reflects its role as an urban carcinogen in air-polluted environments. When individuals already with lung disease are exposed to higher levels of nitrogen dioxide, the chances of malignancy development increase dramatically.

The study confirmed that individuals residing in areas with more concentrated NO_2 levels had twice the risk of lung cancer, once again highlighting the adverse effects of air pollution on vulnerable populations. These findings call for more research into the extent to which long-term exposure to air pollutants influences the onset of lung disease. In addition to NO2, other environmental pollutants, such as heavy metals and volatile organic compounds, have been linked to rising instances of lung cancer, particularly in urban centers where high pollution rates are reported. In India, for instance, there is a visible trend where an increasing number of cases of lung cancer among non-smokers have been noted, which is largely attributed to exposure to toxic airborne pollutants. Genetic vulnerabilities in certain populations increase this risk, with environmental and individual vulnerabilities interacting in a multifaceted manner. While statistics highlight these catastrophic tendencies, policymakers should implement stringent regulatory policies aimed at reducing rates of pollution using eco-friendly methods. In conclusion, minimizing environmental pollutants is not only critical in the prevention of lung disease but also in promoting public health overall (Figure 3.18).

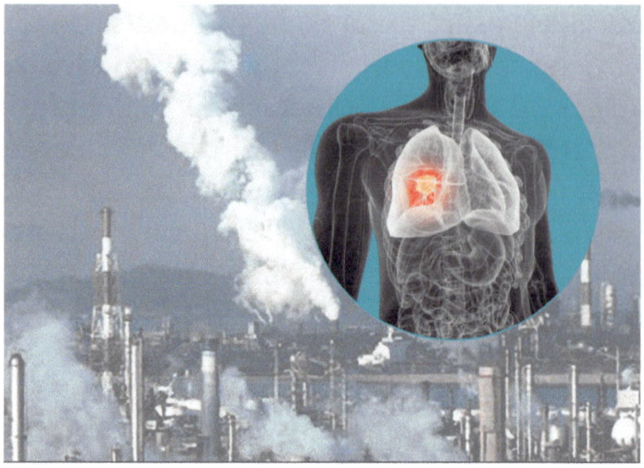

Figure 3.18. Environmental pollutants for lung cancer.

Source: https://www.oncoplus.co.in/wp-content/uploads/2025/02/How-Air-Pollution-Increases-the-Risk-of-Lung-Cancer.png.

3.5.3. Genetic Factors

In ILDs and lung cancer, genetic factors are very relevant in inducing disease and susceptibility prognosis. The genetics underlying such conditions may determine how people respond to environmental insults, such as toxins or microbes. Genetic variation, for instance, may influence the ability of lung cells to recover from damage inflicted by carcinogens, thus predisposing them to malignant transformation. In addition, inflammatory reactions may be influenced by genetic susceptibility, which plays a critical role in ILD pathogenesis and lung cancer. Acquiring information about these genetic determinants will aid in developing effective target therapies and risk stratification methods, highlighting the necessity of thoroughly studying the genome and understanding its impact on lung health. The dynamic interaction between the tumor microenvironment and genetics also adds to the complexity of lung disease progression. Genetic mutations within lung cells do not function as solitary agents; instead, they interact complexly with other stromal components, including inflammatory and immune cells, fibroblasts, and extracellular matrix molecules. Interaction between neoplastic cells and the tumor microenvironment is critical because it influences cancer and ILD behavior. Most crucially, alterations of the gene expression of these cells have the potential to induce differential cytokine and growth factor secretion, as highlighted in recent publications. The tumor microenvironment would then augment the effects of genetic predispositions, which in turn could dictate the fate of patients. Studies on these interactions could provide insight into potential therapeutic targets and biomarkers and hence enhance clinical handling of these diseases. Moreover, the evolution of genomic technologies, such as epigenetic profiling, is shedding light on the intricate interaction between environmental and genetic factors responsible for lung disease. Epigenetic modifications are influenced by the combination of genetic susceptibility and environmental exposure and can change gene expression without altering the underlying DNA sequence. This adds another layer of complexity in deciphering ILDs and lung cancer. Investigation of lung cell epigenetic profiles can provide insight into how specific genetic markers for poorer outcomes predispose patients. Studies have found that there are specific epigenetic profiles associated with severity in lung disease and potential cancer transformation. These findings stress the necessity for additional research integrating genetic analysis and epigenetic settings to create successful prevention and therapeutic strategies in the fight against ILDs and lung cancer (Borok et al., 2016; Castelo-Branco et al., 2019).

Test Your Knowledge

1. What are the risk factors for use smoking and tobacco?
2. What are the environmental pollutants for lung cancer?

3.6. The Link Between Interstitial Lung Diseases and Lung Cancer

Learning Outcome

1. Increased cancer risk in ILD patients;
2. Mechanisms linking ILDs to lung cancer;
3. Clinical implications for patient management.

The intricate relationship between ILDs and cancer of the lungs is a relevant diagnostic and therapeutic issue in the clinical setting. ILD patients possess a high predisposition to the development of lung cancer later on; hence, full observation and early detection are the most important considerations. The subchronic inflammation and fibrotic processes characteristic of ILDs predispose them to malignancy because chronic damage to alveolar elements will promote cellular mutation. As well, studies have established that various ILDs, including idiopathic pulmonary fibrosis, will significantly enhance the risk of lung cancer formation, and there is a causative relationship that merits enhanced surveillance in these cohorts. This connection not only highlights the urgency of appropriate clinical evaluation in ILD patients but also fosters more work on the intrinsic mechanisms that unite these diseases. Diagnostic innovation plays a crucial role in elucidating the connection between ILDs and lung cancer, particularly through sophisticated technologies such as cryobiopsy and magnetic resonance imaging (MRI). Cryobiopsy has also been shown to be a potential technique, and the diagnostic yields in lung cancer and ILDs are better due to the ability of cryobiopsies to collect larger and more intact tissue samples (Griff et al., 2019). The evident morphological differences detected through cryobiopsies, compared to traditional techniques, provide clearer insights into the underlying pathological changes between ILD and lung cancer (Griff et al., 2019). Similarly, though the clinical usefulness of MRIs in ILDs is under investigation, their capacity to provide additional functional information regarding lung mechanics and perfusion can assist us in understanding how ILDs increase the risk of lung cancer in patients (Hebestreit et al., 2011).

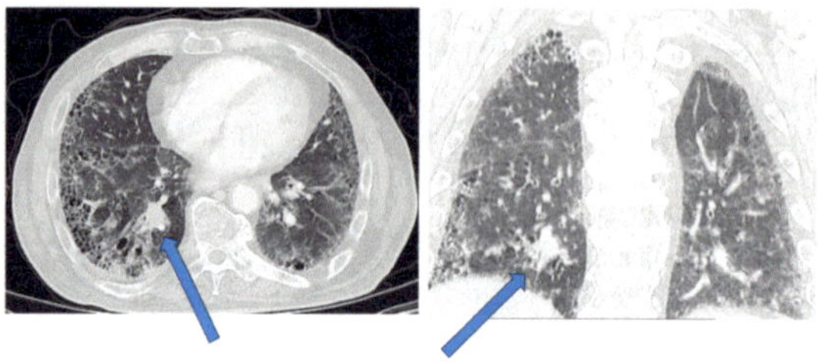

Figure 3.19. The link between interstitial lung diseases and lung cancer.

Source: https://pub.mdpi-res.com/cancers/cancers-16-02837/article_deploy/html/images/cancers-16-02837-g001.png?1723553478.

Such advancements necessitate integration with clinical practice to achieve optimal patient outcomes. Also, the interplay of environmental and genetic risk factors complicates the association of ILDs with lung cancer. Occupational lung carcinogen exposure to substances such as asbestos and silica has been attributed to both conditions, and there is a rationale for targeted risk assessment in exposed populations. There is also a genetic factor, with tumor suppressor gene mutations causing a shared susceptibility to ILD and lung cancer. As additional research comes to light, elucidating these complicated relationships will be critical to developing preventive interventions and individualized treatment regimens. Addressing the ILDs' role in malignancy development is a key area of focus in respiratory medicine that will necessitate interdisciplinary collaboration to increase awareness and improve clinical outcomes for risk-prone patients with malignancies of long-standing lung inflammation (Figure 3.19).

3.6.1. Increased Cancer Risk in ILD Patients

The association of ILD and an increased risk of lung cancer has been the focus of significant interest due to the common pathophysiological underpinnings driving both processes. ILDs, with their progressive inflammation and fibrosis of lung parenchyma, create an environment unfavorable for the growth of malignancies. For instance, the chronic inflammation induced by ILD can induce cellular change and mutational events that predispose to lung cancer, demonstrating the close interrelationship between these respiratory diseases. Studies have shown that patients with conditions such as idiopathic pulmonary fibrosis have a significantly increased risk of lung cancer, and therefore, more vigilant surveillance and early detection are necessary in this patient group. As knowledge grows, this two-fold risk must be addressed through clinical assessment and treatment planning. Furthermore, the prognosis for lung cancer patients with ILD is also complex, much of which is aggravated by the underlying lung pathology and ensuing decrease in pulmonary status. Lung cancer therapies, including chemotherapy and radiotherapy, add to the complexity of these patients' risk through their compromised respiratory status. There is evidence of enhanced mortality in combined progressive fibrosing ILDs and lung cancer patients, since therapeutic regimens have been shown to precipitate acute exacerbation of lung disease (Cadranel et al., 2022). This necessitates careful caution when designing treatment strategies, since the choice of therapeutic interventions should balance therapeutic effectiveness against the risk of lung function worsening. As practice progresses, research is required to determine standardized guidelines that provide the best possible care for these vulnerable patients. Beyond the known relationship between ILD and lung cancer, there is a requirement to understand the broader implications of chronic respiratory disease on overall health outcomes. Research indicates that a number of chronic respiratory disorders, including ILD, are associated with increased risk factors for other health complications, including severe infections like COVID-19 (Bauer et al., 2022). This multifaceted risk presents a unique challenge to healthcare professionals, who must reconcile intricate patient histories and comorbidities when developing overarching management strategies. As the body of evidence expands, the role of multidisciplinary care in managing both ILD and lung cancer becomes more evident. This highlights the need for collaborative care to address the multifactorial etiology of these diseases while maintaining overall quality of life.

3.6.2. Mechanisms Linking ILDs to Lung Cancer

The complex relationship between ILDs and lung cancer has accelerated in recent years, with researchers trying to sort out the pathophysiological mechanisms of the association. Chronic inflammation is a predominant characteristic of both diseases, suggesting that the long-standing inflammatory state induced by ILDs, such as idiopathic pulmonary fibrosis, predisposes individuals to the development of lung cancer. There is an inflammatory cytokine and growth factor release due to lung injury, resulting in a deranged process of wound healing that can be involved in fibrotic transformation and, eventually, carcinogenesis. The action of oxidative stress has come under scrutiny especially, since it has the potential to cause DNA damage and induction of mutagenesis, hence rendering the malignant transformation of affected lung tissue by ILDs increasingly likely. Clarifying these inflammatory mechanisms is key in explaining the mechanism of ILDs and increased lung cancer risk. Besides chronic inflammation, dynamics of epithelial-mesenchymal transition (EMT) are also critical in creating the association between ILDs and lung cancer. In ILDs, particularly fibrotic disease, improper activation of EMT-promoting pathways with epithelial cells converting into mesenchymal phenotypes such as the one explained above takes place. This change not only gives rise to fibrosis but also increases the risk of malignancy, because EMT is associated with tumorigenesis and metastasis. ILD dysregulation of wound healing provides a platform that is conducive to genetic mutation and subsequent tumorigenesis. The literature has demonstrated that growth factors, including TGF-β1, play a key role in this process by promoting fibrosis and tumorigenicity (Pendergraft et al., 2016). By the clarification of EMT mechanisms in ILDs, we can elucidate the complicated interactions involved in putting lung cancer at risk. Furthermore, the biochemical processes responsible for ILD development are also likely to trigger lung cancer by causing dysregulation of apoptosis and cell cycle control. The long-term exposure of lung tissue to pro-inflammatory mediators creates an environment in which the normal cell control mechanisms are disrupted. For instance, overexpression of some of the proteins involved in cell survival and the repression of apoptosis in fibrotic lung tissue pave the way for the survival of cells whose genetic material has been modified. This synergistic process amplifies the susceptibility of epithelial cells lining the airways for malignant transformation. Also, the crosstalk of oxidative stress with chronic inflammation could lead to the development of mutations in addition to causing further damage to cellular integrity to enhance tumorigenesis associated with ILDs (Pendergraft et al., 2016). Understanding such cellular processes is vital for the development of targeted therapies to reduce lung cancer risk in patients with ILDs.

3.6.3. Clinical Implications for Patient Management

Effective treatment of patients with ILDs who are at risk for lung cancer demands an integrated approach to therapy. The physicians must consider the shared risk factors and pathophysiologic mechanisms that complicate disease treatment. Tobacco use and environmental exposures are the central causes of both ILDs and lung cancer, and intensive tobacco cessation programs are indicated. Moreover, with overlapping presentations such as chronic cough and dyspnea, differentiation between worsening of the disease in ILDs and potential malignancy development must be made. Screening protocols have to consider risk assessments that balance against the detection of early lung cancer and potential harm from unjustified intervention.

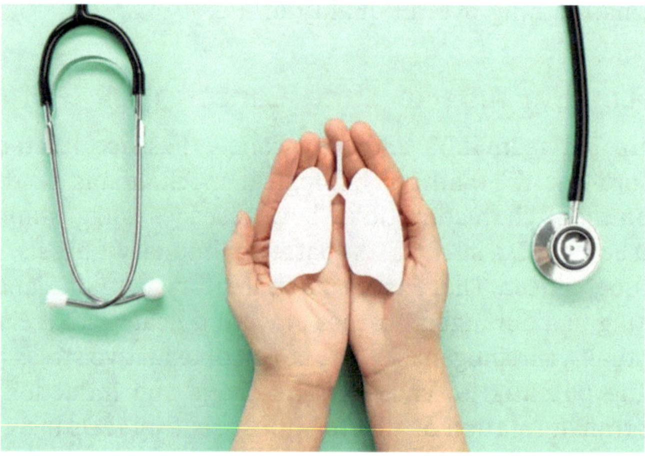

Figure 3.20. Clinical implications for patient management to lung cancer.

Source: https://www.acumenresearchandconsulting.com/reportimages/d065227b9d1391e78f29a27cd5621f9f.webp.

Clinical decision-making must involve a consideration of symptomatology, imaging diagnosis, and patient history to devise a focused management plan that targets both ILD and malignancy risk at the same time, hence optimizing patient outcomes (Umutoni et al., 2024). The application of advanced high-tech imaging technologies, such as HRCT, is crucial for monitoring ILD progression and diagnosing lung cancer. Regular screening is crucial for early detection of incipient malignancies, especially among high-risk populations. Agreement on criteria to initiate HRCT screening, however, remains lacking and depends on clinical judgment from patient-specific risk factors. In individuals with autoimmune disease, even the theoretical potential for spontaneous ILD development independent of disease activity makes management even more challenging (Esposito et al., 2024). This mandates a vigorous follow-up regimen comprising pulmonary function testing and symptom scoring to monitor changes in lung function. Multidisciplinary treatment is critical; collaboration among pulmonologists, oncologists, and radiologists can facilitate optimal management plans that leverage multiple specializations to manage both lung function and cancer risk effectively. Also, treatment modalities for ILD patients with accompanying lung cancer should be specially aligned, given the unique interrelation between the two conditions. Immunosuppressive drugs may be warranted in situations where autoimmune-associated ILD leads to considerable impairment of pulmonary function, but their introduction must be balanced against their potential for augmenting lung cancer risk (Esposito et al., 2024). In addition, novel antifibrotic therapies are promising for controlling ILD, but their advantages must be balanced against possible adverse effects and drug interactions, particularly in patients undergoing cancer therapy. Lastly, an ongoing discussion with the patient regarding their preferences and concerns about care is required, allowing them to be active participants in their own management. Having defined procedures in place for monitoring the effect of treatment and adverse events helps to ensure that patient care is dynamic and responsive to the changing environment of their health needs (Umutoni et al., 2024) (Figure 3.20).

Test Your Knowledge

1. What are the mechanisms linking ILDs to lung cancer?
2. What are the clinical implications for patient management?

Summary

The research on ILDs and their potential involvement with lung cancer suggests that a holistic approach should be undertaken to understand these complex diseases. ILDs such as idiopathic pulmonary fibrosis (IPF) severely impair lung function and life, having a tendency to lead towards a severe prognosis for the patient. Median survival rate in IPF is unfortunately low, between three to five years, and this emphasizes the necessity for developing effective treatment strategies (Collard et al., 2017). With awareness of the multifaceted complexity of ILDs, including co-occurrence of comorbidities like lung cancer, clinicians are able to develop better customized and integrated management plans with the purpose of improving the outcome of patients. Moreover, the converse relationship between ILDs and lung cancer suggests that some clinical predictors might be able to reveal the onset of malignancy in patients suffering from these lung conditions. Results indicate that while the progression of disease may be halted by some interventions, for example, antifibrotic therapy for IPF, they might instead influence the risk of developing concomitant cancers (Collard et al., 2017). These complex relationships must be explored further so as to uncover how treatment practices can diminish or enhance the risk of lung cancer among patients with ILD. These dynamics will not only inform treatment guidelines but also enhance prevention strategies in clinical care. Ultimately, the overlap between ILDs and lung cancer is an appeal for continued research and collaboration among clinicians. Current evidence on the correlation of rheumatoid arthritis interstitial lung disease (RA-ILD) with therapy considerations highlights a necessity to re-evaluate therapeutic approaches on an ongoing basis. With advances in diagnostic methods and the discovery of novel therapeutic agents, early intervention and vigilance for potential malignancy will become highly important. Management of ILDs in conjunction with lung cancer treatment strategies will probably lead to better prognosis not only in patients with IPF but in patients faced with the entire range of interstitial diseases. The multi-modal strategy will probably enlighten significant correlations and promote better disease management among the affected groups.

In exploring the relationship between ILDs and lung cancer, certain key points are outlined that reiterate their connection. ILDs represent a collection of pathologies localized mainly to the lung parenchyma and possibly leading to complications like cancer development. Interestingly, these illnesses entailed chronic inflammation, which plays a role in generating an environment for malignant transformation. Furthermore, the occurrence of such symptoms as dyspnea and fatigue among ILD patients can significantly impair their quality of life, thereby making it essential to look at ILDs not only as lung diseases but as multifaceted conditions that are capable of predisposing people to lung cancer (Boland et al., 2013). The interplay among these diseases highlights the need for healthcare providers to develop comprehensive management plans that include regular screening for malignancy and the treatment of ILDs. In addition, the psychosocial components of chronic lung disease management cannot be overlooked. ILD and lung cancer patients have similar concerns, including pain, distress, and social isolation from their illnesses (Boland et al., 2013). Thus, the incorporation of palliative and supportive care is essential for improving patients' quality of life in totality. New guidelines advocate for the fact that palliative care should not be limited to those with end-stage diagnoses but should encompass all individuals afflicted with life-limiting illnesses. This shift in emphasis highlights the emerging value placed on early intervention in palliative care to promote symptom management, quality of life, and even survival in patients with multifaceted comorbidities, such as ILDs with lung cancer. Understanding immune mechanisms in the pathogenesis of lung disease is also essential. Certain biomarkers have been identified in recent research, which can improve our understanding of macrophage function in lung pathology. Macrophage gene expression kinetics are important not just for the analysis of ILDs but also for understanding their potential course to lung cancer. The identification of universal biomarkers also indicates the interconnectedness of several lung diseases, and the potential promise of prognostic markers to inform therapeutic choices. Continued research in these areas is necessary for the design of therapies that take into consideration the complexities of ILDs and how they are capable of predisposing patients to lung cancer, and eventually leading to improved results in those patients.

KEY TERMS FROM THIS CHAPTER

- Adenocarcinoma
- ALK rearrangement
- Bronchoscopy
- Connective tissue disease-associated ILD
- EGFR mutation
- Ground-glass opacities
- High-resolution CT (HRCT)
- Honeycombing
- Hypersensitivity pneumonitis
- Idiopathic pulmonary fibrosis (IPF)
- Interstitial fibrosis
- Large cell carcinoma
- Non-small cell lung cancer (NSCLC)
- Paraneoplastic syndromes
- Reduced diffusion capacity (DLCO)
- Restrictive lung pattern
- Sarcoidosis
- Small cell lung cancer (SCLC)
- Squamous cell carcinoma
- TNM staging

CRITICAL THINKING QUESTIONS

1. **What is the most common form of idiopathic interstitial pneumonia?**
   a. Cryptogenic organizing pneumonia (COP)
   b. Desquamative interstitial pneumonia (DIP)
   c. Idiopathic pulmonary fibrosis (IPF)
   d. Acute interstitial pneumonia (AIP)
2. **Which HRCT (High-Resolution CT) finding is most characteristic of usual interstitial pneumonia (UIP)?**
   a. Ground-glass opacities with upper lobe predominance
   b. Honeycombing in subpleural, basal regions
   c. Nodular opacities in centrilobular regions
   d. Consolidation in middle lobe only
3. **Which of the following is a known occupational cause of ILD?**
   a. Smoking
   b. Silica dust exposure
   c. Viral infections
   d. Obesity
4. **Which type of lung cancer is most strongly associated with smoking?**
   a. Adenocarcinoma
   b. Small cell lung cancer (SCLC)
   c. Bronchioloalveolar carcinoma
   d. Carcinoid tumor
5. **What is the most common type of lung cancer in non-smokers?**
   a. Squamous cell carcinoma
   b. Adenocarcinoma
   c. Small cell carcinoma
   d. Large cell carcinoma

Short Answer Questions

1. What are Interstitial Lung Diseases (ILDs), and how are they broadly classified?
2. Describe the general pathophysiological mechanism underlying ILDs.
3. List occupational and environmental exposures that can cause ILDs.
4. What high-resolution CT (HRCT) findings are typical in idiopathic pulmonary fibrosis (IPF)?
5. What factors influence prognosis and survival in lung cancer?

Answer to Critical Thinking Questions

1. (c); 2. (b); 3. (b); 4. (b); 5. (b).

References

1. Königshoff, M. (2011). Lung cancer in Pulmonary Fibrosis: Tales of Epithelial Cell Plasticity. *Respiration*, *81*(5), 353–358. https://doi.org/10.1159/000326299Adegunsoye, A., Boctor, N., Chung, J. H., DiGeronimo, R., et al. (2019). Diagnostic test interpretation and referral delay in patients with interstitial lung disease. https://core.ac.uk/download/323068477.pdf (accessed on 30th June 2025).

2. Agostini, C., Cinetto, F., Milito, C., Pulvirenti, F., et al. (2019). Appropriate lung management in patients with primary antibody deficiencies. https://core.ac.uk/download/237174843.pdf (accessed on 30th June 2025).

3. Alfaro, T. M., Alfieri, V., Antoniou, K., Bargagli, E., et al. (2019). Research highlights from the 2018 ERS International Congress: Interstitial lung diseases. https://core.ac.uk/download/187749048.pdf (accessed on 30th June 2025).

4. Alfaro, T. M., Alfieri, V., Antoniou, K., Bargagli, E., et al. (2020). Research highlights from the 2018 ERS International Congress: Interstitial lung diseases. https://core.ac.uk/download/340488777.pdf (accessed on 30th June 2025).

5. Althobiani, M. A., Folarin, A., Hurst, J. R., Jacob, J., et al. (2024). Interstitial lung disease: A review of classification, etiology, epidemiology, clinical diagnosis, pharmacological and non-pharmacological treatment. https://core.ac.uk/download/603470194.pdf (accessed on 30th June 2025).

6. Assaad, S., Friedman, M. B., Kratzert, W. B., Perrino, A. C., et al. (2018). Assessment of pulmonary edema: Principles and practice. https://core.ac.uk/download/145643671.pdf (accessed on 30th June 2025).

7. Assadi, M., Bahtouee, M., Eftekhari, M., Javadi, H., et al. (2015). 99mTc-MIBI lung scintigraphy in the assessment of pulmonary involvement in interstitial lung disease and its comparison with pulmonary function tests and high-resolution computed tomography: A preliminary study. https://core.ac.uk/download/52205651.pdf (accessed on 30th June 2025).

8. Assassi, S., Fischbach, M., GENISOS Study Group, Gonzalez, E. B., et al. (2011). Predictors of fatigue severity in early systemic sclerosis: A prospective longitudinal study of the GENISOS cohort. https://core.ac.uk/download/323073807.pdf (accessed on 30th June 2025).

9. Bauer, T., Geerdes-Fenge, H., Blum, G., Gottlieb, J., et al. (2022). Risk assessment for patients with chronic respiratory conditions in the context of the SARS-CoV-2 pandemic: Statement of the German Respiratory Society with the support of the German Association of Chest Physicians. https://core.ac.uk/download/554061856.pdf (accessed on 30th June 2025).

10. Baye, F., Goswami, C. P., Gurung, G., Jackson, C., et al. (2017). Gene expression profiles among murine strains segregate with distinct differences in the progression of radiation-induced lung disease. https://core.ac.uk/download/83049943.pdf (accessed on 30th June 2025).

11. Bellotti, C., De Francesco, G. P., Lavra, L., Magi, L., et al. (2018). Galectin-3: One molecule for an alphabet of diseases, from A to Z. https://core.ac.uk/download/153369169.pdf (accessed on 30th June 2025).

12. Bjerg, A., Stallberg, B., Modena, E., Clini, E., Herth, F. J. F., Vogiatzis, I., Coolen, J., et al. (2015). Clinical highlights: Messages from Munich. https://core.ac.uk/download/54009225.pdf (accessed on 30th June 2025).

13. Boland, J., Martin, J., Ross, J. R., Ross, J., et al. (2013). Palliative care for people with non-malignant lung disease: Summary of current evidence and future direction. https://core.ac.uk/download/151156967.pdf (accessed on 30th June 2025).

14. Borok, Z., Laird-Offringa, I. A., Marconett, C. N., Stueve, T. R., et al. (2016). The importance of detailed epigenomic profiling of different cell types within organs. https://core.ac.uk/download/323063483.pdf (accessed on 30th June 2025).

15. Brown, K. K., Cottin, V., Currow, D., Danoff, S., et al. (2023). Progressive pulmonary fibrosis: An expert group consensus statement. https://core.ac.uk/download/622653485.pdf (accessed on 30th June 2025).

16. Busby, A., Creamer, P., Dixey, J., Kiely, P., et al. (2019). Is incident rheumatoid arthritis interstitial lung disease associated with methotrexate treatment? Results from a multivariate analysis in the ERAS and ERAN inception cohorts. https://core.ac.uk/download/287581915.pdf (accessed on 30th June 2025).

17. Cadranel, J., Funke-Chambour, M., Kewalramani, N., Machahua, C., et al. (2022). Lung cancer in patients with fibrosing interstitial lung diseases: An overview of current knowledge and challenges. https://core.ac.uk/download/527937990.pdf (accessed on 30th June 2025).

18. Castelo-Branco, P., da Cunha, B. R., Domingos, C., Henrique, R., et al. (2019). Cellular interactions in the tumor microenvironment: The role of secretome. https://core.ac.uk/download/232150565.pdf (accessed on 30th June 2025).

19. Ciulei, G., Coste, S. C., Cozma, A., Fabian, A., et al. (2020). Imatinib-induced interstitial pneumonitis–A literature review and case report. https://core.ac.uk/download/304672916.pdf (accessed on 30th June 2025).

20. Collard, H. R., & Oldham, J. M. (2017). Comorbid conditions in idiopathic pulmonary fibrosis: Recognition and management. https://core.ac.uk/download/323072212.pdf (accessed on 30th June 2025).

21. Creel, M. E. (2008). Gender differences in survival in idiopathic pulmonary fibrosis and following lung transplant. https://core.ac.uk/download/12209464.pdf (accessed on 30th June 2025).

22. Crooks, M. G., & Hart, S. P. (2015). Coagulation and anticoagulation in idiopathic pulmonary fibrosis. https://core.ac.uk/download/151161837.pdf (accessed on 30th June 2025).

23. Daccord, C., & Maher, T. M. (2016). Recent advances in understanding idiopathic pulmonary fibrosis. https://core.ac.uk/download/77013578.pdf (accessed on 30th June 2025).

24. Dang, D., Das, S., Ghosh, P., Prince, J., et al. (2020). Computational approach to identifying universal macrophage biomarkers. https://core.ac.uk/download/323064949.pdf (accessed on 30th June 2025).

25. Dołęga, J., Hudzińska, P., Krzykawski, K., Maciejczyk, A., et al. (2024). The role of pulmonary rehabilitation and physical activity in the prevention, treatment and management of respiratory diseases–A comprehensive review. https://core.ac.uk/download/636385575.pdf (accessed on 30th June 2025).

26. DuCasse, D. S. (2013). Survey of the knowledge and confidence of respiratory therapy students regarding tobacco smoking and respiratory diseases. https://core.ac.uk/download/71424716.pdf (accessed on 30th June 2025).

27. Esposito, A. J., & Ajam, A. (2024). Detection and management of autoimmune disease-associated interstitial lung diseases. *The American Journal of Managed Care, 30*(7 Suppl), S114–S121. https://www.semanticscholar.org/paper/d04a5b87383d2f9ca732e5d1491d074e1179c1c7 (accessed on 30th June 2025).

28. Fenech, M., Gouder, C., & Montefort, S. (2012). Interstitial lung disease in Malta. https://core.ac.uk/download/46602323.pdf (accessed on 30th June 2025).

29. Fioret, D. (2012). *Idiopathic Pulmonary Fibrosis: Diagnosis, Management, and the Search for a Cure.* https://core.ac.uk/download/143833847.pdf (accessed on 30th June 2025).

30. Geelhoed, J. J. M. (M.), Tak-van Jaarsveld, N. C. (N.), Van Manen, M. J. G. (M.), Wijsenbeek-Lourens, M., et al. (2017). Optimizing quality of life in patients with idiopathic pulmonary fibrosis. https://core.ac.uk/download/154411139.pdf (accessed on 30th June 2025).

31. Griff, S. (2019). Einfluss der Art der Materialgewinnung auf die Diagnosefindung in der Lungenpathologie. https://core.ac.uk/download/222573993.pdf (accessed on 30th June 2025).

32. Guzik, T. J., Mohiddin, S., Dimarco, A., Patel, V., Savvatis, K., Marelli-Berg, F. M., Madhur, M. S., et al. (2020). COVID-19 and the cardiovascular system: Implications for risk assessment, diagnosis, and treatment options. *Cardiovascular Research, 116*, 1666–1687. https://doi.org/10.1093/cvr/cvaa106 (accessed on 30th June 2025).

33. Hebestreit, A., Kluge, A., Kluge, A., Kluge, A., Bankier, A. A., Henderson, A. C., Brody, A. S., et al. (2011). MRI of the lung (3/3)—Current applications and future perspectives. https://core.ac.uk/download/28969132.pdf (accessed on 30th June 2025).

34. Karimi, R. (2014). Pulmonary manifestations in smoking-related diseases: Clinical studies with emphasis on chronic obstructive pulmonary disease and rheumatoid arthritis. https://core.ac.uk/download/70341173.pdf (accessed on 30th June 2025).

35. Kobayashi, Y., Ishiguro, T., Kagiyama, N., Sumi, M., & Takayanagi, N. (2024). Prognostic impact of pulmonary diseases in 952 patients with thoracic and/or abdominal aortic aneurysm. *Journal of Clinical Medicine, 13*. https://www.semanticscholar.org/paper/46dfbea085ffaaddba0141775c06927c03bcab18 (accessed on 30th June 2025).

36. Murray, C. J. L., Ikuta, K. S., Sharara, F., Swetschinski, L. R., Robles Aguilar, G., Gray, A. P., Han, C., et al. (2022). Global burden of bacterial antimicrobial resistance in 2019: A systematic analysis. *The Lancet, 399*, 629–655. https://doi.org/10.1016/s0140-6736(21)02724-0 (accessed on 30th June 2025).

37. Ndaba, N. A. (2017). Compensable occupational lung diseases in living miners and ex-miners in South Africa, 2003–2013. https://core.ac.uk/download/188772232.pdf (accessed on 30th June 2025).

38. Pendergraft, B. (2016). The effects of smoking on the calcification of the aortic valve. https://core.ac.uk/download/72841045.pdf (accessed on 30th June 2025).

39. Suhasini, G., Reddy, K. S., Madhulekha, R., & Ugandhar, T. (2024). Emerging epidemic: Non-smoker lung cancer in India's urban centers. *International Journal for Research in Applied Science and Engineering Technology*. https://www.semanticscholar.org/paper/39ae9166e1a52825e5ebcc99f81473b25c7df643 (accessed on 30th June 2025).

40. Umutoni, D., Owolabi, M. S., & Waheed, S. (2024). Unraveling the complex interactions among lung cancer, COPD, cardiovascular disease, and pulmonary fibrosis: Overlapping

risks, converging pathways, and integrated care approaches. *BIOMED Natural and Applied Science*. https://www.semanticscholar.org/paper/615c2d0c5c9cfe98356694a7ea0ac4453a9ac3c1 (accessed on 30th June 2025).

41. Yoon, H., Kim, S. Y., & Song, J. W. (2024). Association between high levels of nitrogen dioxide and increased cumulative incidence of lung cancer in patients with idiopathic pulmonary fibrosis. *European Respiratory Journal, 63*. https://www.semanticscholar.org/paper/b95e0bef1a7ab412d78f9c0bc09bf9d162836e4e (accessed on 30th June 2025).

42. Yu, H. Y., Lee, C. Y., Hu, Y. C., Lin, L. G., Chao, Y., & Li, C. P. (2025). Treatment rechallenge is safe and leads to better survival in pancreatic cancer patients with interstitial pneumonitis. *BMC Cancer, 25*. https://www.semanticscholar.org/paper/03ef94c5ac12dc6be7b949ce272740f78aacca04 (accessed on 30th June 2025).

43. Zimmerman, W. F. (2025). Health requirements for advanced coal extraction systems. https://core.ac.uk/download/pdf/42863125.pdf (accessed on 30th June 2025).

PULMONARY NEOPLASMS OTHER THAN BRONCHOGENIC CARCINOMA

4

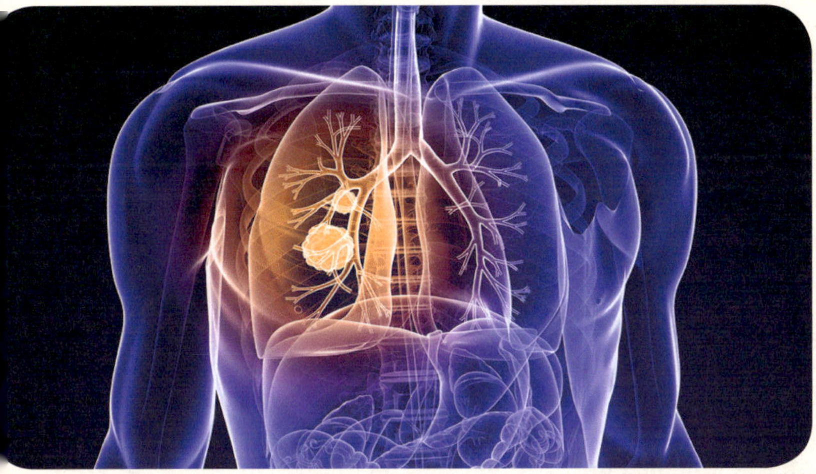

LEARNING OBJECTIVES

After studying this chapter, you will be able to:

1. List the types of pulmonary neoplasms
2. Explain the epidemiology of non-bronchogenic pulmonary neoplasms
3. Explore the pathophysiology of pulmonary neoplasms
4. Illustrate clinical presentation and diagnosis
5. List the treatment options
6. Define prognosis and outcomes

Introduction

The topic of pulmonary neoplasms extends beyond the originally described bronchogenic carcinoma to include a heterogeneous group of tumors in the pulmonary structure. These neoplasms, less common than bronchogenic carcinoma, have a spectrum of characteristics that warrant distinct diagnostic and therapeutic approaches. The diversity of pulmonary neoplasms includes both benign and malignant neoplasms, each presenting with different diagnostic and management dilemmas for the clinician. Improvements in diagnostic methods, as well as the evolution of new therapeutic approaches, have attained better patient outcomes in patients with these diseases. It is essential to comprehend the different pulmonary neoplasms and associated behavior for planning adequate treatment, which is finally associated with survival and quality of life in patients. An important aspect of treating pulmonary neoplasms is understanding the complexity of the tumors. For instance, the prognosis and treatment of mediastinal tumors vary based on the histologic type and anatomical location in the thoracic cavity. Certain tumors, e.g., thymic tumors and neurogenic tumors, may have different implications compared to other neoplasms, e.g., carcinoid tumors or lymphomas. The mediastinum, where significant structures are found, is at the center of the management of these tumors, and postoperative complications directly relate to the nearby vital structures. Proper understanding of the scope of pulmonary neoplasms has been highlighted in current literature to enable early intervention that minimizes morbidity and optimizes patient outcomes (Rodríguez et al., 2018; Jaikaran et al., 2009). Also, the pattern of cancer therapy is being revolutionized, particularly with the incorporation of neo-adjuvant treatment to various neoplasms. Although techniques such as chemotherapy and radiotherapy are traditionally applied to bronchogenic carcinoma, their application in other pulmonary neoplasms will have to be put through careful scrutiny. It is clear that neo-adjuvant treatments can alter the response of the tumor and can affect surgical options and postoperative morbidity. As pointed out by recent research, the relationships among surgical techniques and preoperative treatments should be constantly reevaluated, especially concerning post-operative morbidity within the framework of complex surgical cases (Rodríguez et al., 2018; Jaikaran et al., 2009). Ongoing research of the matters at issue is imperative, as it provides better insight into the pulmonary neoplasms other than bronchogenic carcinoma, eventually leading to optimized patient care and improved survival rates.

Definition of Pulmonary Neoplasms

Pulmonary neoplasms are a diverse group of tumors of the lungs or the surrounding anatomical structures. Pulmonary tumors can be separated into benign and malignant neoplasms, among which malignant neoplasms demand special concern due to their malignancy and metastatic tendency. While bronchogenic carcinoma, the most common cancer of the lung, draws attention and dominates the discussion, many other neoplasms of the lung exist, including carcinoid tumors, mesotheliomas, and metastatic tumors from cancers that originate in other organs. Primary versus secondary (metastatic) neoplasms influence treatment and predictive outcomes and, therefore, are important to differentiate at the time of presentation. In addition to recognizing the different types of pulmonary neoplasms, their clinical presentation, as well as diagnostic workup, needs to be considered. They have a vastly varying spectrum of symptoms, ranging from chronic cough and unexplained weight loss to more ominous ones such as hemoptysis or dyspnea. Imaging modalities, particularly computed tomography (CT), play a crucial role in identifying and describing such tumors. As highlighted in studies, CT features may be helpful in differential diagnosis, distinguishing one mediastinal mass from another, thus enabling clinicians to treat accordingly. For instance, while CT may identify a solitary middle mediastinal mass, this would be indicative of metastatic illness as opposed to lymphoma; the paramount role of imaging in disease management and decision-making by clinicians is illustrated by this (Glazer et al., 1987).

The epidemiology of lung neoplasms is also heterogeneous and influenced by numerous factors, including geography, occupational exposures, and genetic susceptibility. Some groups, for instance, have wildly differing incidences of some lung cancers. Retrospective evidence from studies illustrates bronchogenic carcinoma to be prevalent in Europeans but remarkably rare in Bantu miners in South Africa, illustrating the multifaceted interplay between environmental risk factors and cancer pathology. These disparities justify the pursuit of etiologic factors underlying such discrepancies, such as occupational silica dust exposure, which has a role in the development of several types of neoplasms (Hurwitz et al., 1951). As a rule, knowledge of the complex nature of pulmonary neoplasms requires more than semantic definitions, and a complete examination of their origin, path, and consequences to patient health is justified (Figure 4.1).

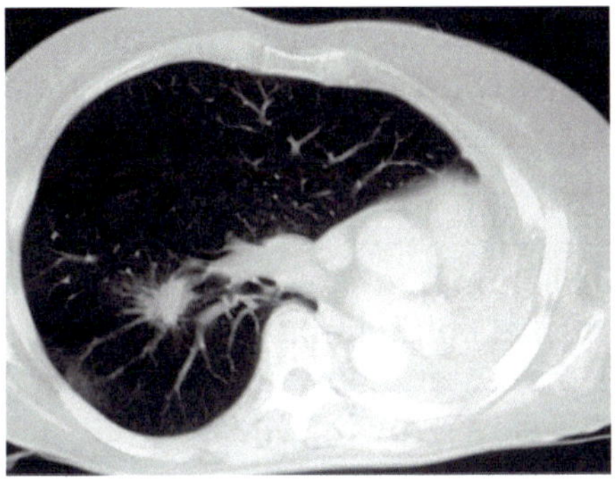

Figure 4.1. Pulmonary neoplasms.

Source: https://external-content.duckduckgo.com/iu/?u=https%3A%2F%2Fstorage.googleapis.com%2Fdl.dentistrykey.com%2Fclinical%2FPulmonaryNeoplasms%2F4_3s20B9780702073113000061.jpg&f=1&nofb=1&ipt=e25e7f854bb2b800945e7434e21a2addc408605baa5cf91850c1b9b621c03282.

Importance of Studying Non-Bronchogenic Neoplasms

The study of non-bronchogenic neoplasms is significant in advancing our knowledge of pulmonary tumors not arising from direct bronchial tissue. These neoplasms, which are a heterogeneous collection of entities such as metastatic tumors, mesenchymal tumors, and benign lesions, are both diagnostic and therapeutic challenges. By appreciating the specific characteristics of these neoplasms, clinicians can differentiate between malignant and benign conditions more effectively and thus enhance patient management. Although constituting a smaller proportion of pulmonary neoplasms compared to bronchogenic cancers, the clinical significance in accurately diagnosing and managing the same is usually high. With their multifarious origin points, interdepartmental synergy involving departments such as oncology, pathology, and radiology is important in arriving at accurate diagnoses and customized treatment protocols that can improve patient outcomes overall (Canadian Medical Association, 1982). Secondly, non-bronchogenic neoplasms tend to be atypical in presentation, making diagnosis more challenging. Compared to bronchogenic carcinomas, which typically have classic symptoms and radiographic findings, these neoplasms can exhibit a wide range of clinical manifestations corresponding to their varied origins. Such diversity requires broad diagnostic strategies, such as sophisticated imaging studies and histopathological analysis, to avoid missing key conditions by clinicians. For example, metastatic disease may manifest as primary lung cancers, and proper knowledge of common metastatic pathways and ability to identify common tumor markers is required. Through diligent study and increased awareness, medical professionals can hone their diagnostic abilities to perfection, ultimately leading to timely interventions that enhance patient survival and quality of life (Anwar et al., 2018). In addition, as the incidence and types of lung neoplasms vary with different risk factors and environmental factors, ongoing research into non-bronchogenic neoplasms is becoming more crucial. Public health issues, such as tobacco use, pollution, and on-the-job exposure, have been linked with various forms of lung neoplasms, so it is becoming more critical that more and more attention be focused on all potential forms of pulmonary tumors. This emphasis not only aids in the interpretation of the etiology and epidemiology of such tumors but also prepares the healthcare system to formulate preventive strategies and sheltered care policies for vulnerable groups. Since investigation endeavors are led by the medical community, a state of scholarly pursuit of research into non-bronchogenic neoplasms will be pivotal in demystifying their nature and developing protocols of appropriate management and treatment (Canadian Medical Association, 1982) (Figure 4.2).

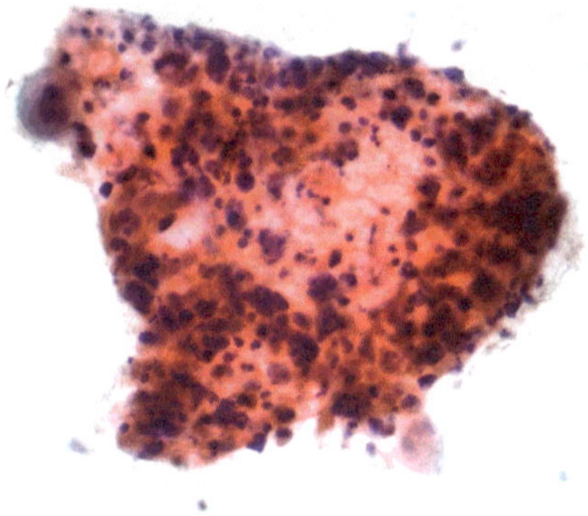

Figure 4.2. Studying non-bronchogenic neoplasms.

Source: https://upload.wikimedia.org/wikipedia/commons/c/c6/Squamous_carcinoma_lung_cytology.gif.

4.1. Types of Pulmonary Neoplasms

Learning Outcome

1. Primary lung tumors
2. Secondary lung tumors
3. Rare pulmonary neoplasms

Among the diverse categories of pulmonary neoplasms, adenocarcinoma is the most prevalent one, a large subgroup of lung cancer. Adenocarcinomas are characterized by glandular differentiation and are prone to occur in the peripheral regions of the lung and often are associated with underlying conditions such as chronic obstructive pulmonary disease (COPD) and environmental carcinogens (e.g., tobacco smoke and asbestos). The histological subtyping is crucial in diagnosing and writing treatment protocols for adenocarcinoma when biomarker expression patterns, such as Thyroid Transcription Factor-1 (TTF-1) and Napsin A, play an integral role in defining tumors. Recent research suggests that Napsin A is superior to TTF-1 in specificity, particularly in the differentiation of adenocarcinoma from other neoplasms of the lung and thus has a greater impact on clinical decision-making as lung cancer pathology continues to evolve (Manibarathi et al., 2018). Another category included within pulmonary neoplasms is neuroendocrine tumors that range from typical carcinoids to aggressive types such as small cell lung carcinoma (SCLC). SCLC develops from disseminated neuroendocrine cells in the bronchial epithelium, leading to distinctive clinical presentations. While usual carcinoids tend to be slow-growing and are well-suited for prognosis, SCLC is notorious for violent growth and early metastasis, making management and treatment challenging. The identification and classification of neuroendocrine tumors largely rely on immunohistochemical markers, where synaptophysin and chromogranin A play decisive roles. Understanding the biological behavior of such tumors is essential for making decisions about appropriate treatment strategies, such as chemotherapy and targeted therapies, that aid in improving patient outcomes (Jaikaran et al., 2009). Lastly, it should be mentioned regarding the metastatic lung neoplasms, where tumors formed from other parts of the body can metastasize to the lungs. The most frequent initial sites are breast, colon, and kidney; the metastases in such organs are likely to manifest as discrete masses or diffuse infiltration of lung parenchyma. Clinical impact of metastatic disease in the lungs necessitates careful assessment and treatment planning. Differential diagnosis between primary pulmonary neoplasms and metastatic lesions is based on complete imaging studies and a detailed review of the patient's history. Furthermore, coordination between oncology, thoracic surgery, and palliative care will be essential. Healthcare professionals should adopt an interdisciplinary approach to assess the extent of disease and tailor therapeutic interventions, recognizing the complexity of managing pulmonary neoplasms outside bronchogenic carcinoma. With continued advances in pulmonary neoplasm knowledge, increasing studies will be necessary to enhance diagnostic accuracy and therapeutic efficacy (Jaikaran et al., 2009).

4.1.1. Primary Lung Tumors

In the setting of pulmonary neoplasms, primary lung cancer is a clinical condition broader than bronchogenic carcinoma. Tumors in this category include a diverse group of histologic types, such as sarcomas and carcinoid tumors, each with distinct natural histories and treatment responses. Among all the various entities, primary pulmonary leiomyosarcoma (PPL) is striking for its rarity and its aggressive behavior. Originating from the pulmonary parenchymal smooth muscle, it has a tendency to resemble other lung tumors; thus, diagnosing and treating it becomes difficult. Even though the majority of patients with primary lung tumors are symptom-free, those who are diagnosed with symptoms have respiratory symptoms, which call for extensive evaluation to differentiate between benign and malignant conditions, as early intervention is crucial to patient prognosis. The treatment of isolated pulmonary nodules (SPNs) is a balancing act, particularly in the case of a primary lung malignancy. Although SPNs are a common radiological presentation, they are mostly benign. This then poses a problem to treating clinicians as they attempt not to subject patients to unnecessary invasive procedures without considering possible curable malignancies that would have become advanced if left untreated. Techniques such as positron emission tomography scanning and percutaneous biopsy have been refined to assist in this process of discrimination. Morphology, growth, and enhancement features of the nodule comprise essential elements in assessing the risk of malignancy represented by SPNs. By employing these strategies, medical clinicians aim to provide timely and accurate diagnoses and thereby enhance patient management and outcomes in cases of primary lung tumors (Quint et al., 2015). Adding to the complexity of the clinical presentation is the fact that some primary lung tumors, including PPL, may have symptoms that mimic other common pulmonary diseases, at times to the point of holding them up. For instance, in a case study, a 21-year-old woman was seen first with milder respiratory disease-dyspnea, only to be later diagnosed with PPL upon completion of a thorough imaging test that revealed a malignant tumor. These cases highlight the importance of maintaining a high index of suspicion and employing full imaging modalities capable of detecting uncommon tumors at an earlier stage. While they are uncommon, these primary lung neoplasms necessitate an aggressive approach, both medically and surgically, and possibly with therapeutic intervention. Finally, the early detection and proper handling of these neoplasms are important, especially with their tendency to result in high morbidity and mortality if diagnosed late (Oscar et al., 2023) (Figure 4.3).

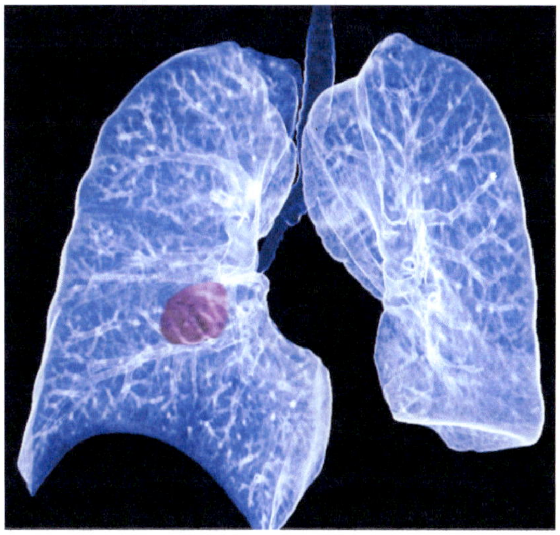

Figure 4.3. Primary lung tumors.

Source: https://www.verywellhealth.com/thmb/PPaqDP88myLUnLh4si-58qhGoCc=/1500x0/filters:no_upscale():max_bytes(150000):strip_icc()/iStock_76754411_XXLARGE-5764b4603df78ca6e42d08ff.jpg.

4.1.2. Secondary Lung Tumors

Secondary lung cancer, also referred to as metastatic lung cancer, occurs when cancer cells from a different location in the body spread to the lungs. Unlike primary lung cancers, which develop in lung tissue, secondary tumors are often advanced disease and may pose formidable challenges to diagnosis and treatment. The most frequent sites of such metastases include the breast, colon, kidney, and other body systems. Clinical presentation can be non-specific, with chronic cough, dyspnea, or weight loss manifesting as the only symptoms, as is characteristic of neoplastic pulmonary symptoms' non-specificity. Such challenges in clinical presentation have made imaging modalities like CT scans vital tools for detecting secondary tumors of the lungs, facilitating better staging and appropriate treatment planning, as evidenced by studies proving the effectiveness of CT in malignancy evaluation (Bhatt et al., 2017). The histopathological presentation of second lung tumors is highly variable depending on their site of origin, which has implications regarding treatment and prognostic considerations. For instance, the development of adenocarcinoma, often originating from breast or colon cancer, typically demonstrates a characteristic appearance on imaging and microscopic examination, which is very critical in appreciating the character of metastatic disease. Unlike primary lung cancers that will normally present with localized neurogenic or squamous characteristics, metastatic lesions often lack regular margins and mixed densities on imaging studies. Doctors must be able to accurately differentiate between primary and secondary tumors, as the treatment would be significantly different. More advanced imaging modalities combined with tissue biopsies can potentially yield an all-round approach to the diagnosis of metastatic lung disease and hence enable patients to be given the most appropriate and effective treatment (Oliveira et al., 2021). The prognosis in patients with secondary lung tumors is typically poor since the original malignancy is typically advanced at the time of diagnosis. Treatment is generally focused on systemic treatments, including chemotherapy and targeted biologic agents, with reduced priorities for surgery. Local treatment, such as radiation treatment, may, however, be applied to manage symptoms or target individual metastases if oligometastatic disease is identified. Because survival rates and overall outcomes are of primary importance, ongoing research to find new treatment drugs and combination regimens needs to be done in order to improve the treatment of secondary lung tumors. The identification of genetic markers and response biomarkers to a variety of treatments is an essential component of this work, with the potential for more personalized care and the enhanced survival in this challenging patient group (Bhatt et al., 2017) (Figure 4.4).

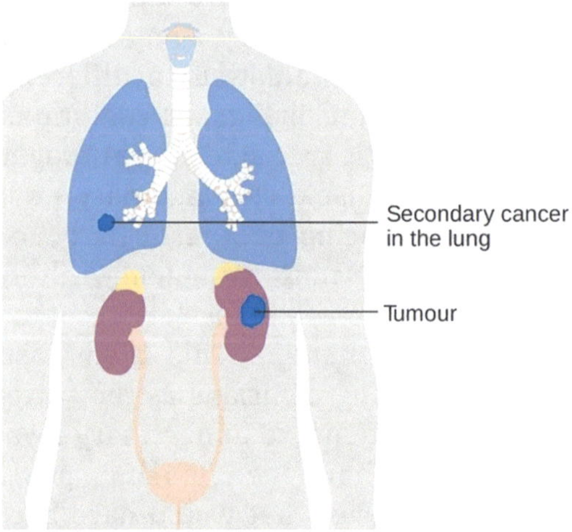

Figure 4.4. Secondary lung cancer.

Source: https://www.news-medical.net/image-handler/picture/2017/8/Diagram_showing_stage_4_kidney_cancer_CRUK_231_680x_.jpg.

4.1.3. Rare Pulmonary Neoplasms

Among all the rare pulmonary neoplasms, bronchial carcinoids are significant as they possess some specific histological characteristics and clinical importance. Initially described as benign, slowly developing tumors, these neoplasms arise from the neuroendocrine cells and constitute around 1-2% of all pulmonary cancers. Their occurrence is very low, with a reported incidence of two tumors per 100,000 population in the US, and they are typically diagnosed in patients of their fifth and sixth decades of life. Unlike more virulent lung carcinomas, bronchial carcinoids are found to have a good prognosis at the time of diagnosis and treatment if detected early. Hence, early detection and awareness gain immense importance in the management of these neoplasms (Bhanot et al., 2013). Their preference for sedentary behavior, however, does not exclude the likelihood of malignancy, highlighting the need for a careful diagnostic approach to separate them from more malignant forms of lung neoplasm. Yet another rare type of pulmonary neoplasm worth mentioning is the occurrence of hypertrophic pulmonary osteoarthropathy (HPOA), which has an extremely close connection with bronchogenic carcinoma and, less often, with other tumors. Although it is most characteristically related to malignant lung disease, HPOA can also be seen in association with other extrathoracic neoplasms, albeit rarely. It has been documented in but a few instances involving soft tissue sarcomas and other cancers such as nasopharyngeal or cervical malignancies (Firooznia et al., 1975). This condition presents especially challenging challenges to clinical management since it can significantly influence the quality of life among individuals with the disease by initiating painful bone and joint symptoms. Understanding the pathophysiology and clinical presentation of HPOA is crucial in the use of therapeutic approaches that, in some instances, involve treatments like vagotomy, intrathoracic or cervical, through which symptomatic relief in patients with this very rare neoplasm is obtained. In addition, unusual neoplasms of the lung often complicate the clinical presentation, as they can present with a broad range of symptoms that might mimic more common pulmonary illnesses. The primary challenge in managing these neoplasms is their diagnostic uncertainty, as many patients may initially present with nonspecific respiratory symptoms or systemic symptoms complicating early detection. For instance, the indolent course of certain tumors like carcinoids may lead to a delay in diagnosis and ultimately affect prognosis. Early detection of such rare entities is necessary for optimal management. With ongoing improvements in medical technology, integrating new imaging modalities and molecular diagnostics into clinical diagnosis will enhance our ability to detect and identify these rare neoplasms, thereby providing personalized therapeutic interventions and optimal patient outcomes in pulmonary oncology (Figure 4.5).

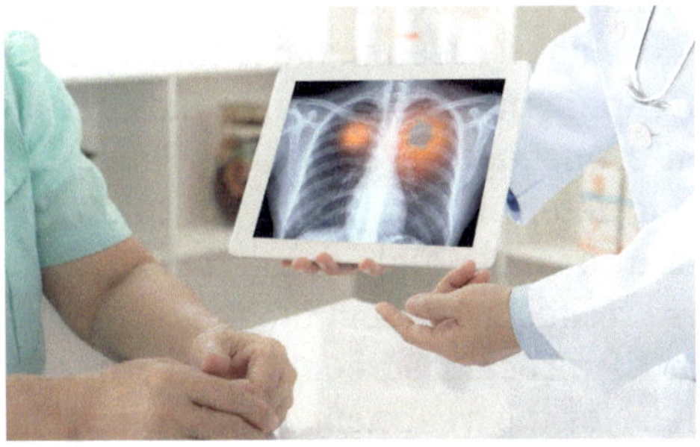

Figure 4.5. Rare pulmonary neoplasms.

Source: https://www.verywellhealth.com/thmb/JyrsT1iKib8U4DdFu6HsmlY2N4c=/1500x0/filters:no_upscale():max_bytes(150000):strip_icc()/GettyImages-1184802628-c2fd505b29474172bbd38021b367a340.jpg.

Test Your Knowledge

1. What are the primary lung tumors?
2. What are the secondary lung tumors?

4.2. Epidemiology of Non-Bronchogenic Pulmonary Neoplasms

Learning Outcome

1. Incidence and prevalence rates
2. Risk factors associated with non-bronchogenic neoplasms
3. Demographic variations in occurrence

Non-bronchogenic pulmonary tumor epidemiology encompasses a range of rare tumors separate from the most prevalent group of bronchogenic carcinoma. These consist of carcinoid tumors, mesotheliomas, and lymphomas, each with its own pattern of prevalence, which is reflective of its different pathophysiology. Carcinoid tumors, for example, represent neuroendocrine tumors that are typically more common in younger populations, while malignant mesothelioma, which has strong links to asbestos exposure, is predominantly seen in older individuals. This demographic diversity implies that neoplasms of non-bronchogenic origin may have specific etiologic determinants worthy of consideration and monitoring in high-risk groups. Awareness of these trends in epidemiology is critical to the design of directed screening and therapeutic regimens for the treatment of such malignancies, given the disparate clinical patterns by which they present compared with bronchogenic tumors. Apart from age and exposure factors, the geographical pattern of non-bronchogenic pulmonary neoplasms also indicates significant regional differences in the rates of incidence. For instance, malignant mesothelioma was more common in the industrialized areas where asbestos exposure was once more frequent. Conversely, carcinoid tumors are more uniformly spread across populations but with some larger rates within specific areas. The allied risk factors of such tumors similarly continue to alter with a change in the environmental exposure, thereby emphasizing constant monitoring in the epidemiologic context. Incorporating intimate knowledge of demographic and geographical factors is vital when formulating public health policies to minimize risks and encourage early detection and treatment. The advent of advances in molecular pathology has also provided insights into the pathogenesis of non-bronchogenic pulmonary neoplasms, with some studies showing that there exists a correlation between some genetic mutations and tumor development in this category. As cited in the literature, understanding the molecular processes involved can lead to increased diagnostic precision coupled with targeted therapy for patients (N/A, 2023).

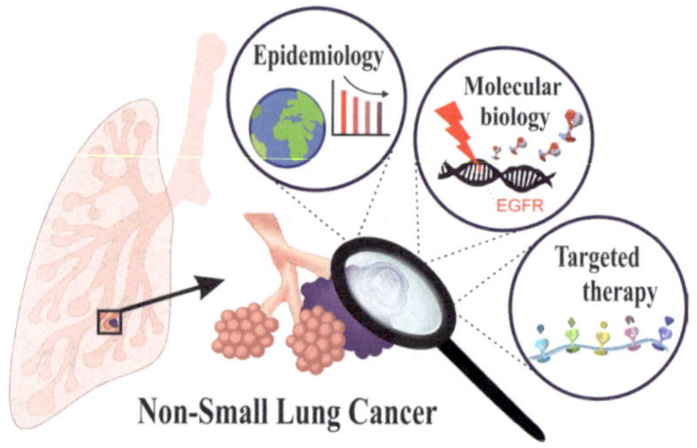

Figure 4.6. Epidemiology of non-bronchogenic pulmonary neoplasms.

Source: https://pub.mdpi-res.com/cancers/cancers-13-04705/article_deploy/html/images/cancers-13-04705-ag.png?1632453999.

The combination of molecular data with epidemiological data can permit finer estimation of risk and enable individualized treatment approaches. Furthermore, guidelines and recommendations suggest that health practitioners apply these results to clinical practice, being sensitive to the context of the individual patient, to enable care that is both science-driven and individualized (Adler et al., 2015). The interface of clinical practice and molecular epidemiology offers promising avenues for maximizing patient outcomes in non-bronchogenic pulmonary neoplasms (Figure 4.6).

4.2.1. Incidence and Prevalence Rates

Understanding the incidence and prevalence rates of lung neoplasms that are not bronchogenic carcinomas is important for estimating the burden of these diseases. The incidence of neoplasms in the lung as a whole is overall low compared to bronchogenic carcinoma, with some subtypes like pulmonary carcinoid tumor and mesotheliomas having different epidemiologic features. Although the majority of lung cancer cases are caused by bronchogenic carcinoma, awareness of the less common forms increases, in part through increased imaging technologies and biomarker investigations. These emerging technologies provide earlier diagnosis, which can influence reported incidence rates. New studies indicate that some groups, including patients with chronic pulmonary disease, may have higher incidence rates of specific neoplasms. This illustrates the commonality of pulmonary and neoplastic risk factors, as evidenced by recent research in COPD and lung carcinomas (Xu et al., 2022). Prevalence rates are also a significant measure in gauging the impact of pulmonary neoplasms, generally considered determinants of the effectiveness of treatment regimens and early detection programs. Non-bronchogenic pulmonary tumors differ in prevalence based on geographical and demographic factors, certain groups experiencing greater rates through exposure to the environment or genetic predisposition. To illustrate, malignant mesothelioma is reported with increasing frequency among asbestos-exposed occupational groups and points toward the necessity for targeted public health actions. Moreover, a number of studies have tracked the increasing incidence of carcinoid tumors, though the neoplasms are uncommon, but underscore the necessity for ongoing surveillance in high-risk groups. These trends also make us mindful of the need for total data collection to know more about such neoplasms and to direct healthcare appropriately, as has been determined by studies that investigate the link between chronic disease and lung cancer incidence (Garc et al., 2015).

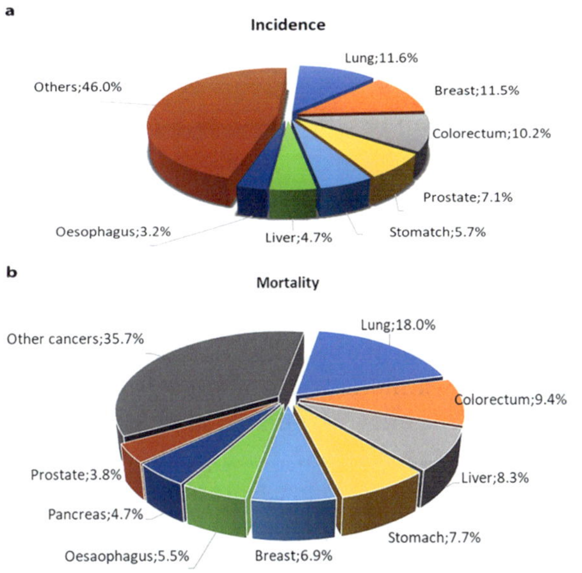

Figure 4.7. Incidence and prevalence rates of pulmonary neoplasms.

Source: https://media.springernature.com/lw685/springer-static/image/chp%3A10.1007%2F978-3-031-22483-6_57-1/MediaObjects/533579_1_En_57-1_Fig1_HTML.png.

Lastly, comparing the incidence and prevalence rates of neoplasms of the lungs excluding bronchogenic carcinoma gives valuable epidemiological data on these and their public health importance. As knowledge of these neoplasms grows, so does the need for proper data collection and assessment. Continuing research into risk factors for pulmonary neoplasms, such as genetic, environmental, and lifestyle, is key to the development of preventions and improvement of patient outcomes. Furthermore, recognition of the patterns of incidence and prevalence can guide health policymakers to apply effective measures by population, ultimately resulting in better screening and treatment. There cannot be an overemphasis on the use of available data in guiding clinical practice because it provides the foundation for subsequent studies and resource planning in the field of pulmonary oncology (Figure 4.7).

4.2.2. Risk Factors Associated with Non-Bronchogenic Neoplasms

Recognition of risk factors of non-bronchogenic neoplasms is crucial in order to improve the prognosis of patients and enhance therapeutic options of these pulmonary malignancies. Non-bronchogenic neoplasms, like rare tumors, including pulmonary spindle-cell carcinoma, have a tendency to present challenges of diagnosis due to their infrequent histologies and mode of clinical presentation. Specifically, those patients who present with illnesses like pulmonary spindle-cell carcinoma may not have the traditional risk factors, such as a history of smoking or environmental exposure, to complicate their clinical management. An example of such a problem case is that of a risk-factor-free young female patient diagnosed with pulmonary spindle-cell carcinoma but with a known condition of neurofibromatosis type 1, demonstrating that genetic predispositions need to be considered when looking for at-risk groups (Fernanda et al., 2025). Besides genetic factors, prior medical history, such as therapies used for other cancers, can play a significant role in the development of non-bronchogenic neoplasms. Patients who receive treatments like bone marrow transplants (BMT) have been found to have secondary tumors, including skin cancers, resulting from the immunosuppression following their treatment. According to an extensive cohort study, there were some risk factors identified for future cutaneous malignant neoplasms, such as sex, age, and some pre- and post-transplant therapies. Specifically, male patients over 50 years who underwent allogeneic BMT were at increased risk for these secondary cancers, which emphasizes the importance of close monitoring and tailored counseling methods (Broman et al., 2024). Furthermore, environmental exposures interacting with genetic susceptibilities cannot be overlooked in the context of risk factors of non-bronchogenic neoplasms. It has been shown that certain occupational exposures might increase the risk of cancer. At the same time, patients with specific genetic syndromes, like neurofibromatosis, might have an elevated likelihood of developing diverse neoplasms, including those of pulmonary origin.

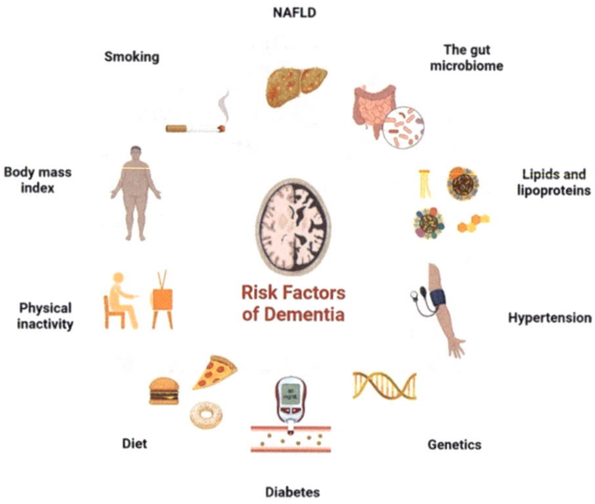

Figure 4.8. Risk factors associated with non-bronchogenic neoplasms.

Source: https://media.springernature.com/lw685/springer-static/image/chp%3A10.1007%2F978-981-99-3746-2_18/MediaObjects/600711_1_En_18_Fig1_HTML.png.

This intricate interaction between genetic predisposition and environmental carcinogenic agents further complicates our understanding of non-bronchogenic lung tumors and further emphasizes the need for targeted study. Identifying these risk factors not only facilitates earlier detection and prevention but also highlights the critical role of individualized methodology in the clinical treatment protocol for patients diagnosed with these rare pulmonary disorders (Figure 4.8).

4.2.3. Demographic Variations in Occurrence

The prevalence of pulmonary neoplasms other than bronchogenic carcinoma demonstrates significant demographic variations that are deserving of investigation. Demographic variables such as age, gender, ethnicity, and geographical position are involved in these variations and affect prevalence rates and also type-specific tumor behavior. For instance, elderly populations would likely demonstrate higher rates of neoplasms, possibly owing to the cumulative effect of years of exposure to carcinogenic agents. Additionally, males have a greater incidence of certain types of pulmonary neoplasms than females, and this might be associated with lifestyle issues, including smoking habits and employment history. These trends in the population are crucial for public health strategy design and the allocation of resources to target certain high-risk groups effectively. Ethnic background is also relevant to the incidence of pulmonary neoplasms. Studies have indicated that specific racial and ethnic populations are particularly vulnerable to specific types of lung tumors. For example, lung cancer occurs more frequently in African American men compared to their Caucasian counterparts, although this disparity is partially accounted for by socioeconomic standing, access to medical care, and differences in smoking habits. Cultural factors also enter into health-seeking behavior, creating disparities in early detection and treatment. Through exploring such demographic disparities, researchers can better understand the origins of the problem and design targeted prevention efforts to reduce the burden of pulmonary neoplasms among groups. Geographic disparities further illustrate the complexity of pulmonary neoplasm rates among differing demographic strata. Regions with high industrial production or recognized environmental carcinogens could be showing greater neoplasm rates, illustrating the influence of environmental factors within the area on health status. For instance, areas with high tobacco production may have higher lung cancer rates due to higher exposure to tobacco and related contaminants. Cities may, alternatively, show contrasting trends of pulmonary neoplasms with varying levels of socioeconomic conditions, such as exposure to health care and public health initiatives. Understanding these geographic variations is significant in framing localized health policy and making sure that interventions are tailored to specific community needs in controlling the incidence of pulmonary neoplasms (Malki et al., 2023; Malki et al., 2023).

Test Your Knowledge

1. What are the incidence and prevalence rates?
2. What are the risk factors associated with non-bronchogenic neoplasms?

4.3. Pathophysiology of Pulmonary Neoplasms

Learning Outcome

1. Mechanisms of tumor development
2. Genetic mutations involved
3. Role of the microenvironment in tumor progression

The pathophysiology of the neoplasms of the lungs encompasses an eclectic collection of neoplasms that do not fit within the scope of the classic classification of bronchogenic carcinoma. The other forms of neoplasms typically arise from non-bronchogenic lung tissue, such as mesenchymal cells, lymphatic tissue, and neuroendocrine cells, and result in varying clinical presentations and behaviors. As a point of illustration, pulmonary sarcomas, which are of mesenchymal cell origin, may exhibit aggressive behavior with predisposition towards early metastasis. Lymphomas, due to their association with the immune system, can occur atypically in pulmonary tissue, especially in immunocompromised patients.

The pathologic mechanisms of these neoplasms are usually associated with complex genetic mutations and disruption of signaling pathways, ultimately culminating in uncontrolled proliferation of cells and tumor development. Such differences must be understood to establish therapy and prognosis distinct from bronchogenic tumors. Additionally, epidemiological trends that regulate the occurrence of other pulmonary neoplasms than bronchogenic carcinoma must be incorporated as an integral part of their pathophysiology. Smoking, occupational exposure to toxic substances, and environmental pollutants are among the significant factors that regulate the development of various non-bronchogenic malignancies. Notably, evidence supports that cigarette smoking is an essential factor in the development of squamous cell carcinomas within solitary pulmonary nodules, whereby the high prevalence of smokers within the patient population with the nodules thus attributes lifestyle factors to disease presentation (Caseiro-Alves et al., 2005). Moreover, the increasing incidence of such infections as tuberculosis has emerged as a significant etiology of lung disease leading to secondary malignancy via inflammatory and fibrotic transformation of lung tissue (Caseiro-Alves et al., 2005). These observations argue for the multifactorial origin of pulmonary neoplasms and the need for directed prevention and screening.

The clinical importance of the diagnosis of pulmonary neoplasms beyond the ambit of bronchogenic carcinoma is great, given the often indolent nature of some of the subtypes and the inherent difficulties of detection. Patients will usually be asymptomatic or present with non-specific symptoms, making early diagnosis and treatment challenging. Research indicates that most solitary pulmonary nodules (SPNs) are benign or caused by infection and that diagnostic procedures such as transthoracic aspiration cytology aid in differentiating malignancies from non-malignant neoplasms (Soumitra et al., 2008).

Even the presence of specific radiological characteristics is significant in risk stratification, as nodule size and the appearance of the margin may predict malignancy. Determination of the spectrum of pulmonary neoplasms beyond bronchogenic carcinoma can maximize clinical vigilance and ensure timely interventions, thereby improving patient outcomes. A syncretic combination of clinical, radiological, and histopathological data is necessary to illuminate the pathophysiological mechanisms that govern these diverse neoplasms (Figure 4.9).

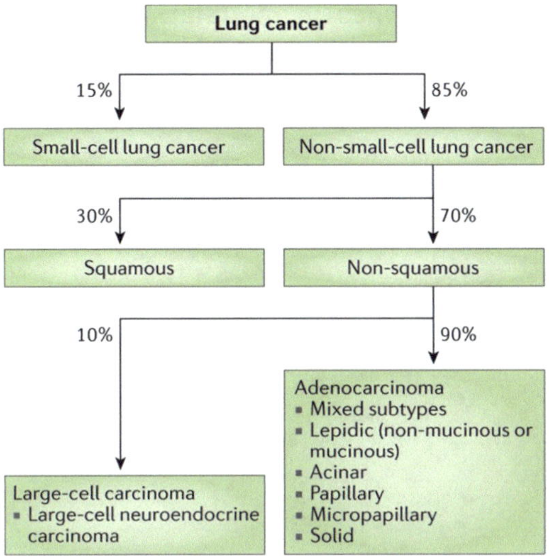

Figure 4.9. Pathophysiology of pulmonary neoplasms.

Source: https://media.springernature.com/m685/springer-static/image/art%3A10.1038%2Fnrdp.2015.9/MediaObjects/41572_2015_Article_BFnrdp20159_Fig1_HTML.jpg.

4.3.1. Mechanisms of Tumor Development

The mechanisms of tumor development are complex and multi-factorial, particularly for pulmonary neoplasms other than bronchogenic carcinoma. Gene mutations supply the substrates of carcinogenesis, with alterations of oncogene, tumor suppressor gene, and DNA repair genes being the primary contributors. Excessive cell growth, for instance, one of the hallmarks of cancer, is produced by tumor suppressor gene mutations. In the lung parenchyma, these genetic alterations are further compounded by various environmental insults such as carcinogen and pollutant exposure to tobacco smoke. This intricate interaction of genetic susceptibility and environmental injury underscores the importance of multifactorial models in the understanding of the pathogenesis of pulmonary neoplasms, which provide valuable insights regarding the target for therapy and prevention. The tumor microenvironment is another crucial element responsible for tumor progression in pulmonary neoplasms. This microenvironment constitutes various cellular components, including immune cells, fibroblasts, and extracellular matrix components, which directly interact with neoplastic cells. These interactions can suppress or promote the growth of neoplasm and metastasis. As an illustration, immune cells within the tumor microenvironment might play a bidirectional role; while some might inhibit tumor expansion, others may promote survival and development of cancer cells through immunosuppressive mechanisms. It has been postulated that evidence indicates the tumor-infiltrating lymphocyte/cytokine equilibrium might be an important factor for defining malignancy of lung tumors. Understanding the complex dialogue between neoplastic cells and their environment is essential for designing new immunotherapies and improving existing treatments in pulmonary neoplasia, as modulating these processes could potentially arrest tumor growth and improve patient prognosis. Inflammation is increasingly recognized as an oncogenic driving force of tumor development in various cancers, including lung cancer. Chronic inflammatory diseases expose the lung tissues to repeated cycles of injury and regeneration, which can result in genetic instability and promote neoplastic cell development. Surprisingly, some of the inflammation biomarkers are typically associated with poorer prognoses in patients with cancer. Elevated levels of inflammatory cytokines and the presence of tumor-associated leukocytes can enhance tumor growth and promote survival by promoting angiogenesis. The movement of immune cells, such as macrophages and neutrophils, also enhances the metastasizing potential of the tumors. New studies have been unlocking the complex signaling pathway of inflammation that gets triggered and their role in the continuum of cancer, marking the importance of targeting inflammatory mechanisms for approaches in modulating pulmonary neoplasms specifically (MDS SS et al., 2023; Gorbokon et al., 2024) (Figure 4.10).

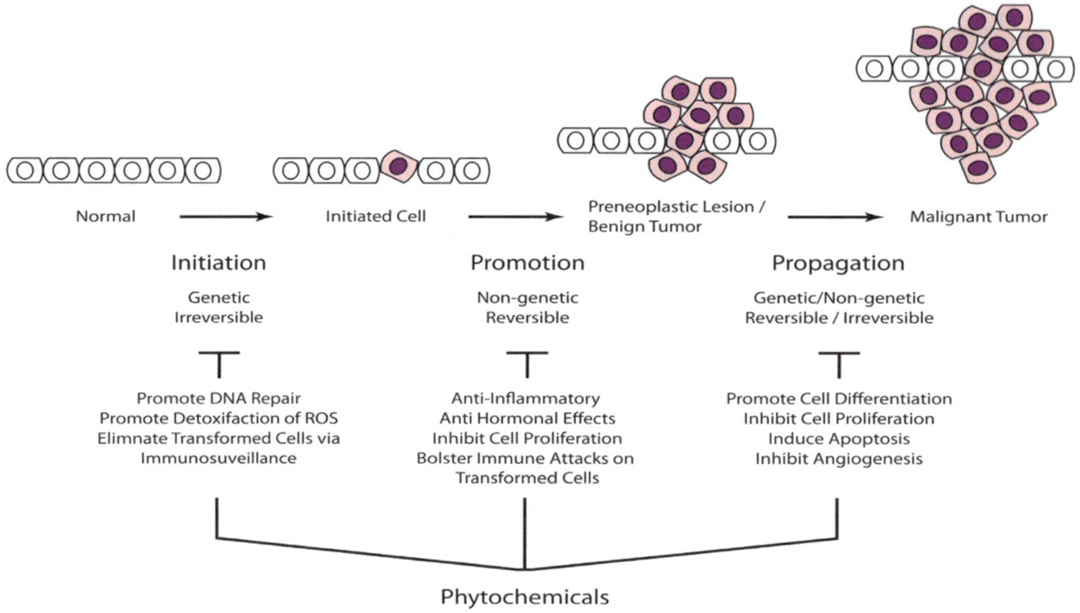

Figure 4.10. Mechanisms of tumor development.

Source: https://www.researchgate.net/profile/Abolaji-Olagunju-2/publication/345178041/figure/fig1/AS:953449411780610@1604331462387/Mechanism-of-Cancer-Development-Sapienza-and-Issa-2016.jpg.

4.3.2. Genetic Mutations Involved

In pulmonary neoplasms outside of bronchogenic carcinoma, the role of genetic mutation has also taken center stage, particularly in the development of adenocarcinomas. Recent reports suggest that atypical adenomatous hyperplasia (AAH) is an early morphological precursor to overt malignant adenocarcinomas. Genetic profiling of AAH is crucial in understanding the mechanism of lung cancer development, and this can provide new horizons for early detection strategies. Mutations in major oncogenes and tumor suppressor genes are known to change cellular signaling pathways, leading to tumor cell growth in these lesions. With increasing evidence, describing these specific genetic alterations can lead to more effective diagnostic methods and treatment plans tailored to the unique genetic characteristics of lung cancers, thereby enhancing patient outcomes (Kolin et al., 2000). Besides, the mutation frequency of different forms of lung neoplasms has varied. For instance, a newly developed population-based investigation revealed a high increase in adenocarcinoma among women, associated with some changes in genetics related to tobacco exposure and environmental factors (Mäkitaro et al., 1999). These mutations can influence the histology of the tumor, affecting its biological behavior as well as its sensitivity to treatment. The presence of some mutations, such as those of the epidermal growth factor receptor (EGFR), is of importance for targeted therapy in some subtypes of lung cancer. Information regarding these genetic factors is not only important for prognosis but also for developing individualized therapeutic approaches that consider the mutational signature of the given tumor, thus enhancing the treatment provided to individuals with pulmonary neoplasms. Finally, the pileup of genetic mutations in lung neoplasms is not just an effect of tumorigenesis but also an expression of a complex interplay between intrinsic genetic predispositions and extrinsic environmental exposures. Cigarette smoking and asbestos are examples of causes linked with particular patterns of mutational changes that potentially propel the formation of varied lung tumors, including non-bronchogenic. Identification of these mutations and their association with specific environmental risk factors is part of planning preventive interventions. For instance, the realization that p53 protein accumulation is central to heavy smoking status can inform risk assessment and early intervention in susceptible populations. Overall, an overall impression of genetic mutations offers a basis for improving methods of prevention and treatment of pulmonary neoplasms aside from bronchogenic carcinoma (Kolin et al., 2000; Mäkitaro et al., 1999) (Figure 4.11).

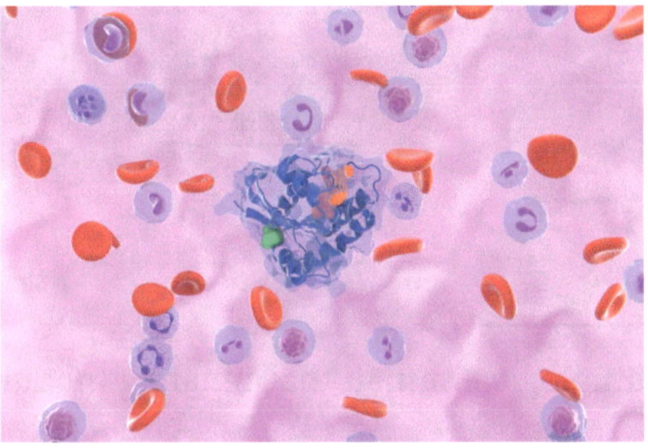

Figure 4.11. Lung cancer gene mutations.

Source: https://www.rockymountaincancercenters.com/hubfs/lung%20cancer%20gene%20mutation.jpeg.

4.3.3. Role of the Microenvironment in Tumor Progression

The tumor microenvironment plays a central role in the occurrence of pulmonary neoplasms, particularly in neoplasms not of bronchogenic carcinoma. It is made up of multiple cellular constituents, extracellular matrix proteins, and signaling factors that, together, create a dynamic environment that promotes tumor growth and progression. Immune cells, fibroblasts in association with the tumor, and endothelial cells interact with one another in complex ways that promote angiogenesis, the creation of new blood vessels needed by the tumor in order to survive. Research indicates that interleukin-8 (IL-8) will significantly enhance the vascularity of neoplasms. Specifically, IL-8 expression correlates with increased angiogenic activity in tumors, which plays a significant role in sustaining rapidly growing masses by guaranteeing plentiful nutrient and oxygen supply (Ochiai et al., 2025). This directs us to the extremely significant interaction between microbial factors and neoplasms, emphasizing that treatment of the microenvironment can be an attractive therapeutic strategy. Moreover, the microenvironment has a direct impact on the invasiveness of tumors and on the metastatic ability of lung neoplasms. Microscopic vascular invasion (MVI) is an excellent prognostic factor for non-small cell lung cancer (NSCLC), among others. It was found that MVI is fairly frequent in early-stage lung cancer and even more prevalent in adenocarcinoma histological subtypes (Asioli et al., 2011). Coexistence of MVI is also linked with larger tumor sizes and the higher likelihood of tumor-infiltrating lymphocytes. These findings also validate the complex interactions between the microenvironment elements, as these may influence the aggressiveness and behavior of the tumor, resulting in poor survival rates. This evidence indicates towards the cell-to-cell interaction within the microenvironment, and the cure may be begun by targeting these interactions for improved patient prognosis. In addition to angiogenesis and invasiveness, the immune microenvironment plays a significant role in promoting tumor development. Tumors are inclined to manipulate the immune response of immune cells in order to evade detection and destruction. Tumor-associated macrophages (TAMs), for instance, exhibit pro-tumorigenic characteristics that support tumor growth rather than attacking it. Such immune evasiveness is likely to be supported by many cytokines and chemokines within the microenvironment that modulate the recruitment and polarization of the immune cells. These movements allow tumors to develop and proliferate, particularly in pulmonary neoplasms with impaired immune responses. Hence, understanding the intricate mechanisms of immune modulation in the microenvironment can provide insights into novel intervention strategies, particularly for resistant tumor types. Generally, targeting the tumor microenvironment and its cellular elements offers new options to enhance therapeutic outcome against different pulmonary neoplasms (Figure 4.12).

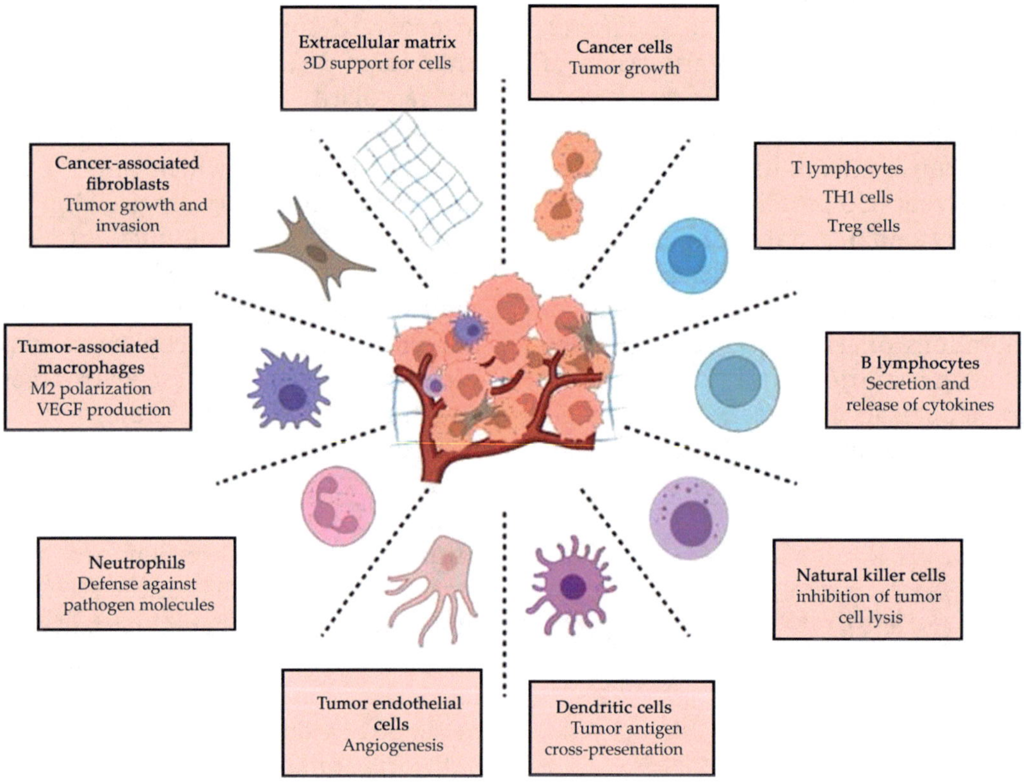

Figure 4.12. Tumor microenvironment complexity: A pathological milieu that innately modulates cancer progression.

Source: https://media.springernature.com/lw685/springer-static/image/chp%3A10.1007%2F978-3-030-80962-1_89-1/MediaObjects/512948_0_En_89-1_Fig1_HTML.png.

Test Your Knowledge

1. What is the mechanism of tumor development?
2. What is the role of the microenvironment in tumor progression?

4.4. Clinical Presentation and Diagnosis

Learning Outcome

1. Common symptoms associated with pulmonary neoplasms
2. Diagnostic imaging techniques
3. Histopathological evaluation methods

The clinical course of pulmonary neoplasms other than bronchogenic carcinoma is important in ensuring early diagnosis and effective management. The patients with such neoplasms may present with varied respiratory symptoms, most commonly cough, hemoptysis, and dyspnea. In particular, pulmonary mucinous cystic carcinomas, even though unusual, typically occur in young individuals who, most often, have recurrent chest infections or pneumonia-type symptoms, which may lead to misdiagnosis. This error emphasizes the significant need for clinicians to be highly suspicious of rare lung tumors when presenting with atypical cases, particularly in the younger population. Early diagnosis of such neoplasms plays a pivotal role in treatment and long-term survival, as total surgical resection is the preferred treatment and often the sole curative therapy for these lesions, with ten-year survival rates of around 53% reported in some cases (Galea et al., 2016). Diagnosis is primarily reliant on an integration of imaging examinations and histopathological examination. Initial exams usually include chest X-rays or computed tomography (CT) scanning, which are particularly useful for detecting solitary pulmonary nodules (SPNs), the initial presentation in a large majority of lung neoplasms. While the majority of SPNs prove to be benign, distinguishing between malignant neoplasm, and benign nodules is of paramount significance, as delayed treatment of malignancies can lead to advanced disease. Radiologic characteristics, such as nodule shape and growth patterns, are crucial to discriminate between these two possibilities. More sophisticated imaging technologies, such as positron emission tomography (PET) and percutaneous biopsy, can further characterize the nature of noted nodules, allowing invasive procedures to be reserved for those at high risk (Quint et al., 2015). The process of multi-modal diagnosis avoids unnecessary interventions for benign disease while rendering rapid and effective management for malignant tumors. Apart from imaging and histology, clinical presentation and history provide significant clues for diagnosis. Such patients presenting with unexplained loss of weight, chronic cough, or hemoptysis must be evaluated urgently to rule out malignancy, including atypical pulmonary neoplasms. Extensive clinicopathological correlation enhances diagnostic yield and informs treatment options. For example, some tumor markers and immunohistochemistry can be crucial in determining the nature of a pulmonary tumor, thereby informing management decisions. Clinicians must remain vigilant, especially in populations usually underrepresented in neoplasm and lung cancer data, such as young adults or non-smokers. Awareness of the variable clinical manifestations of pulmonary neoplasms other than bronchogenic carcinoma can facilitate the provision of optimal patient outcomes through prompt treatment and prudent management strategies.

4.4.1. Common Symptoms Associated with Pulmonary Neoplasms

Other pulmonary neoplasms aside from bronchogenic carcinoma will present in a group of symptoms that, through their tendency to overlap with other pulmonary disease, may lead to repeated misdiagnosis. Among the most common symptoms are respiratory distress manifesting as chronic cough, hemoptysis, and dyspnea. The patient may report, at times, a chronic cough that aggravates with duration, initially, which is normally dismissed as a consequence of a respiratory infection. Notably, certain cancers, i.e., pulmonary mucinous cystic carcinomas, can often be associated with chronic recurrent chest infections, the latter of which can hamper accurate diagnosis. Symptom worsening can significantly impact the quality of life of the patients, rendering correct identification timely for successful treatment, as a particular group of cancers has to be subjected to definitive surgical removal in order to have the best outcomes, hence highlighting the importance of differential diagnosis in symptomatic patients (Galea et al., 2016). The other important sign of pulmonary neoplasms is chest pain, which occurs in various degrees of severity and is secondary to tumor growth and resulting pressure over involved structures. Pain often characteristically localizes or refers to other sites, with a profile similar to conditions such as pneumonia or pleuritis. Systemic signs such as unwanted loss of body weight, weakness, and anorexia can also occur and may be reflective of neoplasms within the lungs. Such systemic symptoms also camouflage the diagnosis to an extent that medical professionals must be highly suspicious, especially in young patients who would otherwise not come in with such prominent systemic symptoms. The uniqueness of such symptoms points to the challenge in diagnosing lung neoplasms beyond the otherwise classical bronchogenic carcinoma (Harken et al., 1966). In addition to the above symptoms, one must remember the occurrence of paraneoplastic syndromes that can be associated with pulmonary neoplasms. Such syndromes are expected to cause a variety of manifestations, ranging from endocrine to hematologic dysfunction, which makes the clinical presentation complicated. For instance, the hypercalcemia symptoms such as nausea, vomiting, and confusion may be caused by other reasons if the oncological etiology is not considered. The intricate interplay between the primary tumor and its metastatic system demands proper evaluation and multidisciplinary treatment in such a case. An awareness of the extensive variety of symptoms of pulmonary neoplasms aids clinicians in making an accurate diagnosis, ultimately resulting in improved patient outcomes through timely and effective treatment procedures (Harken et al., 1966) (Figure 4.13).

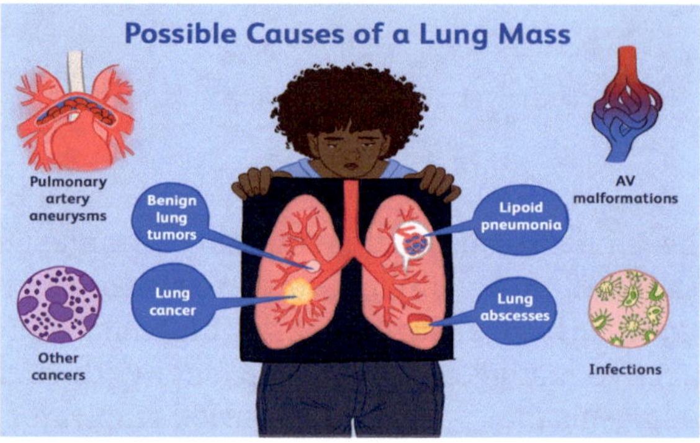

Figure 4.13. Possible causes and diagnosis of a lung mass.

Source: https://www.verywellhealth.com/thmb/2JjQjymbsoqA_6Rt5YqD6789lMg=/1500x0/filters:no_upscale():max_bytes(150000):strip_icc()/lung-mass-possible-causes-and-what-to-expect-2249388-5bc3f847c9e77c00512dc818.png.

4.4.2. Diagnostic Imaging Techniques

Evaluation of pulmonary neoplasms other than bronchogenic carcinoma mostly relies on advanced diagnostic imaging modalities that enhance the discrimination between non-malignant and malignant nodules. Solitary pulmonary nodule (SPN) is a common finding in lung assessment, where most are discovered to be non-malignant, but distinguishing these from potential malignancies is crucial for ensuring early management. Various imaging modalities, including high-resolution CT and MRI, allow the clinician to study the morphology, size, and growth patterns of nodules. Moreover, imaging modalities such as PET allow detection of nodular metabolic activity, thereby increasing diagnostic accuracy. Thus, through an integrative approach of morphologic evaluation and functional imaging, clinicians can make a more effective plan for the treatment of pulmonary nodules and prevention of undue invasive interventions (Quint et al., 2015). In imaging diagnosis, the application of CT scanning is particularly vital for lung lesion characterization and neoplasm staging. Advanced CT technology provides fine-resolution cross-sectional images of the lungs, which can reveal important information about tumor size, location, and related anomalies such as lymphadenopathy or pleural effusion. Research has noted that CT-guided biopsy has become a routine intervention for histopathological examination due to its high sensitivity; however, in 73.33% of the patient population studied in research settings, CT-guided interventions were performed. This technique minimizes risk while providing accurate cellular information on the neoplasm, enabling a logical treatment plan to be formulated. As efficient as it is, the use of CT improves diagnostic accuracy and aids in the critical staging process required to determine patient prognosis and therapeutic intervention (Bhatt et al., 2017). The selection of an appropriate diagnostic imaging modality may significantly impact the clinical implications in evaluating pulmonary neoplasms. Besides CT scans and PET scans, ultrasonography (USG) also has an ancillary role to play, primarily in making biopsies possible when other imaging modalities fail to yield. When nodules have indeterminate features, MRI will be useful, especially for soft tissue discrimination and assessing the involvement of immediately adjacent anatomical structures. Furthermore, new imaging modalities and complementary techniques like depreotide imaging and radiomics are being increasingly investigated because they can potentially provide higher sensitivity and specificity in differentiating between benign and malignant processes. Thus, integration of different diagnostic imaging modalities is of utmost significance in maximizing the diagnostic cascade for pulmonary lesions other than bronchogenic carcinoma, ultimately improving patient outcomes by allowing individualized therapeutic approaches (Quint et al., 2015) (Figure 4.14).

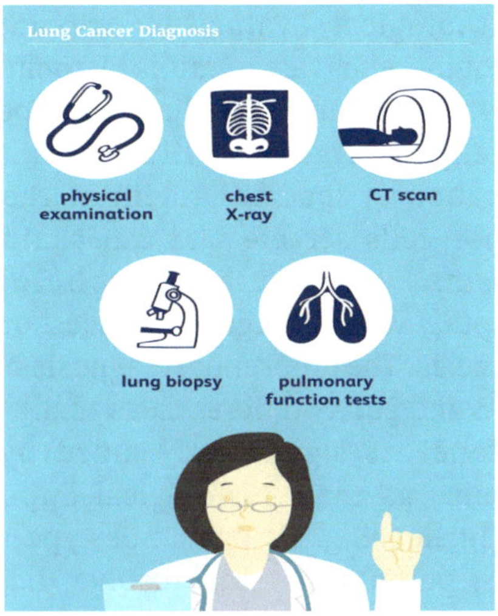

Figure 4.14. Diagnostic imaging techniques pulmonary neoplasms.

Source: https://www.verywellhealth.com/thmb/jY2gGnmo7WFu6qs1P4uWCNsr4b0=/1500x0/filters:no_upscale():max_bytes(150000):strip_icc()/diagnosis_05-ef6311502b9e413fa59c4872492c4a7b.jpg.

4.4.3. Histopathological Evaluation Methods

Histopathologic examination methods are key components in the diagnosis and differentiation of various pulmonary neoplasms, including those that are not bronchogenic carcinomas. The methods primarily involve the macroscopic evaluation of tissue specimens followed by microscopic analysis using light microscopy. The pathologist studies the architecture and cellularity of the neoplasm and assesses tumor type and the presence of important histologic features that may determine prognosis. Such tests not only allow for the identification of neoplastic masses but also typing into specific tumor subtypes, required for the guidance of therapy. In addition, the importance of adequate staging of the tumor cannot be overstressed because it has a direct relationship with treatment intervention and overall patient management. Providing yet another level of diversity to the histopathological evaluation are advanced technologies such as immunohistochemistry (IHC), which enhance the diagnostic potential in challenging situations. IHC allows for the identification of specific protein markers that the tumor cells secrete and can characterize neoplasms otherwise morphologically overlapping with benign processes or other malignancies. The differential diagnosis between sarcomas and poorly differentiated malignancies, for instance, is significantly aided by these techniques, as their histological appearance can be misleading. Using tumor type-specific markers, pathologists can resolve diagnostic uncertainties and facilitate appropriate clinical interventions. As is evident from recent studies, these newer histological technologies have been proven to enhance neoplasm stratification and directly influence treatment outcomes and prognosis of patients. With the diversity of pulmonary neoplasms and heterogeneity in tumor behavior, close histopathological scrutiny is at the core of clinical practice. Techniques like cytogenetic investigations, notably for neoplasms like synovial sarcoma, underscore pathology's progress, directing diagnosis and treatment. For example, the SS18–SSX fusion gene in synovial sarcoma is a marker in tumor diagnosis, as documented in recent publications with careful histopathological investigations and supportive IHC findings. Such concerted work in diagnosis within the histopathological fraternity enhances the ability to identify rare neoplasms that may mimic prevalent ones, leading to comprehensive treatment strategies. So histopathological examination methods not only contribute to diagnosis but also form a significant link between molecular characteristics and clinical work, determining the destiny of oncologic treatment methods in pulmonary neoplasms with the exception of bronchogenic carcinoma.

Test Your Knowledge

1. What are the common symptoms associated with pulmonary neoplasms?
2. What are the histopathological evaluation methods?

4.5. Treatment Options

Learning Outcome

1. Surgical interventions
2. Chemotherapy and targeted therapies
3. Radiation therapy approaches

In treating pulmonary neoplasms other than bronchogenic carcinoma, therapy often depends upon the type and nature of the tumor. Mucoepidermoid carcinoma (MEC) is rare but is most commonly reported as a malignant salivary gland neoplasm, although primary MEC has also been reported in the thyroid gland. Treatment of these cases is typically by surgery, especially for a low to medium-grade tumor with a relatively indolent clinical course. Complications in the form of aggressive clinical behavior with extensive pulmonary metastasis could complicate the treatment further. According to these elements, management strategies would be most effective by involving a multidisciplinary team to determine the optimal intervention for the individual patient to maximize customized treatment modalities

(Mitrache et al., 2024). Large-cell neuroendocrine lung carcinoma (LCNEC) represents another pulmonary neoplasm that has a bad prognosis and limited curative possibilities. The systemic management of metastatic LCNEC demonstrated that the treatment modality impacts the survival of patients significantly. Retrospective analysis in patients showed that immune checkpoint inhibitors were linked with a median overall survival (OS) of 26.4 months versus 9.0 months in patients treated with platinum doublets and only 4.0 months with non-platinum chemotherapy. These results highlight the importance of treating based on disseminated disease characteristics and emphasize the need to prioritize aggressive systemic treatments, which have a profound effect on survival prospects compared to other forms of treatment (Fisch et al., 2021). Furthermore, the treatment of pulmonary neoplasms needs careful blending of locoregional therapy with consideration of systemic therapy. Results show that patients treated with local therapies, such as surgery or radiation, had higher overall survival compared to those receiving no treatment. This hints at the importance of using both methods together. This is particularly relevant in the treatment of oligometastatic disease, where localized therapy can result in better prognostic outcomes. Given the inherent complexities of pulmonary neoplasm management, including differential tumor biology and responsiveness to therapy, clinicians must undertake an extensive treatment strategy. This strategy should include both systemic and local therapies optimally suited to the individual patient, thereby optimizing the likelihood of a successful response and long-term survival.

4.5.1. Surgical Interventions

Surgery is necessary for the management of several pulmonary neoplasms other than bronchogenic carcinoma, including primary pleural tumors and granular cell tumors (GCTs). In solitary fibrous pleural tumors (SFPT), surgery is generally indicated due to the tumor's propensity for bleeding and other adverse effects during primary treatments. A good example of this is depicted in a case where a 41-year-old male patient required a reoperative surgical procedure following successful embolization of the tumor arterial supply following the initial procedure, which was defeated by hemorrhage. This illustrates not only the necessity for surgical procedures but also the elaborate planning involved in handling complicated pleural tumors. Specifically, modern imaging and interventional technologies are part of enhancing surgical results, delivering precise targeting, minimizing perioperative morbidity, and maximizing therapeutic efficacy (Moustafa et al., 2025). Although rare, pulmonary GCTs demonstrate the diverse complexity of neoplasms treated by means of surgical intervention.

The neurogenic tumors may present with diverse symptoms and typically demand careful endoscopic procedures for diagnosis and treatment. In a multicenter tracheobronchial GCT series, surgical resection was only successful in a subset of the patients, highlighting the benign character of most lesions and the potential for surveillance with small tumors present. However, in situations where complications and symptoms such as airway obstruction or associated malignancies arise, surgical excision becomes necessary to mitigate symptoms and prevent complications. The reliance on surgical treatment in these environments highlights the evolving experience of treating pulmonary neoplasms, where timely diagnosis and proper treatments can make a significant difference in patient outcomes (Lachkar et al., 2023). The implementation of surgical methods in pulmonary neoplasms is more than mere resection of tumors; it is also very much associated with a multidisciplinary approach among oncology, radiology, and pathology. Surgical teams must carefully manage the nuances of each tumor entity with consideration of tumor size, location, and metastatic disease. Preoperative imaging studies also contribute significantly to surgical planning by enabling accurate localization and assessment of operability. Additionally, the development of targeted therapies and molecular markers provides hope for tailored treatment regimens that can improve surgical intervention. Such a multi-modal treatment not only optimizes the surgical outcomes but also optimizes the complete care of pulmonary neoplasms, illustrative of the evolving landscape of thoracic oncology where surgery remains the cornerstone of effective disease control (Moustafa et al., 2025) (Figure 4.15).

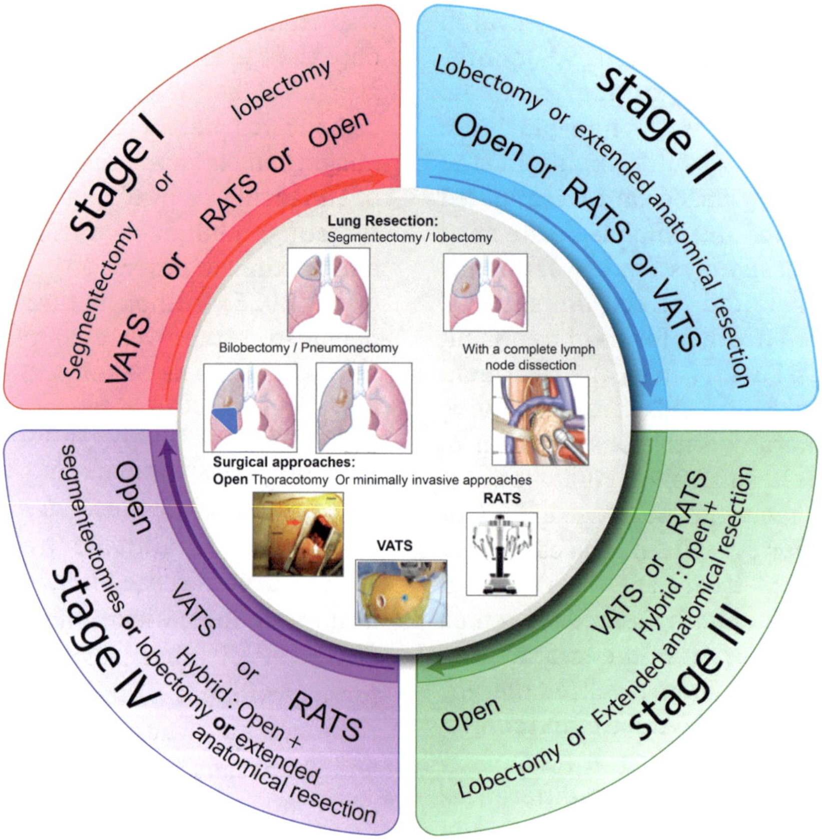

Figure 4.15. The role of surgery in lung cancer treatment.

Source: https://pub.mdpi-res.com/cancers/cancers-13-03711/article_deploy/html/images/cancers-13-03711-ag.png?1627372882.

4.5.2. Chemotherapy and Targeted Therapies

The treatment environment for neoplasms of the lung other than bronchogenic carcinoma has evolved significantly, particularly with the development of chemotherapy and targeted therapy. Chemotherapy, once the standard of cancer treatment, refers to the administration of cytotoxic drugs designed to prevent tumor growth and dissemination. This traditional approach, however, usually exacts a major price in patients through systemic effects, causing far-reaching side effects and detracting from quality of life. In the last few decades, molecular biology has opened the field for therapies that effectively address the molecular and genetic characteristics of tumors, offering an evidence-driven direction to treatment. These new therapeutic modalities aim to address specific pathways and mechanisms unique to cancer cells with the intent of achieving an optimal therapeutic index with minimal side damage to normal tissues, thus increasing patient outcome for a variety of pulmonary neoplasms. As recognized in current literature, small-molecule targeted therapies and antibody-drug conjugates (ADCs) provide highly promising possibilities in the treatment of pulmonary neoplasms. These novel therapies can selectively address cellular dysfunctions frequently observed in neoplastic cells, making therapy more effective with fewer side effects. Application of personalized medicine in the form of targeted therapy has revolutionized a new era in oncology, wherein the treatment can be directed based on the molecular profile of a patient's tumor.

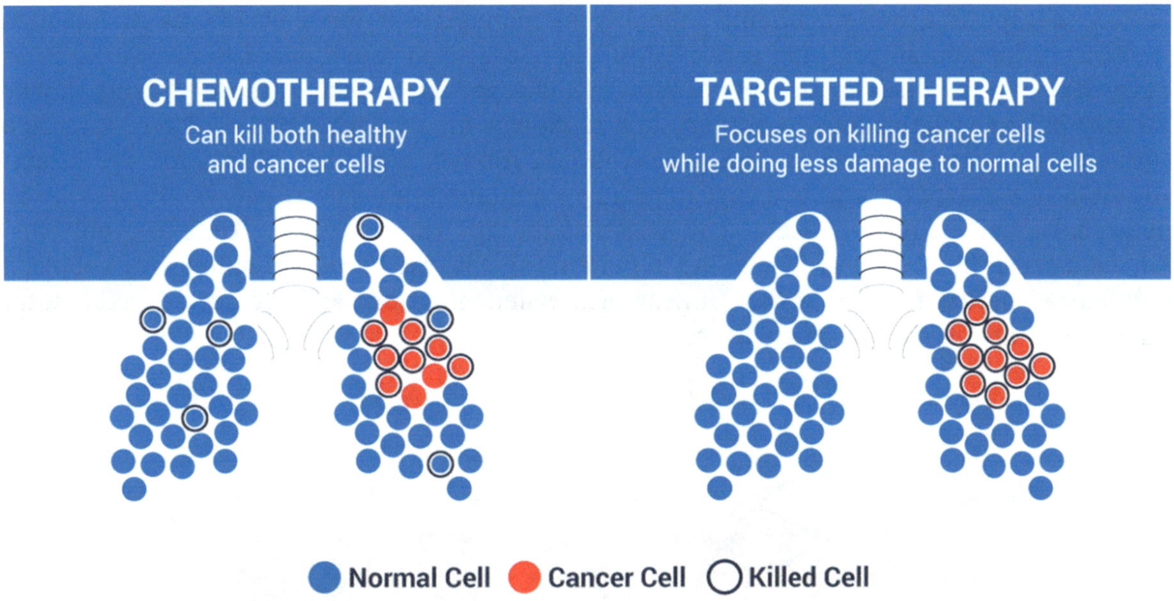

Figure 4.16. Chemotherapy and targeted therapies.

Source: https://external-content.duckduckgo.com/iu/?u=https%3A%2F%2Fwww.medicalcenterturkey.com%2Fwp-content%2Fuploads%2F2021%2F06%2Fchemotherapy-targeted-therapy-1160x609.png&f=1&nofb=1&ipt=8473d8828691dc748dd8a8d94d0460be772f24e50f58be09a2e9f5c6403352e7.

Although traditional chemotherapy remains available, the inclusion of target therapies represents an innovation that holds promise in the management of the complexity that attends various types of lung tumor, including those that do not constitute bronchogenic carcinoma. The evolution of treatment approaches attests to the necessity for ongoing studies and clinical trials to further delineate the interaction between treatment modalities. Interestingly, the ever-changing advancement of targeted therapies continues to highlight the need for further research into molecular alterations that are characteristic of pulmonary neoplasms. Recent evidence reaffirms that the majority of patients possess high burdens of mutations and diverse molecular alterations, which can be the foundation of these new therapeutic agents. For instance, ongoing research on targeted therapy has revealed that existing drugs like erdafitinib, used in the treatment of urothelial carcinoma, have the potential to use chemotherapy and target agents together to achieve the most significant level of treatment. With the research community continually seeking more molecular targets and developing new drugs, the role of combining chemotherapy and target therapies will become ever more significant in the treatment of most pulmonary neoplasms. A broad knowledge base relative to contemporary treatment methods will enhance clinicians' capability to deliver effective patient-centered care. It will also refine the science of oncology, particularly as it relates to lung cancer, ultimately leading to enhanced survival and quality of life (Figure 4.16).

4.5.3. Radiation Therapy Approaches

In the multi-disciplinary management of pulmonary neoplasms other than bronchogenic carcinoma, radiation therapy is a non-negotiable modality of management for a variety of malignancies, particularly in non-small cell lung cancer (NSCLC) and also in those patients who present with primary stages of the disease. The role of radiation is especially crucial in those patients in whom there may be contraindications to surgery due to co-existing comorbidities or where tumors are well-differentiated and localized. The precise application of radiation allows for the selective destruction of cancer cells without engaging their surrounding normal tissue, hence sparing vital structures. Notably, studies indicate that radiation therapy can be used to control symptoms in advanced disease, improving quality of life in patients against the burden of pulmonary neoplasms. This is more relevant in view of the growing acknowledgment of the multifaceted presentations of lung cancer among various patient groups.

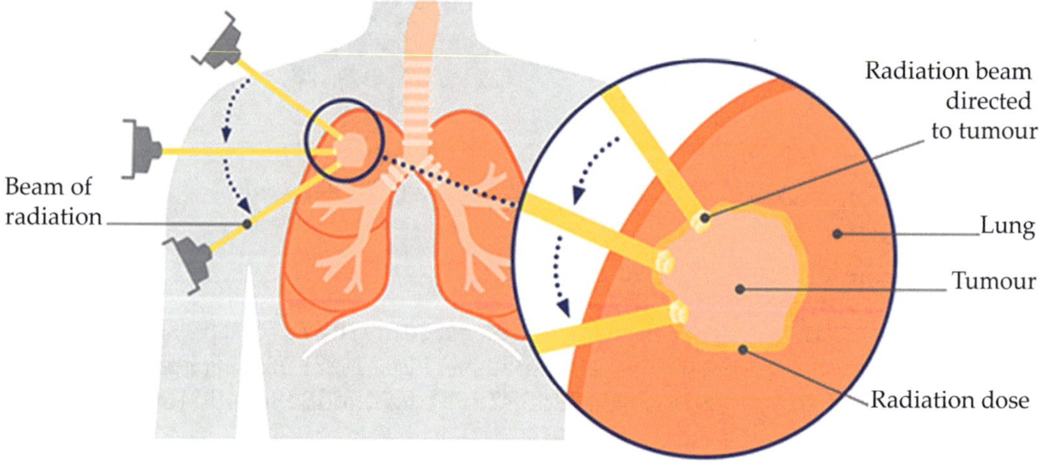

Figure 4.17. Radiation therapy for lung cancer.

Source: https://external-content.duckduckgo.com/iu/?u=https%3A%2F%2Fwww.cancercouncil.com.au%2Fwp-content%2Fuploads%2F2022%2F11%2FStereotactic-body-radiation-therapy-lung.png&f=1&nofb=1&ipt=ba63f2cf3ca7a84dfa2f872a90347bb6d1b15bda8f527b75d0f70a223d638021.

Moreover, the integration of radiation therapy with non-systemic therapies like chemotherapy significantly enhances treatment results for advanced pulmonary neoplasms among patients. For instance, patients who have undergone lung transplants and possess a higher incidence of lung cancer can be managed with radiotherapy to manage malignancies within their transplanted lungs. In these single cases, the application of curative treatments, including lobectomy and radiation to limited cancer, is an integrated model of treatment. Clinical data reveal that many patients treated with chemotherapy plus radiation have enhanced overall survival, even despite grueling with levels of treatment-related toxicity. This subtle interaction between radiation therapy and systemic treatments must be monitored carefully and dosing adjusted carefully to overcome the side effects without compromising optimal therapeutic gain, more so in vulnerable groups such as lung transplant recipients (Du et al., 2015). Last but not least, new evidence suggests the need for individualized radiation approaches in managing pulmonary neoplasms, particularly for preventive intervention against metastatic growth. Prophylactic cranial irradiation (PCI) has been intensively explored not only for small-cell lung cancer but also for NSCLC, in terms of whether it will improve survival and reduce the incidence of brain metastases. While PCI is not part of routine prescription in NSCLC, its recognition as a valuable resource for high-risk patients represents a shift toward more personalized treatment schemes in radiation oncology. This focus on individualized radiation protocols concurs with evolving clinical practice. It underscores the importance of continuing studies to optimize treatment effectiveness for patients with a range of pulmonary neoplasms outside of bronchogenic carcinoma (Feghali et al., 2016) (Figure 4.17).

Test Your Knowledge

1. What are the surgical interventions?
2. What are the radiation therapy approaches?

4.6. Prognosis and Outcomes

Learning Outcome

1. Survival rates for different types of neoplasms
2. Factors influencing prognosis
3. Long-term management and follow-up care

The outlook for pulmonary neoplasms other than bronchogenic carcinoma has incredible variability depending on cancer stage and type at presentation. The two most important subtypes are non-small cell lung carcinoma (NSCLC) and small cell lung carcinoma (SCLC), each with distinct clinical courses and responses to treatment. For instance, with early-stage NSCLC, surgical treatments are most often feasible, significantly improving survival, with median survival rates reaching a maximum of 23.2 months in such cases. Conversely, stage IV has a very dismal prognosis with a median survival of approximately 2.5 months, highlighting the importance of early diagnosis and urgent therapy. The use of chemotherapy, although useful, is qualified by substantial toxicity, especially in those with extensive disease, highlighting the importance of balance between efficacy and quality of life in making treatment decisions. For certain patient groups, including recipients of a lung transplant, the prognosis for neoplasms of the lung may be particularly difficult. Experience has shown that lung cancer arises in a considerable proportion of these patients, frequently at varied stages of development. For example, among 847 transplant patients investigated, only 2% of them developed lung cancer following transplant, and the majority were at stage I or II. Even after the treatments, such as chemotherapy, the outlook is bleak; recipients who had received palliative chemotherapy survived for a median time of only 7.5 months, and there was an excessive amount of severe toxicity. This group presents unique challenges for prognostic assessment, as the overlap of immunosuppression and lung cancer complicates treatment and necessitates ongoing evaluation of survival processes and symptom management procedures (Du et al., 2015). Moreover, pulmonary neoplasms can lead to acute and fatal complications that necessitate urgent medical interventions. Conditions such as massive hemoptysis and obstruction of the central airway not only endanger immediate patient health but also extensively affect long-term prognosis. Emergency treatment typically involves advanced pharmacologic and surgical interventions, which may stabilize the patient's short-term condition but may not cure the associated malignancy. For example, patients with complications of obstructing endobronchial tumors will require rigid bronchoscopy or stent placement to ensure airway patency. Thus, interaction between the acute complications and long-term management plans addresses the complexity of prognosis in pulmonary neoplastic patients and underscores the importance of holistic care that covers both immediate care and long-term considerations (Abramian et al., 2016).

4.6.1. Survival Rates for Different Types of Neoplasms

Survival rates for the various types of pulmonary neoplasms significantly differ based on their histologic types and inherent biological behaviors. NSCLC is the most common type of pulmonary cancer and comprises an estimated 85% of cases. Of NSCLC, the adenocarcinoma and squamous cell carcinoma subtypes of NSCLC have divergent prognoses; for instance, early-stage adenocarcinoma generally has a more favorable five-year survival rate compared to advanced-stage squamous cell subtypes. Conversely, SCLC, although less frequent, is characterized by its virulence and poor survival rates, with a five-year survival rate that typically does not go below 10%, particularly with extensive-stage diagnosis. Determining these correlations is important to modify treatment approaches to optimize long-term management in the event of pulmonary neoplasms other than bronchogenic carcinoma. Survival rates are also very different among lung cancer patients following different treatment modalities. Surgical approaches and biologic interventions have been shown to improve survival in a very important way in patients with localized disease. For instance, patients receiving resection for stage I or stage II NSCLC have been reported to have five-year survival of more than 70%, which underscores the importance of early diagnosis and therapy. Conversely, patients undergoing palliative therapy for lung cancers at an advanced stage might be confronted with survival estimates much lower than the former. In one study of lung transplant patients with lung cancer, those receiving treatment for initial-stage disease showed considerably enhanced survival compared with their counterparts with metastasis, whose median survival wasn't more than a paltry 2.5 months after diagnosis (Du et al., 2015). These differences demonstrate the significant interaction among staging, treatment modality, and patient prognosis within the overall context of pulmonary neoplasms.

Moreover, emerging data on prevention and novel therapies continue to redefine the management paradigm of lung cancer with a greater expectation of improved survival. For instance, prophylactic cranial irradiation (PCI) has been shown to control brain metastases in SCLC, enhance overall survival, and reduce recurrence rate in patients with complete remission (Feghali et al., 2016). However, the intervention remains underutilized in NSCLC despite modest benefits reported in some cohorts. As research into targeted agents and immunotherapies advances, it becomes increasingly important to identify their influence on survival. This change in paradigms of treatment underscores the evolving nature of lung cancer therapy, where ongoing evaluation of survival by different kinds of neoplasms becomes imperative to eventually maximize therapeutic approaches and improve quality of life in patients (Figure 4.18).

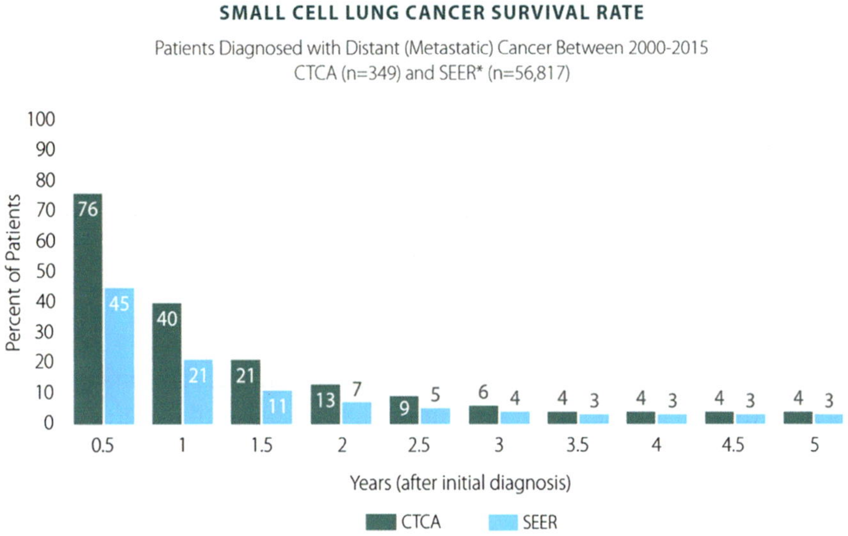

Figure 4.18. Survival rates for different types of neoplasms.

Source: https://external-content.duckduckgo.com/iu/?u=https%3A%2F%2Fcdn.cancercenter.com%2F-%2Fmedia%2Fctca%2Fimages%2Foutcomes%2F2018-winter%2Flung-survival-2018.png&f=1&nofb=1&ipt=34422b9c1f5c317ef3d542b4860e0a780128c93336d3ccbfb5cf1aa7454b6d7b.

4.6.2. Factors Influencing Prognosis

The prognosis for lung neoplasms excluding bronchogenic carcinoma varies based on several variables, including the histologic tumor type, stage at presentation, and the development of metastases. All neoplasms, such as carcinoid tumors, sarcomas, and lymphomas, have differential growth patterns and biological behaviors that significantly influence survival rates for patients. For example, carcinoid tumors, typically low-grade malignancies, have a more favorable prognosis than aggressive histologies like pleomorphic sarcomas or non-Hodgkin lymphoma, both of which can present with unpredictable metastatic potential. Early diagnosis makes it possible to intervene in a timely manner, which is essential for increasing survival rates. The heterogeneity of the histological subtype necessitates the need for individualized therapeutic approaches and emphasizes the importance of accurate diagnostic methods in maximizing outcomes for the patients. The general state of the patients' health, particularly whether they have comorbidities such as obesity or chronic pulmonary diseases, is another crucial prognostic factor. Studies indicate that patients with metabolic disorders can also experience a multi-aspect interaction between their health status and cancer prognosis. Interestingly, while obesity has been associated with lower surgical risk in some patients with lung cancer, it, paradoxically, leads to higher hospital readmission rates after treatment due to complications. Specifically, there is evidence that obesity per se is linked with lower lung cancer risk, with a relative risk of 0.72 reported in some populations. The duality emphasizes the need to consider metabolic health in an individual patient when evaluating prognosis and tailoring follow-up care strategies, thus encouraging a more integrated approach to the management of cancer (Malki et al., 2023). Moreover, the management of pulmonary neoplasms is significantly influenced by developments in molecular profiling and targeted agents that are increasingly at the forefront of treatment regimens. The molecular characteristics of tumors can unmask therapeutic gene alterations, enabling customized treatment regimens that lead to improved prognosis. For instance, tumors with specific mutations can be tolerated satisfactorily by targeted drugs, eventually culminating in enhanced survival. In non-small cell lung carcinoma, for instance, biologically targeted treatments have transformed patient management by taking on the tumors' specific genetic profile. Hence, the incorporation of molecular diagnostics not only assists in the development of therapeutic strategies but also plays an important role in prognostic assessment. This necessitates ongoing research and integration of novel biomarkers in patient evaluation (Malki et al., 2023).

4.6.3. Long-Term Management and Follow-Up Care

Long-term care and follow-up of patients with non-bronchogenic carcinoma pulmonary neoplasms are vital components in the provision of maximum results. After surgical operations, such as bronchial sleeve resection, the patient is often placed under routine monitoring schedules to assess for complications and disease recurrence. Of utmost significance are surgical anastomotic complications, particularly for those receiving neoadjuvant therapies. Studies demonstrate that the complexity of surgery in conjunction with prior chemoradiotherapy may elevate the risk of adverse outcomes, necessitating an extensive analysis of postoperative complications and their influence on long-term survival. This underlines the necessity of an individualized follow-up regimen with intermittent imaging studies and clinical follow-up to facilitate early treatment in case of complications such as pulmonary infections or anastomotic leaks, as highlighted in the present literature (Rodríguez et al., 2018).

Longitudinal follow-up is equally indispensable in taking care of the psychosocial issues in patients diagnosed with pulmonary neoplasms. Diagnosis and treatment of any cancer bring out fear and extreme emotional distress, which, if not handled, can interfere with recovery and quality of life. Long-term care, therefore, should include psychosocial care measures that manage these conditions. Support groups and counseling programs have been identified to effectively provide patients with coping mechanisms for dealing with the emotional impacts of diagnosis and surgery. Hence, integrating mental health services into the follow-up system not only helps with emotional well-being but may also enhance medical regimen compliance, therefore overall health outcomes for this group of patients (Hillinger et al., 2017). Furthermore, examination of survival information can potentially determine long-term consequences of different treatments and management strategies. Clinical trial evidence of evolutionary origin shows variable outcomes depending on tumor histologic type, presentation stage at diagnosis, and treatment modalities used, including neoadjuvant therapy application. For instance, patients undergoing bronchial sleeve resection without anastomosis coverage after neoadjuvant chemotherapy have presented desirable survival rates, reflecting a need to obtain further data collection and analysis for this group. Regular follow-up and monitoring enhance the medical profession's understanding of long-term care requirements, which allows for improved treatment protocols. Last but not least, this evidence-based approach not only informs clinical practice but also ensures patients receive the optimum level of care during their journey of recovery (Rodríguez et al., 2018) (Figure 4.19).

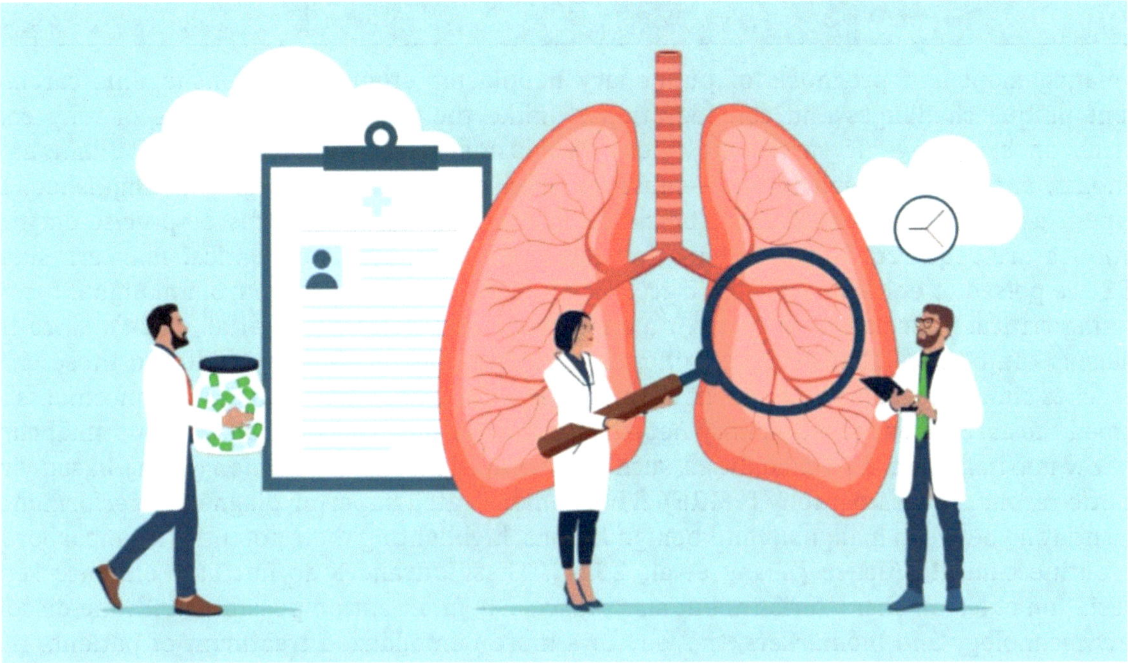

Figure 4.19. Long-term management and follow-up care of pulmonary neoplasms.

Source: https://i0.wp.com/www.denvaxindia.com/blog/wp-content/uploads/2024/04/Lung-Cancer-Treatment-1.png?fit=1107%2C632&ssl=1.

Test Your Knowledge

1. What are the survival rates for different types of neoplasms?
2. What are the factors influencing prognosis?

Summary

The management and prognosis of pulmonary neoplasms other than bronchogenic carcinoma present unique challenges and considerations. Unlike the ubiquitous emphasis of lung cancer research on bronchogenic carcinoma, these neoplasms—e.g., adenocarcinoma, squamous cell carcinoma, and other benign lesions—must be precisely characterized and distinguished. Each subtype is associated with distinct biological behaviors and clinical patterns, so precise diagnostic techniques are required. New evidence indicates that immunohistochemical markers such as TRPS1 are poised to enhance diagnostic accuracy in differentiating benign from malignant lesions, providing critical information for patient management and therapy (Liu et al., 2024). Since these neoplasms can be accompanied by significant morbidity, their pathology is vital to those clinical approaches aimed at maximizing patient outcomes. Besides, imaging technology advancements have reshaped the assessment of pulmonary neoplasms into non-invasive methods with optimal clinical workflow maximization. New modalities, such as intravoxel incoherent motion (IVIM)-based virtual magnetic resonance elastography (vMRE), have demonstrated superior diagnostic performance in differentiating between malignant and benign lesions, highlighting their potential for incorporation into routine clinical practice (Zhang et al., 2024). These advances do not only enhance refined appreciation of lesion characteristics but also make early intervention possible. With the discovery of new technology and biomarkers, the way to a more personalized treatment of patients is laid out. In the end, the treatment of pulmonary neoplasms other than bronchogenic carcinoma will require multi-mechanistic approaches, merging extensive pathological evaluation with sophisticated imaging modalities. Subsequent research into the molecular and genetic underpinnings of the neoplasms will continually enhance diagnostic accuracy and therapeutic results. Integration of novel biomarkers and imaging modalities into clinical decision matrices will be critical in optimizing treatment plans, optimizing patient management, and maximizing survival in this diverse group of pulmonary neoplasms. By expanding the scope beyond bronchogenic carcinoma, we can better understand these associated entities and their roles in patient care in oncology.

The diagnosis of pulmonary neoplasms other than bronchogenic carcinoma reveals a multiform pattern of tumor heterogeneity grossly affecting diagnosis and management. Unlike bronchogenic carcinoma with its well-established association with smoking and environmental exposure, these neoplasms encompass an assortment of histologic patterns like mesenchymal neoplasms, primary sarcomas of the lung, and metastases. The etiologic heterogeneity of the tumors necessitates meticulous clinical evaluation and advanced imaging modalities for accurate identification. Further, molecular profiling is increasingly being recognized as a valuable resource to delineate targeted genetic mutations of such neoplasms that may have the potential to guide therapeutic decisions. Additional research into this spectrum of lung cancers highlights the importance of adopting a differential diagnosis model responsive to their unique nature and presentation, thus impacting treatment regimens and patient outcomes. In addressing the pathogenesis and associated risk of pulmonary neoplasms, researchers emphasize the interdependence of heterogeneous funds for medical advancement. For instance, substantial investment by institutions such as Cancer Research UK illustrates the significance of charitable contributions in supplementing government investment into overall research initiatives. The evaluation of diverse funding modes has highlighted the mutual interdependence between public and philanthropic sector assistance, reiterating that a decrease in government support could harm not only research deliverables but also broader public health efforts against lung cancer. By the development of a collaborative research approach, spectacular advances can be made in the understanding of the pathophysiology of such tumors, thus paving the way for new treatment approaches aimed at improving patient outcomes (Crane et al., 2014). In addition, studies in inhalation toxicity in the context of pulmonary tumors have yielded vital insights in carcinogenicity and in methodologies of risk assessment. Past comparisons between inhalation test results and intraperitoneal studies have shown varying levels of predictive value for different materials, highlighting the limitations of relying solely on intraperitoneal outcomes for drawing inhalation conclusions. With certain fibrous materials, there is concordance among the results of the two tests, while differences may indicate misclassifications of carcinogenicity. The cautionary criticism of such findings indicates a conservative approach to risk assessment and advises a cautionary interpretation of toxicological information. Therefore, it is apparent that although intraperitoneal testing may be useful in exoneration, it is not a substitute for direct evidence from inhalation experiments in human health hazard estimation of pulmonary neoplasms (Bevan et al., 2016).

KEY TERMS FROM THIS CHAPTER

- Adenoid cystic carcinoma
- Carcinoid tumor
- Endobronchial tumors
- Inflammatory myofibroblastic tumor
- Metastatic lung tumors
- Pleuropulmonary blastoma
- Pulmonary blastoma
- Pulmonary hamartoma
- Pulmonary paraganglioma
- Solitary fibrous tumor
- Benign pulmonary nodules
- Clear cell tumor (sugar tumor)
- Granular cell tumor
- Lymphangioleiomyomatosis (LAM)
- Mucoepidermoid carcinoma
- Primary pulmonary meningioma
- Pulmonary chondroma
- Pulmonary lymphoma
- Sarcomatoid carcinoma
- Synovial sarcoma

Critical Thinking Questions

1. **Which of the following is the most common benign lung tumor?**
   a. Pulmonary hamartoma
   b. Carcinoid tumor
   c. Inflammatory pseudotumor
   d. Lipoma
2. **Which pulmonary neoplasm is most likely to cause carcinoid syndrome?**
   a. Small cell carcinoma
   b. Pulmonary hamartoma
   c. Typical carcinoid tumor
   d. Adenocarcinoma
3. **What is the typical location of a pulmonary carcinoid tumor?**
   a. Peripheral lung parenchyma
   b. Apices of the lungs
   c. Central bronchi
   d. Pleura
4. **Which pulmonary tumor is associated with asbestos exposure and involves the pleura?**
   a. Squamous cell carcinoma
   b. Pulmonary hamartoma
   c. Malignant mesothelioma
   d. Large cell carcinoma
5. **Which of the following best differentiates a typical from an atypical pulmonary carcinoid tumor?**
   a. Presence of necrosis and higher mitotic rate
   b. Location in the lung
   c. Smoking history
   d. Calcification on imaging

Short Answer Questions

1. What are the main categories of pulmonary neoplasms other than bronchogenic carcinoma?
2. What is a pulmonary hamartoma, and how is it typically diagnosed on imaging?
3. How do typical and atypical pulmonary carcinoid tumors differ in histology and prognosis?
4. What is the relationship between asbestos exposure and malignant pleural mesothelioma?
5. What are common symptoms of pulmonary neoplasms other than bronchogenic carcinoma?

Answer to Critical Thinking Questions

1. (a); 2. (c); 3. (c); 4. (c); 5.(a)

References

1. Abramian, O., Kolman, D., & Abramian, E. (2016). Oncological airway emergencies in the critical care unit. In *InTech eBooks*. https://doi.org/10.5772/65082Abreu Oliveira, A. L., Alves, C. C., Barroso, I. C., Cabral, I., et al. (2021). Pulmonary adenocarcinoma in dogs: Surgical treatment with real-time video-thermometry. https://core.ac.uk/download/482728979.pdf (accessed on 30th June 2025).
2. Adler, Y., Charron, P., Imazio, M., Badano, L. P., Barón-Esquivias, G., Bogaert, J., Brucato, A., et al. (2015). 2015 ESC guidelines for the diagnosis and management of pericardial diseases. *European Heart Journal, 36*, 2921–2964. https://doi.org/10.1093/eurheartj/ehv318 (accessed on 30th June 2025).
3. Al Feghali, K. A. (2016). Prophylactic cranial irradiation in patients with non-small-cell lung cancer: Systematic review and meta-analysis of randomized controlled trials. https://core.ac.uk/download/650448101.pdf (accessed on 30th June 2025).
4. Alhaj Moustafa, M., Ghanem, A., Hammad, B., Badawy, M. H., Reda, R., Gupta, R., Jeon, E. Y., et al. (2025). Incidentally discovered rare case of solitary fibrous pleural tumor (SFPT) during residency medical clearance examination. *New Emirates Medical Journal*. https://www.semanticscholar.org/paper/2ec6080446536f00cfcdfef05ea99224eac4da84 (accessed on 30th June 2025).
5. Anwar, M., Gorog, D. A., & Gue, Y. X. (2018). A rare cause of myocardial infarction with non-obstructive coronary arteries: Case report of ST-segment elevation myocardial infarction caused by a mediastinal mass. https://core.ac.uk/download/287582241.pdf (accessed on 30th June 2025).
6. Asioli, S., Bruna, M. C., Buffoni, L., Filosso, P., et al. (2011). Significance of the presence of microscopic vascular invasion after complete resection of stage I–II pT1-T2N0 non-small cell lung cancer and its relation with T-size categories: Did the 2009 7th edition of the TNM staging system miss something? https://core.ac.uk/download/pdf/81977092.pdf (accessed on 30th June 2025).
7. Bevan, R., Drummond, G., & Harrison, P. (2016). A comparison of the results from intra-pleural and intra-peritoneal studies with those from inhalation and intratracheal tests for the assessment of pulmonary responses to inhalable dusts and fibers. https://core.ac.uk/download/287581187.pdf (accessed on 30th June 2025).
8. Bhanot, D., Akidiva, S., & Hagan, S. F. (2013). Bronchial carcinoid as a cause of hemoptysis. *Radiology, 6*, 34–38. https://www.semanticscholar.org/paper/b45cac25b4628bc9822a48e0b6c48adc76bcdae9 (accessed on 30th June 2025).
9. Bhatt, A., Chitara, M., Desai, E., Diwanji, P., et al. (2017). Diagnosis and staging of lung carcinoma with CT scan and its histopathological correlation. https://core.ac.uk/download/543135767.pdf (accessed on 30th June 2025).
10. Broman, K., Meng, Q., Holmqvist, A., Balas, N., Richman, J., Landier, W., Hageman, L., et al. (2024). Incidence of and risk factors for cutaneous malignant neoplasms after blood or marrow transplant. *JAMA Dermatology*. https://www.semanticscholar.org/paper/33b158950ecdf74734b40f5944e5befa444aeb87 (accessed on 30th June 2025).

11. Canadian Medical Association. (1982). *Volume 25, Index*. https://core.ac.uk/download/215388092.pdf (accessed on 30th June 2025).
12. Carmona Flores, O., Guerrero Gómez, A., & López Alvarado, M. I. (2023). Primary pulmonary leiomyosarcoma: Review of the literature and case report. https://core.ac.uk/download/570905621.pdf (accessed on 30th June 2025).
13. Caseiro-Alves, F., Curvo-Semedo, L., & Teixeira, L. (2005). Tuberculosis of the chest. https://core.ac.uk/download/61494133.pdf (accessed on 30th June 2025).
14. Crane, P., Farrell, C., Garau, M., Grassano, A., et al. (2014). Exploring the interdependencies of research funders in the UK. https://core.ac.uk/download/30608686.pdf (accessed on 30th June 2025).
15. Du, L., Elson, P., Hashemi-Sadraei, N., Pennell, N., et al. (2015). Lung cancer treatment outcomes in recipients of lung transplant. https://core.ac.uk/download/70384568.pdf (accessed on 30th June 2025).
16. Firooznia, H., Seliger, G., Genieser, N., & Barasch, E. (1975). Hypertrophic pulmonary osteoarthropathy in pulmonary metastases. *Radiology, 115*(2), 269–274. https://www.semanticscholar.org/paper/1e9f8f352ca82993b1435673dc1bc9906c5c3279 (accessed on 30th June 2025).
17. Fisch, D., Bozorgmehr, F., Kazdal, D., Kuon, J., Klotz, L., Shah, R., Eichhorn, F., et al. (2021). Comprehensive dissection of treatment patterns and outcome for patients with metastatic large-cell neuroendocrine lung carcinoma. *Frontiers in Oncology, 11*. https://www.semanticscholar.org/paper/aee2488f0de95b821df919f40fd79e7e20f4d965 (accessed on 30th June 2025).
18. Galea, J., Montefort, S., Schembri, K., Sladden, M., et al. (2016). Recurrent chest infections in two young non-smoker men. https://core.ac.uk/download/46604249.pdf (accessed on 30th June 2025).
19. García Fandiño, M. I., May, L., Cole, T. J., Goh, Y. S. B., Pei, A., Dhorai Raja, B., Bin Zaman, M., et al. (2015). Electronic poster presentations, gynae-oncology. *Journal of Obstetrics and Gynecology Research, 41*, 143–163. https://doi.org/10.1111/jog.12890 (accessed on 30th June 2025).
20. Glazer, G. M., Gross, B. H., Pennes, D. R., Rebner, M., et al. (1987). CT evaluation of mediastinal masses. https://deepblue.lib.umich.edu/bitstream/2027.42/26707/1/0000257.pdf (accessed on 30th June 2025).
21. Gómez García, L. F., Morel, S., & Alvarado McDougal, M. (2025). A rare non-smoking-related spindle cell carcinoma of the lung: A case report. *Cureus, 17*. https://www.semanticscholar.org/paper/0820ffe8e33e5a782c55bf4c8a255672c4d3355b (accessed on 30th June 2025).
22. Gorbokon, N., Baltruschat, S., Lennartz, M., Luebke, A., Höflmayer, D., Kluth, M., Hube-Magg, C., et al. (2024). PAX8 expression in cancerous and non-neoplastic tissue: A tissue microarray study on more than 17,000 tumors from 149 different tumor entities. *Virchows Archiv, 485*, 491–507. https://www.semanticscholar.org/paper/5ea6a7a9d1c0625c93f47fa313c372c23ef975a0 (accessed on 30th June 2025).
23. Harken, K. (1966). Bronchogenic adenocarcinoma in the dog. https://core.ac.uk/download/38907912.pdf (accessed on 30th June 2025).
24. Hillinger, S., Kestenholz, P., Opitz, I., Schneiter, D., et al. (2017). Sleeve resections with

unprotected bronchial anastomoses are safe even after neoadjuvant therapy†. https://core.ac.uk/download/85219640.pdf (accessed on 30th June 2025).

25. Hurwitz, C. (1951). Primary carcinoma of the lung in Bantu miners: An Anthro pathological study in the etiology of the disease. https://core.ac.uk/download/429725505.pdf (accessed on 30th June 2025).

26. Jaikaran, G. K. (2009). Case series of mediastinal masses: A single institutional experience. https://core.ac.uk/download/235659745.pdf (accessed on 30th June 2025).

27. Kara, A., Gelen, V., & Kara, H. (2023). *Molecular Histopathology and Cytopathology*. IntechOpen eBooks. https://doi.org/10.5772/intechopen.105300 (accessed on 30th June 2025).

28. Keerthi, N. S., Vyshak, U. S., Mohapatra, A., Kudva, R., & Sanjai, N. (2022). A rare case of metastatic synovial sarcoma initially masqueraded as bronchogenic carcinoma: A case report. *Journal of Clinical Images and Medical Case Reports*. https://www.semanticscholar.org/paper/107ce111470e76c04d5cff5b5d6fa733afe2fab3 (accessed on 30th June 2025).

29. Kolin, A., Chapman, A. D., Cooper, C. A., Henschke, C. I., Taylor, D., Sterner, D. J., Fearon, E. R., et al. (2000). Early glandular neoplasia of the lung. https://core.ac.uk/download/pdf/3185231.pdf (accessed on 30th June 2025).

30. Lachkar, S., Roger, M., Vergnon, J., Crutu, A., Febvre, M., Mehdaoui, A., Gervais, R., et al. (2023). Endoscopic resection of tracheal and bronchial granular cell tumors: A national multicenter retrospective study. *Respirology, 28*, 794–797. https://www.semanticscholar.org/paper/26c5a3301d379e25cf0b04601a6ce45b871473bb (accessed on 30th June 2025).

31. Liu, B., Zhou, H., Tan, L., Siu, K. T. H., & Guan, X. Y. (2024). Exploring treatment options in cancer: Tumor treatment strategies. *Signal Transduction and Targeted Therapy, 9*. https://www.semanticscholar.org/paper/3a13839be741a1e040fbf5c2a0ee1a8388fafae2 (accessed on 30th June 2025).

32. Liu, Y. A., Aung, P., Wang, Y., Ning, J., Nagarajan, P., Curry, J., Torres-Cabala, C., et al. (2024). TRPS1 expression in non-melanocytic cutaneous neoplasms: An immunohistochemical analysis of 200 cases. *Journal of Pathology and Translational Medicine, 58*, 72–80. https://www.semanticscholar.org/paper/264fef08045d360ea25763638f18fe41857ab2fb (accessed on 30th June 2025).

33. Mäkitaro, R. (1999). A population-based study of lung cancer and benign intrathoracic tumors. https://core.ac.uk/download/628862297.pdf (accessed on 30th June 2025).

34. Malki, A., Sami, W., & Shaik, R. A. (2023). Association between metabolically healthy obesity and metastasis in lung cancer patients–A systematic review and meta-analysis. https://core.ac.uk/download/591830997.pdf (accessed on 30th June 2025).

35. Manibarathi, R. (2018). Comparison of napsin A versus thyroid transcription factor 1 in the typing of lung carcinoma. https://core.ac.uk/download/235669009.pdf (accessed on 30th June 2025).

36. Mitrache, M., Terzea, D., Sîrbu, A., & Fica, S. (2024). Aggressive primary thyroid mucoepidermoid carcinoma with extensive pulmonary involvement. *Biomedicines, 12*. https://www.semanticscholar.org/paper/99852d88f5f54dfbbea43a2ab0b9c47916623ea3 (accessed on 30th June 2025).

37. Ochiai, A., Koch, A. E., Feinberg, A. P., Richards, B. L., Graham, C. H., de Marco, D., Fan, D.,

et al. (2025). Transfection of interleukin-8 increases angiogenesis and tumorigenesis of human gastric carcinoma cells in nude mice. https://core.ac.uk/download/pdf/8037733.pdf (accessed on 30th June 2025).

38. Parvez, M., Islam, M. K., Tapan, M. T. B., & Yeasmin, F. (2023). Histopathological evaluation of malignant adult renal tumors: A study of specialized tertiary care center. *Global Academic Journal of Medical Sciences*. https://www.semanticscholar.org/paper/56752ea3bfde0f390d6a8f67f772efde33c65f07 (accessed on 30th June 2025).
39. Quint, L. E. (2015). Work-up of the solitary pulmonary nodule. https://deepblue.lib.umich.edu/bitstream/2027.42/111300/1/40644_2015_Article_13.pdf (accessed on 30th June 2025).
40. Rodríguez Pérez, M. (2018). Impact of neoadjuvant therapy on adverse events following sleeve resection of the lung. https://core.ac.uk/download/240469516.pdf (accessed on 30th June 2025).
41. Shah, S., Sonwani, I., Harikrishna, K., & Kaur, M. (2023). WBC & their role in tumor microenvironment (TME) of oral squamous cell carcinoma: A review. *International Journal of Scientific Research*. https://www.semanticscholar.org/paper/bb5c20c287cd57572431da32aeddf13f71ab77d8 (accessed on 30th June 2025).
42. Shang, S., Zhang, L., Liu, K., Lv, M., Zhang, J., Ju, D., Wei, D., et al. (2024). Landscape of targeted therapies for advanced urothelial carcinoma. *Exploration of Targeted Anti-tumor Therapy, 5*, 641–677. https://www.semanticscholar.org/paper/5ec384eaeeb5aafa984caf1d73ceac057460720e (accessed on 30th June 2025).
43. Sinha Roy, S. (2008). A study of solitary pulmonary nodule in 50 cases. https://core.ac.uk/download/235663792.pdf (accessed on 30th June 2025).
44. Xu, L., Wang, P., Zhang, Y., Wang, M., Li, Y., & Dang, W. (2022). Study on chronic obstructive pulmonary disease and lung cancer: Web of Science-based bibliometric and visual analysis. *International Journal of General Medicine, 15*, 7523–7534. https://doi.org/10.2147/ijgm.s370781 (accessed on 30th June 2025).
45. Zhang, S., Du, Y., Liang, T., Zhang, X., Guo, Y., Yang, J., Li, X., et al. (2024). Diagnostic efficiency of intravoxel incoherent motion-based virtual magnetic resonance elastography in pulmonary neoplasms. *Cancer Imaging, 24*. https://www.semanticscholar.org/paper/14860045d04dcf3520891fc2e0339adceea6deec (accessed on 30th June 2025).

SARCOIDOSIS AND PULMONARY VASCULITIDES

5

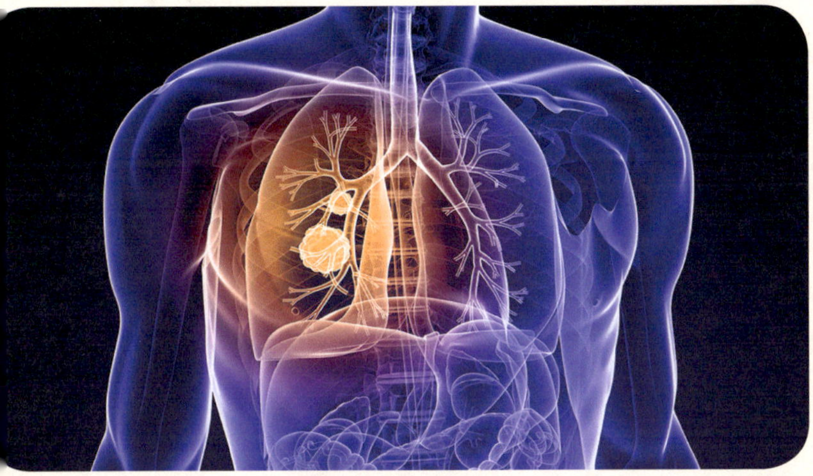

LEARNING OBJECTIVES

After studying this chapter, you will be able to:

1. Understand the pathophysiology of sarcoidosis
2. Illustrate the clinical presentation of sarcoidosis
3. List the treatment options for sarcoidosis
4. Give an overview of pulmonary vasculitides
5. Explore clinical manifestations of pulmonary vasculitides
6. Explain the management strategies for pulmonary vasculitides

Introduction

The introduction of the topic of sarcoidosis and pulmonary vasculitides is essential to understanding the complexity associated with these diseases, particularly what these diseases do with regard to breathing well-being. Sarcoidosis is characterized by the formation of granulomas within the tissues, most commonly the lungs, and it can be potentially very debilitating. Approximately 20% of patients can develop advanced pulmonary sarcoidosis that causes severe respiratory failure or even death (Gupta et al., 2023). The interaction between sarcoidosis and pulmonary vasculitis highlights the necessity for extensive research, as these two entities can coexist and complicate the clinical presentation of one another. Furthermore, understanding the epidemiological patterns of sarcoidosis and its potential transformation into serious cases is significant, particularly given the current lack of standard treatment methods for patients with advanced disease presentation. Greater awareness of pulmonary vasculitides of sarcoidosis has driven developments in clinical perception and management guidelines. Pulmonary vasculitides are characterized by inflammation of the pulmonary vasculature, having the potential to aggravate the complex pathophysiology of sarcoidosis. Recent conference debates, including the 2015. AASOG conference, have highlighted the importance of personalized treatment and increasing awareness of these interconnected complex conditions (Nabeel et al., 2020). There is currently evidence supporting multidisciplinary treatment in the management of sarcoidosis when it is accompanied by pulmonary vascular complications. These approaches not only consider pharmacologic therapy but also involve input from pulmonary disease experts and others as needed, thereby optimizing treatment for affected patients. Furthermore, addressing the therapeutic and prognostic situation of sarcoidosis and pulmonary vasculitides is crucial to optimize patient outcomes. Advanced pulmonary fibrosis as the leading cause of death in sarcoidosis, studies still explore novel therapeutic targets, including antifibrotic therapy (Gupta et al., 2023). The complexity in the management of sarcoidosis, especially where pulmonary vasculitis is the case, necessitates an in-depth understanding of disease pathophysiology. Further, advances in genomic and immunology studies propose avenues for targeted interventions, which further expand our therapeutic armament against such debilitating diseases. Thus, incorporation of new evidence into practice is essential in order to enhance optimal care for patients and improve quality of life in patients with sarcoidosis and related pulmonary diseases (Figure 5.1).

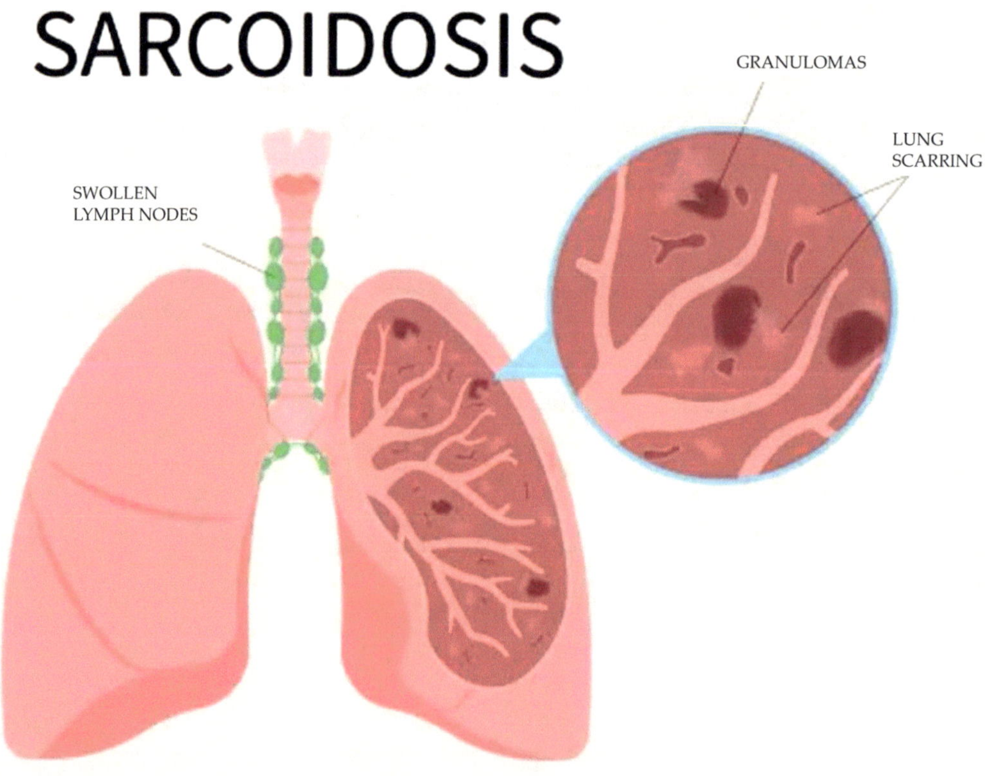

Figure 5.1. Sarcoidosis.

Source: https://www.carehospitals.com/ckfinder/userfiles/images/sarcoidosis.webp.

Definition of Sarcoidosis

Sarcoidosis is a body-wide inflammatory disorder characterized by the presence of granulomas, which are masses of inflammatory cells occurring in small quantities and frequently becoming situated within various organs. The precise etiology of sarcoidosis remains obscure, although it is considered to represent an exaggerated immune response against environmental antigens in genetically predisposed individuals. Frequently involving the lungs, skin, and lymph nodes, sarcoidosis can cause a wide variety of clinical manifestations. Symptoms may vary from cough, asthenia, fever, and dyspnea to markedly impair the quality of life in infected individuals. In some instances, there is spontaneous resolution, whereas in others, there is chronic progression leading to permanent organ damage. The heterogeneity of presentation complicates the diagnosis, necessitating advanced knowledge of the disease definition in combination with a wide range of diagnostic approaches beyond routine laboratory testing (Albano et al., 2021). The diagnosis of sarcoidosis may be challenging, as diagnosis is extensive in the majority of cases, involving clinical history, imaging examinations, and histopathologic documentation of granulomatous inflammation. Radiographic imaging, particularly chest X-rays and high-resolution computed tomography (CT) scans, are valuable in assessing the extent of pulmonary involvement. In most cases, however, bronchoscopy with transbronchial biopsy is used to obtain tissue specimens for histological examination, which can confirm the presence of non-caseating granulomas diagnostic of sarcoidosis. More recent developments, such as the use of 18F-fluorodeoxyglucose positron emission tomography (FDG PET), have also been found to enable increased diagnostic sensitivity for the identification of active inflammatory lesions. This technology has been utilized not only in malignancies but also in systemic diseases like sarcoidosis, highlighting the importance of multimodal diagnostic approaches (Albano et al., 2021). One needs to know about the relationship between sarcoidosis and pulmonary vasculitides because both can demonstrate overlapping symptoms and affect the lung vasculature. Though sarcoidosis typically manifests as granulomatous inflammation, pulmonary vasculitides such as Takayasu arteritis are linked to a more complex phenomenon of vessel ischemia and inflammation, possibly with or without granulomas. Both need to be managed early to prevent severe complications, particularly when vasculopathy leads to parenchymal lung damage or systemic organ failure. Therefore, it is significant to understand the unique features of sarcoidosis within the context of the broader pulmonary vasculitides in order to be able to diagnose and treat them appropriately; both can lead to significant morbidity and mortality if left untreated, particularly in high-risk groups, such as young women with Takayasu arteritis.

Definition of Pulmonary Vasculitides

Pulmonary vasculitides is a category of diseases where inflammatory changes occur in the blood vessels of the lungs. The disease may present as a primary condition or as a secondary phenomenon of other systemic diseases, where it usually reflects underlying pathogenic mechanisms. Inflammation can occur in vessels of any size with attendant varied clinical manifestations and sequelae. The complexity of pulmonary vasculitides is further increased by their potential for overlap with other inflammatory or autoimmune conditions, making differential diagnosis more challenging and requiring appropriate clinical evaluation. While the distinction between such diseases becomes increasingly finer, definitions of large and medium vessel vasculitis, for example, must be further established to further define understanding and treatment regimens in clinical practice (Lötscher et al., 2022). Diagnostic imaging plays a pivotal role in the identification of pulmonary vasculitides, as it allows clinicians to see and assess vascular alterations in the lungs. Later technological developments in positron emission tomography (PET) have improved diagnostic capabilities for these illnesses, thereby facilitating early treatment. In particular, [F-18] FDG PET/CT imaging is a valuable aid in the evaluation of inflammation in pulmonary vasculitis. This imaging technique not only aids in diagnosing the extent of vascular involvement but also in differentiating between infectious and inflammatory processes, which are superficially similar in presentation and thus extremely therapeutically tricky. Thus, the awareness that imaging possesses in the setting of pulmonary vasculitides significantly enhances the clinician's diagnostic armamentarium (Albano et al., 2021). In addition, the clinical implications of pulmonary vasculitides extend beyond the initial diagnosis and treatment; they encompass the management of long-term outcomes as well as potential complications. Along with the recognition of new types of vasculitides, achieving complete knowledge of their pathophysiology is essential. To create uniform clinical practices and improve patient results, future research needs to focus on establishing specific, worldwide accepted definitions of these illnesses. Besides, an interdisciplinary discussion among rheumatologists, pulmonologists, and radiologists is imperative in streamlining diagnostic and management approaches. By doing this, there is promise of developing targeted therapies that directly address the unique issues posed by pulmonary vasculitides, eventually realizing a better quality of care for patients impacted by them (Lötscher et al., 2022) (Figure 5.3).

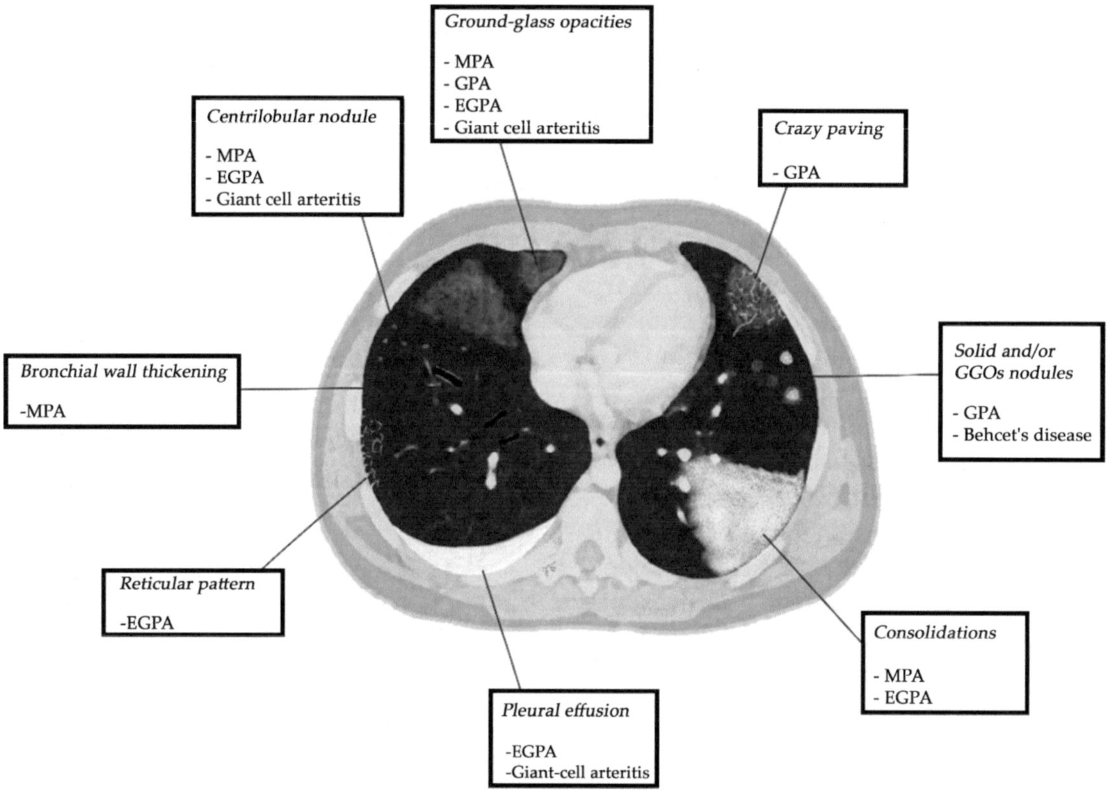

Figure 5.2. Pulmonary vasculitides.

Source: https://www.mdpi.com/diagnostics/diagnostics-11-02318/article_deploy/html/images/diagnostics-11-02318-g001.png.

Importance of Studying These Conditions

The analysis of conditions like sarcoidosis and pulmonary vasculitides is very important in clinical medicine because of their multifaceted nature and serious effect on pulmonary health. Both these conditions may come with overlapping symptoms like shortness of breath and persistent cough, so exact diagnoses are crucial for appropriate treatments. Understanding of the pathophysiology of such diseases not only allows for the recognition of the multi-factorial interaction between the immune system and lung tissue but also contributes to the process of creating targeted therapies. Also, as discussed in recent literature, diseases involving systemic autoimmune disorders have extra-pulmonary complications like sensorineural hearing loss, significantly bringing to the fore an overall understanding of their systemic consequences (Adelchi et al., 2018). This depth of research forms the basis for improved patient management and outcomes and, in turn, the quality of care provided to the affected individuals. Also, studies into sarcoidosis and pulmonary vasculitides can illuminate the broader relevance of autoimmune diseases to general health and well-being. The interlinking of systemic disease and pulmonary involvement makes the clinical picture more complex, and it is therefore important that healthcare providers are cognizant of these associations. For instance, greater awareness of how autoimmune disease may result in audiological and vestibular symptomatology may prevent misdiagnosis and enable early intervention (Adelchi et al., 2018). In addition, as research and technology advance in the field of rheumatology, detection of co-morbidities and common symptoms can enable clinicians to make informed decisions on treatment regimes. This multi-faceted approach not only optimizes treatment effectiveness but also profoundly improves patient quality of life by addressing many aspects of these interconnected diseases. Ultimately, the significance of studying sarcoidosis and pulmonary vasculitides is in developing new therapeutic modalities that address these complex diseases. Therapeutic investigation of corticosteroids and other immunosuppression is imperative in the context of the extensive variability of presentation of these conditions. As recent literature has emphasized, the integration of systemic disease considerations into treatment guidelines can enhance patient outcomes and inform best practices in managing rheumatic disorders. Through continued research and education, healthcare providers are able to better comprehend and deal with these intricate diseases, thus improving diagnostic precision and more effective individualized treatments. Through being proactive in these endeavors, the medical community is better able to provide assistance to patients who are faced with dealing with sarcoidosis and pulmonary vasculitides.

5.1. Pathophysiology of Sarcoidosis

Learning Outcome

1. Immune response and granuloma formation
2. Genetic predisposition and environmental triggers
3. Impact on lung function and systemic health

The pathophysiology of sarcoidosis is characterized by the dysregulated triggering of the immune system, leading to the development of non-caseating granulomas almost exclusively within the lungs but potentially in other organs. This granulomatous inflammation arises as a result of an interplay between genetic susceptibility factors and environmental stimuli, such as infectious pathogens or particulate matter, that provoke an overactive immune response. The characteristic of the condition is the presence of granulomas formed by activated T lymphocytes and macrophages in inflamed tissues, which can compromise normal tissue architecture. The pathophysiologic mechanism is significant to know because it not only accounts for sarcoidosis's clinical presentation but also aids in differentiating it from granulomatous diseases with similar presentations.

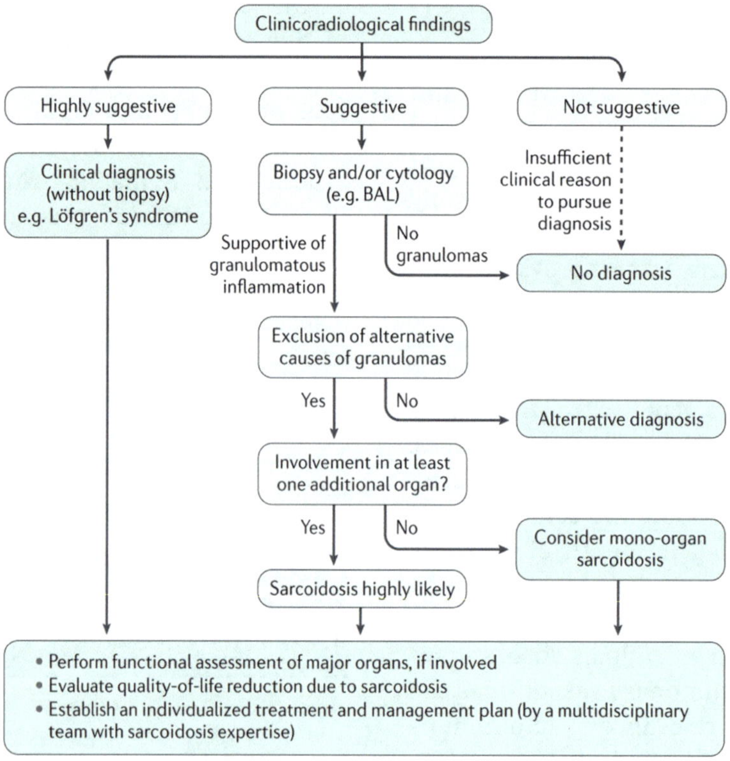

Figure 5.3. Pathophysiology of sarcoidosis.

Source: https://media.springernature.com/lw685/springer-static/image/art%3A10.1038%2Fs41572-019-0096-x/MediaObjects/41572_2019_96_Fig8_HTML.png.

As the immune response continues uncontrolled, it can culminate in fibrosis and major compromise of lung function, leading to morbidity in patients. The inflammatory milieu in sarcoidosis is facilitated by dysregulation of various cytokines and chemokines, which is pivotal in the disease's pathophysiology. Key mediators such as tumor necrosis factor-alpha (TNF-α) and interleukin-6 (IL-6) trigger the inflammatory process and contribute to the maintenance of the granulomas. The secondary resultant inflammatory process may also have systemic implications, such as complications in the form of pulmonary hypertension and cardiac involvement, which are usually added to the clinical picture. The interaction between the adaptive and innate immune responses also worsens the pathophysiology, as the immune system's machinery continues to react even after the removal of the initial stimulus. The interactions indicate that the prospect of untargeted therapies actually worsening the condition rather than improving it exists. Conversely, certain treatments such as TNF-α antagonists have been encouraging for more severe cases, underlining the importance of better unraveling the underlying mechanisms. However, the link between sarcoidosis and pulmonary vasculitides further underscored the importance of making inroads into the pathophysiology regarding systemic disease. The vascular manifestation of sarcoidosis can manifest as pulmonary vasculitis, or inflammation of the blood vessels that obstructs circulation and oxygenation. This cross-talk can enhance other pulmonary symptoms and may result in systemic complications. The immune-mediated inner ear disease, for instance, illustrates how systemic autoimmune aspects of the disease can overlap with sarcoidosis to generate other audiovestibular manifestations in patients. Moreover, identifying such associations is of paramount importance for optimal management, as treatment regimens may need a holistic approach to address both sarcoidosis and any concomitant autoimmune phenomena. Through their study of such intricate interactions, clinicians can improve diagnostic accuracy and maximize therapeutic outcomes in patients with sarcoidosis and associated diseases (Figure 5.3).

5.1.1. Immune Response and Granuloma Formation

The immune reaction is crucial in the pathogenesis of granuloma formation, particularly in conditions such as sarcoidosis. Suppose the body encounters persistent antigens such as microorganisms or environmental triggers. In that case, the body develops a complex immune reaction characterized by macrophage and T cell activation, as well as many cytokines. This excessive immune reaction leads to the clustering of activated macrophages, which become multinucleated giant cells, forming the typical granulomas of sarcoidosis. The granulomas are an immune response to wall off the causative agents, but can lead to tissue injury and organ failure in a seeming paradox. The interaction between immune system activation and regulatory pathways is significant, as their imbalances can similarly lead to the appearance of other non-infectious granulomatous diseases, reflecting the complexity of lung diseases mediated by the immune system. Granuloma formation is most prominent in pulmonary vasculitides, with the immune response potentially targeting the blood vessels directly, leading to inflammation and tissue injury. In most cases, the mechanisms involved in granuloma formation are similar to those for vasculitis. While the primary immune response may be against a specific antigen, the resultant granulomas will inadvertently continue inflammation in nearby tissues and cause a loop of damage and healing. This occurs in those with a clinical presentation suggesting both pulmonary vasculitides and sarcoidosis. Subclinical granulomatous inflammation can often be concomitant with vascular involvement, complicating the diagnostic approach and management of such patients. Clinical features, serology, and imaging modalities must be weighed with care to discriminate between these closely interconnected processes and provide site-specific therapeutic measures. Non-infectious granulomatous lung disease has a heterogeneous nature, necessitating a good grasp of their pathophysiology to allow correct diagnosis and treatment. As noted in research, management of such conditions can be challenging in the context of the overlapping presentation and imaging characteristics. Non-infectious granulomatous lung disease is a group of disorders characterized by granulomatous inflammation (Franks et al., 2021). Notably, presentations with granulomatous inflammation with deep morphea demonstrate the complexity and susceptibility to misdiagnosis in such conditions. Furthermore, a mistaken diagnosis of these conditions can hold up proper treatment, which could result in permanent pulmonary injury. Understanding the immunological basis and the consequent tissue architecture changes is crucial for effectively addressing these lung diseases, leading the way to progress in both comprehension and therapeutic intervention (Figure 5.4).

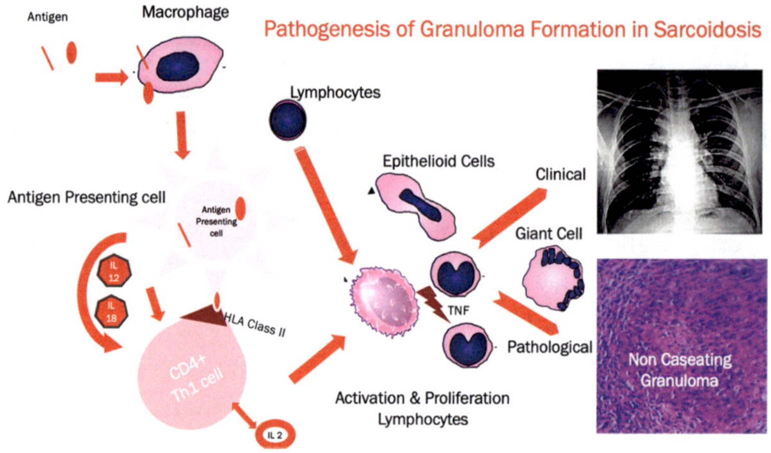

Figure 5.4. Pathogenesis of granuloma formation in sarcoidosis.

Source: https://www.researchgate.net/profile/Dhruv-Talwar-3/publication/357206231/figure/fig1/AS:1103426008166400@1640088669602/Pathogenesis-of-granuloma-formation-in-sarcoidosis.png.

5.1.2. Genetic Predisposition and Environmental Triggers

The interplay between genetic predisposition and environmental stimulation is the key to the pathogenesis of sarcoidosis and other pulmonary vasculitides. Genetic dispositions can enhance one's susceptibility to these diseases, which often affect particular populations, suggesting a possible genetic component. These would include mutations in genes responsible for the immune response that result in an exaggerated inflammatory reaction to environmental antigens, a pathogenetic mechanism alleged in sarcoidosis. Environmental challenges, such as exposure to infectious pathogens, toxins, or workplace exposures, can also enhance genetic susceptibility. Thus, an understanding of this dual effect is necessary in order to identify high-risk groups and for potential preventive measures aimed at reducing exposure to known environmental stimuli. New evidence now makes it clear how complex the pathways involved in gene interaction with environmental exposures are to manifest as diseases like pulmonary vasculitides. There is also a strong connection with autoimmune reactions and these conditions, with a tendency to cause severe inflammation of small to moderate-sized vessels. ANCA, for example, has also been implicated in the causation of granulomatosis with polyangiitis (GPA), indicating that genetic susceptibility contributes to the autoimmune component. The genetic susceptibility of some groups to autoimmunity provides a context to assess environmental determinants, such as infections or toxins, which, in susceptible individuals, trigger disease. Thus, a global review of both genetic and environmental factors reveals superior information regarding the mechanisms of sarcoidosis and pulmonary vasculitides. Greater exploration of the interaction between environmental exposures and genetic susceptibility has the potential to carry significant implications for prevention and management of such diseases. With the discovery of some genetic markers that can offer risk, healthcare providers can target prevention measures specifically. Further, awareness of environmental exposures, such as occupational and lifestyle factors, would facilitate focused education and intervention strategies. The evolution of treatment models, including biologics against select immunopathologic pathways, is an adaptation to enhanced insight into disease mechanisms at both the genetic and environmental levels. Thus, the integration of genetic information with environmental health principles can potentially enhance our capacity to combat sarcoidosis and pulmonary vasculitides, ultimately leading to improved patient outcomes and quality care (Figure 5.5).

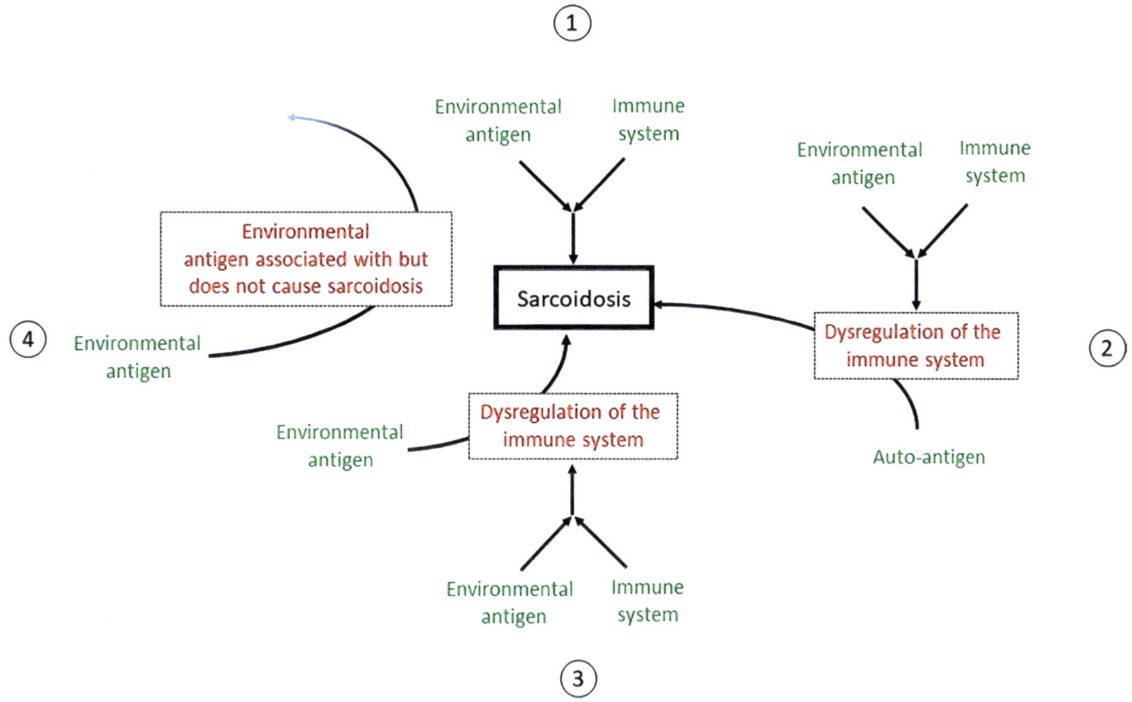

Figure 5.5. Environmental triggers of sarcoidosis.

Source: https://www.frontiersin.org/files/Articles/539872/fimmu-11-01340-HTML/image_m/fimmu-11-01340-g001.jpg.

5.1.3. Impact on Lung Function and Systemic Health

The association between sarcoidosis and pulmonary vasculitides threatens lung function and general health in serious ways. Sarcoidosis patients usually present with granulomatous inflammation of the lung's structures, which appears as patterns of obstructive and restrictive lung disease. These pathological changes may extend to reduced vital capacity and impaired gas exchange, thereby exacerbating dyspnea and exercise intolerance. The systemic nature of sarcoidosis, with potential multisystemic involvement, underscores the double burden faced by patients. Furthermore, the heterogeneity of disease course complicates clinical management, with clinicians requiring a multidimensional strategy to address differences in presentation. Emphasized in the literature, acute presentation might require emergent treatment, while chronic disease courses require appropriately managed long-term strategies for healing and lung function preservation (Chairman et al., 2019). In patients with pulmonary vasculitides, the same lung function impairments will be present. The diseases have a tendency to lead to pulmonary vasculature vasculitis, which compromises blood flow and lung tissue oxygenation. This resultant hypoxia itself may further predispose patients to other systemic complications like cardiovascular disease. As interstitial lung disease (ILD) has a tendency to occur with rheumatologic disease, lung function testing is critical in evaluating patients' overall health (Cassone et al., 2021). It is important to recognize that the impact on lung function is not just limited to respiratory symptoms; overall well-being is also likely to decline due to reduced physical activity and increased healthcare utilization. For this reason, therapeutic interventions must be instituted that overcome both pulmonary and systemic consequences for optimal patient health. Therapeutic interventions for improving pulmonary function and systemic well-being in sarcoidosis and pulmonary vasculitides often utilize immunosuppressive medications. Mycophenolate mofetil (MMF), for instance, has been utilized as a possible alternative to cyclophosphamide for rheumatologic ILD-related treatments (Cassone et al., 2021). Its therapeutic application in treatment protocols highlights the need to balance efficacy with side effects, reflecting the complexity of managing such conditions. In light of the great overlap of lung pathology in sarcoidosis and pulmonary vasculitides, it is still important for healthcare professionals to individualize therapeutic treatment regimens according to patient needs. Successful management of lung function by such individualized therapies not only enhances respiratory symptoms but also facilitates improved systemic health, ultimately resulting in a better quality of life for those involved.

Test Your Knowledge

1. What is an immune response and granuloma formation?
2. What is genetic predisposition?

5.2. Clinical Presentation of Sarcoidosis

Learning Outcome

1. Common symptoms and signs
2. Diagnostic criteria and methods
3. Staging and classification of the disease

Sarcoidosis is an extrapulmonary granulomatous condition with the formation of noncaseating granulomas in many organs, with the lung being the most frequent site. Sarcoidosis can have an extremely diverse clinical presentation and, as a result, be misdiagnosed or its diagnosis delayed. Symptomatic respiratory features are cough, dyspnea, and chest pain, which appear after the onset of the disease. Furthermore, systemic signs such as fever, weight loss, and weakness may be observed in the patients. Interestingly, the clinical presentation is extremely variable depending on the severity of organ involvement, and some patients may be asymptomatic with severe pulmonary compromise. This necessitates a thorough clinical evaluation and, in most cases, imaging studies to determine the extent of lung involvement and any other systemically related findings, ultimately guiding clinical decision-making in treatment strategy for the affected individuals. In pulmonary vasculitides, the clinical presentation may also be complicated by overlapping syndromes with sarcoidosis. Conditions such as antineutrophil cytoplasmic antibodies (ANCA)-associated vasculitis (AAV) usually present with lung involvement that presentations in sarcoidosis can imitate. For instance, GPA may lead to pulmonary nodules and diffuse infiltrates, while microscopic polyangiitis (MPA) may present with interstitial lung disease (ILD). The prevalence of ILD is particularly significant among MPA patients, where it can occur in up to 45% of cases. Overlapping features such as these underscore the importance of differential diagnosis in clinical presentation because response to therapy can be highly variable based on etiology. Hence, extensive examinations such as high-resolution computed tomography (HRCT) scans are crucial in distinguishing between these two conditions to facilitate proper treatment of sarcoidosis as opposed to pulmonary vasculitides of AAV. The linkage between sarcoidosis and pulmonary vasculitides extends beyond their presentation, involving presumptive pathophysiologic mechanisms in vascular dysregulation. In vasculitis, inflammatory responses against vascular elements can enhance the clinical course of patients with sarcoidosis and result in augmented atherosclerosis and cardiovascular risk. Immune complexes, endothelin-1, and other inflammatory mediators are key to determining how these diseases can overlap and impact treatment. Certain inflammatory pathways, such as those involving immune complex-induced inflammation, have the potential to initiate vascular changes of clinical importance in both sarcoidosis and AAV. Such interaction, along with varying patient clinical presentations, supports the necessity of using a multimodal system of diagnosis and treatment, thereby ultimately improving patient prognosis in this complex clinical environment (Figure 5.6).

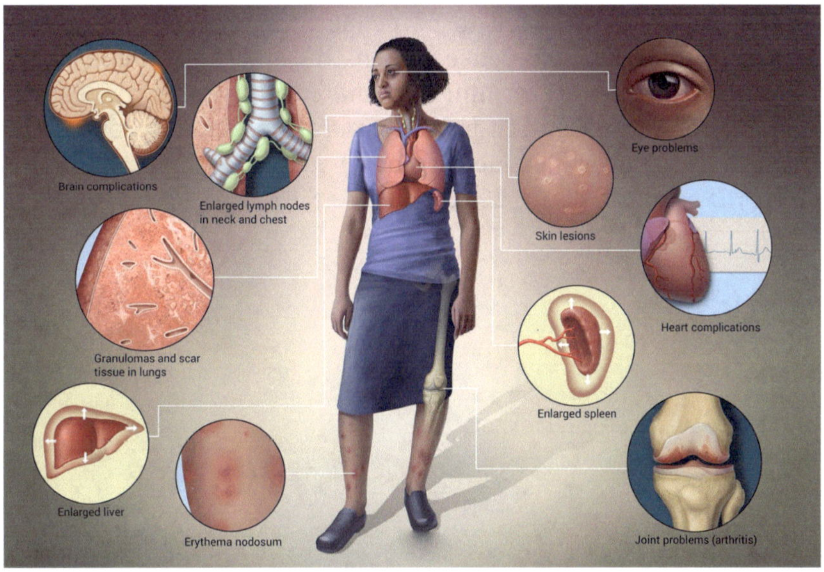

Figure 5.6. Clinical presentation of sarcoidosis.

Source: https://internal-medicine.ecu.edu/pulmonary/wp-content/pv-uploads/sites/500/sarcoidosis1a_Symptoms_600.jpg.

5.2.1. Common Symptoms and Signs

The presentation of sarcoidosis clinically can be highly unpredictable and prone to making diagnosis complicated in most situations. Presenting symptoms are typically a persistent cough, chest pain, and dyspnea, which gradually develop over an extended time frame. The patients also have systemic symptoms like weakness, fever, and weight loss, since the disease is inflammatory. In approximately 90% of the cases, pulmonary involvement is encountered, and many respiratory complaints ensue, which are frequently misinterpreted as more common respiratory diseases. Such similarity may lead to delays in appropriate diagnosis and treatment. Awareness of these common respiratory symptoms is crucial for clinicians because they play a significant role in earlier diagnosis of sarcoidosis and the initiation of therapeutic intervention before the development of serious complications. Outside of respiratory symptoms, individuals with pulmonary vasculitides such as GPA also experience a range of otorhinolaryngologic symptoms, and they may occur as presenting symptoms of the disease. Nasal obstruction, facial pain, and frequent epistaxis are typical findings that indicate upper respiratory tract involvement. Most importantly, the catastrophic effect GPAs have on nasal structures, such as septal perforation of the nose, cannot be overlooked since it signifies granulomatous destruction of nasal cartilage. With GPA characteristically presenting in these ENT symptoms and signs in 70-100% of patients, an eye to the upper respiratory tract is mandatory for correct diagnosis. Moreover, histological examination is pivotal in GPA diagnosis, focusing on the interrelation of specific symptoms and disease pathophysiology (D'aguanno et al., 2018; Vincentiis et al., 2016). Beyond pulmonary and ENT symptoms, systemic symptoms are a significant characteristic of sarcoidosis and pulmonary vasculitides. Malaise, loss of weight, and arthralgia are the usual presentations for the patient. These systemic presentations typically reflect the bodys systemic inflammatory response, so sarcoidosis is challenging to differentiate from other autoimmune diseases like GPA. Clinical presentation can take the form of inflammatory phenomena within numerous organ systems that need to be properly managed by a multidisciplinary team. Physicians need to realize that the occurrence of constitutional symptoms along with findings in the lungs can guide proper diagnosis. This unifying, shared-symptoms concept, therefore, can, in a significant way, facilitate early intervention provision and, as such, improve patient outcomes and minimize the occurrence of long-term sequelae that, in turn, may, as a result of delayed diagnosis (Vincentiis et al., 2016; D'aguanno et al., 2018) (Figure 5.7).

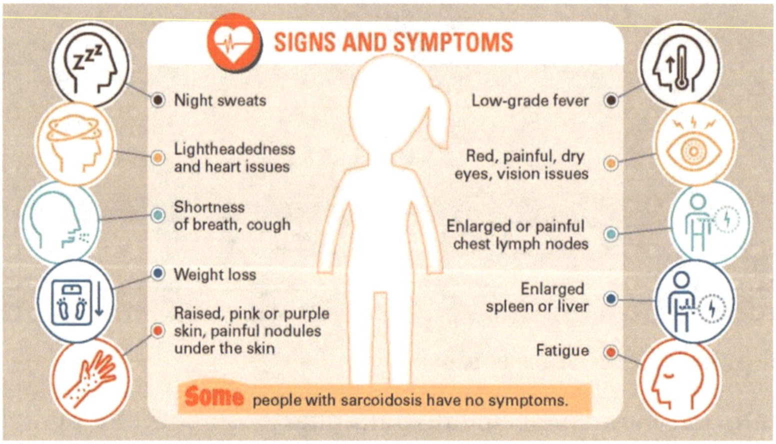

Figure 5.7. Common symptoms and signs of sarcoidosis.

Source: https://www.nationaljewish.org/NJH/files/d6/d67f94b4-61ca-42a3-93bf-3f18d8c6eb8b.jpg.

5.2.2. Diagnostic Criteria and Methods

Diagnosis procedures and criteria for sarcoidosis and pulmonary vasculitides are crucial in arriving at accurate diagnoses and allowing effective management plans. Clinical examination, medical history, and imaging studies are often employed to diagnose sarcoidosis. The practice is usually initiated by physicians using chest X-rays, which often reveal characteristic bilateral hilar lymphadenopathy in patients with sarcoidosis. Finally, high-resolution computed tomography (HRCT) scans provide a more precise picture of interstitial lung disease patterns and can identify the presence of granulomas, which is typical of sarcoidosis. Furthermore, serum biomarkers such as angiotensin-converting enzyme levels may also establish the diagnosis, albeit not specific in isolation. Collectively, these approaches enhance the diagnostic specificity of sarcoidosis and differentiate it from pulmonary vasculitis and other interstitial lung diseases (Antoniou et al., 2009). For pulmonary vasculitides, i.e., GPA, the diagnosis is also multifactorial. Diagnosis typically involves a combination of clinical evaluation, laboratory examinations, and histopathological examinations. The detection of ANCA is a significant serological marker of GPA and aids in the diagnosis with clinical presentation. Histology of tissue biopsy can further define the disease by proving necrotizing granulomatous inflammation. Treatment consists of a multidisciplinary team of specialists from various specialties such as rheumatology, pulmonary medicine, and otorhinolaryngology. This fusion offers comprehensive care, whereby early diagnosis and treatment are crucial in averting severe complications that accompany pulmonary vasculitis (Vincentiis et al., 2016). An early and precise diagnosis of sarcoidosis and pulmonary vasculitides is crucial due to their similarity in clinical presentation and potential for high morbidity. Differential diagnosis between them depends on the identification of their unique diagnostic markers and clinical images. Continuing technical improvements of imaging modalities and laboratory studies enhance our ability to differentiate sarcoidosis from pulmonary vasculitis forms, and therefore optimally guide patient management. Continuing research into pathogenic processes of these diseases also emphasizes the need for more discriminating diagnostic criteria that acknowledge such subtleties. With our growing knowledge, good diagnostic criteria and methods remain essential for clinicians to institute timely and specific therapies to maximize patient survival and quality of life (Antoniou et al., 2009; Vincentiis et al., 2016) (Figure 5.8).

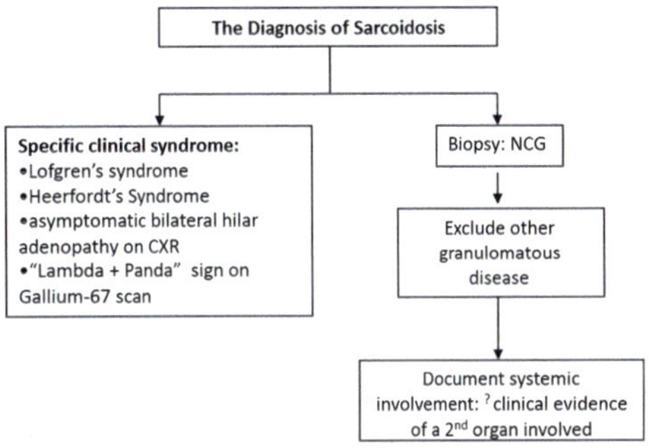

Figure 5.8. Diagnostic criteria and methods of sarcoidosis.

Source: https://www.researchgate.net/publication/267933310/figure/fig1/AS:601767075147785@1520483859476/The-diagnostic-algorithm-for-sarcoidosis.png.

5.2.3. Staging and Classification of the Disease

The staging and classification of conditions like sarcoidosis and pulmonary vasculitides assist in identifying useful treatment regimens and predicting patient outcomes. Disease classification systems create a framework for describing disease severity and the extent of presentation. In sarcoidosis, the Löfgren syndrome is an acute presentation that has a particular prognosis and symptom complex in relation to the chronic presentations that can appear with pulmonary fibrosis and continued lung injury. Accurate staging, often necessitated by high-resolution computed tomography (HRCT), enables the clinician to identify disease progression and modify management. New methods, including lung ultrasound (LUS), hold the promise of associating with established imaging methods and providing prospective and non-invasive assessments of disease severity and activity, and thus enhancing the general classification systems (Amoroso et al., 2015). For pulmonary vasculitides, and for GPA in particular, staging of disease requires imaging and clinical measures to establish disease activity. Assessment of aortic inflammation by PET scans also better characterizes cardiovascular manifestations of GPA and other vasculitides. This imaging technique, which measures aortic FDG uptake quantitatively, has high variability among differing states of disease. For instance, GPA patients have higher uptake levels than healthy controls, which also corresponds to systemic involvement and the severity of the disease. Vasculitides classification also includes renal involvement markers, which require focus in monitoring symptoms that could portend worsening in disease states (Bucerius et al., 2015). The interplay of different classification systems and staging methods mirrors the sophisticated nature of the diagnosis and treatment of sarcoidosis and pulmonary vasculitides. With new evidence revealing novel diagnostic variables and imaging methods, doctors are increasingly faced with integrating these findings into prevailing paradigms. Early detection and precise staging emphasis represents an important factor for preventing irreversible organ damage and optimizing therapeutic impact. Furthermore, recent studies aim to harmonize classification standards across various environments, benefiting the homogeneity of treatment modalities and easing interoperability among clinical practitioners. These advancements eventually work towards an individualized and targeted approach to such complex diseases, which improves quality of care for the concerned patients (Figure 5.9).

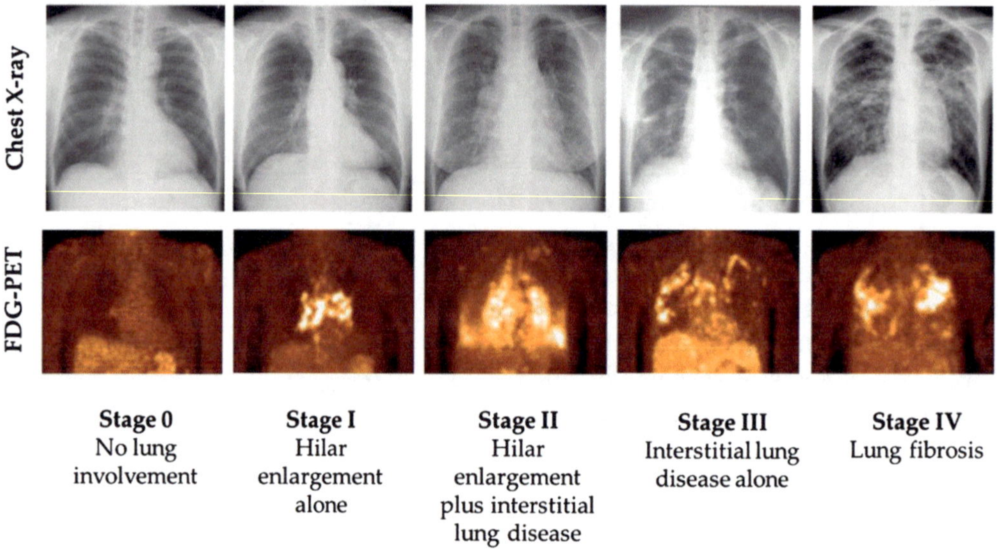

Figure 5.9. Staging and classification of the disease of sarcoidosis.

Source: https://pub.mdpi-res.com/medicina/medicina-61-00342/article_deploy/html/images/medicina-61-00342-g003.png?1739785951.

Test Your Knowledge

1. What are the common symptoms and signs of sarcoidosis?
2. What are the staging and classification of the disease?

5.3. Treatment Options for Sarcoidosis

Learning Outcome

1. Pharmacological interventions
2. Role of corticosteroids
3. Emerging therapies and clinical trials

The treatment of sarcoidosis is primarily based on the severity of the disease and its impact on organ function. Where sarcoidosis is asymptomatic or mildly symptomatic, watchful waiting is the policy of choice, which may result in spontaneous resolution without therapy. Where significant symptoms or organ impairment exist, glucocorticoids remain the first line in treatment. These corticosteroids cannot only reduce inflammation and suppress the immune response but also relieve underlying symptoms without causing further injury to target organs. When the disease becomes more severe and glucocorticoids fail or cannot be used because of their intolerable side effects, other immunosuppressive medications, such as methotrexate or azathioprine, may be employed to manage the disease with minimal side effects. Comorbidity also needs to be treated in sarcoidosis, particularly when pulmonary involvement occurs. Recent evidence indicates that the confluence of sarcoidosis with the pulmonary vasculitides can make management plans more complex.

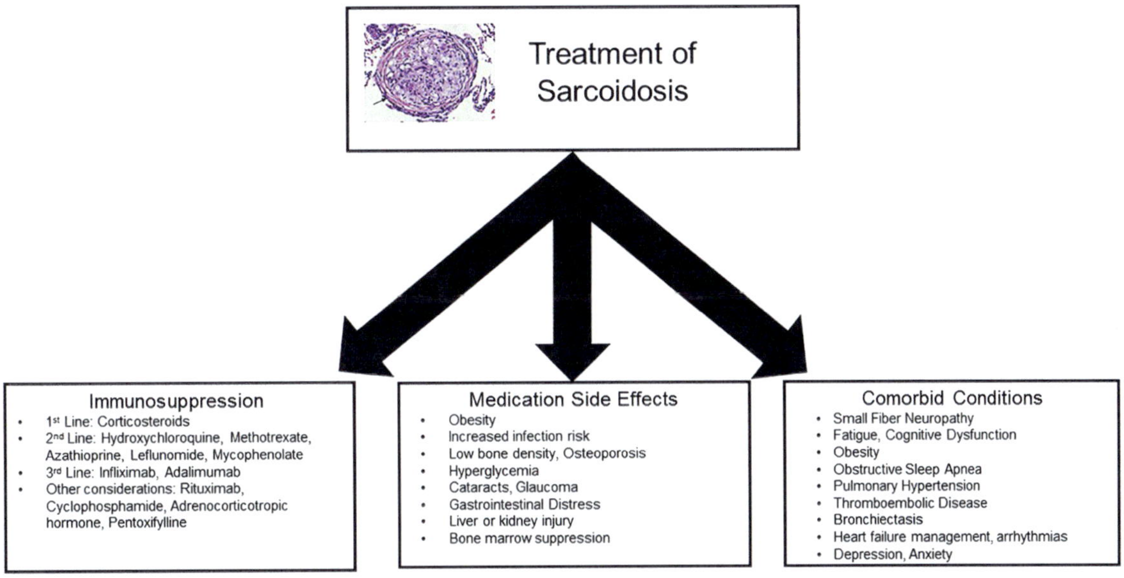

Figure 5.10. Treatment options for sarcoidosis.

Source: https://www.frontiersin.org/files/Articles/545413/fimmu-11-545413-HTML-r1/image_m/fimmu-11-545413-g002.jpg.

For instance, the development of ANCA-associated vasculitis, such as GPA or microscopic polyangiitis (MPA), requires a combined management plan for both sarcoidosis and its vascular component. Patients with interstitial lung disease (ILD) due to ANCA-associated vasculitis generally require specific treatment modalities, since these diseases have a direct effect on respiratory status and quality of life. A sensitive assessment of these two impairments makes it possible to develop a multiple-faceted treatment plan to improve patient outcomes (Cassone et al., 2020). Because sarcoidosis and its management are complex, clinical practice guidelines recommend an individualized approach. Therapeutic decisions need to be made in the context of the individual patient's clinical findings, organ system involvement, and overall health status, as well as anticipated complications. Immunosuppressive therapies, while potentially helpful, are more risky and involve a delicate balance between control of disease and avoidance of side effects. Close observation is necessary to maximize therapeutic approaches, particularly in at-risk individuals for pulmonary fibrosis or other complications. An effective management plan is also coupled with patient education, in which patients are informed about the nature of their condition and the need to comply with prescribed interventions. Such harmonious interaction between patients and healthcare practitioners is important in establishing improvement in quality of life and sustained control of disease (Dörner et al., 2007) (Figure 5.10).

5.3.1. Pharmacological Interventions

Pharmacotherapy of sarcoidosis and pulmonary vasculitides is essential in the management of disease activity and symptom relief. Corticosteroids, such as prednisone, have been the cornerstone of treatment for sarcoidosis due to their very effective anti-inflammatory properties. Corticosteroids exert their action by suppressing the immune system, thereby inhibiting granuloma formation and inflammation in the lungs. Nevertheless, long-term corticosteroid therapy is generally limited by significant side effects, necessitating alternative forms of treatment. Recent studies have established that steroid-sparing drugs, such as methotrexate and azathioprine, can potentially provide efficacy in the management of sarcoidosis with less corticosteroid exposure. Furthermore, interprofessional models that adopt a multidisciplinary discussion (MDD) approach have provided increased diagnostic yield and treatment plans, facilitating personalized pharmacologic strategies through patient-specific profiles (Khalifa et al., 2022). In pulmonary vasculitides, a broader range of pharmacologic agents are employed, such as biologics and immunosuppressants. Immunotherapies like rituximab and tocilizumab target specific components of the immune system and have been shown to be effective in conditions like GPA (Wegeners granulomatosis). Both function to inhibit the actions of B-cells and pro-inflammatory cytokines, respectively, thereby reducing vascular inflammation and damage. Disease-modifying antirheumatic drugs (DMARDs) are also employed for the therapy of underlying autoimmune processes in pulmonary vasculitides. This multifaceted treatment emphasizes personalized medicine, where pharmacologic treatments are appropriately selected based on patient-specific parameters, including disease severity and prior treatment response. The ability to tailor these interventions carries broad implications for long-term patient benefit. Examining the function of complement systems in sarcoidosis and pulmonary vasculitides offers additional therapeutic options for pharmacological treatment. Dysregulation of the complement system has been recognized as an important aspect of autoimmune-inflammatory lung diseases, and evidence exists that it contributes to inflammation and fibrosis. Complement system-targeting therapies may also be employed as adjuvant therapy alongside standard therapy. New therapies, such as complement inhibitors, have the potential to provide new strategies for managing complex pulmonary diseases, particularly in those patients not responsive to conventional therapies. For instance, evidence pointing towards the activation of complement systems with interstitial lung disease (ILD) enables the identification of new therapy avenues that balance pharmacological intervention with current research outcomes (Chimenti et al., 2023). Through investigating such innovative therapies, clinicians are able to provide improved management options for patients with sarcoidosis and pulmonary vasculitides, hopefully improving health-related quality of life (Figure 5.11).

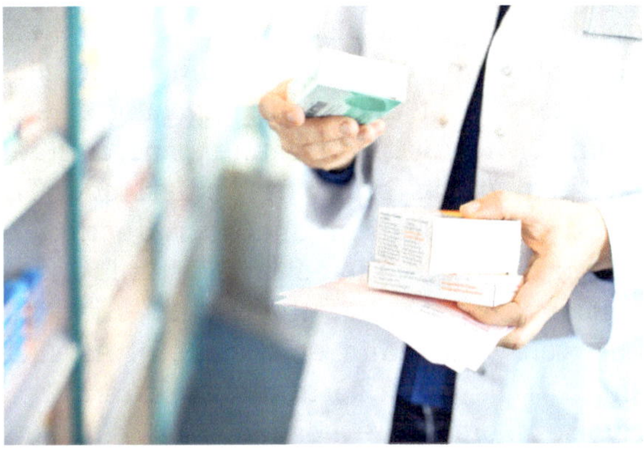

Figure 5.11. Pharmacological interventions for sarcoidosis.

Source: https://www.stopsarcoidosis.org/wp-content/uploads/iStock-537309906.jpg.

5.3.2. Role of Corticosteroids

Corticosteroids form the cornerstone of therapy for sarcoidosis and the pulmonary vasculitides due to their potent anti-inflammatory effect. Corticosteroids are the first choice of treatment in sarcoidosis when the disease causes marked pulmonary symptoms or organ damage. Corticosteroids exert their effect by regulating gene expression to suppress inflammatory cytokines, thus reducing granuloma formation and regulating the immune response. While useful, chronic corticosteroid therapy must be weighed against potential side effects, including osteoporosis, diabetes, and susceptibility to infection. Corticosteroid therapy has been shown in clinical trials to benefit symptoms and function in the lung. Still, careful regulation of dosages must be achieved to prevent risk, particularly in patients prone to pulmonary complications or underlying disease. In the pulmonary vasculitides, particularly the GPA, corticosteroids are pivotal in inducing disease remission. The standard therapeutic regimen is usually a combination of glucocorticoids and other immunosuppressants, i.e., cyclophosphamide. Not only do the two target the acute inflammatory response processes that cause tissue damage, but they also significantly improve the prognosis for individuals. The additive effect of corticosteroids abolishes the perilous presentation of vasculitis in the form of lung and renal damage, resulting in morbidity and mortality. Increasing evidence supports conservative titration of corticosteroid dosage in both induction and maintenance therapy to effectively treat the illness while avoiding excessive side effects. Their addition to the therapeutic arsenal is a testimony to their crucial role in determining outcomes in pulmonary vasculitides. While useful, corticosteroids are to be employed with regard to long-term effects and the risk of eventual requirement for alternative modalities. In those individuals who experience an adverse effect or do not respond favorably to standard corticosteroid therapy, the creation of drugs such as mycophenolate mofetil (MMF) represents a worthwhile alternative. MMF, which has fewer side effects compared to cyclophosphamide, is a suitable option for the management of interstitial lung disease caused by rheumatologic diseases and may be administered in combination with corticosteroids in a bid to maximize therapeutic efficacy. While its application in rheumatoid disease-related interstitial lung disease remains based on scarce evidence, its utilization marks an evolving strategy for pulmonary disease management. With the evolving disease field, further research must be carried out to optimize corticosteroid use and explore adjunct therapies to improve patient outcomes in sarcoidosis and vasculitides.

5.3.3. Emerging Therapies and Clinical Trials

New treatments and ongoing clinical trials are a significant field in the treatment of sarcoidosis and pulmonary vasculitides, especially considering the issues implied by these diseases. Standard treatment is often predicated on corticosteroids; however, there exists an acute need for more targeted treatments aimed at the processes of pathophysiology without the debilitating side effects of chronic steroid use. Present clinical trials have compared several immunomodulatory agents and biologic agents that may decrease inflammation and fibrosis. These advances not only have the potential for improved patient outcomes but also promise to enhance the quality of life for patients with chronic respiratory symptoms. With the advancement of science, it is essential that physicians stay abreast of these developments to create treatment regimens based on the latest information about therapy efficacy and patient response to new treatments. Cures like the monoclonal antibodies and small-molecule inhibitors are on the verge of becoming leading players in the therapy of pulmonary diseases, e.g., sarcoidosis and pulmonary vasculitides. For instance, the effectiveness of new systemic hormonal and cytotoxic treatments, as well as radiotherapy, has been documented in the case of pulmonary carcinoid tumors, which points to the potential of similar approaches in treating sarcoidosis (Danielle et al., 2025). In addition, the creation of inhaled formulations, especially treprostinil, has revolutionized treatment for pulmonary hypertension in association with interstitial lung diseases (PH-ILDs) (Genecand et al., 2025). Following the total evaluation of patients, multimodality management remains central, as novel treatments are subject to increasingly detailed evaluation of their appropriateness and efficacy relative to specific patient factors and disease severity. Given the evolving nature of both the treatment of sarcoidosis and pulmonary vasculitides, clinical trials are an important way of demonstrating new treatments. These experiments not only establish the efficacy and safety of potential drugs but also examine the optimal administration routes and dosing schedules. The interplay of the underlying lung disease with newly introduced treatments necessitates that their effects be clearly understood. The relentless innovation and introduction of treatments, e.g., inhaled treprostinil, enable clinicians to maximize therapeutic strategies effectively (Genecand et al., 2025). As such, clinical trials continue to move forward, they promise an era where individualized treatments can lead to better symptom control, a reduction in exacerbations, and overall better patient health with the presence of complex pulmonary diseases (Figure 5.12).

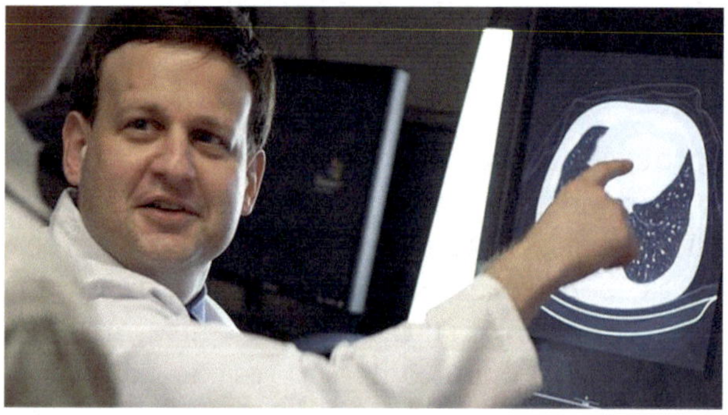

Figure 5.12. Emerging therapies and clinical trials for sarcoidosis.

Source: https://www.mountsinai.org/files/MSHealth/Assets/HS/Locations/Respiratory-Institute/MSHS-NJRI-Respiratory-Sarcoidosis-2col-770x420.jpg.

Test Your Knowledge

1. What are the pharmacological interventions of sarcoidosis?
2. What is the role of corticosteroids?

5.4. Overview of Pulmonary Vasculitides

Learning Outcome

1. Definition and types of pulmonary vasculitides
2. Pathophysiological mechanisms involved
3. Risk factors and epidemiology

The spectrum of pulmonary vasculitides refers to a heterogenous group of diseases causing inflammation of blood vessels within the lung. They may affect both medium and large vessels and have serious morbidity unless properly diagnosed and managed. With ongoing research, particularly in imaging, the range of presentations of these diseases is better known. For instance, conditions previously identified as classic large vessel vasculitis, such as giant cell arteritis, may have characteristic intracranial disease, illustrating the diversity and complexity of pulmonary vasculitides. The progressive refinement of disease definitions has led to more conditions being identified within this category, underscoring the necessity for a comprehensive diagnostic approach involving clinical history and imaging features (Lötscher et al., 2022).

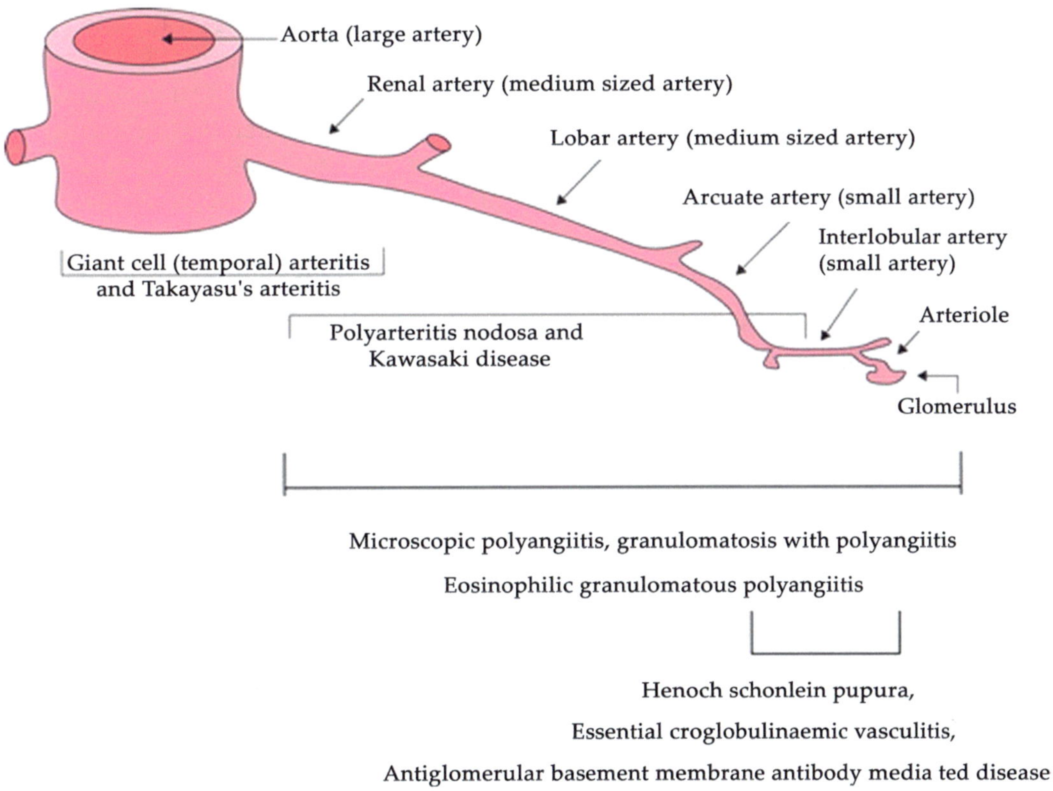

Figure 5.13. Overview of pulmonary vasculitides.

Source: https://www.tandfonline.com/cms/asset/c31e5cb2-9354-4729-91c1-e18e4317e804/iedg_a_697895_f0001_b.jpg.

Differential diagnosis is critical in diagnosing pulmonary vasculitides because pulmonary vasculitides and other lung diseases share similar clinical presentations. It can be challenging to differentiate pulmonary vasculitis from diffuse parenchymal lung diseases (DPLD) as both conditions involve inflammation of the lungs. It requires a complex process with scrupulous attention to clinical history and assessment. In acute cases, such as diffuse alveolar hemorrhage, rapid assessment is necessary to implement early interventions. Chronic ones, on the other hand, will allow for more conservative measures in an outpatient setting. The heterogeneity of clinical presentations requires clinicians to remain vigilant and reactive in their diagnostic strategy to entertain all the potential causes of pulmonary symptoms (Chairman et al., 2019). Furthermore, clinicians need to understand the pathophysiology of sarcoidosis and pulmonary vasculitides' interaction. Sarcoidosis itself might masquerade or coexist with other pulmonary vasculitides, making the clinical presentation confused. Both diseases might present with overlapping symptomatology, such as respiratory impairment and chronic cough, making it imperative to evaluate them to rule out one from the other thoroughly. In certain instances, sarcoidosis might cause inflammation in the vasculature, resulting in a diagnosis of primary pulmonary vasculitis. This highlights the need for an interdisciplinary approach, through concerted action by pulmonologists, rheumatologists, and radiologists, to untangle the complex nature of such diseases. With evolving diagnostic technologies, the ability to properly diagnose and treat pulmonary vasculitides and their overlap with conditions such as sarcoidosis will continue to grow, ultimately resulting in improved patient outcomes in this vexing area of medicine (Figure 5.13).

5.4.1. Definition and Types of Pulmonary Vasculitides

Pulmonary vasculitides are a heterogeneous group of disorders characterized by inflammation of the lung vessels and potentially with severe morbidity and mortality if untreated. They are typically divided based on the size of the vessels that are involved, which may be large, medium, and small, and due to a wide range of underlying etiologies, including systemic autoimmune diseases as well as infections. Knowing the term pulmonary vasculitides is necessary to make an accurate diagnosis and appropriate treatment. Notably, their multifactorial etiology is compounded by frequent overlap with other inflammatory disorders. Therefore, they must be carefully evaluated and differentially diagnosed to distinguish them from numerous mimics with concomitant respiratory symptoms (Lötscher et al., 2022). Of the pulmonary vasculitides, the most frequent are GPA, eosinophilic granulomatosis with polyangiitis (EGPA), and microscopic polyangiitis (MPA). The small-vessel vasculitides are particularly significant because they directly impact the pulmonary system, leading to complications such as interstitial lung disease and alveolar hemorrhage. Giant cell arteritis (GCA), a large-vessel vasculitis, may also impact pulmonary structures, but it does so less so. A nuanced recognition of these categories is able to facilitate clinicians in recognizing symptom patterns and guide necessary imaging and laboratory tests towards an effective treatment strategy that may include immunosuppressive therapies (Albano et al., 2021). The contribution of advanced imaging modalities to the assessment of pulmonary vasculitides cannot be overestimated. New imaging technology advances, such as PET/CT scans, have improved significantly detection and characterization of vasculitic processes in the lung. This is particularly important because classic histopathologic confirmation is not always available. The improvement in imaging accuracy has enabled the description of new disease manifestations, necessitating updated information about pulmonary vasculitides. With increasingly sophisticated differential diagnosis, as highlighted by modern literature, an interdisciplinary process of imaging, histopathology, and clinical correlation is required to optimize patient care in the context of pulmonary involvement in sarcoidosis and other vasculitides (Lötscher et al., 2022).

5.4.2. Pathophysiological Mechanisms Involved

The pathophysiologic mechanisms of pulmonary vasculitides and sarcoidosis are multifactorial and complex, with a component of immune dysregulation and genetic predisposition. Sarcoidosis is characterized by the development of non-caseating granulomas, which is triggered by an inappropriate immune reaction to as-yet-unknown antigens. The ensuing inappropriate immune response leads to the deposition of immune cells, namely macrophages and T lymphocytes, resulting in inflammation and tissue injury in the lungs. The role of cytokines and chemokines in the process cannot be overstated, as they are the ones that recruit and activate inflammatory cells. Moreover, recent research has shown that the complement system can also play an important role in sarcoidosis, with implications for both innate and adaptive immunity, which aids in driving the disease (Chimenti et al., 2023).

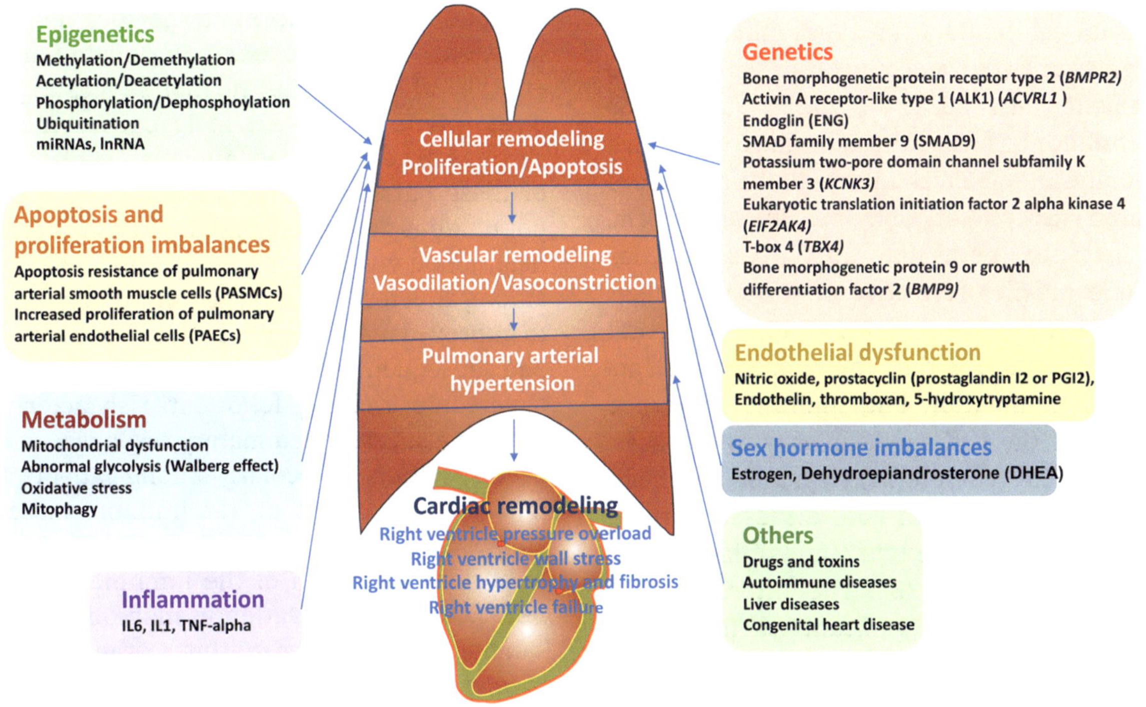

Figure 5.14. The pathophysiological mechanisms underlying pulmonary vasculitides.

Source: https://external-content.duckduckgo.com/iu/?u=https%3A%2F%2Fwww.researchgate.net%2Fpublication%2F357829931%2Ffigure%2Ffig1%2FAS%3A1114586170306560%401642749459596%2FMajor-pathophysiological-mechanisms-that-lead-to-vascular-remodeling-increased-pulmonary.png&f=1&nofb=1&ipt=7c4ef3636ff31abf7c25d4f656c8ba658590845670e2fb2b5c68508e55ce572a.

An understanding of such mechanisms is crucial, as they are the basis of targeted therapy aimed at modulating the immune response and controlling systemic manifestations. Pulmonary vasculitis, by contrast, is a heterogeneous group of disorders that lead to inflammation of the blood vessels of the lungs. It can be secondary to systemic vasculitis syndromes, such as GPA or

Microscopic Polyangiitis, which share the exact underlying pathophysiologic mechanisms. At the core of these illnesses is the production of autoantibodies, specifically anti-neutrophil cytoplasmic antibodies (ANCA), which are associated with neutrophil stimulation and consequent vascular injury. The resulting oxidative stress and inflammatory cascade lead to pulmonary hemorrhage, lung parenchymal damage, and respiratory failure. Similar to sarcoidosis, dysregulation of the immune system is a unifying theme in these diseases. Previous work has cited the role of cytokines in the vasculitic process, underscoring the potential for modulating these inflammatory processes as a source of new targets for effective treatment (Cassone et al., 2021). Sarcoidosis and pulmonary vasculitides share standard pathophysiologic mechanisms that underscore a shared susceptibility of the respiratory system. For instance, both may encompass similar immune profiles reflective of host responses that have been dysregulated to environmental stimuli. This means that common mechanisms within inflammation and immune tolerance can lead to the pathogenesis of both diseases. Moreover, the complement system has been found to play a part in both diseases, serving as an effector of tissue injury and inflammation (Chimenti et al., 2023). The interaction of the two diseases is significant when creating effective treatment strategies. For instance, the use of immunosuppressive therapies such as mycophenolate mofetil has been examined in sarcoidosis and inflammatory lung diseases, suggesting a corresponding pathological paradigm (Cassone et al., 2021). Through research into such connections, clinicians and researchers can better organize treatment interventions and improve patient outcomes in patients afflicted with these complex respiratory diseases (Figure 5.14).

5.4.3. Risk Factors and Epidemiology

The epidemiology of sarcoidosis also shows significant variation between various populations, and thus age, sex, and ethnicity emerge as the key factors. Sarcoidosis predominantly affects individuals in the 20-40 years age bracket and is found to be more prevalent among women compared to men. Ethnically, the impact is disproportionately felt by African Americans, and the reported incidence rates in them are three to ten times the rate in Caucasians, suggesting a possible genetic predisposition to the development of this disease. Environmental toxins, including occupational risk factors and specific geographic locations, have also been implicated in the etiology of sarcoidosis, further suggesting that both intrinsic and extrinsic causes may be responsible for its development. Identification of these patterns assists in the recognition of populations at risk and emphasizes the need for heightened vigilance, screening, and awareness among affected communities, ultimately leading to improved management choices for sarcoidosis and subsequent complications. The pathogenesis of sarcoidosis closely follows its risk factors and induces a severe inflammatory response. Genetic predisposition, particularly among patients with family backgrounds of autoimmune diseases, suggests the influence of heritable factors. Abnormal activation of the immune system is reflected in the activation of macrophages and T helper (Th) cells, resulting in the formation of a granuloma, which defines the disease. Environmental exposures such as silica dust, mold, and certain infectious pathogens have also been associated with the etiology of sarcoidosis. Indeed, some occupational environments have been implicated in increasing the risk for developing sarcoidosis and thereby highlighting the contribution of both genes and environmental interactions to its pathogenesis. Therefore, identification of such factors can improve early diagnosis and specific intervention, ultimately affecting patient outcomes and management of complications of both pulmonary vasculitides and sarcoidosis. Additionally, comorbid conditions also impact the epidemiological pattern of sarcoidosis, which can aggravate its clinical course as well as complicate its treatment. Specifically, persons who already suffer from respiratory illnesses, including asthma or chronic obstructive pulmonary disease (COPD), will experience augmented morbidity due to superimposed inflammation and symptoms. Differential diagnosis can thus be extremely challenging and necessitates rigorous methods utilizing multidisciplinary teams in order to provide optimal patient care. Moreover, the psychosocial healing from the sickness of developing sarcoidosis also cannot be overlooked because chronic disease is known to lead to psychological distress and fatigue on top of making disease treatment more complex. Current literature emphasizes the importance of valuing the comorbidities and their influence over the course of the disease to support an integrated way of treating patients that includes both physical and psychological factors. Thus, integrating an understanding of risk factor interactions with epidemiological patterns into clinical practice promises to improve the management of sarcoidosis and pulmonary vasculitides in the future.

Test Your Knowledge

1. What are the types of pulmonary vasculitides?
2. Illustrate the Pathophysiological mechanisms involved in pulmonary vasculitides?

5.5. Clinical Manifestations of Pulmonary Vasculitides

Learning Outcome

1. Symptoms specific to pulmonary involvement
2. Diagnostic approaches and imaging techniques
3. Differentiating from other pulmonary diseases

Pulmonary vasculitides are a collection of diseases characterized by inflammatory injury to vessels that leads to robust clinical features, particularly in lung tissue. The manifestations of such a disease can be very heterogeneous and tend to be associated with systemic symptoms such as fever, malaise, and weight loss. Cough, hemoptysis, and dyspnea are common respiratory manifestations, particularly. These symptoms can result from the direct implication of pulmonary parenchyma and bronchi, leading to complications like pulmonary hemorrhage or interstitial lung disease. Awareness of the severity of these manifestations is crucial for facilitating timely diagnosis, as early treatment will significantly improve outcomes in these patients. Imaging modalities, such as computed tomography, play an increasingly critical role in the diagnosis of structural changes associated with pulmonary vasculitides, hence enhancing differential diagnostic accuracy (Lötscher et al., 2022). GPA is a well-documented subset of pulmonary vasculitis with well-defined and characteristic clinical features. Upper and lower respiratory tract manifestations develop typically in patients with GPA and should be carefully evaluated clinically. Notably, the disease may manifest nasally as septal perforation due to necrotizing granulomatous inflammation of the nasal cartilage. The other pulmonary manifestations are hemoptysis and chronic cough due to necrotizing granulomas of lung tissue. In practice, identification of the manifestations, followed by serological assessment for anti-neutrophil cytoplasmic antibodies (ANCA), is essential for proper diagnosis (D'aguanno et al., 2018). Overall, understanding the specific clinical manifestations of GPA is important to the development of optimal treatment protocols that minimize morbidity and potential mortality. Beyond GPA, other etiologies of pulmonary vasculitis are relevant in clinical practice. Microscopic polyangiitis and EGPA represent entities that might share overlapping respiratory symptomatology but can vary widely in terms of pathophysiology and treatment approaches. The complexity of diagnosis of these disparate patterns of pulmonary vasculitis is further compounded by the potential for similar clinical presentations of other disease conditions, necessitating a cautious differential diagnosis. The presence of advanced imaging modalities and more sensitive laboratory tests has enhanced the capability to properly distinguish between vasculitides. Besides, the production of novel disease paradigms, together with uncovering disease imitators, demonstrates the importance of ongoing research and new clinical practice recommendations in this ever-evolving field of research (Lötscher et al., 2022) (Figure 5.15).

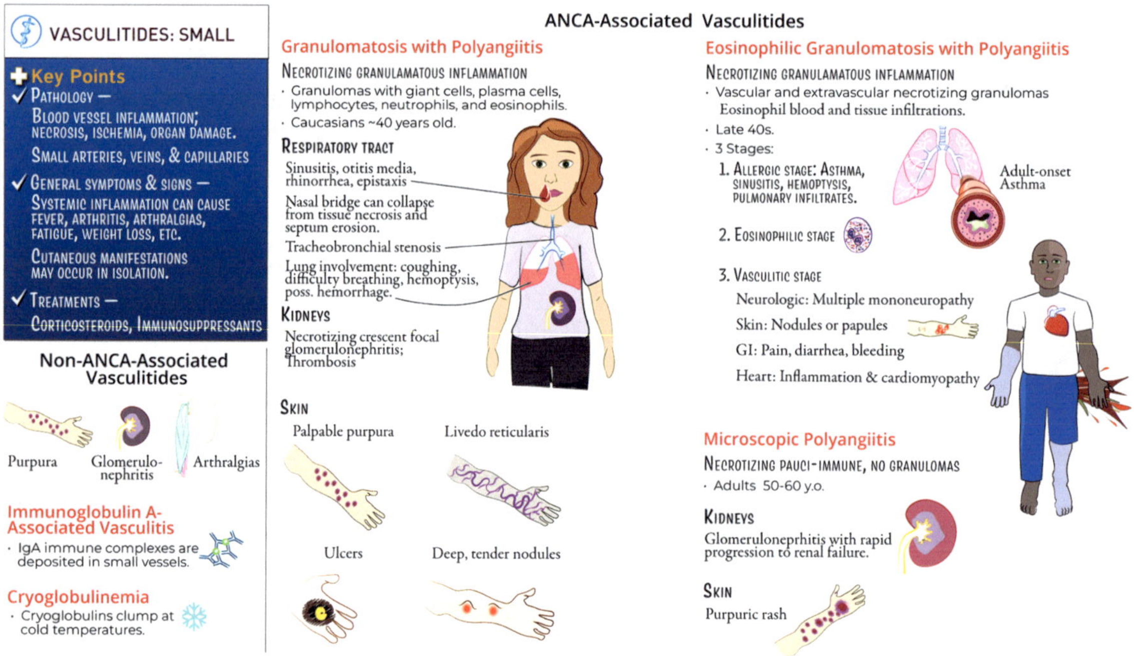

Figure 5.15. Clinical manifestations of pulmonary vasculitides.

Source: https://external-content.duckduckgo.com/iu/?u=https%3A%2F%2Fd1j63owfs0b5j3.cloudfront.net%2Ftutorial%2FfinalImage%2F1639-1689361231230.png&f=1&nofb=1&ipt=efd0251d132826d4f0b5b937555211bfc884fca4c2ce37428b698b7c15792a0f.

5.5.1. Symptoms Specific to Pulmonary Involvement

The respiratory symptoms of sarcoidosis are heterogeneous and play an important role in patient morbidity and mortality. The presentation tends to be insidious, with patients presenting with non-specific respiratory symptoms such as a persistent cough or shortness of breath. As the disease advances, these complaints become more severe, manifesting as wheezing, chest pain, and in severe cases, respiratory failure. The presence of granulomas in the interstitium of the lungs can interfere with lung function, leading to both obstructive and restrictive patterns of lung disease.

In addition, pulmonary sarcoidosis leads to pulmonary fibrosis that enhances the severity of the symptoms and makes treatment more difficult. Early recognition of these types of clinical findings is significant because it may lead to further diagnostic workup, including imaging studies and pulmonary function tests, to determine the extent of lung involvement in sarcoidosis and ultimately guide treatment and patient outcomes. Symptoms in pulmonary vasculitides are more definite and typically mark a more severe course of disease. Conditions such as GPA are defined by a characteristic constellation of pulmonary findings that consist of pleuritic chest pain, hemoptysis, and cough. They are caused by necrotizing granulomatous inflammation that degrades airway integrity, leading to profound respiratory distress. Notably, pulmonary vasculature involvement can also lead to pulmonary hemorrhage, an acute life-threatening complication. In addition, patients may present with concomitant systemic inflammatory signs, such as fever, weight loss, and asthenia, which complicate the clinical presentation. Early identification and differential diagnosis of such symptoms are essential as they decide immediate measures, subsequent to immunosuppressive therapy, and the involvement of multidisciplinary teams for the optimal management of GPA and pulmonary vasculitides. Moreover, the interaction of sarcoidosis with pulmonary vasculitides contributes to the complexity of the process of diagnosing pulmonary involvement. Overlapping presenting features in both entities complicate differential diagnosis. Both entities cause cough and dyspnea, thus complicating clinical diagnosis. Moreover, serious dangers are associated with misdiagnosis of the two disorders, particularly because therapeutic regimens differ substantially; while the treatment of sarcoidosis can be responsive to glucocorticoids as well as disease-modifying agents, such vasculitides as GPA require intense immunosuppressive therapy. The synergy of high-tech imaging modalities and laboratory markers, highlighted by recent research, is pivotal in specifying the specific vascular involvement in such diseases, paving the way towards certain therapeutic interventions which target the individualized pulmonary participation pathophysiology in each disease (Vincentiis et al., 2016; Lötscher et al., 2022) (Figure 5.16).

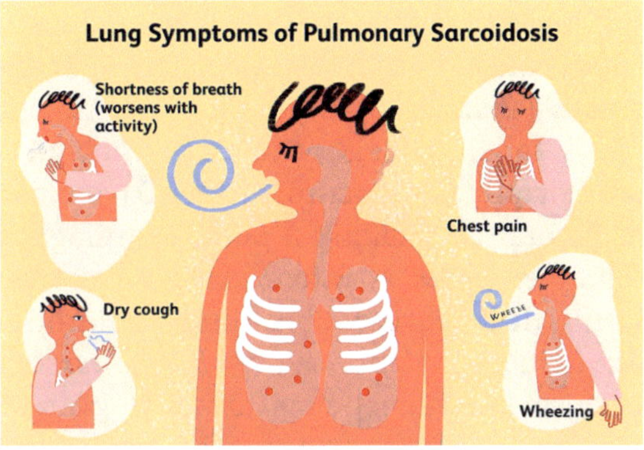

Figure 5.16. Symptoms specific to pulmonary involvement.

Source: https://external-content.duckduckgo.com/iu/?u=https%3A%2F%2Fwww.verywellhealth.com%2Fthmb%2FY-isA-2wutbZBN7oHaZwbl8rDTM%3D%2F1500x0%2Ffilters%3Ano_upscale()%3Amax_bytes(150000)%3Astrip_icc()%2FSarcoidosis-overview-5097521_final-5958ff0e0b2d4528a4f4602bd09a8ccb.jpg&f=1&nofb=1&ipt=038e9f7fe5e91321f00c75429583e4ee5b5635d39fd6cc25e2f87e05722ff7ef.

5.5.2. Diagnostic Approaches and Imaging Techniques

In sarcoidosis and pulmonary vasculitides, imaging modalities play a crucial role in diagnosing the presence and extent of inflammatory disease within the lungs. Chest radiography and CT scanning are established in this use because they provide visual data regarding pulmonary anatomy and can identify characteristic disease patterns for these conditions, such as hilar lymphadenopathy and interstitial infiltrates. Furthermore, advances in diagnostic imaging, namely the use of 18F-fluorodeoxyglucose ([F-18] FDG) positron emission tomography/computed tomography (PET/CT), have dramatically enhanced diagnostic precision. This technology enables clinicians to assess metabolic changes indicative of inflammation, thus to better discriminate between sarcoidosis and infectious diseases as outlined in recent consensus guidelines for its application in inflammatory and infectious diseases (Albano et al., 2021). While imaging is key to diagnosis, the contribution of multidisciplinary discussion (MDD) teams is also pivotal for making a definitive diagnosis in complex cases of interstitial lung diseases (ILDs) like sarcoidosis and pulmonary vasculitides. MDDs typically consist of specialists like pulmonologists, radiologists, and histopathologists who are seated together and review clinical presentations alongside imaging reports. Based on the data analysis, a considerable percentage of patients in MDDs receive definitive diagnoses, reaffirming the importance of this combined process. Even in cases where images are nonspecific, further suggestions can be given regarding diagnostic tests like bronchoscopy or tissue biopsy (Khalifa et al., 2022). By this integrated evaluation process, patients receive precise diagnoses and corresponding treatment plans, enhancing outcomes. Furthermore, the evolving imaging technology environment necessitates constant continuing professional education and standardization of practice. Well-defined guidelines on the use of [F-18] FDG PET/CT and ancillary devices are essential to maximizing their efficiency in the diagnosis of inflammatory disease, as highlighted in the Italian Association of Nuclear Medicine consensus. Standardized protocols apply across various areas, from patient preparation to image acquisition and interpretative criteria. These methods assist in minimizing potential pitfalls and discrepancies during the diagnostic process. Lastly, technological development of imaging modalities, combined with a systemized approach to interpretation and consensus diagnosis via MDDs, significantly enhances the capability to differentiate sarcoidosis and pulmonary vasculitides from other diseases, making it possible to develop effective treatment strategies (Figure 5.17).

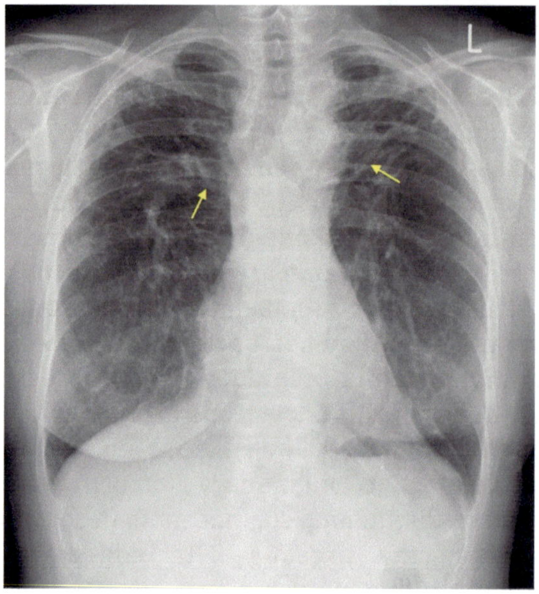

Figure 5.17. Imaging technique for sarcoidosis.

Source: https://external-content.duckduckgo.com/iu/?u=http%3A%2F%2Fwww.svuhradiology.ie%2Fwp-content%2Fuploads%2F2015%2F04%2FSarcoidFibrosis.jpg&f=1&nofb=1&ipt=eca9fcc590f8fdaa84196f9715c402a9b98ef39db6dbfa47b6a1d35364b1b492.

5.5.3. Differentiating from Other Pulmonary Diseases

Sarcoidosis must be differentiated from other pulmonary illnesses of utmost concern during the proper diagnosis and treatment. The illness may imitate the clinical picture of other interstitial lung diseases, and diagnostic challenges could arise. The illness usually begins with nonspecific manifestations like dry cough and exertional dyspnea, which are as frequent in idiopathic pulmonary fibrosis or hypersensitivity pneumonitis. A careful evaluation with a comprehensive patient history and physical exam must be done. More sophisticated imaging techniques, such as high-resolution computed tomography (HRCT) of the chest, are essential in establishing sarcoidosis by showing typical features, like hilar lymphadenopathy and reticular opacities, not typically present in other diseases (Pande, 2025). The mercurial nature of overlapping symptoms demands an orderly approach to minimize the differential diagnosis. Outside of imaging, histopathological examination remains a pillar in the determination of sarcoidosis from other lung conditions. The occurrence of typical non-caseating granulomas in lung biopsies is essential for diagnosing sarcoidosis, but these hallmarks can also occur in some infections or granulomatous disorders. Furthermore, bronchoscopic techniques are commonly employed to obtain tissue for histological analysis, but the yield can be limited in differentiating forms of interstitial lung disease (Pande, 2025). Sarcoidosis, being generally indolent in nature, and other more aggressive pulmonary processes need to be distinguished since they have varying prognostic predictors and treatment strategies. Therefore, clinical, radiological, and pathological data remains essential in forming an accurate diagnosis and reasonable treatment plan. The application of new imaging modalities plays a crucial role in the discrimination between sarcoidosis and other pulmonary diseases, particularly in complex cases. One such example is positron emission tomography/computed tomography (PET/CT), which has proven to be a valuable application due to its ability to detect heightened metabolic activity associated with inflammation. This imaging modality can potentially help quantify disease extent, helping clinicians define the severity of sarcoidosis relative to other inflammatory disorders, such as pulmonary vasculitis. By quantifying metabolic activity, PET/CT can potentially distinguish active sarcoidosis from other diseases that present similarly. Moreover, ongoing research on inflammatory biomarkers may serve to enhance the diagnostic specificity for sarcoidosis further and result in a clearer understanding of its pathophysiological mechanisms relative to other differential pulmonary diseases. The confluence of advanced diagnostic technology and clinical protocol undergirds the need for an integrated strategy in the management of the complexities of such pulmonary diseases.

Test Your Knowledge

1. What are the symptoms specific to pulmonary involvement?
2. What are the diagnostic approaches and imaging techniques?

5.6. Management Strategies for Pulmonary Vasculitides

Learning Outcome

1. Treatment protocols and medications
2. Importance of multidisciplinary care
3. Prognosis and long-term outcomes

Successful management of pulmonary vasculitides, particularly sarcoidosis, requires a strict strategy that balances diagnostic and therapeutic modalities. Therapeutic treatments often begin with a comprehensive assessment by clinical evaluation and imaging modalities. For instance, integrating positron emission tomography-computed tomography (PET-CT) in detecting myocardial involvement among patients with sarcoidosis can serve as a determining factor in selecting personalized immunosuppressive treatment. Moreover, treatment specific to the disease, such as corticosteroids and other immunomodulators, is important in controlling inflammation and preventing further problems. As research has evidenced, early immunosuppressive drug treatment can significantly improve patient outcomes, supporting the necessity of standardized diagnostic routes that address both pulmonary and extrapulmonary difficulties, particularly in those with cardiac manifestations of pulmonary vasculitides (Rossi et al., 2025). Understanding the pathophysiology of SAPH is key to proper management. SAPH, occurring in a high proportion of sarcoidosis, needs to be evaluated thoroughly to identify potential underlying mechanisms such as parenchymal lung disease or left ventricular dysfunction. Current guidelines emphasize the utility of right heart catheterization (RHC) as the investigation of choice for SAPH, with transthoracic echocardiography being a useful screening tool. In addition, the 6-minute walk test (6MWT) is now a significant prognostic indicator, thereby enhancing risk stratification. Treatment methods must correct reversible illness, employ pulmonary vasodilators if required, and treat complications with the use of multidisciplinary approaches. In severe disease, lung transplant is an option to consider, and it is a milestone in therapy for patients with end-stage SAPH with otherwise limited treatments (Liu et al., 2024). An interdisciplinary management with the incorporation of frequent monitoring and follow-up is important for patients with pulmonary vasculitides. Regular monitoring by clinical examination and imaging techniques allows clinicians to assess the efficacy of treatment and evaluate the necessity for adjustment of therapeutic regimens. Patient education about the disease process and compliance with treatment regimens is a significant point in maximizing patient involvement and outcomes. Further, as emerging therapies become part of routine practice, data from multi-centered randomized controlled trials will be essential in further refining management strategies for pulmonary vasculitides of sarcoidosis. A strong research agenda to unravel the intricacies of vascular complications in sarcoidosis can provide insights that optimize therapeutic protocols, leading to improved prognostic outcomes and quality of life for patients with these multifaceted disorders.

5.6.1. Treatment Protocols and Medications

Therapy for sarcoidosis and pulmonary vasculitides typically involves a multi-modal approach, depending on the severity of the disease and the symptomatology presented. First-line treatment may involve corticosteroids, which are potent at reducing inflammation and at suppressing the abnormal immune response characteristic of these diseases. For chronic or severe sarcoidosis, immunosuppressive drugs like azathioprine and methotrexate can be used to reduce the side effects of long-term corticosteroid therapy. This combination of immunosuppressants and steroids aims to balance the regulation of inflammation while minimizing side effects that significantly impact a patient's quality of life. Therefore, it is necessary to monitor the treatment response periodically and adjust protocols accordingly to achieve optimal results. Other imaging techniques such as [F-18]FDG PET/CT have also found space as valuable tools in monitoring the course of sarcoidosis and pulmonary vasculitides.

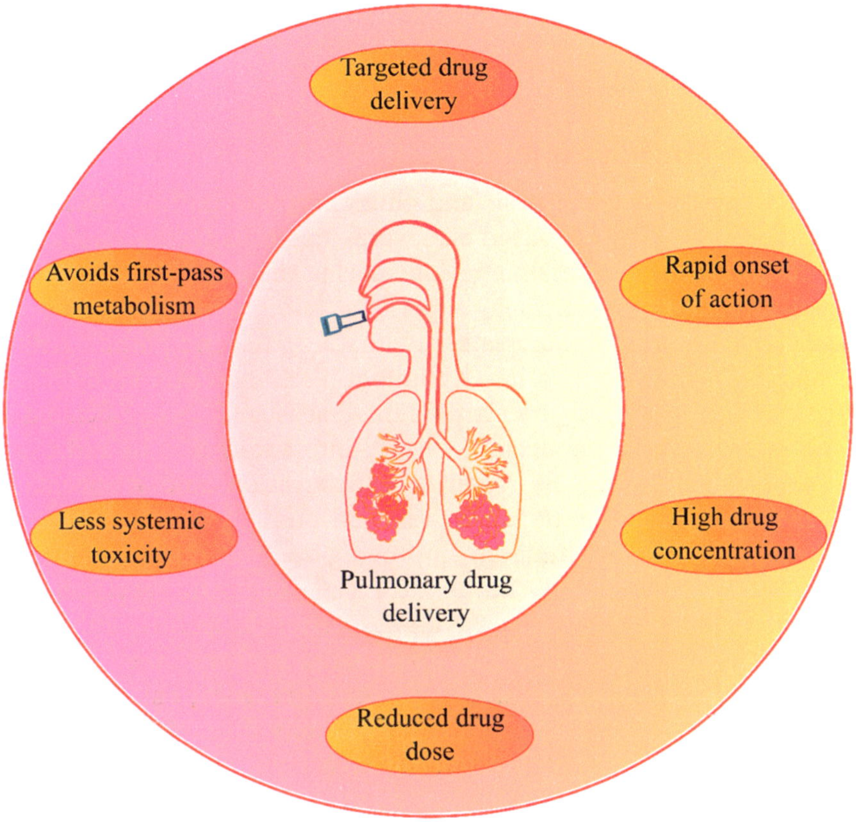

Figure 5.18. Treatment protocols and medications for pulmonary vasculitides.

Source: https://external-content.duckduckgo.com/iu/?u=https%3A%2F%2Fwww.mdpi.com%2Fpharmaceutics%2Fpharmaceutics-13-01077%2Farticle_deploy%2Fhtml%2Fimages%2Fpharmaceutics-13-01077-g001.png&f=1&nofb=1&ipt=3e8b644c3b08689d9b766e7c408280aca1ab101c7d7fe5f115a2b84a038993b2.

The high-resolution visualization potential of [F-18]FDG PET/CT can aid clinicians in determining the magnitude of disease activity, localizing sites of inflammation, and distinguishing between active granulomatous inflammation and fibrosis. The diagnostic accuracy enables improved decision-making for treatment and facilitates more effective tailoring of therapeutic interventions. Growing agreement on the use of [F-18]FDG PET/CT in these inflammatory diseases positions it centrally, not just in diagnosis but also in treatment follow-up, in promoting the new paradigm of management paradigms to provide the best patient outcomes for sarcoidosis and pulmonary vasculitides (Albano et al., 2021). In acknowledging the complex nature of sarcoidosis and pulmonary vasculitides management, multidisciplinary strategies remain vital. The European Association of Nuclear Medicine (EANM) and the Society of Nuclear Medicine and Molecular Imaging (SNMMI) are major stakeholders for the inclusion of nuclear medicine practice into treatment protocols. Through educational programs and the publication of research, these organizations promote practitioners' understanding and application of nuclear medicine techniques that can improve the therapeutic milieu for such diseases. The incorporation of nuclear medicine knowledge can ultimately lead to more personalized and effective treatment approaches, as health care workers strive to identify the best outcomes for patients who have sarcoidosis and pulmonary vasculitides (Buscombe et al., 2021) (Figure 5.18).

5.6.2. Importance of Multidisciplinary Care

Heterogeneity of diseases such as sarcoidosis and pulmonary vasculitides necessitates a care team that uses an interdisciplinary approach based on several medical specialties. Multidisciplinary care teams can provide comprehensive assessments considering the unpredictable presentations of the disease. For instance, sarcoidosis patients may experience both pulmonary and systemic symptoms, necessitating consultation with pulmonologists, rheumatologists, and pathologists to establish the correct diagnosis and implement appropriate treatment plans. A recent study highlights the value of interdisciplinary teams in managing interstitial lung diseases (ILDs) associated with connective tissue disorders, underscoring the importance of well-integrated care to address diverse patient needs effectively (Cerri et al., 2016). By fostering collaboration among specialists, patients are more likely to receive timely interventions and tailored therapies that address both pulmonary and extrapulmonary manifestations, ultimately improving their overall health outcomes. Moreover, integration of several specialties can truly add to increased diagnostic precision for conditions that might overlap in clinical presentation, e.g., ANCA-associated vasculitis. Pulmonary involvement in ANCA-associated vasculitis requires careful differentiation from other ILDs. Rheumatologists and pulmonologists can better diagnose heterogeneous presentations of pulmonary vasculitis by consulting one another. The prevalence of interstitial lung disease in microscopic polyangiitis patients is a good example, where timely detection through a multidisciplinary evaluation can result in immediate and appropriate treatment. Studies find that about 45% of patients with MPA suffer from ILD, which underscores the need for specialist teams to evaluate these complexities in clinical settings (Cassone et al., 2020). Therefore, collective input from multiple healthcare professionals not only improves diagnostic capabilities but also maximizes therapeutic action. Multidisciplinary management can also further improve sarcoidosis and pulmonary vasculitide treatment by being able to tackle the psychosocial aspects of patient management. Chronic respiratory disease often involves not only physical symptoms but also emotional and psychological problems that can undermine compliance with treatment. The integration of mental health professionals into the treatment team enables a holistic approach to treatment aimed at both patient well-being and physical health. These holistic models of treatment can enhance the participation and adherence of patients to treatment programs. The evidence for the harmful effects of pulmonary disease in ANCA-associated vasculitis supports the need for care systems with involvement of psychological well-being (Cassone et al., 2020). Last but not least, multidisciplinary care is not only wholesome but also irreplaceable in providing patients with a comprehensive spectrum of medical care that encompasses all dimensions of health, thereby yielding improved health outcomes and quality of life (Figure 5.19).

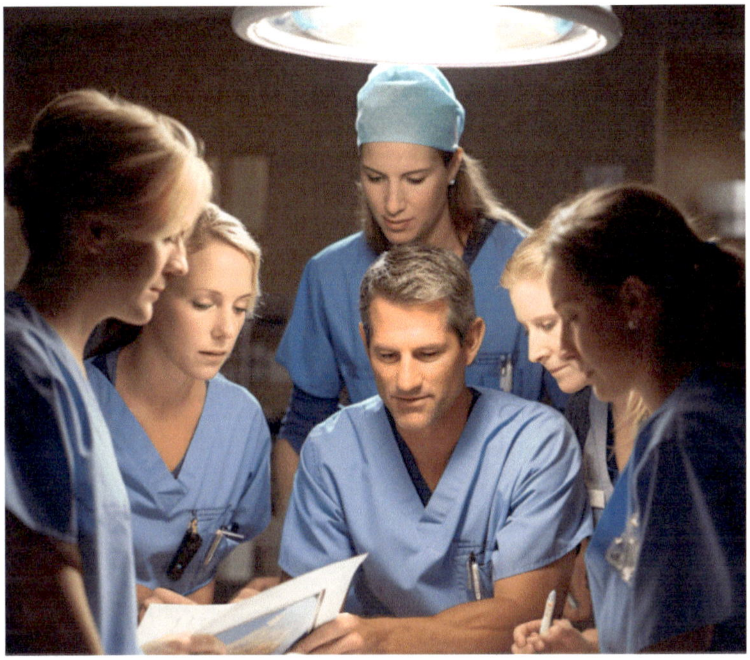

Figure 5.19. The importance of multidisciplinary care.

Source: https://external-content.duckduckgo.com/iu/?u=https%3A%2F%2Fwww.ucmals.com%2Fwp-content%2Fuploads%2F2023%2F07%2Fcc4ed44cc7f3dc592299ee5fac73dd141.png&f=1&nofb=1&ipt=fbb40bd7b485cbcdcd43d8f67241df42f71e8ed29f2697b253d2a3894a5941f8.

5.6.3. Prognosis and Long-Term Outcomes

The prognosis for patients with sarcoidosis and pulmonary vasculitides is inherently uncertain on the basis of several factors, such as disease severity, involved organ systems, and therapeutic options. Of particular interest, cardiac involvement patients, especially in the context of cardiac sarcoidosis, have a more complex prognosis. A retrospective multicenter registry (the ILLUstration registry) had noted that corticosteroid therapy significantly improves long-term prognosis, particularly in patients with preserved left ventricular ejection fraction (LVEF) at presentation, with a lower incidence of severe events such as heart failure and fatal arrhythmias (Wang et al., 2025). This suggests that early intervention and targeted treatment can be crucial in minimizing harm and improving quality of life in these patients. The prognosis in the long run in patients with pulmonary sarcoidosis is typically good but varies according to whether comorbidities are present and the degree of impairment of pulmonary function. Evidence indicates that even though survival is as much as 69.8% at 15 years in certain cohorts receiving surgical interventions for related conditions such as primary pulmonary vein stenosis, the heterogeneity of the patient's health status makes prognosis challenging (Wang et al., 2025). The number of pulmonary veins involved and preoperative severity scores correlate with adverse outcomes. Consequently, careful follow-up and overall management plan are required to ensure maximum long-term success and prevention of sarcoidosis and its pulmonary complications. The prognosis and long-term success of pulmonary vasculitides and sarcoidosis can be significantly influenced by the treatment plan employed and the patient's presentation of the disease. Treatment with corticosteroids, for example, has been highly beneficial in the case of patients with normal LVEF, highlighting the significance of tailored treatment plans (Segawa et al., 2024). Yet, if patients present with multi-organ or critical lung involvement, the prognosis is worse, and multidisciplinary intervention becomes necessary for management. An understanding of the nuances of each patient's situation is vital to healthcare providers because individually tailored interventions can dramatically improve prognosis and general quality of life for this heterogeneous group of patients.

Test Your Knowledge

1. What are the treatment protocols and medications for sarcoidosis and pulmonary vasculitides?
2. What are the importance of multidisciplinary care of sarcoidosis and pulmonary vasculitides?

Summary

The relationship between sarcoidosis and pulmonary vasculitides is complex, which reflects the complexity of interstitial lung disease. Enhanced vulnerability of patients with sarcoidosis to infection, such as COVID-19, poses a critical clinical problem. Clinical studies have indicated that patients with sarcoidosis are at increased risk of developing severe disease upon infection with SARS-CoV-2, and thus, it is necessary for healthcare professionals to be more vigilant. The relative risk ratio of COVID-19 infection among patients with sarcoidosis being 5.86 underscores the necessity of proactive treatment approaches like vaccination and regular assessment of pulmonary function. It is important to recognize this correlation because it guides treatment procedures and helps in reducing the severity of complications of both sarcoidosis and concomitant pulmonary infections (Choi et al., 2025). Moreover, technical improvement in imaging modalities plays a vital role in assessing the progression of sarcoidosis and complications. Comparative effectiveness between chest roentgenogram, CT, and MRI demonstrates an excellent correlation with regard to disease status determination, with MRI having a potential role as an alternative to HRCT in following lung parenchyma changes over time. These modalities not only enhance better diagnostic precision but also lend themselves to a more nuanced understanding of disease evolution. According to studies, the strong correlations found between imaging scores and pulmonary function test results affirm the efficacy of interdisciplinary approaches in comprehensively curing sarcoidosis. By correlating imaging data with clinical assessments, health professionals can optimize care strategies and improve patient outcomes (Griffin et al., 2025). Lastly, management of sarcoidosis and pulmonary vasculitides requires a team approach and an informed strategy with multidimensional management. Collateral efforts in research, patient education, and personal therapeutic management are most important because they all share the common aim of enhancing quality of life in the afflicted population. The increased morbidity and mortality of COVID-19 in patients with sarcoidosis demonstrate the necessity for immediate special guidelines in this group of patients. In addition, sustained research exploring future mechanisms and therapeutic targets is essential because it holds the potential to enhance treatment regimens. Aggressive initiative towards this will provide avenues for improved management strategies and significantly improve the prognosis of patients battling such complex respiratory diseases.

Understanding the complexity of sarcoidosis and pulmonary vasculitis involves a close examination of their key features and molecular diagnostic problems. Sarcoidosis, a granulomatous disease that almost exclusively affects the lungs, can cause an array of widespread respiratory symptoms that have a propensity to mimic other illnesses. The justification for distinguishing sarcoidosis from pulmonary vasculitides, which are inflammatory disorders of the pulmonary vasculature, lies in their distinct treatment approaches and prognoses. Current advances in imaging diagnostics, primarily hybrid [18F]FDG PET, have been a valuable asset for differentiation between them. Clinical practice guidelines indicate that applying this approach has been significantly useful in assessing the inflammatory processes underlying the two diseases and underscores the need for further research into refining interpretative criteria for clinical purposes (Abikhzer et al., 2025). The relationship of sarcoidosis with other pulmonary vasculitides is further complicated by overlap of clinical manifestations, requiring careful planning of treatment protocols. Traditional forms of treatment such as corticosteroids may benefit sarcoidosis but may act inversely on manifestations of vasculitis. The specific patient profiles must be adequately understood for individualized planning of treatment regimens. This emphasizes the importance of modern-day literature, urging the combination of multidisciplinary interventions into patient treatment. The aspects of therapy, including the monitoring of adverse effects and patient responses to therapy, emphasize the significance of ongoing clinical education. A rheumatology text provides learning on how to manage coincident symptomatology among patients, thus equipping clinicians with relevant information for optimum care (N/A, 2021). With each advancing research on sarcoidosis and pulmonary vasculitides, there is an increased need for updated clinical guidelines. Evidence-based studies, particularly using hybrid imaging technologies, are significant in determining the demographic and clinical presentation of these conditions. Not only do they enable more accurate diagnoses, but they also improve outcomes in patients with focused treatments. The inherent difficulties of monitoring the efficacy of treatments and monitoring disease progression remain paramount; thus, research into new diagnostic tools is continually needed. The convergence of future data with clinical practice will ultimately shape best practice and enhance the care of diseases like sarcoidosis and pulmonary vasculitides in general, with an improved sensitive understanding of these complex respiratory illnesses (Abikhzer et al., 2025).

KEY TERMS FROM THIS CHAPTER

- Angiotensin-converting enzyme (ACE)
- Alveolar hemorrhage
- Anti-neutrophil cytoplasmic antibodies
- Bilateral hilar lymphadenopathy
- Bronchoalveolar lavage (BAL)
- Capillaritis
- Erythema nodosum
- Granulomatosis with polyangiitis (GPA)
- Hemoptysis
- Hypercalcemia
- Löfgren's syndrome
- Microscopic polyangiitis (MPA)
- Necrotizing vasculitis
- Non-caseating granulomas
- Pulmonary fibrosis
- Pulmonary hypertension
- Pulmonary nodules
- Uveitis

Critical Thinking Questions

1. Which of the following is the most common pulmonary finding in sarcoidosis?

a. Cavitary lesions

b. Pleural effusion

c. Bilateral hilar lymphadenopathy

d. Apical fibrosis

2. Sarcoidosis is characterized by which type of granuloma?

a. Caseating granulomas

b. Non-caseating granulomas

c. Necrotizing granulomas

d. Suppurative granulomas

3. Which serum marker is commonly elevated in sarcoidosis?

a. Troponin

b. C-reactive protein

c. Angiotensin-converting enzyme (ACE)

d. D-dimer

4. Which of the following is most characteristic of Granulomatosis with polyangiitis (GPA)?

a. Non-caseating granulomas

b. Upper and lower respiratory tract involvement with glomerulonephritis

c. Isolated pulmonary hypertension

d. Pulmonary embolism

5. Which serologic marker is most associated with GPA?

a. ANA

b. c-ANCA (PR3-ANCA)

c. p-ANCA (MPO-ANCA)

d. Anti-dsDNA

Short Answer Questions

1. What is the proposed etiology of sarcoidosis?
2. Describe the characteristic histopathological finding in sarcoidosis.
3. What are the common clinical features of pulmonary sarcoidosis?
4. What are the major types of pulmonary vasculitis affecting the lungs?
5. What are the typical clinical and laboratory features of granulomatosis with polyangiitis?

Answer to Critical Thinking Questions

1. (c); 2. (b); 3. (c); 4. (b); 5. (b)

References

1. Abikhzer, G., Treglia, G., Pelletier-Galarneau, M., Buscombe, J., Chiti, A., Dibble, E. H., Glaudemans, A. W. J. M., Palestro, C. J., Sathekge, M., Signore, A., Jamar, F., Israel, O., & Gheysens, O. (2024). EANM/SNMMI guideline/procedure standard for [18F]FDG hybrid PET use in infection and inflammation in adults v2.0. *European Journal of Nuclear Medicine and Molecular Imaging*, *52*(2), 510–538. https://doi.org/10.1007/s00259-024-06915-3Aggarwal, A., Hata, A., Matsuyama, A., Rodriguez-Pla, A., Valsakumar, A. K., Bagga, A., Gulati, A., et al. (2025). Large vessel vasculitis. https://core.ac.uk/download/pdf/8399944.pdf (accessed on 30th June 2025).
2. Albano, D., Altini, C., Baldari, S., Bartoli, M., et al. (2021). State of the art of 18F-FDG PET/CT application in inflammation and infection: A guide for image acquisition and interpretation. https://core.ac.uk/download/554203023.pdf (accessed on 30th June 2025).
3. Amoroso, A., Barbano, B., Barilaro, G., Gigante, A., et al. (2015). Lung ultrasound in systemic sclerosis: Correlation with high-resolution computed tomography, pulmonary function tests and clinical variables of disease. https://core.ac.uk/download/74319195.pdf (accessed on 30th June 2025).
4. Antoniou, K. M., Birba, G., Bouros, D., Ch., et al. (2009). Epidemiology of interstitial lung diseases in Greece. https://core.ac.uk/download/pdf/82239741.pdf (accessed on 30th June 2025).
5. Aronowitz, D. I., & Hyman, K. (2025). Emerging therapies and current standards in pulmonary carcinoid management. *Current Opinion in Pulmonary Medicine*. https://www.semanticscholar.org/paper/5954eafacdb7bf7e54b6ae6038f630997d98a4fd (accessed on 30th June 2025).
6. Brucato, A., Tombetti, E., Cimaz, R., & Giani, T. (2019). Recurrent pericarditis in children and adolescents. https://core.ac.uk/download/237698546.pdf (accessed on 30th June 2025).
7. Brutsche, M., Böni, C., Daccord, C., Distler, O., et al. (2022). Sarcoidosis - a multisystem disease. https://core.ac.uk/download/592036195.pdf (accessed on 30th June 2025).
8. Bucerius, J., Cohen Tervaert, J. W., van Kroonenburgh, M. J. P. G., Drent, M., Veenman, M., Kemna, M. J., van Paassen, P., et al. (2015). Aortic 18F-FDG uptake in patients suffering from granulomatosis with polyangiitis. https://core.ac.uk/download/191641874.pdf (accessed on 30th June 2025).
9. Buscombe, J., Chiti, A., Christian, P. E., Delbeke, D., et al. (2021). EANM/SNMMI guideline for 18F-FDG use in inflammation and infection. https://core.ac.uk/download/427408084.pdf (accessed on 30th June 2025).
10. Cassone, G., Cavazza, A., Faverio, P., Luppi, F., Manfredi, A., Salvarani, C., Sebastiani, M., et al. (2020). Epidemiology and management of interstitial lung disease in ANCA-associated vasculitis. https://core.ac.uk/download/333570449.pdf (accessed on 30th June 2025).
11. Cassone, G., Erre, G. L., Manfredi, A., Salvarani, C., et al. (2021). Efficacy and safety of mycophenolate mofetil in the treatment of rheumatic disease-related interstitial lung disease: A narrative review. https://core.ac.uk/download/389869978.pdf (accessed on 30th June 2025).
12. Cerri, S., Colaci, M., Della Casa, G., Ferri, C., et al. (2016). Interstitial pneumonia with autoimmune features and undifferentiated connective tissue disease: Our interdisciplinary rheumatology-pneumology experience, and review of the literature. https://core.ac.uk/

download/132771526.pdf (accessed on 30th June 2025).

13. Chairman, D. (2019). Approach to diffuse parenchymal lung disease (interstitial lung disease) for the hospitalist. https://core.ac.uk/download/389643240.pdf (accessed on 30th June 2025).
14. Chikkula, K. V., Jaiswal, A., Kadiri, S. K., Kumar, R., et al. (2023). Anti-neutrophil cytoplasmic antibody-associated vasculitis: A glimpse into the future. https://core.ac.uk/download/591404192.pdf (accessed on 30th June 2025).
15. Chimenti, M. S., Conigliaro, P., De Martino, E., Monosi, A., et al. (2023). Overview on the link between the complement system and auto-immune articular and pulmonary disease. https://core.ac.uk/download/590751785.pdf (accessed on 30th June 2025).
16. Choi, S. I., Jung, W., Jeong, Y., Park, S., Kim, B. K., Lee, S. Y., An, H., et al. (2025). COVID-19 infection and pulmonary sarcoidosis: A systematic review and meta-analysis of morbidity, severity and mortality. *Journal of Thoracic Disease, 17*, 744–752. https://www.semanticscholar.org/paper/b55aa00b263b3695732aa63c4d850ac26108d993 (accessed on 30th June 2025).
17. Christensen, A., Di Loreto, C., Guma, M., Jones, T., et al. (2018). Granulomatous fasciitis followed by morphea profunda: Is granulomatous fasciitis part of a spectrum of deep morphea? A case report and review of the literature. https://core.ac.uk/download/323067040.pdf (accessed on 30th June 2025).
18. Croce, A., D'Aguanno, V., De Vincentiis, M., De Virgilio, A., et al. (2018). Audio-vestibular symptoms in systemic autoimmune diseases. https://core.ac.uk/download/188823057.pdf (accessed on 30th June 2025).
19. D'Aguanno, V., De Vincentiis, M., Falasca, V., Greco, A., et al. (2018). Nasal manifestations in granulomatosis with polyangiitis: A case report and review of the literature. https://core.ac.uk/download/188830239.pdf (accessed on 30th June 2025).
20. De Vincentiis, M., De Virgilio, A., Fusconi, M., Gallo, A., et al. (2016). Clinic manifestations in granulomatosis with polyangiitis. https://core.ac.uk/download/74319070.pdf (accessed on 30th June 2025).
21. Dörner, T., & Guillevin, L. (2007). Vasculitis: Mechanisms involved and clinical manifestations. https://core.ac.uk/download/pdf/7779645.pdf (accessed on 30th June 2025).
22. Factor, P., Sulica, R., & Palmero, V. (2011). Sarcoidosis associated pulmonary hypertension. https://core.ac.uk/download/322403240.pdf (accessed on 30th June 2025).
23. Franks, T. J., Franquet, T., Galvin, J. R., Giménez, A., et al. (2021). Non-infectious granulomatous lung disease: Imaging findings with pathologic correlation. https://core.ac.uk/download/477979917.pdf (accessed on 30th June 2025).
24. Genecand, L., Wacker, J., Guerreiro, I., Lechartier, B., Beghetti, M., Pohle, S., Darie, A. M., et al. (2025). Pulmonary hypertension associated with interstitial lung disease–A review on diagnosis and treatment with a focus on emerging therapies. *Respiration; International Review of Thoracic Diseases*. https://www.semanticscholar.org/paper/610f13fa0fd2c883d54039696a8fd515859d51f4 (accessed on 30th June 2025).
25. Griffin, I., Pasini, R. A., Mehrad, B., Al-An, M. A. Z., Mohammed, T., Gomez Manjarres, D. C., Patel, D., et al. (2025). The evolving role of MRI in pulmonary sarcoidosis: Comparative analysis with PFTs and progression markers. *Sarcoidosis, Vasculitis, and Diffuse Lung Diseases,*

42. https://www.semanticscholar.org/paper/d960854d65ccc049ea1deaaeed0cedd45fed0c86 (accessed on 30th June 2025).

26. Gupta, R., Kim, J. S., & Baughman, R. (2023). An expert overview of pulmonary fibrosis in sarcoidosis. *Expert Review of Respiratory Medicine, 17*, 119–130. https://www.semanticscholar.org/paper/5df799984d1f4cf1731fa197700a0cd9db57bdd3 (accessed on 30th June 2025).
27. Hamzeh, N., Marc, A., & Lisa, A. (2020). Proceedings of the 2015 AASOG conference: Reducing disparities in sarcoidosis through personalized care and increased detection. *Sarcoidosis Vasculitis and Diffuse Lung Diseases, 34*, 264–268. https://www.semanticscholar.org/paper/fd57921c47e500f0e7e1cbc62e1da94e47048e30 (accessed on 30th June 2025).
28. Khalifa, A. (2022). Diagnostic ability of multidisciplinary discussion in interstitial lung diseases and rare lung diseases. https://core.ac.uk/download/599598608.pdf (accessed on 30th June 2025).
29. Kolovou, G., Markousis-Mavrogenis, G., & Mavrogeni, S. (2016). The Sphinx's riddle: Cardiovascular involvement in autoimmune rheumatic disease. https://core.ac.uk/download/pdf/81790073.pdf (accessed on 30th June 2025).
30. Liu, A., Price, L. C., Sharma, R., Wells, A. U., & Kouranos, V. (2024). *Sarcoidosis Associated Pulmonary Hypertension, 12, Biomedicines*. https://www.semanticscholar.org/paper/36c71172f747b02fb51b37d1a19df7eeb64c3c10 (accessed on 30th June 2025).
31. Lötscher, F., Pop, R., Seitz, L., Seitz, M., et al. (2022). Spectrum of large and medium vessel vasculitis in adults: Primary vasculitis's, arthritis's, connective tissue, and fibroinflammatory diseases. https://core.ac.uk/download/541130762.pdf (accessed on 30th June 2025).
32. Pande, J. N. (2025). An approach to interstitial lung disease in India. https://core.ac.uk/download/pdf/287211111.pdf (accessed on 30th June 2025).
33. Rossi, D., Magnano, R., Pezzi, L., Scollo, C., Sacchetta, D., D'Alleva, A., Forlani, D., et al. (2025). Cardiac involvement in sarcoidosis with induced malignant arrhythmias–multimodal management approach. *European Heart Journal Supplements*. https://www.semanticscholar.org/paper/c1d4b6b73b02e09afb0d5fcf11076dff28fd925e (accessed on 30th June 2025).
34. Segawa, T., Taniguchi, T., Nabeta, T., Naruse, Y., Kitai, T., Yoshioka, K., Tanaka, H., et al. (2024). Corticosteroid therapy and long-term outcomes in patients with cardiac sarcoidosis stratified by left ventricular ejection fraction. *European Heart Journal Open, 5*. https://www.semanticscholar.org/paper/13b962556ff9ab153e1c541299f0cc57513d5259 (accessed on 30th June 2025).
35. Wang, Z., & Yang, Y. (2025). Long-term outcomes of individualized repair in patients with primary pulmonary vein stenosis. *Cardiology in the Young*. https://www.semanticscholar.org/paper/03f3427d524ebefb60ce032e852e283f8819bf1e (accessed on 30th June 2025).

LUNGS IN SYSTEMIC DISEASES

6

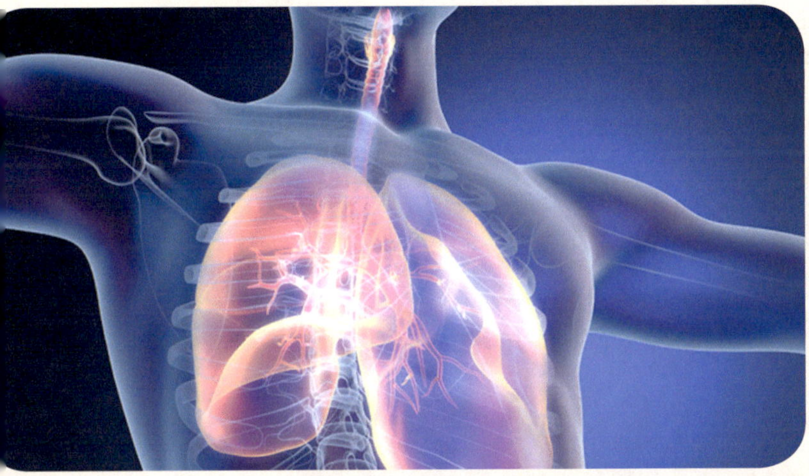

LEARNING OBJECTIVES

After studying this chapter, you will be able to:

1. Give an overview of systemic diseases
2. Define the role of the lungs in systemic diseases
3. Explain autoimmune diseases and lung complications
4. Describe the infectious diseases and lung implications
5. Explore cardiovascular diseases and lung interactions
6. List the metabolic disorders and their effects on the lungs

Introduction

The lungs, which are key respiratory organs, play a pivotal role in a spectrum of systemic diseases, particularly those of an autoimmune nature. Systemic sclerosis (SSc), a prototypic autoimmune systemic disease, is paradigmatic of the interdependent interactions between pulmonary function and systemic pathologies. Characterized by diffuse fibrosis of both the skin and multiple internal organs, SSc constitutes a common cause of interstitial lung disease (ILD) and pulmonary arterial hypertension (PAH). Their development is an important reason for morbidity and mortality in patients affected. Understanding the mechanisms of lung disease in systemic diseases like SSc is relevant because it provides basic insight into disease pathogenesis and therapeutic approaches. One such critical process that has been implicated in SSc lung pathology is endothelial-to-mesenchymal transition (EndoMT). This is an allusion to endothelial cell phenotypic conversion to myofibroblast-like cells, which are pivotal in fibrotic mechanisms that produce lung disease. Participation of these transformed cells in SSc patients lends support to the correlation between aberrant lung architecture and systemic disease. Research has shown that pulmonary endothelial cells from SSc patients also have mesenchymal markers and profibrotic genes, which has been taken as evidence that EndoMT contributes extensively to ILD and pulmonary vascular complications. The extent of EndoMT involvement in the pathogenesis of these conditions is a subject of research, reflecting the systemic disease involvement in lung function (Arciniegas et al., 2016; Jimenez et al., 2016). Investigating the role of the lungs in systemic disease offers a key insight into interactions between local and systemic pathophysiologic mechanisms. Investigating how systemic diseases impact lung function allows scientists to create more targeted therapies to improve pulmonary complications. An in-depth comprehension of the cellular and molecular alterations that happen in the lungs can result in improvements in the clinical care of patients with SSc and associated diseases. More research is required to clarify the exact mechanisms in which the lungs affect systemic disease processes so that this knowledge can improve our prognostic capability and management for patients involved. Hence, investigation of the lungs in systemic disease is not only at the very heart of the explanation of SSc but also critical to the whole specialty of respiratory medicine (Figure 6.1).

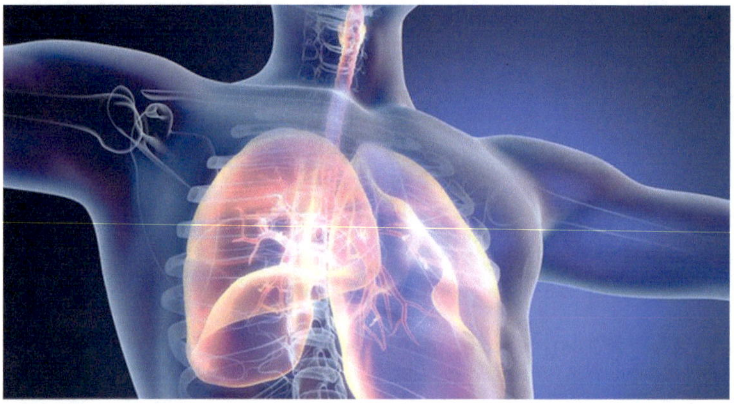

Figure 6.1. Lungs in systemic diseases.

Source: https://www.healio.com/~/media/slack-news/stock-images/pulmonology/l/lungs-5_adobe.jpg?w=800.

Definition of Systemic Diseases

In medical science, systemic diseases are disorder states affecting entire organ systems or the whole body, essentially disturbing homeostasis. Systemic states, as compared to localized diseases involving certain areas, typically arise from underlying reasons such as autoimmune responses, metabolic disturbances, or infections. They manifest in diverse signs and symptoms, with varying severity, which tend to complicate diagnosis due to their diffused state. The identification of systemic illnesses, including diabetes, lupus, and cardiovascular illness, emphasizes the interdependence of body systems and the need for a comprehensive treatment plan. When discussing the lungs alone, one can see how the system's diseases compromise the respiratory system, as seen with pulmonary hypertension or interstitial lung disease, which complicate pre-existing conditions and greatly affect quality of life. Characterization of system diseases is further accentuated by the ability of such diseases to cross-talk with other physiological pathways. An example is metabolic syndrome, which is a combination of obesity, hypertension, and dyslipidemia, where the risk of cardiovascular disease as well as type 2 diabetes is crucial. Evidence has shown that hyperglycemia in relation to metabolic syndrome is associated with increased vulnerability to peri-implant disease, which can complicate dental management and overall health outcomes. Through understanding the interaction between systemic diseases and local manifestations, medical practitioners are capable of enhancing responsiveness to developing complications, particularly those that relate to the lungs. This encounter highlights the need for integrated treatment plans that take into account more than one health condition to ensure patient safety and maximize long-term wellness as suggested by Letizia et al. (2018). Further, having systemic diseases has a tendency to reveal intricate sex-based differences that influence disease prevalence and outcomes. Sexual dimorphism has been proven to play a role in the development of systemic conditions in males and females, affecting the course and severity of diseases. The difference in hormonal and genetic status between sexes necessitates personalized treatment regimens. MicroRNA studies, for instance, have proven their potential in regulating the course of various systemic diseases and shedding light on sex-biased illnesses. As such findings suggest, sex-specific therapeutic methods can enhance effectiveness and reduce complications in systemic lung diseases. Such dynamics are likely to lead to more effective control practice in the care of disorders like asthma or COPD in the context of enhancing disease paradigms as discussed in Eghbali et al. (2014).

Importance of Lung Health in Systemic Diseases

Pulmonary function is important in the pathogenesis and prognosis of systemic disease, illustrating the interdependent nature of respiratory function and body physiology as a whole. Sustained lung inflammation has the potential to have a significant impact on systemic illnesses such as cardiovascular disease, diabetes, and even cancer. The underlying mechanisms for such correlations usually involve inflammatory cytokines that not only affect lung tissue but also circulate throughout the body's bloodstream, impacting other systems. For instance, older adults often experience decreased lung function due to age-related declines in physical performance, which highlights the importance of maintaining healthy respiratory function to enhance overall body resilience. Research shows that the inflammatory profiles observed in the elderly, for instance, high levels of cytokines like interleukin and tumor necrosis factor, are associated with muscle catabolism and compromised physical function, which emphasizes coordination between lung and body health (Addison et al., 2017). Besides, environmental factors, particularly air pollution exposure, contribute significantly to lung health as well as the burden of disease at the systemic level. Particulates such as PM2.5 and PM10 can penetrate lung tissue, cause respiratory distress, and trigger systemic inflammatory processes. Results of thorough research indicate the connection between building height and the dissemination of these pollutants, which shows that indoor air quality is vital to respiratory health in metropolitan cities (Kozlovtseva et al., 2016). This is especially necessary in densely concentrated urban centers where pollutant exposure is higher. Inadequate lung health due to environmental factors can increase vulnerability to systemic diseases, highlighting the need for strict air quality control and interventions to improve respiratory health. Therapy of lung health as a whole is thus essential in order to fight the pervasive impact of systemic diseases. In addition to its direct impact on chronic disease, impaired lung function can lead to significant decreases in quality of life and health care costs. Cross-talk between respiratory status and systemic disease identifies an important target for intervention, especially in high-risk populations, such as the elderly or those with underlying disease. Effective management strategies that optimize lung function can reduce the occurrence of exacerbations from systemic diseases, lower morbidity rates, and enhance the overall quality of life for patients. For example, exercise strategies specifically designed to increase lung function can enhance systemic health, benefiting older patients who are likely to exhibit impaired physical function and increased inflammation. Thus, incorporating lung health into the broader discourse on systemic diseases is paramount to creating holistic treatment strategies to maximize quality of life and promote resilience against age-related decline (Kozlovtseva et al., 2016; Addison et al., 2017) (Figure 6.2).

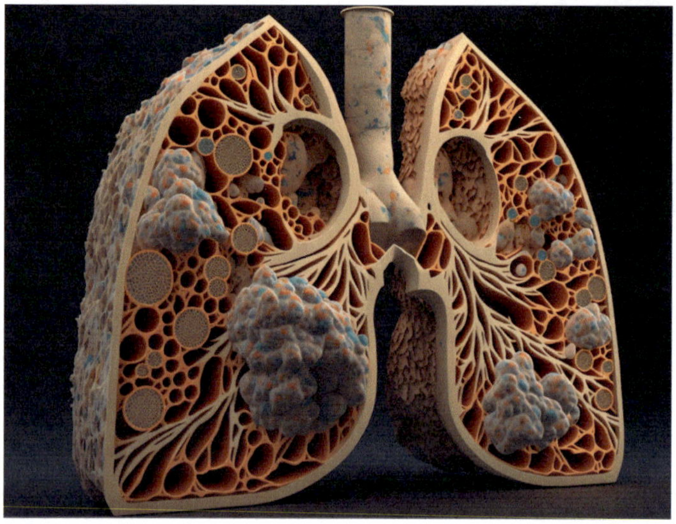

Figure 6.2. Lung health in systemic diseases.

Source: https://external-content.duckduckgo.com/iu/?u=https%3A%2F%2Fuploads-ssl.webflow.com%2F63e131fc226aff56a2f7f30d%2F64a2d8e6122f1f8d7bd2aea5_Interstitial%2520Lung%2520Disease.jpg&f=1&nofb=1&ipt=352baa0eb91035713e72824e1569ee5b0ebc10169fe7c8919c36467e49f62f78.

6.1. Overview of Systemic Diseases

Learning Outcome

1. Common types of systemic diseases
2. Pathophysiology of systemic diseases
3. Impact on multiple organ systems

Systemic diseases embrace a broad range of disorders affecting two or more organ systems, commonly leading to widespread impairment of overall health. Systemic diseases are characterized by their ability to spread throughout the body and thus affect proper physiological functions. Systemic sclerosis, lupus erythematosus, and rheumatoid arthritis are some of the systemic diseases that can have extensive effects on pulmonary health. The lungs, essential for respiration, are the most vulnerable to the impact of such diseases, leading to interstitial lung disease and impaired pulmonary function. The integration of systemic inflammation with the pathology of the lungs emphasizes the need for a holistic understanding of how systemic disease impacts respiratory health, necessitating an interdisciplinary examination of suitable management and treatment regimens. Clinical management of pulmonary disease in systemic illnesses has been shown in studies to be multifaceted, primarily due to the disease's heterogeneity. For instance, scleroderma-associated interstitial lung disease (SSc-ILD) management perfectly captures the dilemma for clinicians.

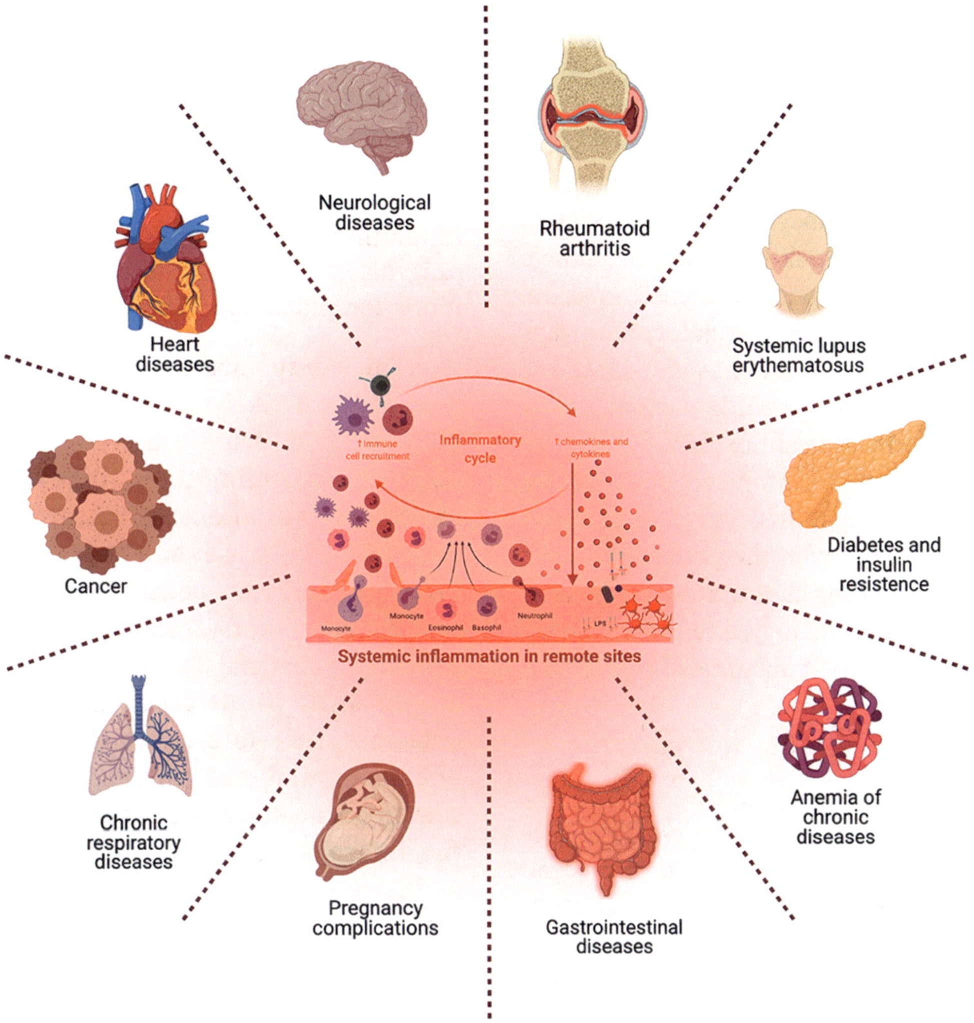

Figure 6.3. Overview of systemic diseases.

Source: https://www.frontiersin.org/files/Articles/709438/fphys-12-709438-HTML/image_m/fphys-12-709438-g003.jpg.

A recent study assessed the efficacy of dasatinib in patients with SSc-ILD and found that, despite the drug being well tolerated, it was not associated with spectacular clinical improvement. In particular, quantitative HRCT revealed distinctive response patterns, stability of lung function in certain patients, and evolving fibrosis of the lungs in others. Such heterogeneity underlies the value of personalized treatments, where individual patient profiles correlate with corresponding treatment outcomes based on mechanisms of disease progression (Bogatkevich et al., 2017). The biochemical environment of systemic diseases further complicates the correlation between lung pathology and systemic inflammation. Oxidative stress plays a key role in numerous respiratory disorders, interfering with cellular signaling and impacting the lung's health. Glutathione (GSH), a major antioxidant, is central to the body's defense system against oxidative damage, controlling numerous physiological reactions, including inflammation. Disruption in the ratio of GSH/GSSG is implicated in the activation of some stress kinases and transcription factors such as Nrf2 and NF-κB, which modulate the lung's response to oxidative stress and inflammation. The comprehension of GSH's regulatory pathways offers therapeutic approaches to systemic diseases relevant to lung health, particularly in strategies for modulating antioxidant production during oxidative stress (Antonicelli et al., 2009). Therefore, the investigation of systemic diseases must be approached from the perspective of a complex understanding that unites the strands of immunology, pulmonology, and biochemistry toward improved patient outcomes (Figure 6.3).

6.1.1. Common Types of Systemic Diseases

Systemic diseases encompass a wide variety of conditions that affect more than one organ system, with profound effects on lung function. Of particular relevance among them are autoimmune diseases such as systemic lupus erythematosus (SLE) and rheumatoid arthritis (RA) due to their inflammatory nature. SLE, for instance, can be associated with pleuritis and pulmonary infiltrates, which manifest as respiratory comorbidities. Similarly, RA also has a connection with interstitial lung disease, involving scarring within the lung tissue, loss of lung function, and global respiratory compromise. The interrelated nature of these systemic diseases highlights the importance of adopting a comprehensive diagnostic and therapeutic approach that considers both systemic observations and local influences on the lung's overall health. Lastly, such conditions highlight the need for interdisciplinary treatment plans to optimize patient outcomes and tailor therapies that address the pulmonary and systemic aspects of such illnesses. Metabolic diseases such as diabetes mellitus also present significant challenges to lung function. Diabetes is related to increased risk for respiratory infections and obstructive sleep apnea to a large degree due to its correlation with obesity. Hyperglycemia is also responsible for inflammatory pathways that may exacerbate lung disease, making the clinical presentation more complicated.

The study further reveals that diabetic patients are likely to present with higher frequencies of acute exacerbations of chronic obstructive pulmonary disease (COPD), indicating the potential interaction between respiratory disease and metabolic disease. Effective diabetes control through lifestyle modification and treatment adherence is not only beneficial for metabolic control but is also likely to yield benefits in respiratory outcomes. Therefore, awareness of the systemic effects of diabetes emphasizes the use of combined healthcare strategies that embrace the interconnectedness of such diseases. In addition, CVD often coincides with systemic disease and carries major implications for pulmonary function.

Such diseases can also lead to pulmonary congestion, thus compromising gas exchange and contributing to secondary respiratory complications. Furthermore, systemic inflammation in CVD can exacerbate underlying lung disease, once again highlighting the two-way interaction between these systems in terms of pathophysiology. Air pollution, or rather the presence of particulate matter (PM2.5), is a key driver that connects cardiovascular and pulmonary health since it causes systemic inflammation and oxidative stress and can result in serious health conditions such as lung cancer and chronic respiratory disease (Liu et al., 2016; Bednarek et al., 2024). Thus, it is of vital importance to approach cardiovascular health for improving lung function, emphasizing the need to incorporate a general strategy while treating patients with systemic lung diseases.

6.1.2. Pathophysiology of Systemic Diseases

The reciprocal relationship between systemic illness and lung disease is a tribute to the multiplicity of pathophysiological mechanisms governing respiratory manifestations of most disease processes. At its nucleus is the induction of inflammatory mechanisms, typically mediated by cytokines such as TNF-alpha. Prolonged exposure to inflammatory mediators might have a widespread impact on lung structure and function, which will further exacerbate respiratory symptomatology. For instance, autoimmune patients regularly exhibit increased TNF-alpha levels that not only lead to intestinal and joint inflammation but also impair the lungs.

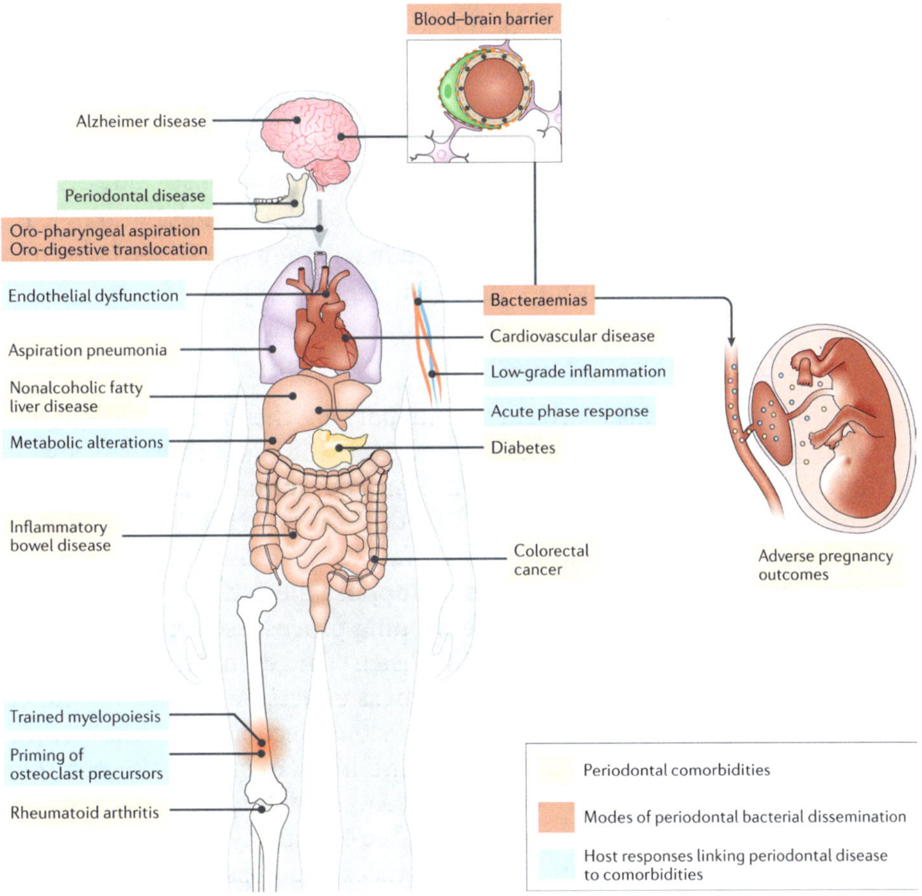

Figure 6.4. Pathophysiology of systemic diseases.

Source: https://media.springernature.com/full/springer-static/image/art%3A10.1038%2Fs41577-020-00488-6/MediaObjects/41577_2020_488_Fig1_HTML.png.

The outcome of studies performed on TNF Delta ARE mice shows that while acute exposure to CS increased lung inflammation, chronic exposure may lead to different immune responses within the lung. This indicates the active inflammatory environment required for understanding the pathophysiology of systemic conditions affecting lung function (Churg et al., 2015). Another equally important part of systemic disease is the action of leukotrienes produced by the 5-lipoxygenase (5-LO) pathway, which is a key mediator of immune response and inflammation. These lipid mediators are particularly involved in acute lung injury (ALI) and systemic inflammatory conditions. Leukotrienes in pathological processes such as shock or ischemia-reperfusion injury mediate uncontrolled recruitment of neutrophils, leading to lung tissue damage. Greater understanding of the role of the 5-LO pathway in neutrophil trafficking offers therapeutic promise for the patient with systemic disease affecting the lungs. Inhibition of the 5-LO metabolites provides the potential for reducing inflammation and dysfunction within the lungs, thereby improving patient recovery in systemic disease with respiratory distress (Cuzzocrea et al., 2009). Furthermore, systemic diseases also portray a multi-determined interdependence, in which the breakdown within one organ system can give rise to or aggravate pathology in another. For example, chronic inflammation in diseases such as rheumatoid arthritis and systemic lupus erythematosus could cause pleuritis or other respiratory complications and also contribute to the clinical complexity. This integral pathology needs to be treated with a comprehensive approach, taking into consideration both the systemic character of the disease and the pulmonary specificity of its manifestations. Therapies need to consider not only the inflammatory biomarkers of the systemic diseases but also the immediate pulmonary effects. Therefore, improving our knowledge of the pathophysiological mechanisms involved will result in more tailored and effective management protocols for patients with the complex effects of systemic diseases on lung function (Figure 6.4).

6.1.3. Impact on Multiple Organ Systems

The lungs are a major gas exchange interface and part of the homeostatic apparatus of the multiorgan system. If systemic disease is a factor, however, one must consider beyond respiratory function to its impact on cardiovascular function, immune status, and even metabolic process. For instance, chronic respiratory diseases (CRD) like COPD can further exacerbate cardiovascular disease through systemic inflammation and hypoxia, further increasing the risk of heart failure as well as hypertension. This interconnectivity goes to support the rationale for an overall approach in envisioning how lung pathologies can initiate cascading processes throughout the body, thereby refuting traditional thinking regarding organ-specific disease and embracing a multi-organ approach in treating systemic disease. Furthermore, systemic illness effects on respiratory function highlight the extent of microbiota in other organ systems. Previous accounts for the protective roles of microbiota have typically emphasized localized immune mechanisms at the cost of the systemic disease effects of these microorganisms. Current research highlights that host microbiota can regulate pathogenic impacts. This preserves a view of "co-immunity" that includes both the host's immune response and microbial contribution towards disease defense. This is particularly relevant in systemic diseases, where dysbiosis can not only impair lung function but also disrupt immune homeostasis. This disruption renders the patient more prone to infection and inflammation throughout the body, thereby supporting the argument that the health of one organ system is interlinked with others. Lastly, an understanding of the aging process provides valuable insight into the multi-systemic impact of pulmonary diseases within the context of systemic diseases. With an aging population in the world, the health burden of aging morbidities, particularly pulmonary in nature, is monumental. The role of extracellular vesicles in tissue repair highlights a promising therapeutic mechanism for reversing the functional decrements of aging and systemic diseases. These vesicles can mediate intercellular communication and epigenetic modification of aging cells, culminating in healthspan improvement and avoiding organ function deterioration. Continued exploration of these mechanisms not only illuminates the complexity of lung pathologies but also guides the design of new therapeutic paradigms. These paradigms address numerous obstacles to multiple organ systems due to aging and systemic disease, resulting in an integrative treatment and management strategy (Figure 6.5).

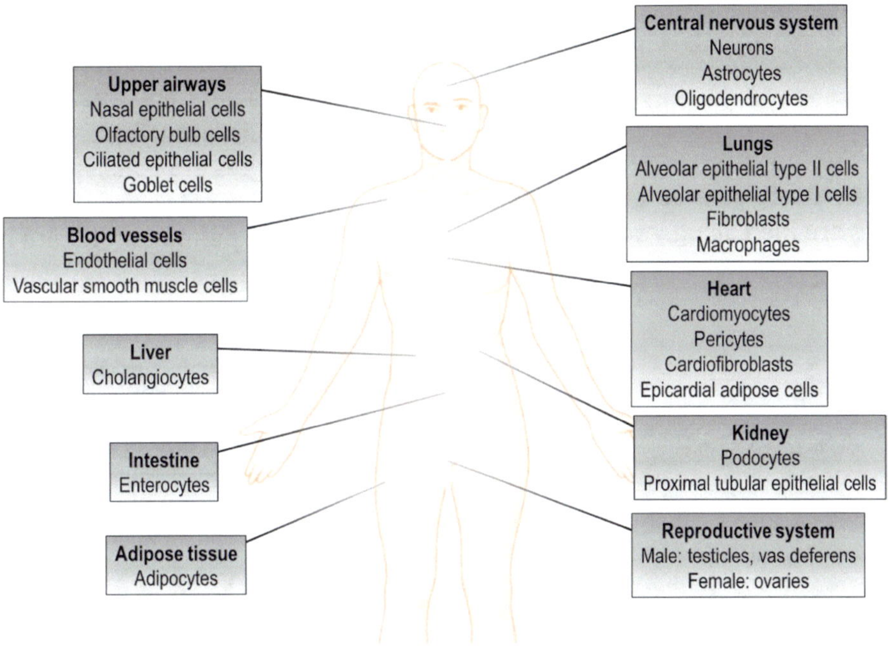

Figure 6.5. The lungs impact on multiple organ systems.

Source: https://www.frontiersin.org/files/Articles/593223/fphys-12-593223-HTML/image_m/fphys-12-593223-g001.jpg.

Test Your Knowledge

1. What are the common types of systemic diseases?
2. What is the pathophysiology of systemic diseases?

6.2. The Role of the Lungs in Systemic Diseases

Learning Outcome

1. Respiratory function and systemic health
2. Mechanisms of lung involvement in systemic diseases
3. Clinical significance of lung assessment

The function of the lungs in systemic diseases goes beyond their basic role as gas exchange organs. The lungs are increasingly recognized as essential participants in systemic inflammatory responses, affecting conditions ranging from autoimmune diseases to cardiovascular disease. For instance, recent studies have illustrated that inflammation within the lungs can potentially exacerbate systemic manifestations of diseases such as systemic lupus erythematosus and rheumatoid arthritis and therefore illustrate the interconnectedness between pulmonary and systemic manifestations of these diseases. Experimental models, such as rat models of induced autoimmune disease, demonstrate that lung pathologies are consistent with alterations in cardiac and renal vasculature, highlighting the importance of pulmonary health in the systemic outcomes of disease.

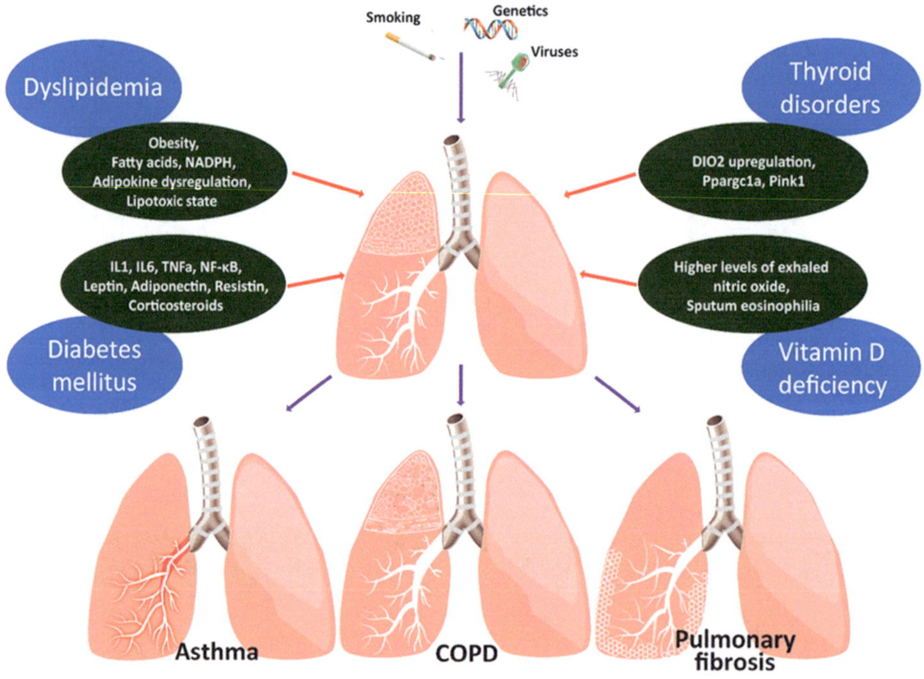

Figure 6.6. The role of the lungs in systemic diseases.

Source: https://www.frontiersin.org/files/Articles/327679/fmed-04-00246-HTML-r1/image_m/fmed-04-00246-g001.jpg.

Such observations highlight the active participation of the lungs in a highly inflammatory terrain, which warrants consideration in further research as well as multimodal treatment and management within the clinic (Iegudina et al., 2017). The intricate interaction between lungs and the immune system is also emphasized by recent evidence for non-neuronal cholinergic transmission. The lungs harbor a special cholinergic pathway that regulates immune responses through neurotransmitters such as acetylcholine (ACh). Research indicates that ACh can polarize dendritic cells to a Th2-inducing phenotype, which plays a critical role in lung inflammatory processes. Activation of muscarinic acetylcholine receptors enhances cytokine release associated with tissue damage and inflammation. The mechanism thus engages ACh in respiratory disease, and dysregulation may be involved in the development of systemic disease. The pathways must be analyzed for an in-depth understanding of the complications of systemic inflammation and disease development (Alcain et al., 2019). Lastly, the lungs are a critical interface between local and systemic disease, with both therapeutic and diagnostic connotations. Lung involvement in systemic disease refutes the long-standing divorce between respiratory medicine and disciplines such as rheumatology and cardiology. Sensation of pulmonary involvement in systemic disease emphasizes multi-disciplinary management of patients. Clinicians need to recognize that lung disease is a precursor to systemic complications and also vice versa. As continued research continues to unravel the molecular and cellular links between the lungs and other organ systems, therapies targeting both pulmonary and systemic features of disease may be an exciting emerging paradigm for enhancing patient outcomes (Iegudina et al., 2017) (Figure 6.6).

6.2.1. Respiratory Function and Systemic Health

Lungs not only facilitate gas exchange but also play a role in general systemic health. The lungs function as an environmental barrier against infection and are part of the immune response. Immunological function is not limited to the pulmonary system; the lungs interact with the microbiota, which influences the immune system and metabolic processes of the body. By providing a microbe-friendly environment, the lungs establish a protective microbiome that helps counteract infections and inflammatory responses. The co-immunity theory emphasizes the complementarity of the body's defense system with that of microbes to demonstrate the interdependency between respiratory health and well-being (Abt et al., 2017). Therefore, any lung health pathos has wide-ranging implications, leading to an immune system that is infected and increased susceptibility to systemic disease. Respiratory illnesses also tend to reveal complex interdependencies with systemic diseases such as cardiovascular disease and diabetes. Lungs are not standalone organs; their physiological status is interrelated with the body's physiological status. For example, COPD not only restricts airflow but can potentially be responsible for systemic inflammation and vascular dysfunction. This systemic consequence can result in worsening cardiovascular diseases, which pose the risk of heart attacks and strokes. Conditions such as hypertension, on the other hand, can induce pulmonary complications, such as pulmonary hypertension. Thus, the intricate relationship between systemic diseases and the lungs underscores the significance of respiratory function as an indicator of health. Respiratory well-being is addressed through a comprehensive understanding of these relationships, as neglecting respiratory issues significantly impacts systemic well-being. In the context of the significance of lung health in systemic disease, it is also essential to examine the role played by environmental factors. Exposure to respiratory irritants and air pollutants may lead to long-term respiratory disease, which, combined with genetic predisposition, increases the likelihood of developing systemic illness. For example, lung function has been shown to be influenced by air quality and can exacerbate pre-existing respiratory diseases, along with other systemic impacts such as oxidative stress and inflammation in the body. Particulate matter research has emphasized the adverse effect of air pollution on lung function and the consequential risk of systemic disease (Alving et al., 2012).

Understanding the mechanisms by which respiratory function interacts with and is influenced by environmental exposure is crucial for developing overarching strategies to improve public health outcomes. Heightened sensitivity and precautions to protect the health of lungs can thus assist in reducing the burden of systemic illnesses in the population (Figure 6.7).

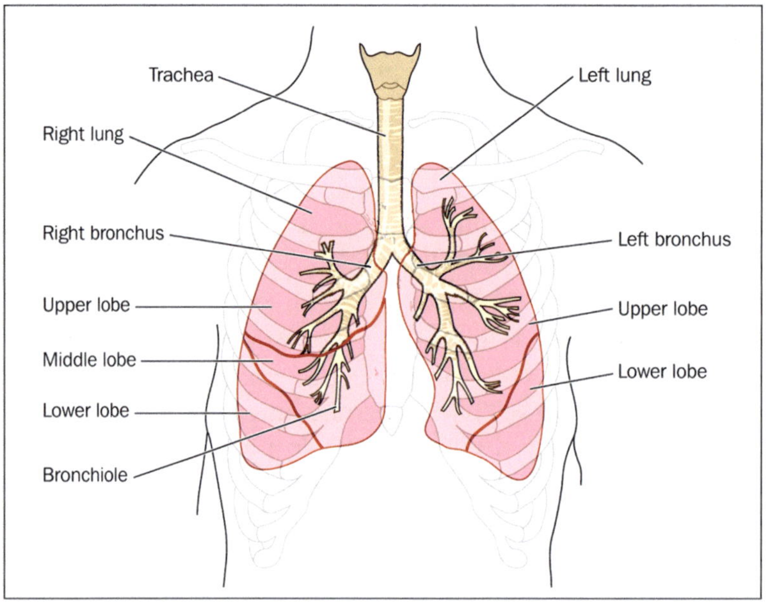

Figure 6.7. Respiratory function and systemic health.

Source: https://www.britishjournalofnursing.com/media/v1ddc1ti/bjon20233213613_f01.jpg.

6.2.2. Mechanisms of Lung Involvement in Systemic Diseases

The interrelationship between systemic diseases and lung disease is irrevocably linked to the pathophysiology of pulmonary hypertension (PH). In systemic diseases such as connective tissue disease, impaired lung function with pulmonary vascular remodeling is usually observed in the lungs. An elevated mean pulmonary arterial pressure (mPAP) of ≥25 mmHg is a key indicator for such vascular remodeling. Current research indicates that typical mPAP is about 14.0 ± 3.3 mmHg, and measurements above 20 mmHg should be of concern. These rises may be due to an elevation in cardiac output or pulmonary wedge pressure instead of merely reflecting vascular disease. Clinicians need this level of understanding because they need to identify the underlying reasons in order to use management measures effectively. Significantly, recognizing pulmonary vascular resistance of ≥3 Wood Units as specific to pre-capillary PH suggests a more targeted definition of lung involvement in systemic disease and the necessity for focused therapeutic approaches (Gérald Simonneau et al., 2018). In addition to vascular changes, the role of cytokines like transforming growth factor-β (TGF-β) is also highlighted in chronic lung disorders associated with systemic disease. TGF-β is a master regulator that acts to control a wide variety of biological processes from inflammation to fibrosis. In diseases such as cystic fibrosis and COPD, polymorphism within the TGF-β pathway has been associated with disease severity. Elevated levels of TGF-β have been correlated with lung function impairment, in large part through inhibition of critical proteins such as CFTR that are crucial to pulmonary homeostasis. TGF-β is also implicated in fibrotic lung tissue remodeling, promoting increased stiffness of the extracellular matrix and further pathological remodeling. Consequently, the TGF-β-mediated processes offer valuable information on mechanisms whereby systemic diseases impact the lung's health, presenting therapeutic targets for modulation (Alastair et al., 2018). The complex interplay between systemic diseases and lung involvement warrants a multidimensional approach to treatment and management. This includes understanding how fibrogenic signals, such as those activated by TGF-β, interact with other inflammatory processes and with cellular environments in the lungs. Clinical evidence suggests that drugs selectively inhibiting TGF-β signaling have therapeutic potential to reverse pathological remodeling events typical of chronic respiratory disease. Broad inhibition of TGF-β is not without risk, with the potential to disrupt multiple important physiological processes, including immune modulation and tissue homeostasis. Hence, the design of selective inhibitors targeting TGF-β's fibrotic functions without compromising its protective role holds promise for improving lung function in systemic disease patients. Generally, there is a need to achieve a thorough understanding of these processes to facilitate therapeutic interventions targeted explicitly at resolving lung pathology among systemic disease conditions (Alastair et al., 2018) (Figure 6.8).

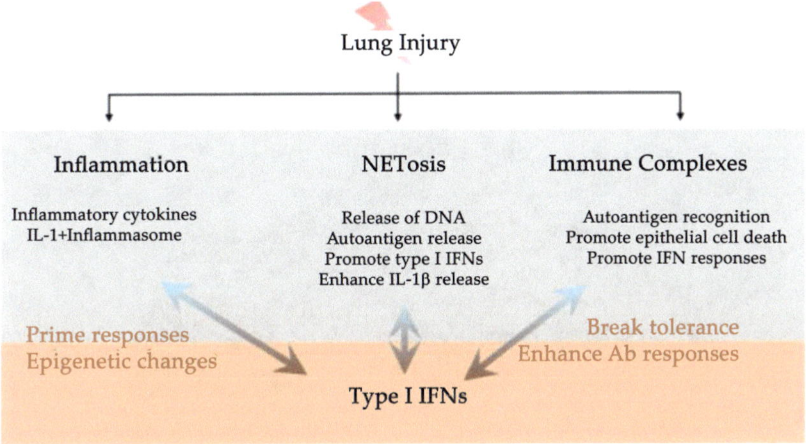

Figure 6.8. The lung in systemic lupus erythematosus.

Source: https://ars.els-cdn.com/content/image/3-s2.0-B9780128145517000453-f45-01-9780128145517.jpg.

6.2.3. Clinical Significance of Lung Assessment

Lung assessment is of major clinical importance in the broader context of systemic disease, serving as a critical diagnostic tool supported by the role of lung function in gas exchange and general physiological homeostasis. It is therefore crucial to the regular operation of various organ systems. In conditions such as systemic sclerosis or scleroderma, where lung disease can lead to significant morbidity, serial pulmonary evaluation becomes more important. According to research, tests such as the Diffusing Capacity of the Lungs for Carbon Monoxide (DLco) estimate future levels of patient fatigue, highlighting the importance of lung function quantification in monitoring disease severity and patient well-being (Assassi et al., 2011). This implies that precise measurement of lung well-being not only enhances clinical care strategies but also reflects the relationship of respiratory function with general disease outcomes. Moreover, systemic inflammatory response can significantly affect lung function, justifying the need for global bronchopulmonary examinations. Various systemic disorders, including neoplasias, present a multifaceted relationship between pulmonary dysfunction and inflammatory processes, potentially making concomitant symptoms such as fatigue and diminished quality of life more complicated. Research indicates that inflammatory responses can spread harmful effects on physical performance via mechanisms that interfere with lung and overall organ function (Dolan et al., 2017). The health professionals should not, thus, ignore the respiratory tests in such cases, as they constitute a key component of understanding the general state of patients with systemic diseases. Careful lung assessment is a key factor in identifying possible interventions that will protect against the harmful effects of systemic inflammation in various stages of disease. Finally, the importance of lung assessment extends beyond short-term respiratory illness, dictating treatment regimens and quality of life in patients with systemic disease. Physicians can use accurate lung function tests and imaging diagnostics to establish baseline lung function and detect temporal changes, providing treatment response data. For instance, a decrease in lung function may prompt adaptation of therapy modalities, illustrating the dynamic nature of systemic disease therapy. With a focus on the clinical usefulness of lung assessment, clinicians can determine focused intervention channels, with the ultimate goal of enhancing patient outcomes and quality of life. Implementing a more comprehensive modus operandi of lung assessment reaffirms its essential role in managing systemic disease, a shift towards patient-centered care based on the interdependence of all bodily systems (Figure 6.9).

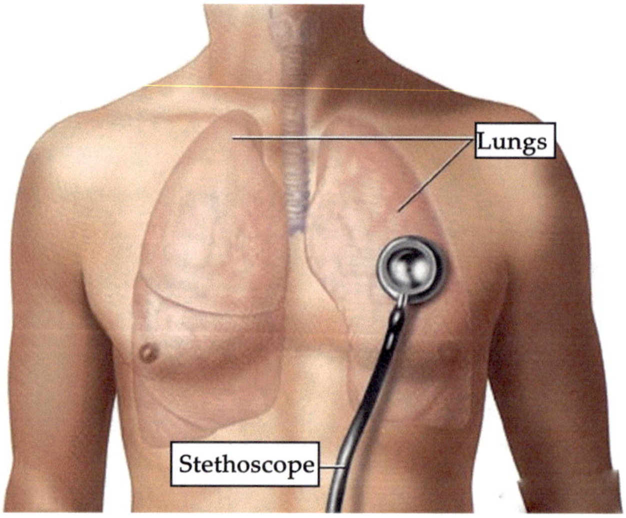

Figure 6.9. Clinical significance of lung assessment.

Source: https://medlineplus.gov/ency/images/ency/fullsize/23267.jpg.

Test Your Knowledge

1. What is the mechanism of lung involvement in systemic diseases?
2. What are the clinical significance of lung assessment?

6.3. Autoimmune Diseases and Lung Complications

Learning Outcome

1. Overview of autoimmune diseases affecting the lungs
2. Specific lung conditions associated with autoimmune diseases
3. Diagnostic challenges in autoimmune-related lung issues

Autoimmune diseases and pulmonary complications are subtly interrelated, as various systemic diseases directly influence respiratory function. Systemic lupus erythematosus, rheumatoid arthritis, and progressive systemic sclerosis are all known to produce severe respiratory illness. These complications have the potential to occur in many different ways, including interstitial lung disease and pulmonary arterial hypertension, which are two of the most commonly occurring complications in patients with connective tissue diseases (CTDs) (Fernandes et al., 2015).

The severity of such conditions necessitates that clinicians be well aware of the thoracic complications that can occur, as management can significantly differ according to the underlying autoimmune condition. By recognizing shared patterns of lung involvement, clinicians can more effectively individualize their management approaches, ensuring patients receive timely and proper interventions for their pulmonary complications.

Racial differences in the expression of autoimmune diseases, especially systemic sclerosis, add to the complexity of lung complications related to these diseases. Research has shown that African American patients with systemic sclerosis have more severe manifestations of the disease when compared to their European American counterparts. A Genome Research in African American Scleroderma Patients (GRASP) cohort study identified that a significant 43% of patients had pulmonary fibrosis and, significantly, this was often associated with severe respiratory dysfunction, e.g., forced vital capacity (FVC) of 50% or less (Boin et al., 2017). These findings emphasized to underscore the significance of considering genetic and environmental factors when determining the extent of pulmonary involvement in autoimmune diseases. Doctors must be aware of these variations to deliver personalized treatment plans that address the individualized requirements of different patient populations.

Impacts of lung complications in patients with autoimmune diseases extend beyond the borders of pulmonary function itself; they have drastic psychosocial consequences that affect overall quality of life. Presentation of respiratory symptoms can be followed by increased morbidity since patients will have limitations in physical functioning, social activity, and overall living. Additionally, the psychological burden of chronic lung disease can exacerbate mental illness, including anxiety and depression, further complicating patient care.

Due to the interconnected nature of physical and mental well-being, both the treatment of the autoimmune disease and the respiratory consequences thereof necessitate a multidisciplinary team to treat both ailments. By adding pulmonologists, rheumatologists, and mental health professionals to the team, clinicians can create an integrated treatment plan that addresses the entire spectrum of needs for patients with the lung complications of autoimmune disorders (Figure 6.10).

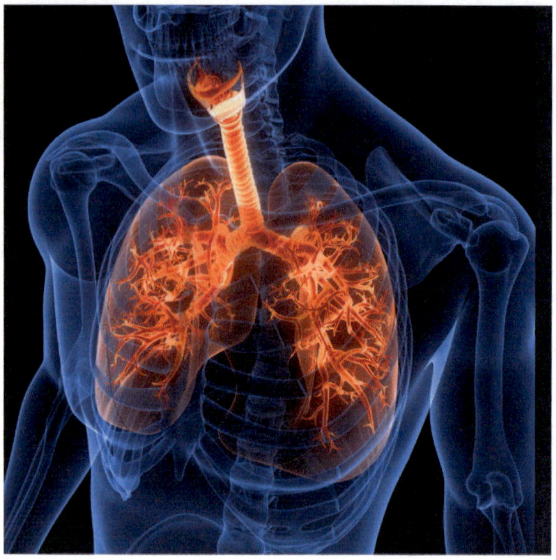

Figure 6.10. Autoimmune diseases and lung health.

Source: https://drmaggieyu.com/wp-content/uploads/2023/09/iStock-1444039822.jpg.

6.3.1. Overview of Autoimmune Diseases Affecting the Lungs

Autoimmune diseases represent a significant category of diseases in which the immune system is turned against the body's own cells, causing inflammation and damage to organs like the lungs. The intricate structure and function of lung tissue render it particularly susceptible to autoimmune attacks. Diseases such as systemic lupus erythematosus (SLE) and rheumatoid arthritis (RA) may result in pulmonary manifestations because both are systemic conditions with inflammatory processes that can be extrapolated to the lung parenchyma. They may appear in different forms, such as pleuritis, interstitial lung disease, and pulmonary hypertension, showing the systemic nature of these autoimmune diseases. Understanding the pathology of these illnesses is crucial, as early detection and treatment can prevent long-term complications and improve the patient's quality of life. Therefore, research clarifying the mechanisms by which these systemic diseases correlate with lung impairment is even more critical. In systemic lupus erythematosus, there has been proven a profound association between particular genetic factors and the respiratory manifestations that characterize the disease. For example, single-nucleotide polymorphisms (SNPs) within genes such as IRF5 and TNPO3 were linked to the etiology of lupus as well as its pulmonary manifestations, such as pleuritis and pulmonary disease. Research demonstrates that genetic mutations within these genes contribute independently to the morbidity of symptoms encompassing both the lungs and the etiology of the disease as a whole, showing the complexity of autoimmune interactions within the body. The significance of these gene correlations is significant in clinical practice, as they have the potential to enable more personalized therapeutic approaches for managing lupus patients' pulmonary-related issues. This underscores the necessity for ongoing research in the genetic origins of autoimmune diseases of the respiratory tract. Furthermore, the interplay between the microbiome, metabolome, and immune function is increasingly recognized as a biological basis for the autoimmune pathogenesis of lung health conditions. It is becoming increasingly clear that changes in the microbiome can potentially modify immune responses to influence predisposition towards autoimmune disease that involves lung tissue (Dorrestein et al., 2014). The diversity of microbial communities in the body is able to modulate inflammation and immune responses to have a beneficial or pathological impact on lung function, depending on the type of interactions involved. This new area of research imparts an integrated approach, through which the realization of how the microbiome, immune system, and lung tissue responses are interconnected could unlock new therapeutic approaches to managing autoimmune illness within the lung. As further research develops, the need will arise to institute targeted interventions that could capitalize on these relationships for the purpose of maintaining lung function in the setting of systemic autoimmune attack (Figure 6.11).

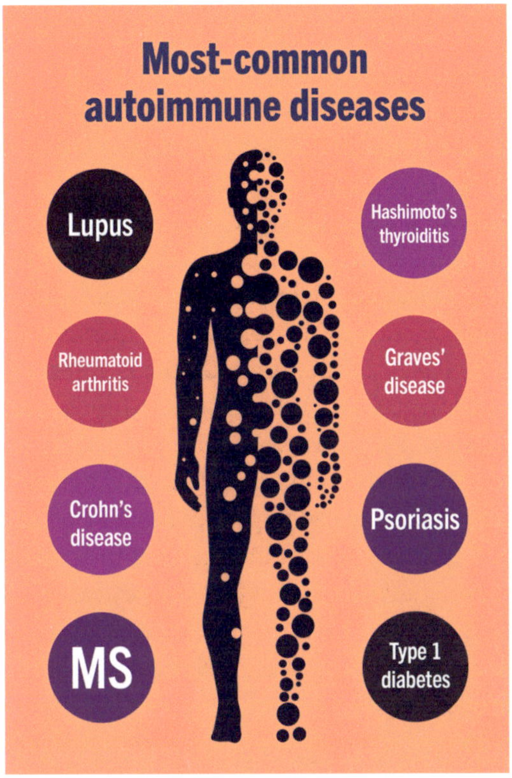

Figure 6.11. Autoimmune diseases affecting the lungs.

Source: https://www.wellmark.com/-/media/sites/blue-magazine/2021-content-marketing/february/most-common-autoimmune-diseases.png?sc_lang=en&hash=A53C0D8E611A27A7166B1F7365079741.

6.3.2. Specific Lung Conditions Associated with Autoimmune Diseases

Autoimmune diseases are characterized by the body's own tissue being attacked by the immune system's erroneous attack, and this can significantly impact lung health. Some lung conditions such as interstitial lung disease (ILD), pulmonary fibrosis, and pleuritis have a connection with autoimmune diseases, one of them being ILD. ILD is a condition that is commonly associated with diseases like rheumatoid arthritis and systemic sclerosis, and has inflammation and scarring within the lungs that causes breathing problems and reduced quality of life. The progressive nature of these conditions mandates early detection and therapy, as timely intervention is capable of slowing down the deterioration in lung function. The patients may have diverse respiratory manifestations based on the complexity of autoimmune pathology and its systemic effects, thereby mandating careful pulmonary assessments in the setting of systemic conditions like autoimmune diseases (Ailal et al., 2020). Various autoimmune diseases can be associated with different pulmonary manifestations. For example, systemic lupus erythematosus (SLE) is usually associated with pleuritis, or inflammation of the pleura over the lungs. This can cause chest pain and dyspnea, worsening the clinical course of the disease. Further, Sjögrens syndrome patients are susceptible to lung infection and airway injury due to autoimmune processes. The interaction between systemic inflammation and localized lung pathology presents a complex challenge for healthcare professionals, as understanding these relationships is essential for managing these entities. Clinicians are required to stay alert when assessing respiratory signs and symptoms in autoimmune patients since prompt identification results in improved outcomes and effective disease management as a whole (Amadi-Obi et al., 2014). Untreated chronic pulmonary involvement in autoimmune disorders can ultimately lead to severe complications like respiratory failure and increased mortality. Chronic inflammation has the potential to lead to lung damage that is irreversible in character, complicating treatment and rehabilitation processes. Patients may also be at increased risk of lung cancers, and therefore careful screening and monitoring are important. The interconnectedness of autoimmune diseases and pulmonary diseases highlights the multifactorial pathogenesis of the conditions, in which immune dysfunction leads to systemic and localized disease.

Understanding of the inherent role of the lungs in systemic disease mandates a holistic treatment approach that recognizes the imperative for integrative management addressing both autoimmune disease and pulmonary sequelae. As the research process continues, a better understanding of such relationships will enhance care for patients in this complex field (Ailal et al., 2020).

6.3.3. Diagnostic Challenges in Autoimmune-Related Lung Issues

The diagnostic challenges in autoimmune-related lung diseases are multifaceted and often compounded by the overlap of presentations of several systemic illnesses. Respiratory symptoms are common in patients and may be mimicked by other lung diseases, such as infection or malignancy, leading to erroneous diagnosis. For instance, the immune checkpoint inhibitor mechanism, which is one of the established therapies for cancer immunotherapy, results in irAEs that can affect the lungs and present as pneumonitis.

The complication is characterized by its late presentation and great variability, therefore necessitating high clinical suspicion among clinicians. Early detection is essential because tardy intervention can be linked with severe outcomes and complicate overall patient management (Abdallah et al., 2017). Therefore, the integration of multidisciplinary approaches in the diagnosis of autoimmune disorder-associated lung complications is crucial to ensure prompt and efficacious management. Additionally, conditions like immunoglobulin G4-related disease (IgG4-RD) pose further diagnostic ambiguity because of their rare and multifaceted presentations. While IgG4-RD selectively affects organs such as the pancreas and salivary glands, pulmonary manifestations can appear with the same symptoms as other lung diseases, e.g., fibrosis or nodular lesions. Histopathological features of IgG4-RD, such as storiform fibrosis and lymphoplasmacytic infiltration, are challenging to diagnose and may require biopsy, a painful process that is harmful to patients (Adelheid et al., 2014). Elevated serum IgG4 levels are useful in diagnosis, but the marker is not consistently found in all patients, and hence, the detection of the disease at its early stage is challenging. Clinicians must thus consider IgG4-RD while evaluating systemic diseases like the lungs, making diagnosis more difficult. The complexities reflect the need for enhanced diagnostic approaches and consistent clinical guidelines for autoimmune-induced lung diseases. Current management practices tend to be based on historic case series and single institutional clinical experiences, generating heterogeneity

in approaches to treatment across institutions. This heterogeneity is most clearly seen in managing immune-related pneumonitis, where early intervention with immunosuppressive therapies has the potential to shape patient outcomes dramatically. As highlighted by the emphasis of present studies and organizational guidelines based on consensus regarding irAEs management, it is vital to possess thorough diagnostics that take patients' general systemic state into account as well (Abdallah et al., 2017). The establishment of strict diagnostic criteria and understanding of the interrelationship of various autoimmune diseases will enhance clinicians' skills to diagnose, document, and manage lung-associated complications effectively, ultimately improving patient care in this crucial section of systemic conditions (Figure 6.12).

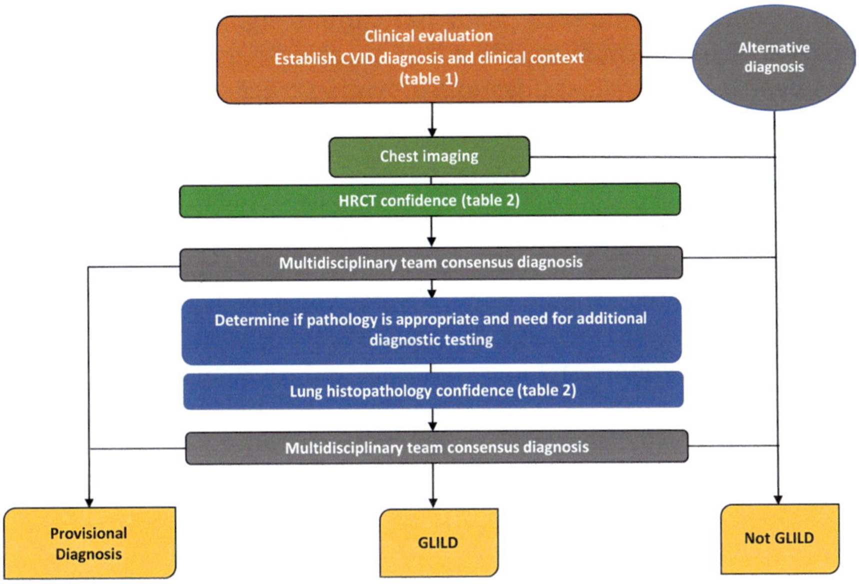

Figure 6.12. Approach to diagnosing and managing granulomatous-lymphocytic interstitial lung disease.

Source: https://www.thelancet.com/cms/10.1016/j.eclinm.2024.102749/asset/ebc90e04-c812-4f19-b81c-11c03841bfe0/main.assets/gr3_lrg.jpg.

Test Your Knowledge

1. Give an overview of autoimmune diseases affecting the lungs.
2. What are the diagnostic challenges in autoimmune-related lung issues?

6.4. Infectious Diseases and Lung Implications

Learning Outcome

1. Overview of systemic infections affecting lung function
2. Impact of lung infections on systemic health
3. Treatment considerations for lung involvement

The interaction of infectious diseases with pulmonary considerations requires a comprehensive understanding of respiratory function in the context of systemic illness. The lungs are not just the predominant site of gas exchange but also a critical organ of the immune system, often acting as the initial line of defense against respiratory pathogens. Infection can profoundly compromise pulmonary function, leading to complications such as pneumonia, acute respiratory distress syndrome (ARDS), and chronic lung disease. As chronic lower respiratory disease was the third most common cause of death in the United States in 2015, it is apparent that imbalances in the pulmonary system can extend beyond the act of breathing to have a systemic impact on well-being around the world and increase the mortality rate of many populations (Miller et al., 2017). Furthermore, the role of the microbiota in maintaining lung tissue health and modulating immunity is of paramount significance when considering how infectious diseases can generate dysbiosis. Resident microbiota not only shape host immunity but also develop a protective barrier against infection, providing crucial protection during infection. This co-immunity model illustrates that lung health is not only dependent upon the innate mechanisms of the immune system but also, to a large degree, upon the microbial communities resident within the respiratory tract (Abt et al., 2017). These interactions highlight the intricate dynamics that inform lung health in systemic disease and have encouraged researchers to explore new therapy interventions that acknowledge the protective role of the microbiota as a potential route towards increasing pulmonary resilience. The impact of infectious disease on lung function calls for interdisciplinarity in treatment and research. An understanding of the pathogenesis of lung disease in the context of systemic infection can guide clinical practices aimed at preventing complications. For instance, studies in nonhuman primates have shed light on the mechanisms through which inhaled microorganisms and exposures can influence the evolution of lung disease. These models have been invaluable for guiding molecular targets for new treatment regimens and for confirming the safety and efficacy of vaccines to prevent lung infections (Miller et al., 2017). With advancing research, the integration of microbiota studies with advanced modeling systems can promise revolutionary treatment that not only cures existing lung illnesses but also eliminates the risk of future respiratory complications due to infections (Figure 6.13).

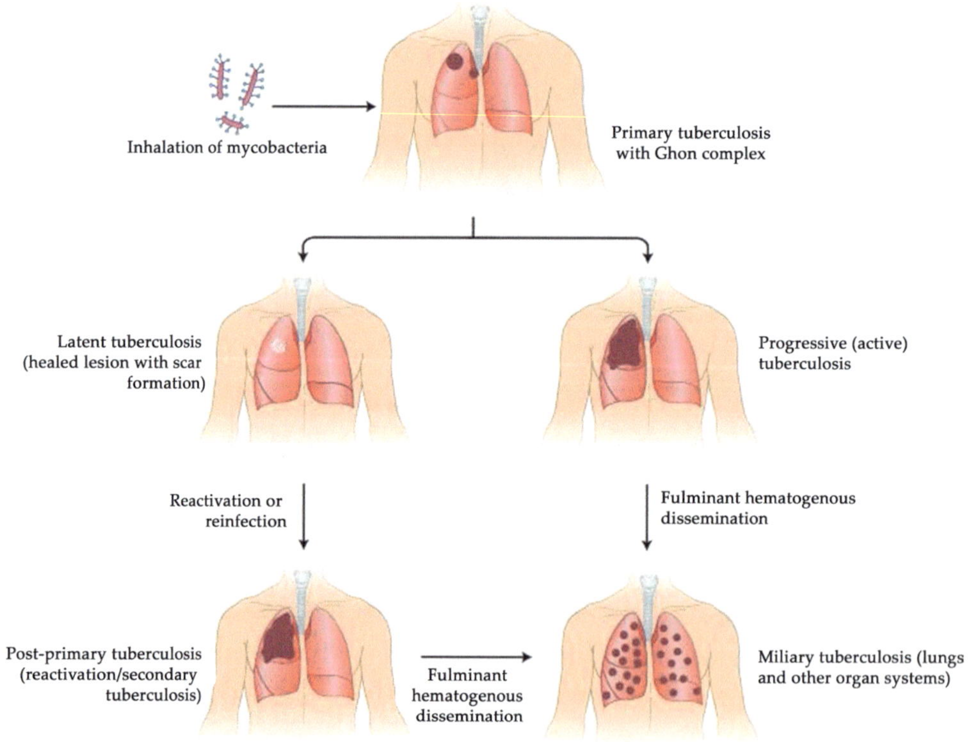

Figure 6.13. Infectious lung disease.

Source: https://media.springernature.com/lw685/springer-static/image/chp%3A10.1007%2F978-3-030-36438-0_1/MediaObjects/370472_1_En_1_Fig9_HTML.png.

6.4.1. Overview of Systemic Infections Affecting Lung Function

Systemic infections, which affect lung function, are generally the outcome of a complex interaction between the causative microbes and the immune response of the host. Systemic infections can lead to dysregulation of immune reactions, compromising lung health when they occur.

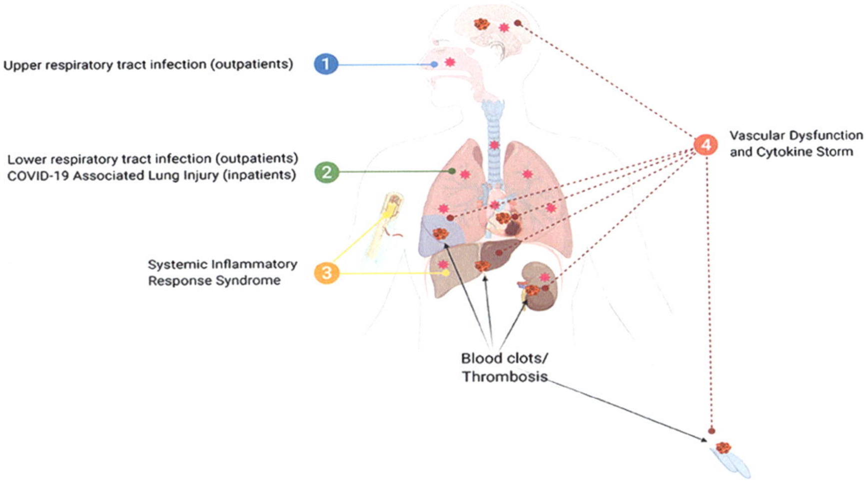

Figure 6.14. Systemic infections affecting lung function.

Source: https://www.frontiersin.org/files/Articles/564628/fimmu-11-01626-HTML/image_m/fimmu-11-01626-g001.jpg.

This dysregulation of immune responses may manifest as inflammation, disturbed gas exchange, or crippling fibrosis of the lungs, ultimately leading to respiratory failure. For instance, bacterial, viral, or fungal infections can trigger secondary complications such as ARDS, which extensively compromises lung function. Pathogens such as Streptococcus pneumoniae and Mycobacterium tuberculosis are notorious for inducing systemic effects that compromise lung integrity. Aside from bacterial infections, viral infections like coronaviruses and the influenza virus reveal how immune responses to pathogens can exacerbate chronic lung ailments or induce new respiratory abnormalities. This highlights the importance of timely identification and treatment in systemic infections affecting pulmonary health. The interaction between systemic infection and lung function is not only concerned with how such infection can exacerbate underlying chronic pulmonary disease. In patients with conditions such as COPD or interstitial lung disease, the presence of a systemic infection can destabilize an already compromised respiratory system. The inflammatory mediators released in response to infection may provoke further deterioration, leading to an increased frequency of exacerbations and associated symptoms. Moreover, systemic diseases, such as systemic sclerosis, tend to present with interdependency of pulmonary and cardiac functions, and lung injury from infection may be indicative of myocarditis or other cardiovascular disease (He et al., 2023). It is essential to appreciate that systemic infection does not act independently but can prolong the multi-organ dysfunction characteristic of systemic illness, thereby adding to the challenges faced by patients with lung dysfunction. Moreover, the intricate interaction between lung function and gut health plays a pivotal role in explaining systemic infections within the lungs. The gut microbiota, through their metabolic byproducts, influence the immune response, which plays a crucial role in fighting systemic infections (Ney et al., 2023). Short-chain fatty acids (SCFAs) produced by gut bacterial fermentation of dietary fiber are significant regulators of the immune response, increasing vigorous defense against lung infection. Dysregulation of gut microbiota can weaken the respiratory system's defense and expose individuals to infection and respiratory disease. As infections along altered immune pathways propagate systemically, understanding these interactions facilitates novel therapeutic possibilities, including the potential use of probiotics or SCFA supplementation to optimize the immune response and preserve lung function in individuals predisposed to systemic infections. Such a holistic knowledge underscores the necessity for interdisciplinary interventions towards managing systemic infections and maintaining optimal lung health (Figure 6.14).

6.4.2. Impact of Lung Infections on Systemic Health

Lung infections often serve as a pivotal component in the broader landscape of systemic health issues. Their impact extends beyond the respiratory system, with evidence suggesting that these infections can exacerbate pre-existing systemic conditions and precipitate new health challenges. In disease states such as cardiovascular disease, diabetes, or chronic inflammatory disease, pulmonary infections may instigate inflammatory pathways that not only amplify local symptoms but also cause systemic inflammation.

This points to the synergistic link between the function of the lung and of the body as a whole, creating the need for comprehensive treatment regimens that include both localized infection and generalized impact. Epidemiological studies have contended that infections of the lungs may be aggravating factors in underlying systemic ailments, highlighting the need to identify these infections as a key determinant of overall health. The role of particulate matter in exacerbating lung infections cannot be ruled out. High levels of air pollutants, excellent particulate matter (PM2.5), have been linked with unfavorable effects on lung functions and increased susceptibility to respiratory infections. The mechanisms of this relationship are diverse, encompassing oxidative stress responses, inflammatory pathways, and lung clearance mechanisms. Such exposures have a tendency to lead to higher susceptibility to infections, with significant impacts on systemic health. Further, the systemic inflammatory response to lung infections can present through various pathways, including increased cardiovascular risk and metabolic disturbances. With growing evidence implicating air quality as contributing to lung health, treatment of lung infections must involve an integrative approach that addresses environmental impacts on respiratory and overall health, as outlined in Liu et al. (2016). The interaction between the human microbiota and lung infections complicates the impact of respiratory diseases on overall health. The resident microbiota play a crucial role in shaping the immune system and providing a protective barrier against pathogens, including those causing lung infections. In current literature, there has been the concept of co-immunity, indicating that the hosts' immune system and the microbiota collaborate to contribute to health outcomes. This mutually supportive relationship postulates that dysbiosis of microbiota through causes like antibiotics or environmental stress could intensify lung infections, later affecting overall bodily health. Strategies for restoring or maintaining a normal microbiota potentially offer new avenues for preventing or modulating the systemic effects of pulmonary infection. This underlines the need for integrated interventions that consider both respiratory and general health dynamics, as outlined in Abt et al. (2017).

6.4.3. Treatment Considerations for Lung Involvement

The treatment of lung disease in systemic diseases such as systemic sclerosis and other fibrosing diseases needs to be multidisciplinary, given the complexities and heterogeneities of these diseases.

Most important to the therapeutic algorithms is the definition of the driving pathophysiologic mechanisms of lung disease. For instance, the excessive production of collagen and connective tissue within the lungs, which occurs in systemic sclerosis, can significantly adversely affect pulmonary function. Existing therapies revolve around modulating these fibrotic processes with diverse agents.

Experimental therapies aim to inhibit the growth factors that lead to fibrosis, such as TGF-β and PDGF, which are known to be critically significant in causing and maintaining fibroblast activation. Understanding these pathways improves the likelihood of developing effective anti-fibrotic drugs, which is a pressing need since very few drugs are available to treat lung involvement in systemic disease (Jimenez et al., 2013). Therapy should also be according to the severity and progression of lung disease, with regular monitoring of pulmonary function. Early identification of pulmonary complications provides an opportunity for early intervention, which can improve clinical outcomes. Pharmacologic interventions, including immunosuppressants and novel antifibrotics, are being studied in greater numbers for secondary lung disease due to systemic conditions. These drugs act by inhibiting the inflammatory process and arresting the progression of fibrosis in the lungs.

Clinical trials of nintedanib and pirfenidone, for example, have been promising in managing fibrosis in pulmonary involvement secondary to systemic sclerosis. In this case, a multidisciplinary treatment approach, including the coordination of pulmonologists, rheumatologists, and other professionals, is required to ensure maximal treatment regimens and tailor interventions based on the patient's profile (Castro et al., 2010). It is also essential in managing lung involvement in systemic diseases to inform and motivate the patient. Patients need to be informed about the disease process, the importance of monitoring respiratory symptoms, and the need to adhere to prescribed therapeutic measures. Pulmonary rehabilitation programs are also extremely effective in enhancing the quality of life for patients with respiratory complications. Pulmonary rehabilitation programs enhance lung function, promote physical activity, and provide psychological care.

Briefly speaking, even as therapeutic treatment of lung involvement in systemic diseases continues to be refined, a combination of pharmacologic treatment, appropriate surveillance, and patient-centered support systems becomes an integral part of overall care. Holistically working on these facets will eventually enhance therapy outcomes of lung complications of systemic diseases (Jimenez et al., 2013) (Figure 6.15).

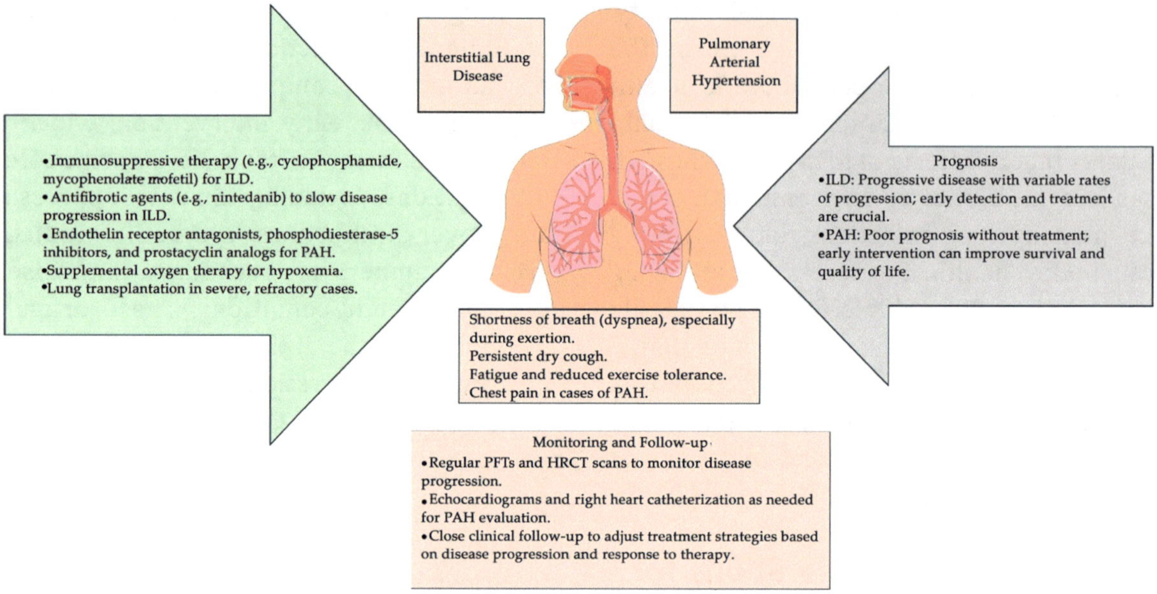

Figure 6.15. Treatment considerations for lung involvement in systemic diseases.

Source: https://www.mdpi.com/sclerosis/sclerosis-02-00014/article_deploy/html/images/sclerosis-02-00014-g003.png.

Test Your Knowledge

1. Give an overview of systemic infections affecting lung function.
2. What are the impact of lung infections on systemic health?

6.5. Cardiovascular Diseases and Lung Interactions

Learning Outcome

1. Relationship between heart and lung health
2. Effects of cardiovascular diseases on lung function
3. Management strategies for coexisting conditions

The dynamic relationship between cardiovascular and lung disease has come into focus in recent years, highlighting the massive contribution of lung disease to cardiovascular endpoints. The heart and lung are closely intertwined by shared mechanisms of inflammation and gas exchange, so systemic disease in one organ can adversely affect the other. For instance, CRD, such as COPD, is prone to inducing systemic inflammation that can fuel cardiovascular diseases like hypertension and heart failure. The mediators released when there is respiratory impairment have the potential to initiate a chain of events that enhance the severity of cardiovascular disease, pointing to the importance of an interdisciplinary treatment approach to these related health issues. Complicating the co-relationship between lung and cardiovascular disease is the influence of environmental determinants such as air pollution. Epidemiologic data suggest a strong association between exposure to particulate matter and cardiovascular morbidity and mortality. Specifically, fine particulate matter (PM2.5) has been established to be causally associated with systemic inflammation that exacerbates disease states such as atherosclerosis and arrhythmias. Because particles that are inhaled penetrate deep into the respiratory system, they can pass into the bloodstream and lead to adverse cardiovascular events, including myocardial infarctions. The intricate interplay between lung function and cardiovascular responses underscores the importance of public health interventions aimed at reducing exposure to air pollutants, thereby mitigating the risk of cardiovascular disease due to compromised lung function (Sioutas et al., 2005). Also significant are the effects of treating patients with co-occurring cardiovascular and respiratory illnesses. Uniform treatment guidelines that take into account the dual nature of these illnesses are critical for enhancing patient prognosis. For instance, drugs used to manage pulmonary symptoms often require careful consideration of their impact on the cardiovascular system. Beta-agonists, which are typically used in the treatment of asthma or COPD, can cause heart rate alterations and other cardiovascular difficulties. Therefore, health care providers must assess the risk-benefit picture of these treatments on a multidisciplinary level. Transdisciplinary integration of care between specialties can enhance patient management, potentially reducing complications arising from the interaction between cardiovascular disease and lung health. Awareness of this dual nature encourages enhanced therapeutic strategies and the system-wide impact of these ailments on the well-being of individuals (Alving et al., 2012) (Figure 6.16).

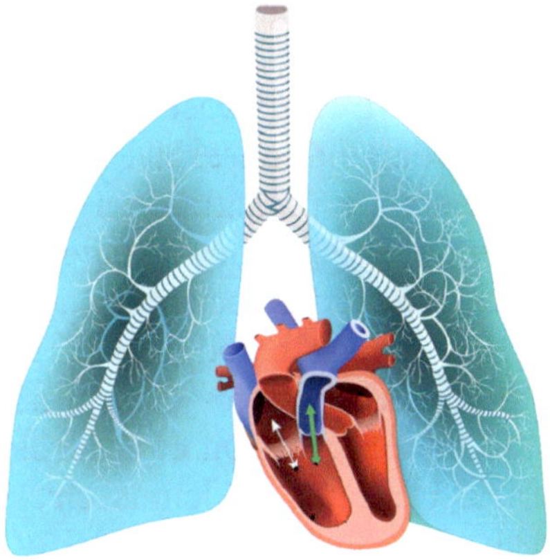

Figure 6.16. Cardiovascular diseases and lung interactions.

Source: https://www.u-tokyo.ac.jp/content/400132085.jpg.

6.5.1. Relationship Between Heart and Lung Health

The intricate interdependence of lung and cardiac health is established through shared pathways in respiratory and cardiovascular physiology. The lungs are responsible for oxygenating blood, an activity with a direct effect on cardiac function. As lung health declines, such as in COPD or asthma, the heart must compensate for increased workloads and stress. This is primarily due to hypoxemia, which can lead to pulmonary hypertension and, in the process, increase the risk of heart failure. Studies have proven that respiratory diseases have the potential to exacerbate cardiovascular disease, increasing the mortality rate of patients with both conditions immensely. It is thus essential to maintain good lung function in a bid to prevent heart complications and thus the two-way interaction between the conditions becomes evident. Environmental conditions, especially air pollution, have significant effects on lung and heart health. Studies have proven that exposure to particulate matter (PM), more so fine particulate matter (PM2.5), has been associated with many adverse health effects, including cardiovascular morbidity. Epidemiologic studies have shown that increased levels of PM correlate with hospitalization for cardiovascular disease and death, implicating that unresolved air pollution can cause systemic inflammation in both the heart and lungs. Respiratory changes in air can lead to increased cardiac ischemia, arrhythmias, and incidents of high blood pressure. Further, this systemic inflammatory response could also hasten the progression of atherosclerosis, which in turn creates a vicious circle where reduced lung function irreversibly affects heart function, with the need for integrated public health interventions for respiratory and cardiovascular risk due to air pollution (Sioutas et al., 2005; Liu et al., 2016). It is critical to clarify the mechanisms between heart and lung health to provide effective therapeutic interventions. The toxic activities of ultrafine particles have the potential to cause oxidative stress and inflammation that adversely affect the respiratory and cardiovascular systems. Such health effects are caused by the size and composition of the particles, which allow them to penetrate deep into lung tissue and the bloodstream. Thus, the interaction of such particles with the cardiovascular system can induce drastic effects, such as myocardial infarction or stroke. This emphasizes that there is a critical requirement for extensive research to explain these mechanisms and their public health relevance. Because heart and lung disease are also found together very frequently, medical approaches must be addressed with an integrated strategy towards diagnosis and care, which encourages an integrated concept of systemic disease and its inter-relationship (Figure 6.17).

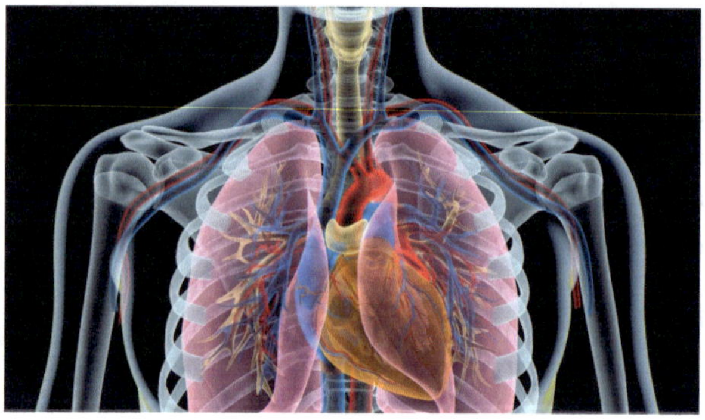

Figure 6.17. Relationship between heart and lung health.

Source: https://cdn.nddmed.com/posts/2023/ndd-blog-the-heart-and-the-lungs-whats-the-connection.webp.

6.5.2. Effects of Cardiovascular Diseases on Lung Function

The interdependence between cardiovascular disease and pulmonary function highlights the complexity of systemic relationships within human physiology. Cardiovascular disease, particularly that leading to heart failure, is capable of triggering pulmonary complications due to the interdependent relationship between the respiratory and cardiovascular systems. As the efficiency of the heart declines, pressures in pulmonary circulation may increase, leading to pulmonary edema and decreased gas exchange capacity.

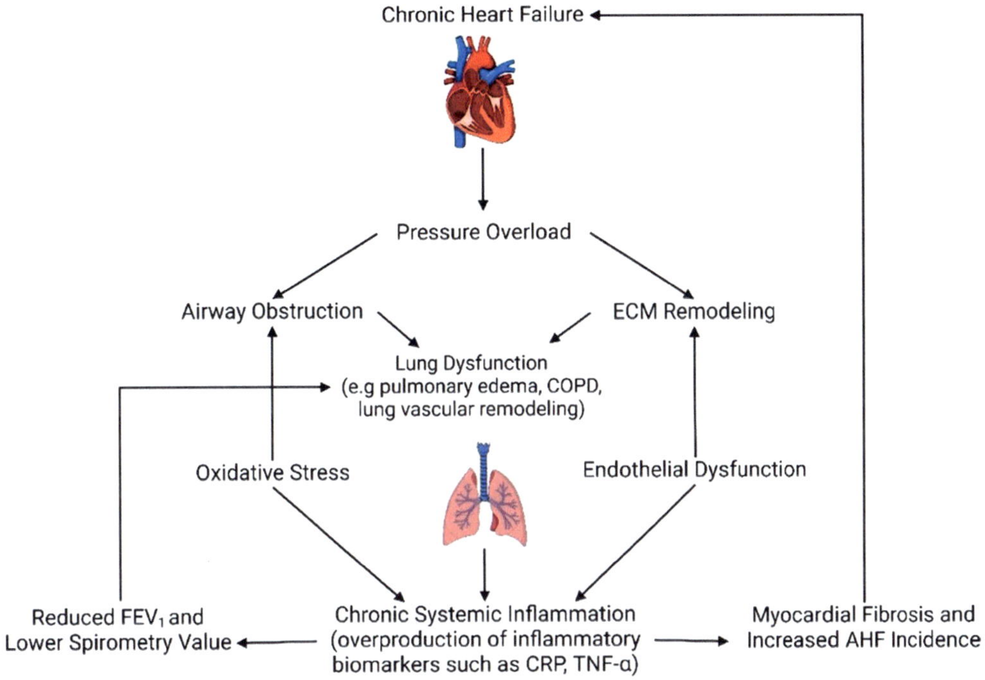

Figure 6.18. Effects of cardiovascular diseases on lung function.

Source: https://www.sciepublish.com/uploads/2024/12/02/0067734306b022460afa54c3951433e6.jpg.

This dysregulation not only helps to exacerbate symptoms of COPD but also leads to acute respiratory failure, where patients experience wheezing, shortness of breath, and reduced exercise tolerance. Evidence shows a high risk of death in patients with both cardiac disease and COPD, making an integrated treatment regimen that considers both systems at once, leading to improved patient outcomes in patients with complicated comorbidities. Evidence also strengthens the systemic effect by indicating that patients with COPD frequently have cardiac comorbidities, further supporting the principle that cardiovascular and respiratory health cannot be divided. As seen through recent studies, individuals with mild COPD experience a greater cardiovascular disease mortality than respiratory insufficiency death itself (André et al., 2019). This poignant reality emphasizes the need for healthcare professionals to address these comorbidities with an integrated treatment strategy. In addition, the shared risk factors of smoking and physical inactivity contribute to the complexity of the clinical picture because they exacerbate the lung as well as cardiac dysfunction. By recognizing the systemic influence of cardiovascular diseases on lung function, therapists can develop targeted interventions, attempting to contain the negative risks that encircle combined systemic failures in patients. The effects of cardiovascular diseases extend to longer-term respiratory conditions, with studies pointing to possible alterations in pulmonary function as a consequence of chronic systemic inflammation. It has been postulated that inflammatory mediators implicated in cardiovascular diseases could decrease the regulation of microRNAs critical to maintaining homeostasis in lung tissues (Eghbali et al., 2014). It can cause a cascade leading to epithelial dysfunction and increased susceptibility to infection, thereby worsening the challenge faced in treating patients with concomitant heart and lung diseases.

As ongoing research continues to deconstruct the interface between microRNA biology and systemic disease, the findings may spearhead the way toward innovative treatment strategies. By leveraging the therapeutic potential of microRNA, clinicians can better address the complex interplay between lung function and cardiovascular health, leading to improved patient outcomes overall (Figure 6.18).

6.5.3. Management Strategies for Coexisting Conditions

The management of conditions accompanying systemic disease involves a multi-disciplinary approach that attempts to comprehend the interactive network of multiple diseases. Systemic disease, such as autoimmune conditions or malignancies, can weaken the lungs and create secondary conditions like bronchiectasis. This disease, with irreversible dilatation of bronchial airways, can significantly impair patients' quality of life, primarily when it is associated with underlying disease like cystic fibrosis or COPD. The management protocols for bronchiectasis must consequently integrate respiratory therapy, drug treatment, and physical rehabilitation. A well-coordinated team of pulmonologists, rheumatologists, and physiotherapists is necessary for the effective implementation of treatment plans that incorporate these varied aspects of treatment. This approach enables custom management responsive to the specific patient's needs and co-morbidities, thus maximizing overall health outcomes (Aksamit et al., 2019). In patients with hematological malignancies undergoing allogeneic stem cell transplantation (allo-SCT), comorbidities such as graft versus host disease (GVHD) pose significant challenges to respiratory function. Ocular GVHD, present in a high proportion of allo-SCT recipients, can lead to secondary conditions causing damage to lung function by inducing systemic inflammation. Treatment of such patients consists of vigilant monitoring and prompt intervention to prevent irreversible consequences. A successful strategy includes intermittent ocular monitoring as well as respiratory monitoring for any early sign of lung involvement. Co-administration of artificial tears with immunomodulatory treatments for ocular complications can effectively counter the effects of GVHD on quality of life and pulmonary function when using systemic immunosuppression.

Through the application of a multimodal method that encompasses ocular and pulmonary presentations of GVHD, health professionals are able to optimize patient care and improve general quality of life (Djalilian et al., 2014). The need for collaborative management approaches is also highlighted by considering the concomitant impact of systemic disease on lung function. Conditions such as rheumatoid arthritis or inflammatory bowel diseases not only involve the immune system but also cause pulmonary complications such as interstitial lung disease, which makes treatment regimens for these patients more complex.

Proper treatment includes continuous screening for pulmonary complications, in addition to targeted therapies that address both the primary systemic disease and resulting pulmonary pathology. Being part of collaborative care with rheumatologists and pulmonologists can enable an integrated treatment such that therapy is sensitive not only to lung complications but also to the systemic effects of the disease. Collaborative care can lead to greater patient satisfaction and better outcomes, and thus an interdisciplinary approach is crucial in addressing patients with coexistent systemic and respiratory disease (Aksamit et al., 2019).

Test Your Knowledge

1. Describe the relationship between heart and lung health.
2. What are the effects of cardiovascular diseases on lung function?

6.6. Metabolic Disorders and Their Effects on the Lungs

Learning Outcome

1. Overview of metabolic disorders impacting lung health
2. Specific lung complications associated with metabolic diseases
3. Importance of integrated care for metabolic and respiratory health

Metabolic disorders exert significant impacts on pulmonary function, often through complex pathophysiological mechanisms. Type 2 diabetes, characterized by insulin resistance and chronic hyperglycemia, illustrates this interaction vividly. Individuals with diabetes frequently exhibit increased inflammation and oxidative stress, which can compromise lung function over time. Such inflammatory responses can lead to respiratory complications, including an elevated risk for COPD and other obstructive lung diseases. These concerns are compounded by the systemic nature of diabetes, where chronic inflammation not only affects metabolic pathways but also leads to alterations in lung physiology, predisposing individuals to pulmonary infections and reduced lung perfusion. Understanding the intricate relationship between metabolic disturbances and lung health underscores the necessity for integrated care strategies that address both systemic and respiratory health in individuals with metabolic disorders. Moreover, obesity, a prevalent metabolic disorder, significantly influences respiratory health, imposing mechanical and inflammatory burdens that alter lung function. Increased adipose tissue leads to a higher prevalence of obesity hypoventilation syndrome and increases the likelihood of developing obstructive sleep apnea, both of which further deteriorate lung function. This relationship is bidirectional; not only does excess weight contribute to respiratory issues, but compromised lung function can also exacerbate metabolic dysregulation, creating a vicious cycle. The inflammation associated with obesity, characterized by the release of proinflammatory cytokines, aggravates the risks of lung diseases and can lead to conditions such as asthma, where airway hyperresponsiveness is exacerbated. As the global pandemic of obesity continues to rise, recognizing its implications on the respiratory system becomes increasingly vital for developing targeted interventions that mitigate both pulmonary and metabolic complications. The interplay between oral health, systemic diseases, and lung function offers additional insight into the multifaceted nature of metabolic disorders and their systemic effects. Specific metabolic disorders can influence oral health, leading to conditions such as halitosis, which has been documented in patients with concurrent systemic diseases. Oral malodor, when associated with systemic issues, can reflect underlying metabolic disturbances and has been shown to impact patients' social and psychological well-being. As discussed, chronic inflammation from metabolic disorders can alter the oral microbiome, leading to periodontal disease and potentially exacerbating lung diseases by facilitating bacterial translocation to the respiratory tract. Addressing oral health as part of comprehensive management for metabolic disorders is critical, as it can serve as a valuable component in preventing the further decline of lung function and overall health in affected individuals, thereby emphasizing the interconnectedness of systemic diseases and their implications for lung health.

6.6.1. Overview of Metabolic Disorders Impacting Lung Health

Metabolic disorders include a wide range of diseases that alter the body's chemical processes, and they have significant consequences for lung health. Obesity, diabetes, and thyroid disease are some examples of diseases that can lead to alterations in lung mechanics and gas exchange. For instance, obesity can raise the pressure of the chest wall and diaphragm, reducing lung volumes and impairing ventilation. This mechanical limitation can then cause hypoxemia and increased work of breathing, which may aggravate underlying pulmonary disease, like asthma or COPD. Also, diabetic patients are susceptible to pulmonary complications due to chronic inflammation and increased oxidative stress, which would damage the lung tissue and lead to impaired lung function over time. Hence, one needs to recognize the interplay between lung health and metabolic disorders to develop efficient treatment strategies. The physiological mechanisms behind the effects of metabolic disorders on pulmonary health are intricate and multi-factorial, comprising complex biochemical pathways. For example, insulin resistance underlying type 2 diabetes leads to inflammatory alterations that affect pulmonary function. Pro-inflammatory cytokines released from adipose tissue exert harmful influences on lung function as well as aggravate existing pathologies. In addition, metabolic derangement characterizing conditions like hyperthyroidism can lead to an increased rate of respiration and altered lung compliance, which will further complicate the respiratory mechanics of such patients. Moreover, metabolic syndrome, with its constellation of obesity, hypertension, dyslipidemia, and hyperglycemia, has been associated with an increased prevalence of respiratory disorders, suggesting that systemic inflammation is the etiological factor behind such a correlation. Study of these interactions provides insight into the mechanisms by which metabolic disease has the potential to cause significant pulmonary complications, which is why multicenter treatment is required for afflicted individuals.

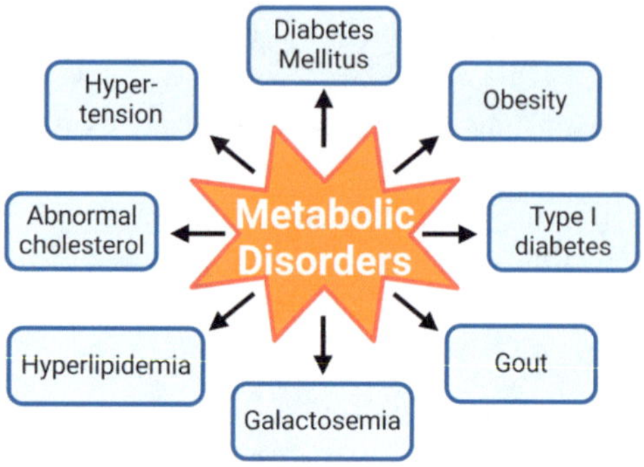

Figure 6.19. Metabolic disorders and their effects on the lungs.

Source: https://external-content.duckduckgo.com/iu/?u=https%3A%2F%2Fwww.mdpi.com%2Fnutrients%2Fnutrients-16-00507%2Farticle_deploy%2Fhtml%2Fimages%2Fnutrients-16-00507-g003.png&f=1&nofb=1&ipt=59bf395971a4722e39a37d6520556132d76d8153c436e66af0ace8dc5bffe090.

Interventions aimed at minimizing the effect of metabolic disease on pulmonary function are key factors in maximizing patient outcomes. Modification of lifestyle, such as losing weight via diet and exercise, can have a significant positive effect on lung function in obese patients and those with concomitant metabolic disease. For instance, the routine of pranayamic breathing can enhance lung function and autonomic control (Austin et al., 2006).

Besides weight management and metabolic control, these therapies can improve the quality of life for patients with respiratory and metabolic disease comorbidities. Pharmacologic therapy for metabolic derangements can enhance lung function and well-being. Being able to comprehend the complex interdependencies between metabolic diseases and respiratory function is vital in creating effective plans that address both systemic and pulmonary problems, ultimately leading to improved patient outcomes for these interrelated conditions (Figure 6.19).

6.6.2. Specific Lung Complications Associated with Metabolic Diseases

The connection between lung function and metabolic disease is a sophisticated but needed area of study, cutting across particularly in terms of the increasing awareness of some of the pulmonary complications with the metabolic pathologies such as diabetes and obesity. In particular, conditions such as preserved ratio impaired spirometry (PRISm) have emerged as significant respiratory disease that encompasses the broader definition of systemic metabolic disease. PRISm is characterized by non-uniform lung function that deviates from typical COPD diagnoses, with a characteristic clinical presentation normally observed in metabolic markers. Recent research has identified that a deficiency in vitamin D is associated with an elevated risk of acquiring PRISm and suggests that maintaining adequate vitamin D can assist in potentially preventing this lung complication, as well as general respiratory health in individuals with metabolic disorders (Lin et al., 2025). Moreover, metabolic dysfunction-associated fatty liver disease (MAFLD) has also demonstrated significant correlations with pulmonary complications, particularly by influencing systemic inflammation and oxidative stress. Pathophysiological mechanisms in MAFLD tend to cause long-term diseases such as chronic kidney disease (CKD) and cardiovascular disease, which also tend to complicate pulmonary complications. For instance, the inflammatory pathways of MAFLD enhance the risk of respiratory complications by contributing to systemic and pulmonary inflammation. Such interconnection points towards the imperatives of understanding the interlinkages between lung function and metabolic disease, as it is realized that satisfactory control of metabolic defects could be critical for averting the worsening of respiratory functions in affected patients (Dayal et al., 2025). The interlinkages between metabolic diseases and lung function present a challenge for medical professionals to embrace holistic management strategies. Treatment of diseases such as obesity, hypertension, and diabetes—both from their direct presentation and respiratory effects—may improve the overall clinical outcome of patients. With the growing recognition of evidence linking vitamin D to lung function in metabolic disorders, modulating interventions toward adequate vitamin D levels may prove beneficial. By acknowledging the two-way interaction among metabolic diseases and lung complications, researchers and clinicians can establish preventive strategies that are directed towards the maintenance of the lung and suppression of systemic conditions more effectively. Promotion of an integrated healthcare approach can not only optimize the quality of life among patients but also reduce the frequency of lung complications in the context of systemic diseases (Lin et al., 2025; Dayal et al., 2025).

6.6.3. Importance of Integrated Care for Metabolic and Respiratory Health

Integrated care is the solution to addressing the complicated interplay of metabolic disorders with respiratory health, particularly in the context of systemic diseases. For the most part, metabolic disorders such as obesity, diabetes, and metabolic syndrome not only jeopardize metabolic function but also adversely affect lung health, with the added risk of respiratory complications like asthma or COPD. These interrelationships require an integrative approach to patient management, where both metabolic and respiratory conditions are considered simultaneously by healthcare providers.

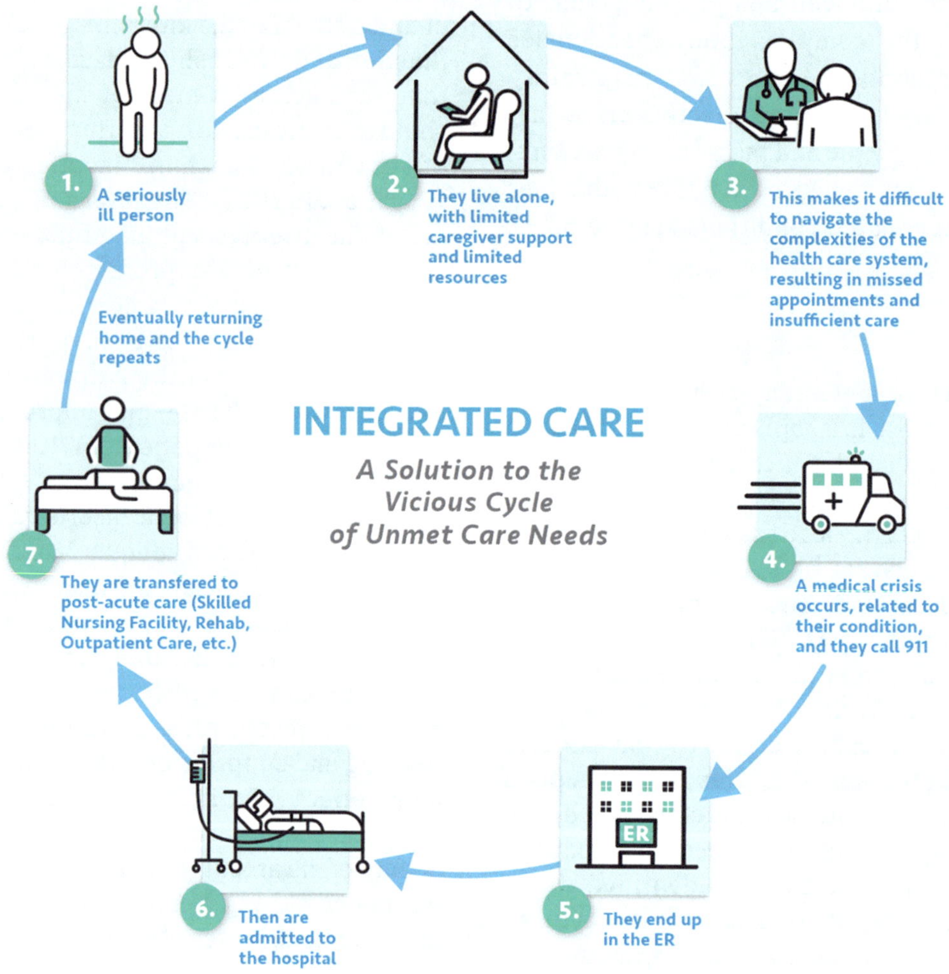

Figure 6.20. Importance of integrated care for metabolic and respiratory health.

Source: https://external-content.duckduckgo.com/iu/?u=https%3A%2F%2Fwww.navianhawaii.org%2Fwp-content%2Fuploads%2F2020%2F07%2Fintegrated-care-chart.jpg&f=1&nofb=1&ipt=60291b4c327127f63e030411607e44a8ec963d500789c19cf78fd29f992b1f51.

There is evidence that coordinated care models drive better health outcomes through more comprehensive patient assessments. This allows interventions to be effectively designed to address multiple risk factors and comorbidities simultaneously, ultimately improving the overall health and quality of life of patients suffering from these interrelated conditions (Humbert et al., 2022). Apart from this, interrelated care models support interdisciplinary coordination, which is crucial in the treatment of patients with overlapping metabolic and respiratory disorders. For example, multi-disciplinary coordination between pulmonologists, endocrinologists, and nutritionists can lead to more effective treatment strategies that provide better control of metabolism, while also assuming the responsibility of the respiratory function. It will significantly improve patient education and adherence to lifestyle modifications, such as physical training and dietary changes, which are essential for managing respiratory and metabolic health. In today's patterns of chronic diseases in the healthcare sector, integration of this kind will play a fundamental role in avoiding systemic disease risk and improving long-term health results (Míkel et al., 2021). Furthermore, encouraging patient-centered care using combined models will be capable of enabling people to be proactively engaged in their health care. By implementing individualized care plans that integrate metabolic and respiratory health issues, healthcare professionals can help patients appreciate their combined health issues and how they will be properly managed. More communication between health care professionals and patients enables an inspiring environment where individuals are motivated to adhere to treatment protocols, exercise, and adopt healthier lifestyles overall. Integrated care not only, therefore, improves clinical handling of systemic illnesses but also results in sustainable and proactive maintenance of health and eventually reduces the burden on the health care systems (Humbert et al., 2022) (Figure 6.20).

Test Your Knowledge

1. What are the specific lung complications associated with metabolic diseases?
2. What are the importance of integrated care for metabolic and respiratory health?

Summary

In summarizing the intricate interaction between lung disease and systemic diseases, it is evident that multifaceted intervention is necessary for both treatment and comprehension. The lungs are not just responsible for respiratory function; they are also critically involved in the pathophysiology of most systemic diseases. Though systemic inflammation and oxidative stress fueled by environmental toxins fuel respiratory disease, these are also involved in the aggravation of other chronic diseases. This highlights the grim reality of the way that compromised lung function can affect the incidence and severity of systemic disease. Ultimately, correction of these interconnected medical conditions needs specialized interventions that cut across multiple medical specialties, emphasizing the lungs' role in systemic health as both an early warning sign and a causative agent in overall wellness (Bednarek et al., 2024). Moreover, evidence proving an association between COPD and cardiac complications highlights the importance of an interdisciplinary care approach. As COPD is projected to become a leading cause of death globally, it is imperative to understand its compatibility with cardiovascular comorbidities. Such conditions are often characterized by similar risk factors and disease processes, requiring treatment modalities that integrate both pulmonary and cardiac care. Existing recommendations assert that addressing comorbidities is likely to improve patient outcomes, especially for those with complex health problems. The interconnected nature of such diseases indicates that ignoring one can negatively impact the control of the other, making a combined approach in treatment more effective to achieve optimal patient care (André et al., 2019). In conclusion, the dynamic relationship between lung disease and systemic disorders illustrates the necessity for more research on pollutant-specific effects and health consequences. The severity of health risks caused by environmental factors enhances the need to implement strong public health policies to address these problems. Plans must prioritize integrated strategies that pair respiratory health with managing chronic conditions, thus improving patient outcomes and health-related quality of life. Emphasis on education and awareness of the systemic effects of respiratory disease can lead to individuals and practitioners both becoming aware of early signs and symptoms that lead to more substantial health consequences. Lastly, a team effort will be crucial in unraveling the health burden offered by both lung diseases and their systemic counterparts (Bednarek et al., 2024; André et al., 2019).

The interconnection between lung function and systemic diseases is complex and multi-faceted, providing important insights into how systemic disease affects the respiratory system. Understanding these relationships is important for effective disease management of conditions such as cardiovascular disease, where respiratory function is a key component. Research has found that exposure to particulate matter (PM), particularly PM2.5 and PM10, has severe cardiovascular implications. It emphasizes that polluters can exacerbate respiratory diseases, leading to increased rates of hospital admissions and deaths (Sioutas et al., 2005). This supports the importance of air quality being seen as a significant factor in pulmonary and cardiovascular disease pathogenesis, forming a clear association between environmental stressors and systemic inflammatory responses. Also, advances in understanding oxidative stress have revealed its significance in systemic disease that encroaches upon the lungs. Synthetic compound use, such as Salen Mn compounds, has been shown to effectively hinder oxidative damage caused by environmental toxins, a sector of highest importance in radiation injury or any other form of injury (Doctrow et al., 2011). Experiments conducted using lung injury models indicate that such compounds can inhibit markers of oxidative stress, paving the way for therapy in chronic diseases. Because oxidative stress has systemic significance for various tissues like the lungs, renal systems, and skin, it becomes necessary to recognize and institute interventions that can increase lung resistance and overall health. Finally, the evidence highlights the significance of holistic principles in clinical practice for addressing systemic diseases relevant to lung health. With the awareness of the interconnectedness of systemic and pulmonary conditions, healthcare practitioners can design more integrated management strategies aimed at the root causes of disease rather than just treating symptoms. Prevention in reducing exposure to harmful pollutants, as well as antioxidant therapy, can play an influential role in patient outcomes when managing chronic cardiovascular and respiratory disease (Sioutas et al., 2005; Doctrow et al., 2011). In summary, a deep understanding of these relationships is critical for improving both study and clinical treatments in addressing the challenges posed by systemic diseases affecting lung health.

KEY TERMS FROM THIS CHAPTER

Amyloidosis
Capillaritis
Goodpasture syndrome
Hypersensitivity pneumonitis
Lupus pneumonitis
Pulmonary alveolar proteinosis
Pulmonary embolism
Pulmonary hypertension
Sarcoidosis
Vasculitis-associated lung disease
Bronchiolitis obliterans
Diffuse alveolar hemorrhage
Granulomatous inflammation
Interstitial lung disease (ILD)
Pleural effusion
Pulmonary edema
Pulmonary fibrosis
Rheumatoid lung disease
Scleroderma lung disease

Critical Thinking Questions

1. **Which systemic autoimmune disease is classically associated with "honeycomb lung" fibrosis?**
   a. Rheumatoid arthritis
   b. Systemic lupus erythematosus
   c. Systemic sclerosis (scleroderma)
   d. Sjögren's syndrome
2. **Which lung manifestation is commonly seen in patients with rheumatoid arthritis?**
   a. Bronchiectasis
   b. Pulmonary arterial hypertension
   c. Caplan syndrome (rheumatoid pneumoconiosis)
   d. Alveolar hemorrhage
3. **Which pulmonary complication is most commonly associated with systemic lupus erythematosus (SLE)?**
   a. Pulmonary embolism
   b. Diffuse alveolar hemorrhage
   c. Pulmonary fibrosis
   d. Sarcoidosis
4. **In which systemic disease is pulmonary alveolar proteinosis most commonly seen?**
   a. Systemic lupus erythematosus
   b. Dermatomyositis
   c. Rheumatoid arthritis
   d. None of the above; it is usually idiopathic or secondary to hematologic disorders
5. **Which systemic vasculitis commonly involves the lungs and is associated with p-ANCA positivity?**
   a. Granulomatosis with polyangiitis (GPA)
   b. Microscopic polyangiitis (MPA)
   c. Eosinophilic granulomatosis with polyangiitis (EGPA)
   d. Takayasu arteritis

Short Answer Questions

1. What are the common pulmonary manifestations of rheumatoid arthritis?
2. Describe the typical lung involvement seen in systemic lupus erythematosus.
3. What pulmonary complications are commonly associated with systemic sclerosis?
4. What is the general approach to diagnosing lung involvement in systemic diseases?
5. Which systemic diseases are commonly associated with pulmonary arterial hypertension?

Answer to Critical Thinking Questions

1. (c); 2. (c); 3. (b); 4. (d); 5. (b)

References

1. Puzanov, I., Diab, A., Abdallah, K., Bingham, C. O., Brogdon, C., Dadu, R., Hamad, L., Kim, S., Lacouture, M. E., LeBoeuf, N. R., Lenihan, D., Onofrei, C., Shannon, V., Sharma, R., Silk, A. W., Skondra, D., Suarez-Almazor, M. E., Wang, Y., Wiley, K., . . . Ernstoff, M. S. (2017). Managing toxicities associated with immune checkpoint inhibitors: consensus recommendations from the Society for Immunotherapy of Cancer (SITC) Toxicity Management Working Group. *Journal for ImmunoTherapy of Cancer*, *5*(1). https://doi.org/10.1186/s40425-017-0300-zAbt, M., Algburi, A., Altenhoefer, A., Altier, C., Anderson, J., Annuk, H., et al. (2017). Protective microbiota: From localized to long-reaching co-immunity. https://core.ac.uk/download/223236091.pdf (accessed on 30th June 2025).

2. Addison, M., Bandeen-Roche, K., Buford, T., Calvani, R., Cesari, M., De Martinis, M., et al. (2017). Systemic inflammation, body composition, and physical performance in old community-dwellers. https://core.ac.uk/download/98345726.pdf (accessed on 30th June 2025).

3. Ailal, F., Al-Herz, W., Bousfiha, A., Casanova, J. L., et al. (2020). Human inborn errors of immunity: 2019 update of the IUIS phenotypical classification. https://core.ac.uk/download/323074666.pdf (accessed on 30th June 2025).

4. Aksamit, T., Maglione, M., & Santamaria, F. (2019). Pediatric and adult bronchiectasis: Specific management with coexisting asthma, COPD, rheumatological disease and inflammatory bowel disease. https://core.ac.uk/download/pdf/237170250.pdf (accessed on 30th June 2025).

5. Alcain, J. M., Candolfi, M., Geffner, J. R., Gori, S., et al. (2019). Acetylcholine-treated murine dendritic cells promote inflammatory lung injury. https://core.ac.uk/download/287880884.pdf (accessed on 30th June 2025).

6. Allocca, G., Menozzi, G., Grossi, G. B., et al. (2018). Oral malodor in special care patients: Current knowledge. https://core.ac.uk/download/159636738.pdf (accessed on 30th June 2025).

7. Alving, W., Asano, K., Basu, S., Fubini, B., Bosquillon, C., Brain, J. D., Brown, J. S., et al. (2012). Toxicity of lunar dust. http://arxiv.org/abs/1206.6328 (accessed on 30th June 2025).

8. Amadi-Obi, A., Arida, A., Cortes, A., Fox, A., Jager, A., Peters, A., Rothova, A., et al. (2014). Autoimmune and autoinflammatory mechanisms in uveitis. https://core.ac.uk/download/29416272.pdf (accessed on 30th June 2025).

9. André, S., Areias, V., Boléo-Tomé, J. P., Cardoso, J., et al. (2019). COPD and cardiovascular disease. https://core.ac.uk/download/225163131.pdf (accessed on 30th June 2025).

10. Antonicelli, L., Aoki, T., Arfsten, D., Aruoma, O. I., Asti, A., Ault, J. G., Azzi, A., et al. (2009). Environmental toxicity, redox signaling and lung inflammation: The role of glutathione. https://core.ac.uk/download/28978002.pdf (accessed on 30th June 2025).

11. Arciniegas, E., Beon, K., Cooley, B. C., Del Galdo, F., Falke, L., Gabrielli, A., Gilbane, J. M., et al. (2016). Endothelial cells expressing endothelial and mesenchymal cell gene products in lung tissue from patients with systemic sclerosis-associated interstitial lung disease. https://core.ac.uk/download/83049879.pdf (accessed on 30th June 2025).

12. Assassi, S., Fischbach, M., GENISOS Study Group, Gonzalez, E. B., et al. (2011). Predictors of fatigue severity in early systemic sclerosis: A prospective longitudinal study of the GENISOS cohort. https://core.ac.uk/download/323073807.pdf (accessed on 30th June 2025).

13. Austin, M. A., Benson, P. J., Bhargava, R., Bhattacharya, S., Bijlani, R. L., Brown, R., Busek, Z., et al. (2006). Physiology of long pranayama breathing: Neural respiratory elements may provide a mechanism that explains how slow deep breathing shifts the autonomic nervous system. https://core.ac.uk/download/131210060.pdf (accessed on 30th June 2025).

14. Bednarek, S., Bychowski, M., Górski, M., Homza, M., et al. (2024). *The Air We Breathe: Exploring the Multifaceted Impacts of Air Pollution on Health and Disease.* https://core.ac.uk/download/636386041.pdf (accessed on 30th June 2025).

15. Bogatkevich, G. S., Du, S., Ganguly, B. J., Goldin, J., et al. (2017). Novel lung imaging biomarkers and skin gene expression subsetting in dasatinib treatment of systemic sclerosis-associated interstitial lung disease. https://core.ac.uk/download/323078738.pdf (accessed on 30th June 2025).

16. Boin, F., Carns, M., Chung, L., Criswell, L. A., et al. (2017). Clinical and serological features of systemic sclerosis in a multicenter African American cohort: Analysis of the genome research in African American scleroderma patient's clinical database. https://core.ac.uk/download/323074312.pdf (accessed on 30th June 2025).

17. Castro, S. V., Jimenez, S. A., & Piera-Velazquez, S. (2010). Role of growth factors in the pathogenesis of tissue fibrosis in systemic sclerosis. https://core.ac.uk/download/83050041.pdf (accessed on 30th June 2025).

18. Churg, A., D'Hulst, A. I., Oberholzer, A., Ananthakrishnan, A. N., Chassaing, B., Vuillemenot, B. R., et al. (2015). The effect of cigarette smoke exposure on the development of inflammation in lungs, gut and joints of TNFΔARE mice. https://core.ac.uk/download/55798655.pdf (accessed on 30th June 2025).

19. Cuzzocrea, S., Rossi, A., & Sautebin, L. (2009). Involvement of leukotriene pathway in the pathogenesis of ischemia-reperfusion injury and septic and non-septic shock. https://core.ac.uk/download/55023705.pdf (accessed on 30th June 2025).

20. Dayal, U., Soni, U., Bansal, S., Aggarwal, K., Chennupati, C., Kanagala, S., Gupta, V., et al. (2025). MAFLD: Exploring the systemic effects beyond liver. *Journal of Community Hospital Internal Medicine Perspectives, 15,* 42–48. https://www.semanticscholar.org/paper/e1346b007d7c62e6245ed06977f2052740c3110f (accessed on 30th June 2025).

21. Djalilian, A. R., Eslani, M., Mehravaran, S., Nassiri, N., et al. (2014). Ocular graft versus host disease following allogeneic stem cell transplantation: A review of current knowledge and recommendations. https://core.ac.uk/download/28948118.pdf (accessed on 30th June 2025).

22. Doctrow, S. R., Fish, B., Hill, R. P., Huffman, J., et al. (2011). Salen Mn complexes mitigate radiation injury in normal tissues. https://core.ac.uk/download/213079025.pdf (accessed on 30th June 2025).

23. Dolan, R. D., Horgan, P. G., McMillan, D. C., McSorley, S., et al. (2017). How and why systemic inflammation worsens quality of life in patients with advanced cancer. https://core.ac.uk/download/82958762.pdf (accessed on 30th June 2025).

24. Dorrestein, P. C., Knight, R., & Mazmanian, S. K. (2014). Finding the missing links among metabolites, microbes, and the host. https://core.ac.uk/download/33113984.pdf (accessed on 30th June 2025).

25. Eghbali, M., & Sharma, S. (2014). Influence of sex differences on microRNA gene regulation in disease. https://core.ac.uk/download/323079075.pdf (accessed on 30th June 2025).

26. Elias, P. M., & Man, M. Q. (2019). Could inflammaging and its sequelae be prevented or mitigated? https://core.ac.uk/download/323062598.pdf (accessed on 30th June 2025).

27. Fernandes, O., Figueiredo, L., Leal, C., Lourenço, A., et al. (2015). Thoracic manifestations of connective tissue diseases. https://core.ac.uk/download/71738721.pdf (accessed on 30th June 2025).

28. Hawtrey, S. (2013). Two genetic effects at the IRF5/TNPO3 locus are independently associated with the development of specific lupus symptoms. https://core.ac.uk/download/43645373.pdf (accessed on 30th June 2025).

29. He, H., Tong, X., Ning, Z., Zhou, J., Du, C., Wang, Y., Xu, D., et al. (2023). POS1277 lung function associated with subclinical myocardial impairment in systemic sclerosis: A cardiac magnetic resonance study. *Annals of the Rheumatic Diseases*. https://www.semanticscholar.org/paper/34f7ca800be4e3025d35840a7832b0f292a8654c (accessed on 30th June 2025).

30. Humbert, M., Kovács, G., Hoeper, M. M., Badagliacca, R., Berger, R. M. F., Brida, M., Carlsen, J., et al. (2022). 2022 ESC/ERS guidelines for the diagnosis and treatment of pulmonary hypertension. *European Respiratory Journal, 61*, 2200879. https://doi.org/10.1183/13993003.00879-2022 (accessed on 30th June 2025).

31. Iegudina, Y., Mikuksts, V., Syniachenko, O., Yakovlenko, O., et al. (2017). Types of angiopathy in experimental autoimmune disease in rats. https://core.ac.uk/download/301580717.pdf (accessed on 30th June 2025).

32. Izquierdo, M., Merchant, R. A., Morley, J. E., Anker, S. D., Aprahamian, I., Arai, H., Aubertin-Leheudre, M., et al. (2021). International exercise recommendations in older adults (ICFSR): Expert consensus guidelines. *The Journal of Nutrition Health & Aging, 25*, 824–853. https://doi.org/10.1007/s12603-021-1665-8 (accessed on 30th June 2025).

33. Jimenez, S. A., & Piera-Velazquez, S. (2016). Endothelial to mesenchymal transition (EndoMT) in the pathogenesis of systemic sclerosis-associated pulmonary fibrosis and pulmonary arterial hypertension: Myth or reality? https://core.ac.uk/download/129190893.pdf (accessed on 30th June 2025).

34. Jimenez, S. A., Mendoza, M. D., Fabian, A., & Rosenbloom, J. (2013). Strategies for anti-fibrotic therapies. https://core.ac.uk/download/83049954.pdf (accessed on 30th June 2025).

35. Kozlovtseva, E. Y., Loboyko, V. F., & Nikolenko, D. A. (2016). Monitoring of fine dust pollution of multistory buildings air environment as an adoption factor of town-planning decisions. https://core.ac.uk/download/pdf/82606330.pdf (accessed on 30th June 2025).

36. Letizia, C., Papi, P., Petramala, L., Pilloni, A., et al. (2018). Peri-implant diseases and metabolic syndrome components: A systematic review. https://core.ac.uk/download/153368842.pdf (accessed on 30th June 2025).

37. Lin, T., Huang, S., Zhou, F., Shen, X., & Mao, H. (2025). Association between vitamin D levels and preserved ratio impaired spirometry: An investigation of mediating roles of systemic inflammation and metabolic indicators. *Frontiers in Nutrition, 12*. https://www.semanticscholar.org/paper/f700f9a217580694e5c238b24648bb6e77260d11 (accessed on 30th June 2025).

38. Liu, S., Mu, L., Xia, T., Zhang, Y., et al. (2016). Pulmonary diseases induced by ambient ultrafine

and engineered nanoparticles in twenty-first century. https://core.ac.uk/download/323076917.pdf (accessed on 30th June 2025).

39. Lopes, A. A. (2015). Oxygen transport: A physiologically-based conceptual framework for the promotion of functionality. https://core.ac.uk/download/541043686.pdf (accessed on 30th June 2025).

40. Miller, L., Pinkerton, K., Royer, C., Schelegle, E., et al. (2017). Nonhuman primate models of respiratory disease: Past, present, and future. https://core.ac.uk/download/323069778.pdf (accessed on 30th June 2025).

41. Ney, L. M., Wipplinger, M., Grossmann, M., Engert, N., Wegner, V., & Mosig, A. (2023). Short chain fatty acids: Key regulators of the local and systemic immune response in inflammatory diseases and infections. *Open Biology, 13.* https://www.semanticscholar.org/paper/884aaed89d75f079945b40338e7ac12687829fcf (accessed on 30th June 2025).

42. Neytchev, O., Panagiotou, N., Selman, C., Shiels, P., et al. (2018). Extracellular vesicles, ageing, and therapeutic interventions. https://core.ac.uk/download/160606189.pdf (accessed on 30th June 2025).

43. Simonneau, G., Montani, D., Celermajer, D. S., Denton, C. P., Gatzoulis, M. A., Krowka, M. J., Williams, P., et al. (2018). Hemodynamic definitions and updated clinical classification of pulmonary hypertension. *European Respiratory Journal, 53,* 1801913. https://doi.org/10.1183/13993003.01913-2018 (accessed on 30th June 2025).

44. Sioutas, C., Desai, M. M., Diaz-Sanchez, D., Godleski, J. J., MacNee, W., McGrath, J. J., Pekkanen, J., et al. (2005). Potential role of ultrafine particles in associations between airborne particle mass and cardiovascular health. https://core.ac.uk/download/pdf/3798552.pdf (accessed on 30th June 2025).

45. Stewart, A. G., Thomas, B. J., & Koff, J. L. (2018). TGF-β: Master regulator of inflammation and fibrosis. *Respirology, 23,* 1096–1097. https://doi.org/10.1111/resp.13415 (accessed on 30th June 2025).

46. Wöhrer, A., Oppl, B., Pieringer, H., Parzer, I., Zwerina, J., & Reis, P. (2014). IgG4-related disease: An orphan disease with many faces. https://core.ac.uk/download/pdf/81907024.pdf (accessed on 30th June 2025).

OCCUPATIONAL AND ENVIRONMENTAL LUNG DISEASES

7

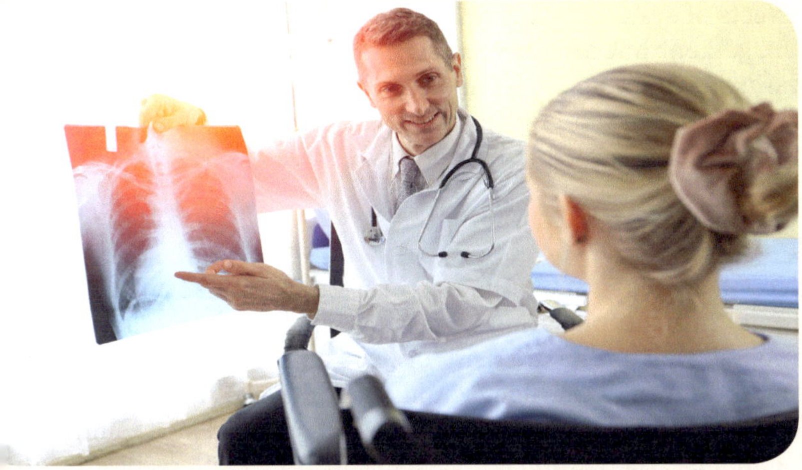

LEARNING OBJECTIVES

After studying this chapter, you will be able to:

1. Explain the types of occupational lung diseases
2. Describe the types of environmental lung diseases
3. List the risk factors for occupational lung diseases
4. Focus on the risk factors for environmental lung diseases
5. Discuss the symptoms and diagnosis
6. Understand the treatment and management

Introduction

The increasing prevalence of occupational and environmental lung disorders reiterates the importance of knowledge and information regarding the varied etiological agents that cause pulmonary morbidity. The diseases are primarily attributed to the inhalation of toxic substances at the workplace, along with environmental toxins. These include pre-existing conditions, genetics, and age, which can influence individual susceptibility to diseases like interstitial lung diseases (ILDs). These are a collection of disorders of the lung tissue influenced by both occupational and environmental exposure. As acknowledged in recent studies, the inflammatory and fibrotic responses initiated by such exposures also highlight the complex interface between the external environment and the patient's condition, which deserves a multi-faceted approach to prevention and diagnosis within the medical field (Partida-Zavala et al., 2018). Diagnosis of lung diseases related to hypersensitivity typically relies heavily on extensive histories of exposure delineating environmental and occupational sources, which can provide insight into likely causative agents. Such a disease is hypersensitivity pneumonitis (HP), and learning from clinical databases is crucial for its effective management and research. Steps to classify HP types reveal variations in presentation, ranging from acute to chronic, informing treatment plans and defining the social and occupational histories of affected individuals. While cryptogenic and occupational etiologies remain the priority, obtaining such detailed exposure history is essential for elucidating the complex aetiologies of the diseases and for extending accurate diagnosis and management (Walters et al., 2018). The respiratory system is a first-line defense mechanism against environmental insult, and damage by occupational exposure can lead to a spectrum of lung disease. Immune responses, including cell types like M2 macrophages during repair and remodeling, play an integral role in promoting lung diseases such as ILDs and fibrosis. Grasping the underlying pathophysiologic mechanisms can influence treatment strategies and therapeutic maneuvers aimed at neutralizing the detrimental effects of systemic inflammation caused by inhaled particles. The issue involves not only clinical management but also advocating for legislation related to air quality and occupational health standards. Addressing these intricacies ensures the integrity of worker health and highlights the imperative to pursue ongoing research on the risks associated with occupational as well as environmental factors (Partida-Zavala et al., 2018).

Definition of Occupational Lung Diseases

Occupational lung diseases are a collection of respiratory illnesses resulting from exposure to hazardous atmospheres or toxic materials through inhalation in occupational settings. They can be acute or chronic based on the duration as well as the intensity of exposure. Occupational lung diseases such as pneumoconiosis, asthma, and chronic obstructive pulmonary disease (COPD) can be caused by exposure to dust, fumes, chemical agents, and other respiratory irritants. The definition of occupational lung disease outlines the intrinsic correlation between occupational and respiratory health, indicating that intervention through protective measures is necessary to counteract harmful exposures. The determinants of occupational hazard-related respiratory diseases are significant in the formulation of effective policies and workplace safety measures for the decrease in incidence levels of such diseases, with the resulting improvement in public health outcomes (Shyamali et al., 2019). The work-related lung disorders can further be categorized in a more specific etiological sense, both environmental and genetic. Exposure to substances such as asbestos, silica, and some heavy metals during employment has been found to result in some pulmonary conditions. Exposure to heavy metals, for example, is a critical public health concern because these chemicals are not only toxic but also accumulate in organisms, leading to more extensive environmental contamination (Ali et al., 2019). Previous developments in research have highlighted how these determinants interact and therefore result in the necessity to act against environmental determinants as well as occupational exposure. Such a multi-factorial framework allows for an improved understanding of lung disease pathology. This is important for developing interventions explicitly targeted at vulnerable groups. In addressing occupational lung diseases, surveillance systems and workplace interventions should be both effective and implemented. Interventions such as air monitoring for quality, enforcement of personal protective equipment wear, and training for handling safe procedures play a vital role in preventing exposure to harmful substances. Early detection and preventive care for respiratory diseases also go a long way in better health outcomes for the population affected. The global burden of occupational lung disease underscores the need for an integrated approach that brings together scientific inquiry and public health programs. By encouraging collaboration among employers, employees, and health professionals, we can create healthier workplaces, minimize the risks of occupational lung diseases, and thus contribute to improved community health (Shyamali et al., 2019) (Figure 7.1).

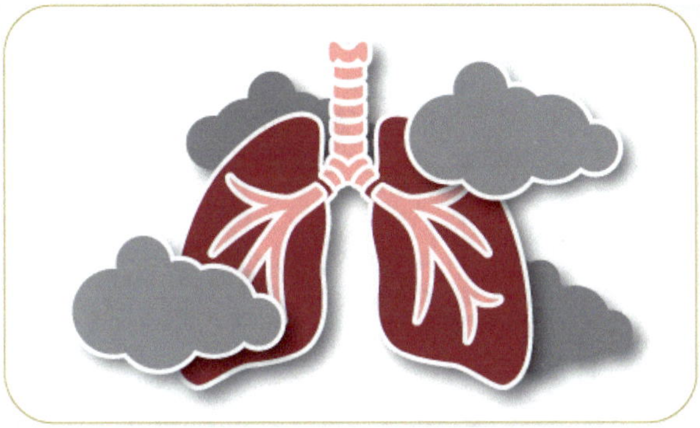

Figure 7.1. Occupational lung disease.

Source: https://external-content.duckduckgo.com/iu/?u=https%3A%2F%2Fwww.oakwoodsolicitors.co.uk%2Fwp-content%2Fuploads%2F2023%2F06%2FLungs-Diagram.png&f=1&nofb=1&ipt=d1315ed6bdff03fc0798ae89c6828ae20f280673bca7f18fb0728e6033184c6b.

Definition of Environmental Lung Diseases

Environmental lung diseases are a broad category of respiratory illness produced by exposure to harmful materials in the environment. The diseases are characterized by alterations in the normal function of the lungs and can be due to a range of environmental stimuli, such as pollutants, chemicals, and biological agents. Most importantly, perhaps, these diseases can affect individuals of all geographic and demographic backgrounds, which suggests their ubiquity. For instance, repeated exposure to ambient outdoor air pollution, such as particulate matter and ground-level ozone, has been linked to chronic respiratory diseases, including asthma and COPD. Furthermore, environmental lung disease is also important due to its added contribution to increased morbidity and mortality among vulnerable groups of people, such as children, the elderly, and those with pre-existing illnesses. The definition of environmental lung diseases also includes diseases arising from exposures to some occupational hazards, where the persons are most likely to be subjected to toxic chemicals in the workplace. These include exposure to asbestos fibers, silica, and other gases, resulting in pneumoconiosis and occupational asthma. Therefore, the overlap of occupational and environmental determinants necessitates a synergistic approach towards prevention and intervention strategies. More studies have emphasized the importance of public awareness and education on environmental hazards, coupled with stringent laws regulating emissions from industrial and urban sources. These programs are beneficial not only in curbing exposure to hazardous chemicals but also in improving public health through better air quality.

The link between environmental exposures and respiratory disease, thus, remains a significant area of study within the broad framework of occupational health. Recent studies have found new risks, such as electronic smoking, that further complicate the investigation of environmental lung disease. The Centers for Disease Control and Prevention (CDC) has documented the rising occurrence of lung injuries associated with vaping products, prompting increased caution among healthcare professionals and public health officials. Identification of such risk is crucial since the population is being exposed to emerging environmental threats through vaping, which can be added to traditional tobacco-related risk by other toxic components. This progress towards such environmental lung disorders, such as e-cigarette or vaping product use-associated lung injury (EVALI), demonstrates the role for ongoing research and public health measures for addressing multifaceted respiratory harms. Consideration of these aspects is essential in the development of efficient prevention programs that can adapt to the dynamic nature of environmental exposure (David et al., 2019; Donald et al., 2022) (Figure 7.2).

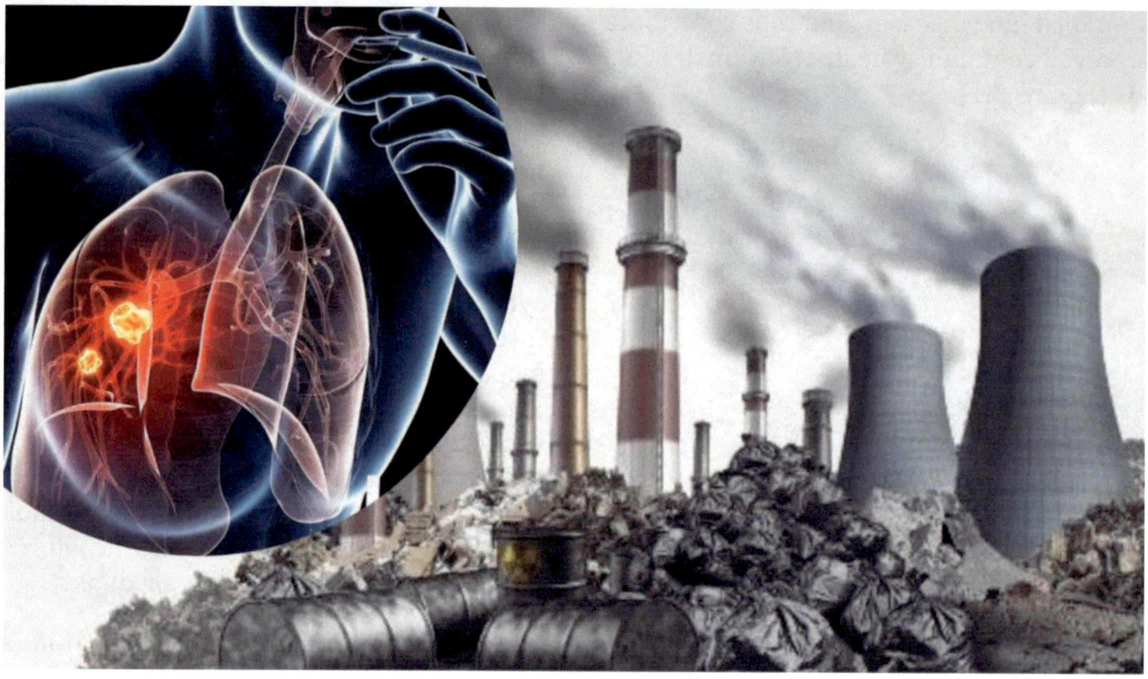

Figure 7.2. Environmental lung diseases.

Source: https://external-content.duckduckgo.com/iu/?u=https%3A%2F%2Fst1.thehealthsite.com%2Fwp-content%2Fuploads%2F2022%2F11%2FLung-Cancer-3.jpg&f=1&nofb=1&ipt=38d3ac1c9f399507984f350dda1e1e514744608da2cd92028433fc71f80e85ac

Importance of Studying Lung Diseases in Relation to Public Health

Foraging into lung disease research is also imperative to enhance public health programs, especially in occupational and environmental etiologies. Lung diseases are a large category of diseases encompassing asthma, COPD, and lung cancer, and they impose significant global health burdens. Chronic respiratory diseases (CRD), according to current world health statistics, are responsible for millions of deaths worldwide each year and have a significant impact on quality of life. Understanding the intricate risk factors of such conditions, where exposures and occupational hazards are concerned, is what equips public health professionals with the knowledge required to reduce morbidity and mortality levels in populations that are afflicted by them. As there are prospective preventive interventions and treatment modalities, the need for appropriate research on such factors assumes priority in advancing healthcare policy and health promotion initiatives at the community level. The study of lung disease also demonstrates the pressing convergence of social determinants and health disparities. Vulnerable populations—e.g., marginalized communities and workers in risky jobs—are generally disproportionately affected by respiratory conditions due to environmental exposure and lack of appropriate health care. A study of lung cancer is a case in point, with most instances being reported among never-smokers, clearly demonstrating the role of extrinsic factors such as air pollution and workplace exposure (Elvin et al., 2021). Such disparities necessitate that the public health response target reduction of exposure risk, improved access to healthcare services, and enhanced community awareness of the necessity for preventive treatment. Moreover, resolving these inequalities also improves general population health, as it is crucial to identify and highlight those most affected by environmental degradation and working conditions. Lastly, with global warming and industrialization, the necessity to study lung diseases as part of public health becomes even more pressing. Increased air pollution and changing occupational settings pose new hazards that may complicate respiratory conditions. The Global Burden of Disease Study illustrates how chronic respiratory disease has surged over the past decades, emphasizing the global necessity of advancing cleaner air initiatives and enhanced occupational health practices (Wassim et al., 2020). Through further research in the area, policymakers are able to develop targeted interventions that reduce the health impact of exposures that occur in the workplace and the environment. This investment not only seeks to counteract the effects of existing respiratory illness but also enables a proactive approach towards preventing the development of future health crises related to lung disease, ultimately contributing to a healthier population.

7.1. Types of Occupational Lung Diseases

Learning Outcome

1. Asbestosis
2. Silicosis
3. Coal workers' pneumoconiosis

Occupational lung diseases are one of the key problems in those workplaces where employees are exposed to various dangerous substances. Among them, pneumoconiosis is one of the key categories, which is induced by inhaling mineral dusts. Pneumoconiosis is typically seen in mining and construction industries and could lead to progressive lung damage and respiratory impairment. Coal workers' pneumoconiosis, or black lung disease, is a targeted syndrome attributed to long-term coal dust exposure. As the condition advances, it may lead to debilitating symptoms, such as a chronic cough and impaired lung function. Current research emphasizes increased monitoring and regulation of occupational dust exposure in an effort to prevent such risk and preserve workers' health. Thus, preventive measures to reduce the exposure of toxic dust are still critical in preventing pneumoconiosis and improving occupational health results (Mkorombindo et al., 2022). Another significant category of occupational lung disease is from chemical exposure, that is, in construction, manufacturing, and agricultural industries. Chemical pneumonitis is caused by employees inhaling harmful vapors, gases, or mist, leading to inflammation of the lung tissue. There are some agents, such as isocyanates in polyurethane manufacturing or asbestos in older structures, which are highly toxic, resulting in the likes of reactive airway dysfunction syndrome or even lung cancer. Furthermore, such chemical exposure results in cumulative effects, causing chronic lung disease in the long term. The demand for robust safety measures and training in chemical danger identification and response is vital to safeguard laborers from such detrimental health consequences. There is a need for enhanced awareness and interventions to mitigate instances of occupational lung disease caused by chemicals and prevent workers' respiratory health (El-Rahman et al., 2018). In addition to chemical and dust exposure, occupational lung disease may also be caused by biological agents, especially in animal husbandry, health care, and agricultural sectors. Hypersensitivity pneumonitis is an illness caused by the inhalation of organic dust, mold spores, or animal proteins, leading to an immune response that results in undue respiratory distress. Workers in such professions are at a higher risk from repeated exposure, which tends to cause chronic inflammation and irreversible damage to the lungs. For instance, farmers may get exposed to organic dust containing allergens from hay, grain, and animal dung, which can exacerbate respiratory illnesses. Understanding the role of biological agents in occupational lung disease is essential in the development of good prevention strategies, including ensuring a well-functioning ventilation system and the enforcement of best management practices in the workplace. Through massive educational interventions, employers can boost the resilience of workforces to such climatic issues and strengthen the health outcomes (Mkorombindo et al., 2022) (Figure 7.3).

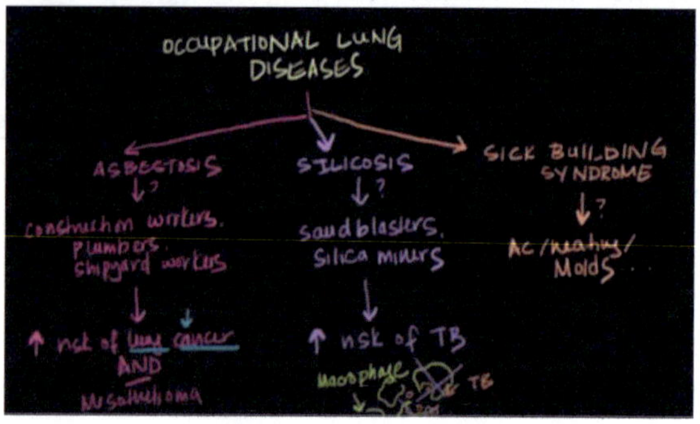

Figure 7.3. Types of occupational lung diseases.

Source: https://external-content.duckduckgo.com/iu/?u=https%3A%2F%2Ftse3.mm.bing.net%2Fth%2Fid%2FOIP.0R8sO3QVRFnsJAPoAxXRyAHaEP%3Fr%3D0%26pid%3DApi&f=1&ipt=ad478572213c880a794ebb8ec9f8b9c792b0889fc2309b2ba417472a11e72ec7

7.1.1. Asbestosis

Asbestosis is a serious disease in the realm of occupational lung diseases that is primarily linked with the inhalation of asbestos fibers. These fibrous minerals, once favored for their insulating properties in the construction and shipbuilding industries, have become a major factor behind chronic respiratory ailments. The disease results from inflammation and fibrosis of lung tissue caused by long-term exposure to asbestos, leading to a restrictive lung disease that causes breathing difficulty. As the disease progresses, patients can exhibit chronic cough, chest pain, and worsening dyspnea, significantly impairing their quality of life. Clinical assessment generally identifies characteristic pulmonary fibrosis on imaging studies, and a great deal of suspicion is typically required, especially for those with asbestos exposure histories, as early identification is crucial for management strategies aimed at slowing the disease process. The overall implications of asbestosis extend beyond personal health, being critical environmental and occupational health concerns. As argued in current literature, ambient and occupational poisons are the cause of several lung disorders, including asbestosis, and the evidence points to the importance of comprehensive preventive measures. Because asbestos exposure is often everyday in specialized work environments, effective policies and regulations must prevent risks. Education campaigns to enlighten workers on risks posed by asbestos, combined with vigorous enforcement of occupational safety standards, can substantially reduce instances of asbestosis. Also, understanding the histopathological patterns of asbestosis, like lung tissue fibrotic changes, makes it easier for doctors to differentiate it from other diffuse parenchymal lung diseases (DPLDs), hence enhancing diagnosis and treatment (Ahmad, 2024). In asbestosis management, treatments are usually geared towards symptomatic relief and prevention strategies for health improvement, as opposed to reversing lung damage. The availability of antifibrotic drugs represents a significant advancement in the management of most fibrotic lung disorders; nevertheless, their application in asbestosis is limited since the disease is predominantly expressive rather than active inflammation. Nonetheless, pulmonary rehabilitation becomes an intrinsic part of management, improving lung function, enhancing physical capacity, and enhancing overall patient well-being. Furthermore, the knowledge of occupational air toxicants, like asbestos, on respiratory health underscores the importance of ubiquitous public health measures that prioritize employee well-being and environmental excellence. As highlighted in recent research, the interlink between occupational exposure and respiratory illness underscores the importance of preventive measures to effectively combat asbestosis and other illnesses (Nishida et al., 2022) (Figure 7.4).

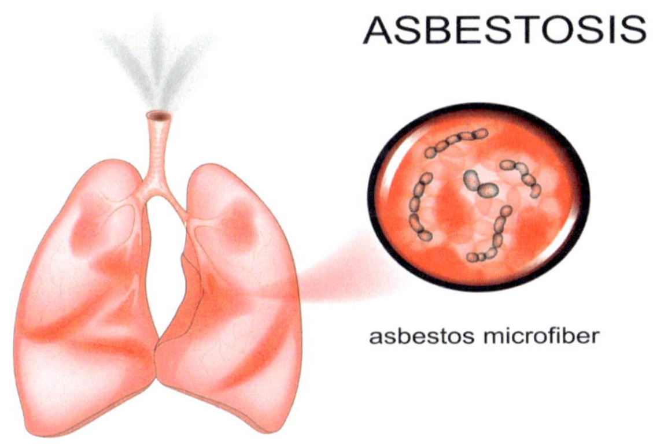

Figure 7.4. Asbestosis.

Source: https://www.pintas.com/wp-content/uploads/2020/09/lung-cancer-what-is-the-life-expectancy-of-someone-with-asbestosis-scaled.jpg.

7.1.2. Silicosis

Among the occupational lung diseases, silicosis is a significant public health problem among miners, construction workers, and stone processors. The reversible illness is caused by long-term inhalation of respirable crystalline silica dust, leading to different pulmonary abnormalities. The interplay among duration, exposure intensity, and latency period, from several years to decades, accounts for the complexities of the disease. Current research underscores that silicosis is characterized by inflammatory responses, leading to the formation of silicotic nodules and progressive pulmonary fibrosis in lung tissues. The ensuing alterations in the pathological conditions lead to compromised pulmonary function and a high rate of morbidity among the afflicted individuals with a substantial impact on their quality of life and working capacity (Handra et al., 2023). Preventive measures are crucial in the battle against silicosis because there are limited treatment options, and they are primarily ineffective in reversing lung damage. Reducing exposure to silica dust by ensuring good workplace practice, such as application of dust control measures, use of personal protective equipment, and promoting respiratory health programs, is an important control measure. Moreover, taking into account risk determinants like socio-economic status and genetic predisposition enhances awareness of the disease's epidemiology. New evidence further suggests that silicosis diagnosis might be difficult since overlapping symptoms with other pulmonary diseases make it difficult to distinguish it from diseases like sarcoidosis (Thillai et al., 2020).

Prevention and early intervention methods are required to reduce the onset of this debilitating disease since it has no treatment. While research continues into new treatments for silicosis, interest is growing to move ahead with antifibrotic, cellular, and immunomodulatory treatments. Preliminary evidence has indicated areas of therapy that have the potential to alleviate some of the disease's disabling effects, but these options must be studied further to validate their efficacy and safety in the clinical setting. This absence of effective treatment emphasizes the importance of prevention and early diagnosis, allowing for targeted intervention before widespread lung injury occurs. Employers' and workers' awareness about silicosis is most critical, as educating exposed workers on the potential hazards of silica exposure can make working environments safer. With an immaculately coordinated effort that is centered on prevention, research, and awareness, the effect of silicosis can significantly decrease, ultimately protecting the health and well-being of employees in different industries (Handra et al., 2023) (Figure 7.5).

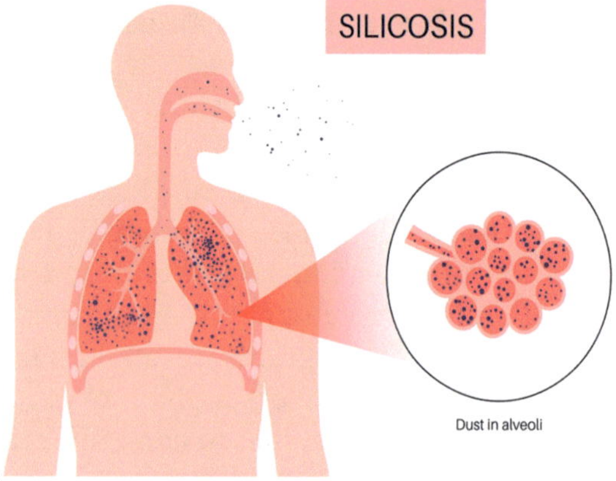

Figure 7.5. Silicosis.

Source: https://res.cloudinary.com/cognitives-s3/image/upload/c_fill,dpr_auto,f_auto,fl_lossy,g_face:auto,h_1515,q_auto,w_1979/v1/cog-live/n/1271/2024/Feb/19/x2PA4Cr47bFVp6zEL8Zt.jpg.

7.1.3. Coal Worker's Pneumoconiosis

Coal workers' pneumoconiosis (CWP), or black lung disease, is a disabling occupational respiratory disease caused exclusively by the inhalation of coal dust. It is not a solitary medical condition but a significant public health burden among miners in an energy-intensive industry that heavily relies on coal mining. CWP is characterized by progressive pulmonary fibrosis, which causes decreased lung capacity and chronic respiratory symptoms. The insidious nature of this disease, combined with long latency, results in high underreporting and missed diagnosis among affected patients at the right time. For the majority of miners, the outcome exceeds health impairments, typically manifesting as permanent disability, reduced quality of life, and premature mortality, thus highlighting the need for extended occupational protection measures and health monitoring schemes in coal mining operations (Nguyen, 2024). The presence of CWP highlights severe loopholes in occupational health laws and enforcement, particularly in developing countries with poorly regulated mining operations. Despite advances in industrial protective measures across many industrialized nations, there is an ominous trend of increasing CWP cases in most areas, such as Eastern Europe and parts of Asia. As illustrated in recent studies, including those on the mining sectors in Poland, the incidence of pneumoconiosis among coal miners has dramatically increased, accounting for a significant percentage of diagnosed occupational diseases (Mocek, 2023). This trend requires stringent health tests, occupational monitoring for dust inhalation, and implementation of protective measures to guard the respiratory tract of miners. Comprehensive measures should emphasize not only health education of workers but also the obligation on the part of mines to adhere to health acts and prevention practices (Mocek, 2023). Prevention of CWP should incorporate multi-disciplinary action involving technology, policy reform, and education. Current diagnostic techniques such as high-resolution computed tomography and regular spirometry tests can facilitate early identification of respiratory deficiencies among miners, allowing for effective interventions. Apart from this, stringent health and safety guidelines placed on the mining sector can encourage mining firms to adopt better dust-suppressing technologies and maintain a secure working environment. Public policy interventions have to be led by robust epidemiological evidence capable of underpinning effective legislative measures aimed at reducing the burden of CWP. As such, awareness among miners about coal dust exposure risks is also crucial to encourage a safety culture in the industry, thereby maximizing worker compliance with prescribed health practices and hence decreasing the occurrence of CWP (Nguyen, 2024) (Figure 7.6).

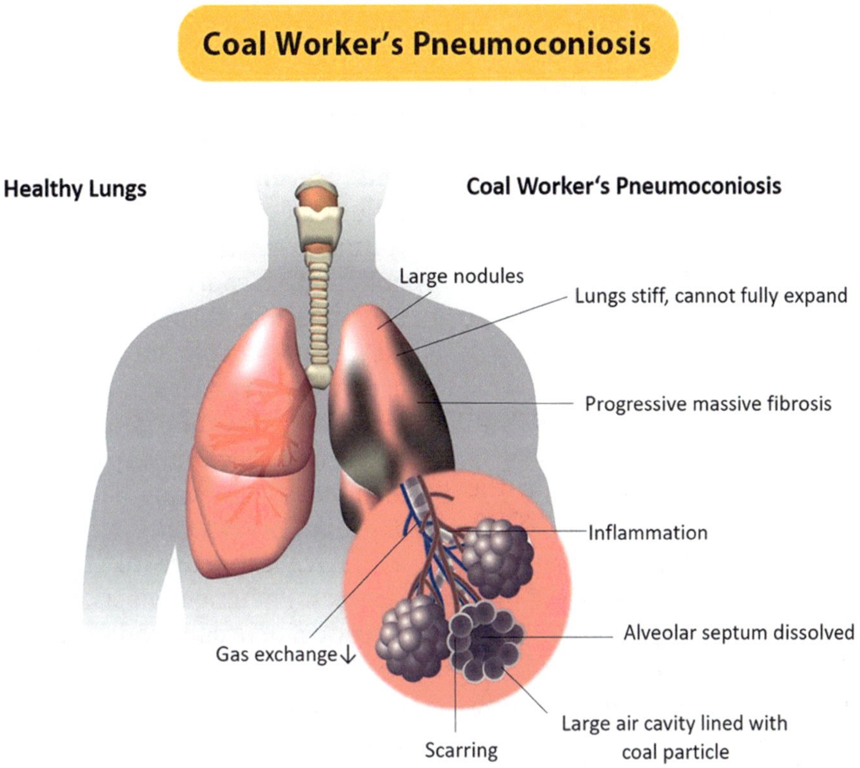

Figure 7.6. Coal worker's pneumoconiosis.

Source: https://cdn-images.prepp.in/public/image/aaecb4e27a6bba256e6ed29703f60aeb.png?tr=w-485,h-402,c-force.

Test Your Knowledge

1. What is asbestosis?
2. What is silicosis?

7.2. Types of Environmental Lung Diseases

Learning Outcome

1. Asthma
2. Chronic obstructive pulmonary disease (COPD)
3. Lung cancer is related to environmental factors

Environmental lung disease is a category of conditions caused by exposure to a range of pollutants and toxic substances found in the air, water, and soil. A good example is COPD, which can result from prolonged exposure to airborne toxicants such as particulate matter, ozone, and volatile organic compounds. Such airborne toxicants are typically industrial by-products and traffic exhaust, and with time, they significantly impair lung function. In addition, environmental allergens such as mold and pollen can exacerbate respiratory problems in individuals with underlying conditions such as asthma, which shows the complex interplay of the various environmental factors and lung health. With more importance now being given to these problems, it has become increasingly necessary to study the specific categories of environmental lung disease in order to develop effective prevention and intervention strategies that can help enhance public health as well as air quality management. Another significant group of environmental causes of lung diseases are those brought about by heavy metal use, particularly industrial outlet and occupational. Cadmium, for example, is a poisonous agent that naturally concentrates in the environment as well as among environmental pollutants because of human actions such as mining and cigarette production. Epidemiological studies have established a relationship between exposure to cadmium and several lung conditions, such as chronic bronchitis and lung cancer, establishing its toxic impact on lung health. The oxidative stress from inhaling cadmium can lead to inflammatory responses that might result in chronic airway disease. The growing number of studies on the health risk of cadmium exposure underscores the need for control and preventive strategies, especially in the industrial environment where such exposure is routine (Genchi et al., 2020). Besides industrial pollutants, airborne suspended biological agents also present threats to environmental lung diseases. Histoplasmosis and pneumoconiosis are two major classifications with pathogen exposure and inorganic dust inhalation as determining factors, respectively. Histoplasmosis, an illness caused by the fungus Histoplasma capsulatum, typically affects individuals with excessive exposure to infected soil, such as farmers. Pneumoconiosis, on the other hand, is a product of occupational dust exposure to silica or asbestos inhalation, leading to progressive lung damage with fibrosis and scarring. Both diseases underscore the importance of preventing diverse environmental causes of lung disease, emphasizing the need for continuous monitoring and intervention to protect high-risk groups from developing serious long-term health issues. As research continues to elucidate the mechanism and impact of these diseases, an integrated approach to occupational and environmental health becomes increasingly important.

7.2.1. Asthma

Asthma is a significant public health problem, a chronic inflammatory disease of the airways, chiefly characterized by wheezing, shortness of breath, chest tightness, and cough. Its increasing prevalence is attributed to genetic predispositions and environmental exposures that, in turn, interact multiplicatively to aggravate respiratory outcomes. The incidence of asthma is most common in populations undergoing rapid industrialization and urbanization, where exposure to allergens and pollutants is heightened. Increasing evidence now points to exposures in early life contributing to developing susceptibility to asthma, with implications that environmental-based interventions can make a substantial difference in disease prevention and management. It is worth understanding the biopsychosocial background of asthma so that effective prevention strategies can be created, especially as morbidity due to the condition remains a problem in most societies across the globe (Toril et al., 2018). The multifactorial nature of asthma means a set of risk factors that are likely to be both occupational and environmental in nature. Historical precipitating factors such as air pollution, exposure to secondhand smoke, indoor allergens (e.g., mold and dust mites), and occupational irritants contribute to exacerbated asthma symptoms. Occupational exposure, particularly in the healthcare, agricultural, and construction sectors, is causally linked to exacerbated asthma symptoms from repeated exposure to irritants and sensitizers. Simultaneously, early childhood exposure to a number of environmental conditions, including high levels of biodiversity or low microbial diversity, has been associated with a lower incidence of asthma and allergy. The intriguing relationship warrants continued exploration of the mechanism by which shifts in the environment influence breathing health, particularly how lower microbial exposures might lead to increased allergic and asthmatic responses (Vos et al., 2017). Secondly, ongoing research into epigenetic control presents a fascinating avenue towards the understanding of asthma development and persistence. Epigenetic marks, in turn influenced by exposures to the environment, can have long-term effects on gene expression that do not alter the fundamental DNA sequence. Thirdly, the fact that certain epigenetic modifications are heritable keeps open the possibility that environmental exposures affecting one generation could determine asthma susceptibility in subsequent generations. This intergenerational basis of asthma raises the call for comprehensive public health approaches considering historical environmental contexts and biological susceptibilities. As the global battle against the rising challenge of asthma progresses, an amalgamation of evidence from molecular biology, environmental science, and social determinants of health will be critical in formulating complex prevention and management plans (Toril et al., 2018) (Figure 7.7).

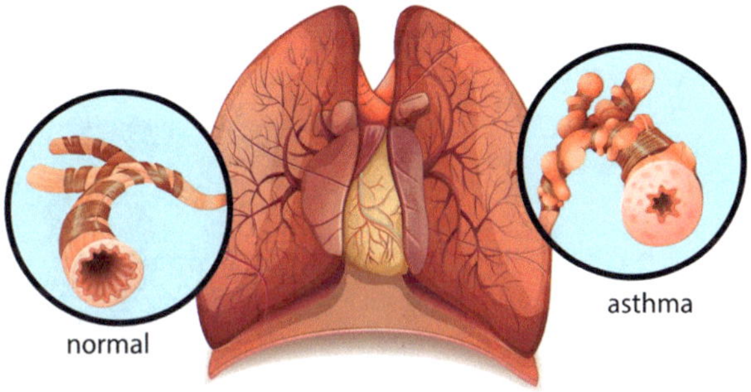

Figure 7.7. Asthma.

Source: https://external-content.duckduckgo.com/iu/?u=https%3A%2F%2Fpedilung.com%2Fwp-content%2Fuploads%2F2018%2F06%2Fasthma-lungs-1024x586.jpg&f=1&nofb=1&ipt=3a06061b60acc83f13c2e689e7306aae920149b99b517b30a9a17393691ade06.

7.2.2. Chronic Obstructive Pulmonary Disease (COPD)

COPD is among the most common causes of morbidity and mortality worldwide, as evidenced by the complex interplay between occupational and environmental exposures that result in its etiology. Predominantly characterized by progressive airflow limitation, COPD generally results from the interaction of prolonged exposure to noxious gases and particles, primarily smoking and the work environment. Employments that subject workers to dust, chemicals, and fumes significantly increase the risk of COPD onset, and therefore, enforcing effective occupational health legislation and policies is of prime importance. As the background against which growing recognition of these correlations is made, it is essential that public health measures give consideration to prevention of occupational exposures and to promotion of smoking cessation programs, particularly in high-risk subjects in occupations that are most likely to be engaged in extraction, construction, and manufacturing. Clinical manifestations of COPD extend beyond lung function, affecting patients' quality of life and overall well-being.

As the disease progresses, patients acquire disabling symptoms that interfere with daily living, in most instances causing increased use of healthcare and expense. The heterogeneity of COPD, expressed as its various phenotypes and comorbidities, complicates management schemes and individualized treatment regimens. Currently, the importance of proper lung function tests is emphasized in guidelines, as they can demonstrate the extent of airflow obstruction and monitor disease progression.

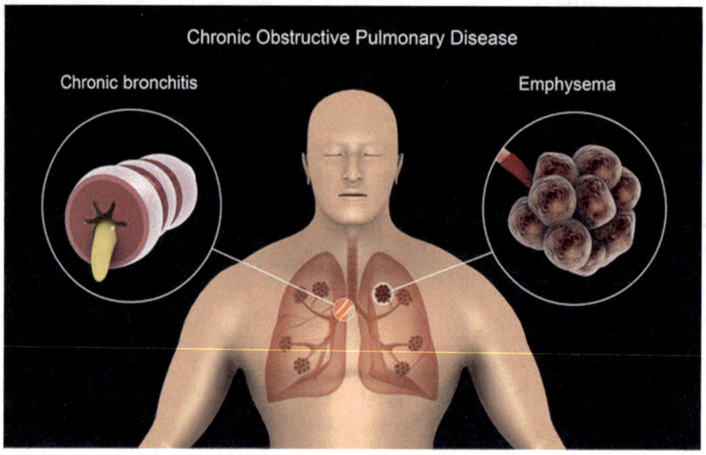

Figure 7.8. COPD: Chronic obstructive pulmonary disease.

Source: https://www.healthvermont.gov/sites/default/files/styles/max_650x650/public/image/COPD%20illustration.jpg?itok=GlYZ77NU.

Proper interpretation of the tests, as was presented in the latest revisions of American Thoracic Society and European Respiratory Society guidelines, is of crucial significance to clinicians for providing proper conclusions and making proper decisions, maximizing patient management, and following evidence-based guidelines (Stanojevic et al., 2021). Environmental determinants play a significant role in the etiology of both COPD and the pathophysiological foundation. Environmental exposure to pollutants, such as particulate matter and smoking, can lead to airway and parenchymal structural modifications as well as chronic inflammation. In industrialized and urban areas, high prevalence rates of COPD have been correlated with air quality. Additional research must examine the interactions between environmental and genetic factors in detail, as such work may shed significant light on the etiology of COPD. Elucidation of the interaction between genetic susceptibilities and noxious exposures could point to high-risk groups and thus guide the development of appropriate targeted interventions in disease prevention and control. Therefore, integration of genetic and environmental research holds great promise for enriching our knowledge about COPD as well as optimizing clinical outcomes (Shyamali et al., 2019) (Figure 7.8).

7.2.3. Lung Cancer Related to Environmental Factors

Lung cancer is a life-threatening public health issue globally, primarily because of environmental causes together with lifestyle choices. The World Health Organization reported that lung cancer was the most common cancer diagnosed, accounting for almost 2.5 million new cases in 2022, further maintaining its status in cancer epidemiology (Bray et al., 2024). While the most frequently underscored cause of tobacco smoking is number one, environmental exposures play a gigantic role in the incidence of lung cancer. Second-hand smoke, outdoor ambient air pollution, and indoor household combustion emissions are some of the exposures that harm lung health. An understanding of the multi-factorial causality of lung cancers calls for a wide vision, keeping in view environmental health, particularly as urbanization and industrialization keep increasing these hazards, mostly among exposed people. In addition, it has been reported that a considerable percentage of the occurrence of lung cancer happens among nonsmokers at an average of 15% to 25% of total cases (Elvin et al., 2021).

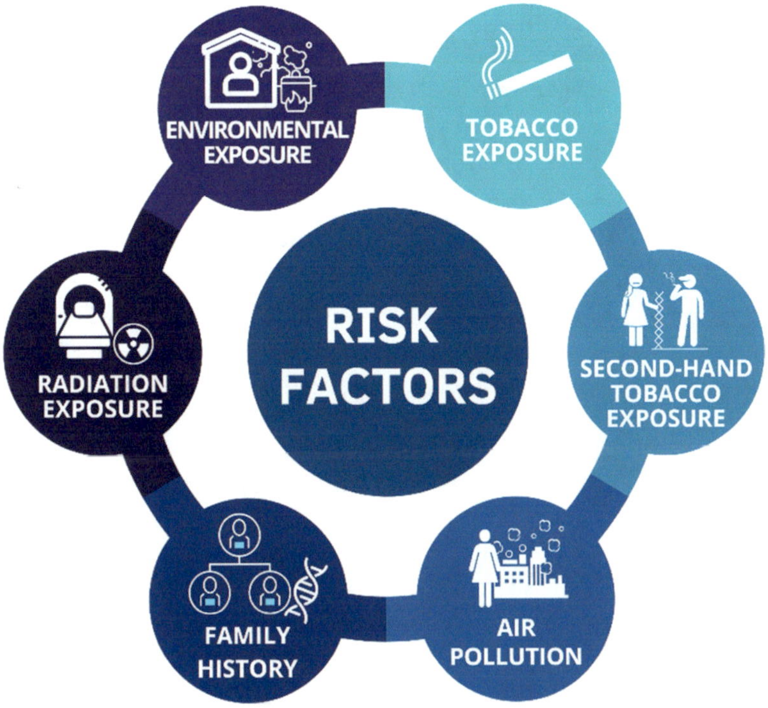

Figure 7.9. Lung cancer related to environmental factors.

Source: https://external-content.duckduckgo.com/iu/?u=https%3A%2F%2Fwww.clinical-lung-cancer.com%2Fcms%2Fattachment%2F040141aa-4590-47b6-a90c-5956ff7e1777%2Fgr1_lrg.jpg &f=1&nofb=1&ipt=221c33e0e917cd91fe7a8377b38b9e23f0aa743cf593a0d884e16bb9eb72e777.

These examples point to the undeniable role of environmental causes in lung carcinogenesis, and their mechanisms have to be the focus of diligent inquiry. Many pollutants, ranging from radon exposure within the home to particulate pollution due to industrial emissions, have been established as carcinogens. The International Agency for Research on Cancer further incorporates that environmental risks depend on their characteristic epidemiological patterns, particularly among never-smokers who have different clinicopathological presentations and molecular characteristics from smokers. This nuanced comprehension encourages a critical dialogue on prevention programs, with strong emphasis on the imperative to reduce environmental carcinogens as part of an intense public health agenda. Essentially, this acknowledgment of the connection between lung cancer and the environment fundamentally challenges public health policy and occupational health practice. Combating pollution by enforcing stringent control over industrial waste and banning smoking in public spaces can mitigate some of these hazards. Moreover, increasing awareness about residential burning of coal or other combustible materials is equally important, particularly among low-income families where such practices may be prevalent (Elvin et al., 2021). As the world grapples with rising lung cancer rates, multi-dimensional and proactive steps in both medical and environmental spheres are essential. This dual-pronged strategy not only alleviates the present lung cancer burden but also helps prevent future events, thereby maximizing public health gain and quality of life across populations (Figure 7.9).

Test Your Knowledge

1. Explain about chronic obstructive pulmonary disease (COPD).
2. What is lung cancer?

7.3. Risk Factors for Occupational Lung Diseases

Learning Outcome

1. Exposure to hazardous materials
2. Duration and intensity of exposure
3. Occupational safety measures and regulations

Occupational lung diseases like pneumoconiosis, COPD, and other interstitial lung diseases are serious public health issues due to exposure to causative agents primarily at the workplace. Long-term exposure to airborne particulate matter, chemicals used in industries, and biological agents is a significant risk factor for these diseases. Occupations like construction, mining, and agriculture expose workers to silica, asbestos, and organic dusts, which are recognized as the main causes of lung pathologies. An example is the inhalation of crystalline silica, which can lead to silicosis, a condition characterized by progressive lung fibrosis. It is crucial to identify such risk factors since it enables occupational safety regulators and doctors to implement preventive measures, which optimize workers' health and reduce the incidence of occupational lung diseases in the working populations, as reported by the increasing health burden documented worldwide in studies like the Global Burden of Disease Study 2017 (Wassim et al., 2020). In addition to environmental exposures, intrinsic characteristics such as a history of smoking, gender, and underlying diseases play very important roles in the etiology of occupational lung diseases. Smoking especially synergizes with occupational exposures to promote their adverse effects, as it speeds up inflammation and loss of lung function. It has been shown that smoking among high-risk occupational workers has much higher respiratory disease rates compared to non-smoking workers. Gender difference affects vulnerability as well; for instance, women are differently exposed and may have different extents of severity from the same occupational exposure. Additionally, employees with asthma or other chronic respiratory illnesses may be more vulnerable to occupational exposure; thus, particular health evaluation and intervention measures should be targeted in such populations (Vos et al., 2017). Emphasizing these risk factors can inform case-specific plans for monitoring health and improve preventive measures in occupational health. Effective worksite interventions and health policies are essential to mitigate risk factors associated with occupational lung diseases. Suppressing effective regulatory systems that enforce standard limit requirements for harmful substances and proper ventilation systems can significantly reduce exposure hazards. Also, awareness sessions that teach workers about the dangers of inhalational exposures and the importance of personal protective equipment can allow them to take active measures for their health. Further, regular health screenings and surveillance among exposed industries are essential in early detection and treatment of respiratory disease. With the rising number of chronic respiratory disease burden in the world, these interventions will be responsible for improving occupational health effects and reducing the undue costs associated with lung disease due to occupational settings (Wassim et al., 2020).

7.3.1. Exposure to Hazardous Materials

Exposure to harmful substances remains a high-priority topic in occupational and environmental lung disease, having a significant impact on public health. The extensive presence of air pollutants, particularly those resulting from natural disasters such as bushfires, underscores the need for proper control. During the 2019–2020 bushfires in Australia, high levels of particulate matter, PM2.5, which can readily penetrate the lungs, were emitted. Studies have shown that an increase in PM2.5 levels is associated with increased mortality and hospitalization due to respiratory disease, particularly among vulnerable populations such as the elderly and those with pre-existing health conditions. Such findings highlight the need for subtle public health interventions to mitigate exposure during prolonged pollution episodes, enabling individuals to make pragmatic decisions about their daily habits and health care during periods of elevated air quality alerts (Vardoulakis et al., 2020). Beyond particulate matter, the threat presented by heavy metals as harmful substances cannot be overlooked. Metals like lead, mercury, and cadmium are well known for their toxicity, primarily through bioaccumulation within ecosystems and food chains. The contaminants usually emanate from anthropogenic sources, such as industrial activities and mining, which disrupt natural biogeochemical processes and thus contaminate the environment. Heavy metals have a peculiar persistence since they tend to accumulate in living tissues over extended periods, thus representing serious threats to the health of consumers, including humans. This is of utmost importance to food safety and the potential for chronic illness following inhalation and ingestion of the poisons. The understanding of exposure to heavy metals and their impact on lung health highlights the need for continued monitoring and regulation to restrict public exposure and protect vulnerable groups (Ali et al., 2019). Besides, higher rates of lung diseases associated with exposure to toxic materials are compounded by a lack of preparedness and awareness among communities. The majority of individuals are not aware of the health risks posed by widespread air pollutants, including particulate matter and heavy metals in the environment. Educational campaigns in public health are crucial for raising awareness about the pathways of exposure and the cumulative effects these poisonous substances have on lung function. With enhanced environmental health literacy, communities will realize their exposures and be in a position to take preventive actions to protect their respiratory health. Lastly, comprehensive policy systems are needed that bring together environmental regulation and public education initiatives to minimize exposure risks as well as increase community resistance against occupational and environmental lung diseases. This multi-faceted approach has the ultimate aim of safeguarding both public and individual health effectively in the face of escalating environmental hazards (Figure 7.10).

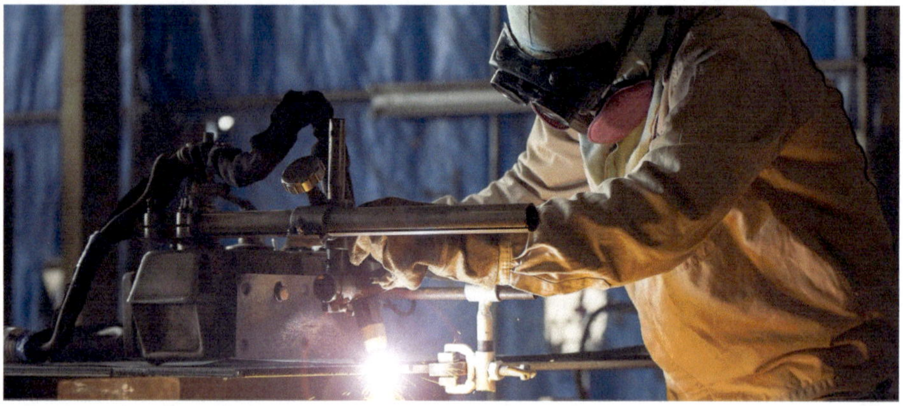

Figure 7.10. Exposure to hazardous materials for occupational lung diseases.

Source: https://www.lungcancercenter.com/app/uploads/2020/08/LC-Occupational-Exposure_2800x1800-scaled.jpg.

7.3.2. Duration and Intensity of Exposure

When occupational and environmental lung diseases are investigated, the duration and intensity of exposure to the causative noxious agent are significant factors underlying the development and causation of the disease. Higher durations of exposure are usually linked to higher risk of developing diseases such as COPD and lung cancer. It has been found that laborers with ongoing exposure to respiratory irritants, such as asbestos or silica, have significantly higher probabilities of developing lung-related diseases. For instance, construction or mining laborers may be exposed for decades, thereby making them vulnerable. The identification of these factors enables the development of more informed policies and measures to reach high-risk segments and counteract the harmful impact of occupational diseases. When the subtlety of exposure time conflicts with personal vulnerability, a complex appreciation is necessary to develop effective intervention and educational outreach strategies. Not only does the severity of exposure increase the susceptibility to respiratory illness, but it also affects the rate at which the lung function declines with high levels of particulate matter, for example. The severity of exposure becomes as important an area of study as the duration one spends in contaminated environments. Studies have proven that environments with high rates of air pollution or dense industrial emissions significantly contribute to morbidity among affected communities. Urban metropolises with heavy traffic and industry are paradigmatic sites where the interaction between intensity and duration creates a poisonous intersection for lung health. Institutions concerned with public health need to place the highest priority on interventions that mitigate not only chronic exposure but also manage to decrease peak levels of exposure that can result in abrupt health crises. Through comparative exposure intensity analyses, researchers can better determine the routes towards lung pathology and more effectively suggest targeted regulatory interventions. Furthermore, lung cancer statistics underscore the marked impact of both exposure duration and intensity within occupational environments. As indicated by existing evidence, lung cancer represents one of the most prevalent types of cancer globally and a major contributing cause of cancer mortality, particularly among exposed workers from high-risk occupational backgrounds.

The International Agency for Research on Cancer has continually documented the relationship between occupational exposure and increased incidences of lung cancer, particularly in industries such as construction and manufacturing, where harmful chemicals are prevalent. Public health measures must address these links by establishing cleaner environments and providing assistance to workers who may be exposed. Understanding the dynamics of exposure duration and intensity provides a basis for establishing targeted strategies to prevent and control environmental and occupational lung diseases, thereby promoting improved public health outcomes (Bray et al., 2024; Bray et al., 2018).

7.3.3. Occupational Safety Measures and Regulations

Workplace health and safety acts and policies are important in minimizing the occurrence of lung diseases resulting from dangerous workplace conditions. Effective regulation centers on the identification and management of workplace hazards that can lead to respiratory illnesses, providing better working conditions. The legislation is often grounded on comprehensive risk assessments that help develop specific safety protocols corresponding to employment activities and exposure rates. For example, screening programs for workers can assist in the early detection of lung health hazards and enable employers to introduce corrective action before further damage occurs. As noted in Gauci et al. (1997), attention should be on avoiding harmful exposures instead of mere detection of health effects after exposure, which stresses the need for proactive management in occupational health. In conjunction with preventive measures, regulatory frameworks that ensure adherence to safety standards play a crucial role in safeguarding employees' health. When businesses adhere to standards provided by occupational safety organizations, they make substantial contributions toward minimizing instances of lung disease. Such regulations tend to require the distribution of personal protective equipment (PPE), efficient ventilation systems, and periodic training of employees on handling hazardous chemicals. The role of the enforcement agencies cannot be emphasized enough, as they see to organizational compliance with statutory requirements. Therefore, Kriebel et al. (2011) highlight the importance of case studies that reveal the impact of non-regulatory complacency and the resulting health consequences on workers, clearly implying that an effective regulatory environment is essential for maintaining occupational health. Apart from this, constant education and training regarding occupational safety practices are of extreme significance to ensure maximum compliance and foster employee awareness. Measures to educate employees about best practices in exposure control to airborne hazards are both preventive and educational. Occupational pulmonary diseases like pneumoconiosis and other respiratory ailments are often covered in training programs to enable employees to know what they need to do for self-protection. By establishing a safety culture in workplaces and encouraging active participation in safety programs, workers can become integral in the enforcement of occupational safety laws. Through a collaborative effort in health and safety, occupational and environmental lung diseases can be effectively curbed, highlighting the importance of stringent occupational safety rules and measures (Figure 7.11).

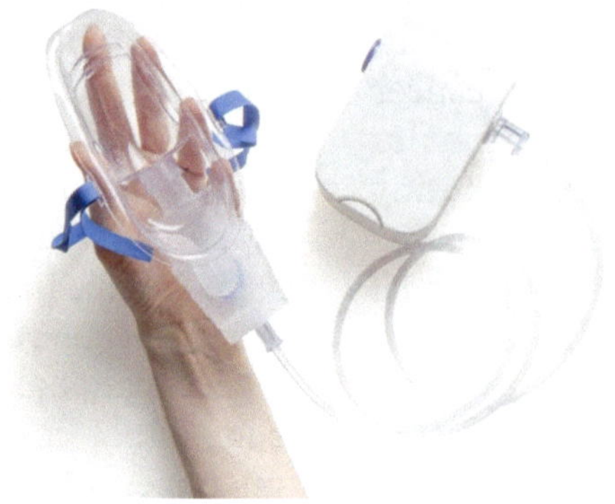

Figure 7.11. Occupational safety measures and regulations for occupational lung diseases.

Source: https://workhealthsolutions.com/wp-content/uploads/2021/10/mockup-graphics-2WlwSXFw7Kk-unsplash-1024x683.jpg.

Test Your Knowledge

1. What is the duration and intensity of exposure?
2. What are the occupational safety measures?

7.4. Risk Factors for Environmental Lung Diseases

Learning Outcome

1. Air pollution sources
2. Indoor air quality issues
3. Socioeconomic status and health disparities

The interaction between environmental exposure and lung function is an intricate and multifactorial process, underscoring the importance of understanding various risk factors for environmental lung diseases. Inhalation of air pollutants, particularly in urban areas, is a primary cause of respiratory diseases such as asthma and COPD. The primary sources of these pollutants are automotive emissions, industrial discharges, and the burning of fossil fuels. These harmful substances in the environment can also induce inflammation and exacerbate existing conditions or induce new respiratory diseases. Demographic factors also enhance the effect of these diseases, as certain groups like children and the elderly are particularly vulnerable because of their developing or compromised respiratory functions. Thus, a comprehensive prevention strategy for air pollution is crucial in reducing the incidence of these occupational and environmental respiratory diseases (Yatera et al., 2024). In addition to that, occupational exposures remain a significant risk factor, especially in industries handling toxic substances. Workers in the construction, mining, and manufacturing sectors are regularly exposed to dust, particulate matter, and chemical vapors, which adversely affect lung health. Prolonged exposure can lead to a number of diseases, from harmless pneumoconiosis to dangerous respiratory conditions like lung cancer. The factors of risk within the work environment are not static; they may heavily rely on industry, compliance with regulations, and occupational health measures. Thus, it is crucial to identify the exact environmental and occupational factors that render one susceptible to lung disease. This recognition can lead to targeted preventive measures, including improved occupational safety regulations and health monitoring programs that will ultimately enhance worker health outcomes and reduce the socioeconomic burden of these disorders (Moretta et al., 2024). The convergence of environmental and occupational lung diseases is a public health challenge that confronts policymakers and clinicians in more than one dimension. Chronic respiratory conditions such as COPD, with powerful environmental and occupational determinants, underscore the importance of an overall prevention and management approach. Other than their physical manifestations, the degree to which they impact general health status, including comorbidities such as depression and anxiety, underscores the importance of addressing mental health as much as respiratory care. Effective management is an interdisciplinary approach that borrows from expertise in pulmonology, occupational health, and psychology to create an integrated understanding of how occupational and environmental risk factors overlap to affect lung health. Through research and intervention priorities that take these overlapping areas into account, society can progress toward more effective prevention and treatment of occupational and environmental lung diseases (Moretta et al., 2024) (Figure 7.12).

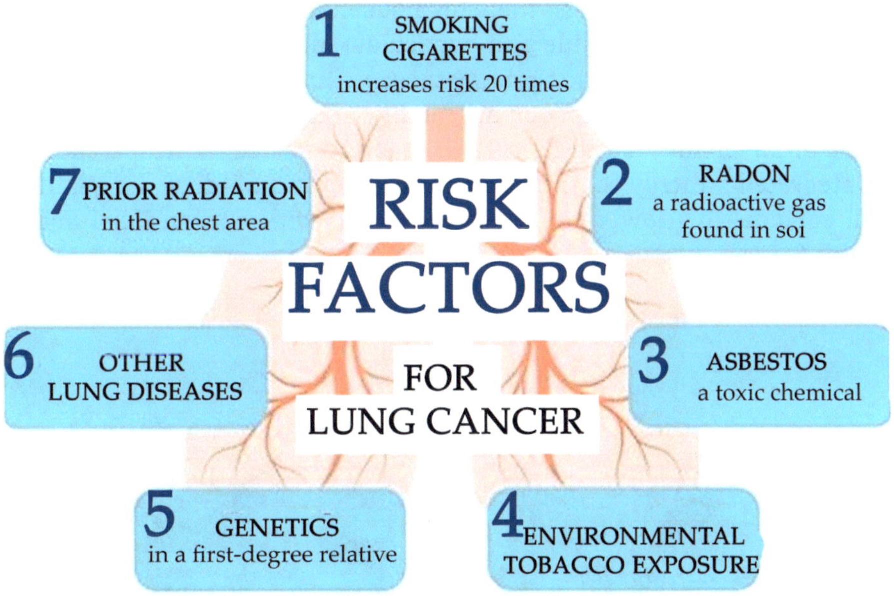

Figure 7.12. Risk factors for environmental lung diseases.

Source: https://www.medschool.lsuhsc.edu/lungcancer/images/riskfactorsforlc.bmp.

7.4.1. Air Pollution Sources

Air pollution sources contribute significantly to the advancement of occupational and environmental lung disease, and there are numerous sources of varying types impacting the air. Industrial operations are among the significant culprits, releasing air toxicants such as particulate matter (PM), sulfur dioxide (SO_2), and volatile organic compounds (VOCs). These chemicals emanate from activities such as combustion, chemical manufacturing, and mining, subjecting workers and communities to hazardous airborne substances. Second, cars are a major cause of air pollution, particularly in cities, with traffic congestion causing elevated emissions of nitrogen oxides (NOx) and fine particles. Prolonged exposure to these has been linked with respiratory ailments like asthma and COPD, indicating the need for stringent regulation and control measures to contain their adverse impacts on public health. Farm activities also contribute to air pollution, affecting occupational and environmental health. Fertilizers and pesticides emit ammonia into the air, which can combine with other air pollutants to form toxic particulate matter. Livestock farming, especially large-scale production, emits methane and volatile organic compounds, exacerbating air quality problems. Moreover, farm burning operations—often employed to minimize foliage—emit smoke and particulate matter that may travel into surrounding regions, affecting the air quality for agrarian workers as well as nearby populations. The impact of such aerial toxins is considerable, as evident from the increasing incidence of respiratory ailments among agrarian workers and individuals living near agricultural activities. It is necessary to tackle the multifactorial determinants of air pollution to preserve lung health and foster healthier living conditions. Lastly, indoor air pollution is a significant but often overlooked cause of respiratory disease, stemming from an array of sources such as home cleaning chemicals, mold, and secondhand tobacco smoke. In most cases, individuals are exposed to indoor contaminants at concentrations even greater than those of outdoor air contaminants. For instance, burning fossil fuels for household space heating and cooking releases hazardous products like carbon monoxide and particulate matter, which exacerbate or cause lung disease. Also, suboptimal home ventilation retains these pollutants, augmenting their harmful effect on lung function. The intersection of indoor air quality and occupational exposures underscores the complex nature of air pollution and its role in respiratory health. Researchers emphasize the necessity for an integrated strategy to mitigate both indoor and outdoor air quality, as addressing these sources can considerably lower the risks associated with occupational and environmental lung disease (Figure 7.13).

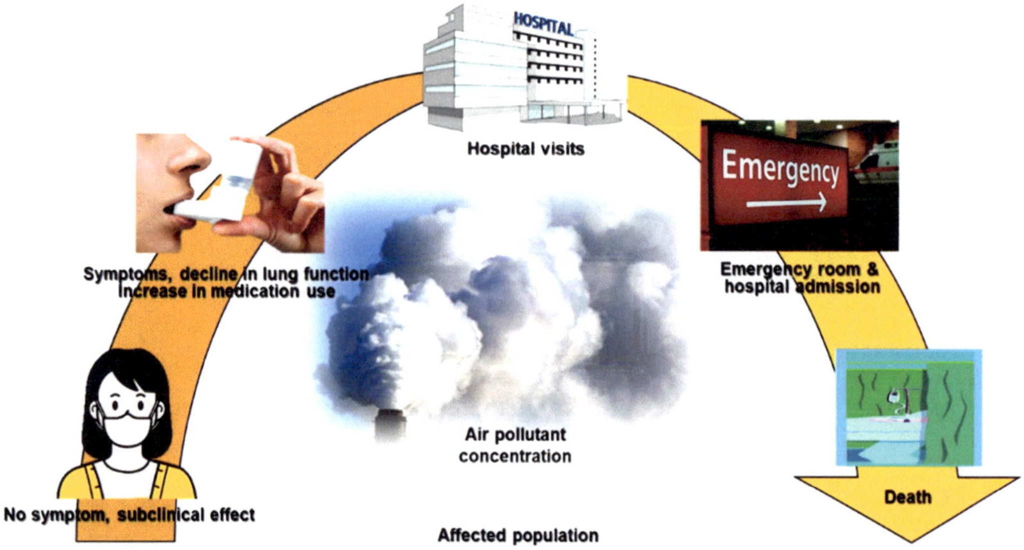

Figure 7.13. Air pollution sources for environmental lung diseases.

Source: https://pub.mdpi-res.com/ijerph/ijerph-18-09905/article_deploy/html/images/ijerph-18-09905-g001.png?1632303018.

7.4.2. Indoor air Quality Issues

The contribution of indoor air quality (IAQ) as a factor for determining respiratory health is increasingly recognized in occupational and environmental lung disease environments. A considerable majority of the population remains indoors for considerable durations, and consequently, the pollutants in these environments become vital for their overall well-being. Low IAQ is related to a number of adverse health effects, particularly among vulnerable populations such as the elderly and children. Indoor air contaminants, including volatile organic compounds, mold, and particulate matter, are well-known triggers and exacerbants for respiratory conditions such as asthma and COPD. Further, certain indoor spaces may have inadequate ventilation, leading to the build-up of harmful substances. It is important to address these indoor air quality issues as much for improving individual health outcomes as for reducing the overall burden of indoor pollution-related lung disease. The present study calls for indoor air quality to be considered a modifiable risk factor for respiratory illness. It has been proposed in several studies that some indoor pollutants contribute to a significant proportion of respiratory morbidity. For example, allergen exposure to house dust mites, cat and dog dander, and cockroach feces may aggravate diseases such as asthma, particularly in sensitized individuals. In addition, indoor air pollution from fuel combustion, predominantly in poorly ventilated housing, is a central concern because it results in exposure to toxic emissions, which form crippling respiratory ailments. More data have indicated that even among nonsmokers, domestic air pollution can contribute to a higher prevalence of COPD. This highlights the importance of interventions to improve IAQ and restrict exposure to established hazards in the domestic environment. Indoor air quality and lung disease are becoming more accepted as global public health issues. Since air pollution has been established to be the most urgent environmental risk to health, cutting indoor air pollution cannot be overemphasized (Liu et al., 2023). Measures for improvement of IAQ such as the incorporation of high-efficiency particulate air (HEPA) filters and ensuring good ventilation are the basic elements of proper public health intervention. In addition, ongoing research on the influence of allergens and toxins on lung function will shed further insight into the dynamics of such interactions and inform future preventive measures. The focus on improving indoor air quality is particularly relevant in high-risk areas where groups may face simultaneous adversity from both indoor and outdoor pollution. Solving IAQ issues not only enhances respiratory health but also complements general well-being and quality of life among individuals from all walks of life (Liu et al., 2023) (Figure 7.14).

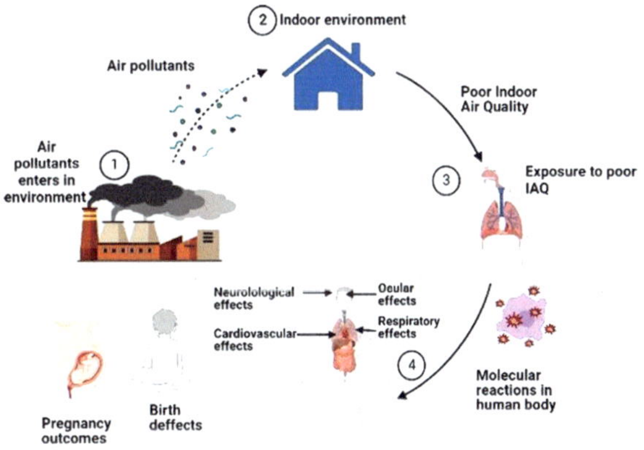

Figure 7.14. Indoor air quality issues for environmental lung diseases.

Source: https://ars.els-cdn.com/content/image/1-s2.0-S0048969723007799-ga1.jpg.

7.4.3. Socioeconomic Status and Health Disparities

Socioeconomic status (SES) is a predictor of health conditions, particularly occupational and environmental respiratory diseases. Workers with lower SES experience greater exposure to hazardous materials and occupational hazards.

Such workers are likely to experience long-term respiratory illnesses such as asthma, COPD, and lung cancer. This is exacerbated in industries where safety is not adequate, that is, where the workers do not have protective clothing. Besides, lower SES individuals frequently lack access to healthcare and thus experience delayed diagnosis and intervention. These hindrances persist to create a cycle of adverse health outcomes, confirming that socio-economic status is inherently linked to the risk of developing and progressing lung diseases. In light of rising interest in health equity as a public health priority, it is not only critical but also urgent to address these disparities to improve the health of vulnerable groups. Additionally, the overlap of SES with environmental elements renders differences in lung disease much more difficult. Economic deprivation areas have higher levels of air and industrial pollution, both of which are toxic to the respiratory tract. For instance, economically disadvantaged neighborhoods are more likely to be situated near freeways or factories, exposing them to higher concentrations of airborne toxins. Consequently, patients in these environments may have higher rates of occurrence of respiratory disorders than their more affluent neighbors. Furthermore, limited access to parks and recreation facilities can restrict physical well-being, further adding to health inequalities. The realization of the profound impact of environmental disparity on the occurrence of lung diseases is crucial to inform effective public health interventions in an attempt to reduce the burden of disease in the most vulnerable communities. Finally, addressing the complex relationship between health disparities and socioeconomic status requires tackling policy reform along with community engagement. Improving workplace safety policies, strengthening environmental regulations, and increasing healthcare access are all among those actions that can significantly mitigate occupational and environmental lung disease risk. In addition to empowerment measures, including health risk and preventive education within communities, these mechanisms can promote resilience among high-risk groups. Successful interventions will also need to acknowledge the principal role that social determinants of health, such as education and income, have in shaping an individual's capacity for attaining good health. By accepting multi-faceted strategies informed by the intricacies of SES, public health initiatives can create a more inclusive atmosphere that minimizes health disparities and provides healthier futures for all, especially in at-risk populations.

Test Your Knowledge

1. What are the air pollution sources?
2. What are the indoor air quality issues?

7.5. Symptoms and Diagnosis

Learning Outcome

1. Common symptoms of lung diseases
2. Diagnostic methods and tools
. Importance of early detection

Recognition of occupational and environmental lung disease symptoms is essential for early detection and effective management. These symptoms—chronic cough, wheezing, breathlessness, and chest tightness —may be worsened by the presence of certain irritants or allergens in the environment or workplace. For instance, individuals exposed to asbestos can manifest pleural effusion and dyspnea decades later, highlighting the latent development of these conditions. Moreover, the chronic nature of the majority of occupational lung disease, e.g., pneumoconiosis, requires healthcare professionals to obtain meticulous patient histories with occupational exposure. Identification of such symptoms in high-risk populations can enable early medical intervention, improving the overall health status and decreasing chronic complications of continued exposure to harmful substances. Diagnosis should be achieved using the appropriate diagnostic process to properly identify occupational and environmental lung diseases. Techniques such as spirometry and peak expiratory flow rate (PEFR) testing are greatly used to assess lung function abnormalities because they provide objective data on respiratory status. A study that included patients with abnormal lung function showed a high sensitivity rate for both spirometry and PEFR in the screening of asthma, indicating their reliability as diagnostic tools (Saltanat et al., 2022). Nonetheless, the specificity of these tests is still a concern, and spirometry has a more negative predictive value than PEFR. Thus, clinicians need to understand that even with the effectiveness of these screening tests, they must be integrated with thorough patient assessments, including symptom assessment and work history, to arrive at a concrete diagnosis. Advanced imaging techniques have also taken center stage in the diagnosis of interstitial lung diseases, the majority of which arise due to occupational and environmental exposure. For instance, computed densitometry (CD) is a new imaging modality that quantitatively measures lung tissue density, providing invaluable information about the extent of lung involvement in pneumoconiosis and pulmonary fibrosis. The ability to correlate changes in lung density with clinical manifestations and other findings enhances the overall understanding of disease pathogenesis and progression (Basanets et al., 2022). Further, the standardization of CT scanning protocols and the potential reduction in radiation dosage during these tests emphasize developments in diagnostic methods. By applying these measures, healthcare professionals can enhance effective disease diagnosis, better inform treatment planning, and reduce the dangers of occupational and environmental lung diseases.

7.5.1. Common Symptoms of Lung Diseases

Lung diseases are a broad spectrum of disorders with many symptoms, having a significant impact on patients' quality of life. The common symptoms of lung diseases typically include chronic cough, dyspnea, wheezing, tightness in the chest, and sputum production. The signs and symptoms may be present as a result of a wide range of environmental and occupational exposures such as exposure to harmful agents, particulate matter, or toxic gases. For instance, occupational respiratory diseases like asbestosis and silicosis commonly present with chronic cough and increasing dyspnea, frequently worsening on exertion. Prompt recognition of these symptoms by employers and health care providers is extremely crucial since early diagnosis can significantly improve control and outcome in patients, especially those with a history of exposure to respiratory irritants or toxic emissions. In addition to the above, clinical presentation of lung disease can also include systemic symptoms that reflect underlying pulmonary diseases. Tiredness, weight loss, and fever can be associated with primary respiratory symptoms, reflecting the development of acute exacerbation or secondary diseases such as pneumonia. Compromised lung function can also lead to worsening exercise tolerance, making physical activity more difficult and contributing to psychological distress. Research has shown that people exposed to high air pollutants tend to have reduced pulmonary function, which relates to greater respiratory symptoms (Ta et al., 2022).

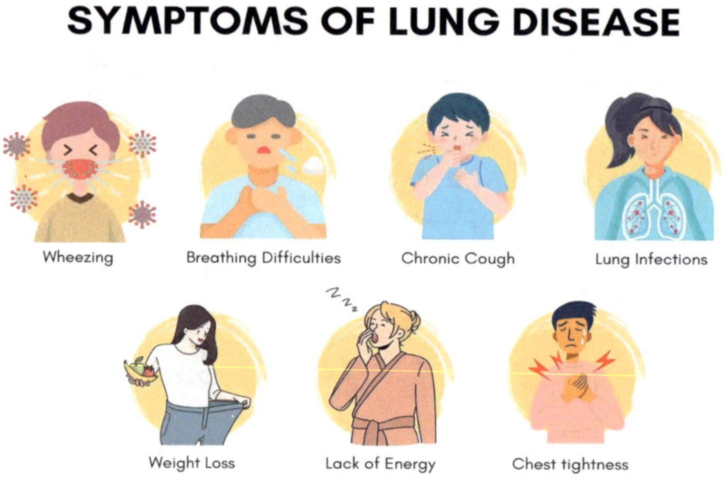

Figure 7.15. Common symptoms of lung diseases.

Source: https://www.drsheetusingh.com/wp-content/uploads/2018/03/Symptoms-of-Lung-Disease-Dr.-Sheetu-Singh.webp.

The interdependence emphasizes the need to monitor lung health for those working in demanding environments or living in high-air pollution regions to mitigate long-term outcomes from lung function loss. Diagnosis and discrimination of lung disease symptoms are essential not just for diagnosis but also for treatment. Patients with exercise intolerance and breathlessness, for instance, can undergo pulmonary function tests, thereby allowing intervention to be tailored. Respiratory diseases common in post-9/11 military populations, for example, include asthma and presentations of distal lung disease that occur with wheezing and chest tightness. Reductions in diffusion capacity have also been strongly associated with distal lung diseases, which emphasizes the importance of detailed assessments to capture the whole range of deployment-related respiratory diseases (Krefft et al., 2020). By understanding the common signs and their significance for lung health, physicians can better personalize treatment regimens, ultimately improving outcomes for those compromised by occupational and environmental lung disease (Figure 7.15).

7.5.2. Diagnostic Methods and Tools

Occupational and environmental lung disease diagnosis employs various techniques and instruments to accurately identify the presence of disease-causing agents and assess the resulting pulmonary status. Traditional diagnosis usually includes medical history questionnaires, chest X-rays, and pulmonary function tests. These diagnoses identify lung impairment and provide clinicians with valuable information for recognizing patterns associated with environmental exposure. However, advances in technology have enabled the development of molecular diagnostics that will result in more sensitive and specific testing. For instance, robust approaches such as real-time reverse transcription polymerase chain reaction (RT-PCR) have revolutionized the identification of viral pathogens, which is now a significant diagnostic option for infectious lung illnesses, including occupational exposures to viral agents (Zekhnini et al., 2025). Another promising diagnostic method in pulmonary medicine is the use of laser-induced breakdown spectroscopy (LIBS) for the assessment of elemental contamination of lung tissue. This novel method has the potential to provide in situ quantitation of toxic elements, such as titanium, which can result from occupational exposure. The analytical technique has been highly confirmed for its reliability and accuracy relative to conventional methods, such as inductively coupled plasma mass spectrometry. When relating elemental concentrations to effects on health, LIBS more effectively shows how specific environmental pollutants are responsible for causing respiratory disease. This intersection of advanced technologies is a critical step forward in occupational lung disease diagnosis and treatment because it allows direct measurement of exposure levels in human samples (Gardette et al., 2024). In addition to such analytical advances, the use of large databases and epidemiological research is also critical in understanding the larger context of lung disease in occupational and environmental determinants. These databases enable researchers and medical professionals to trace trends, identify vulnerable populations, and ascertain the association between exposures and disease incidence levels. Moreover, bringing diagnostic machinery into direct contact with results from such studies promotes a patient-oriented treatment approach as well as disease avoidance. Overall, the combination of traditional methods with modern diagnostic tools and large research databases enables clinicians to be well-prepared to manage and diagnose occupational and environmental lung diseases efficiently, ultimately improving outcomes for target group patients (Figure 7.16).

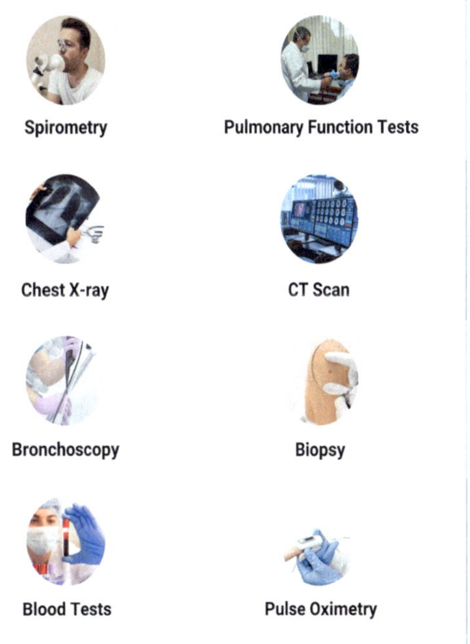

Figure 7.16. Diagnostic methods and tools of occupational and environmental lung diseases.

Source: https://images.drlogy.com/assets/uploads/img/admin/health_blog/editor-img/lung_diseases_diagnosis_-_drlogy.webp.

7.5.3. Importance of Early Detection

Early detection is crucial for avoiding the irreparable impact of occupational and environmental lung disease. Early detection of such diseases allows for timely intervention and treatment, significantly improving the patient's outcome. For instance, screening schemes tailored to a given workplace hazard can facilitate the detection of individuals at risk prior to the development of signs. Such practices must be incorporated into occupational health policies since they promote prevention and sustain worker well-being. The allocation of resources to early detection programs not only complies with public health policies but also enhances the importance of worker safety. By adhering to guidelines for managing dangerous exposure, companies can implement effective early detection plans instead of reactive measures that occur when health issues arise (Gauci et al., 1997). Early diagnosis is particularly crucial in insidious onset conditions like mesothelioma. The cancer does not present in its earlier stages and therefore comes with a poor prognosis. Accurate estimation of past asbestos exposure—a pre-requisite to the development of screening programs—can significantly enhance the likelihood of diagnosing mesothelioma at an earlier stage. Experience indicates that construction of strong individual reconstruction procedures is beneficial in risk apportionment. By using in-depth assessments to evaluate past exposure, health workers can identify individuals with high risks and arrange for them to be enrolled in targeted screening programs. Because there exists a favorable correlation between measurements and estimated exposure levels, the development of such measurement techniques can transform early detection work and ultimately lead to improved treatment and control of those affected (Blyth et al., 2017). In addition to patient-specific endpoints, the broader interests of efficient early detection also extend to public health. With occupational lung diseases being identified more accurately, there is the possibility of more effective resource allocation in prevention and treatment. Early detection enables medical personnel to obtain data that can inform workplace safety interventions and training programs, thereby reducing the incidence of these diseases in the long term. Exposure of workers to fewer hazardous substances can significantly lower the incidence of diseases such as pneumoconiosis, asbestosis, and lung cancer. Moreover, developing a work culture focused on early detection and health surveillance can have beneficial knock-on effects, improving employees' general well-being and productivity levels. Early detection is hence not only an individual-care measure but also a core component of occupational health practice (Gauci et al., 1997).

Test Your Knowledge

1. What are the common symptoms of lung diseases?
2. What are the diagnostic methods and tools of lung diseases?

7.6. Treatment and Management

Learning Outcome

1. Medical treatments available
2. Lifestyle changes and preventive measures
3. Role of rehabilitation programs

It takes a comprehensive approach with both medical therapy and preventive interventions to treat and control occupational and environmental lung diseases. Removing exposure to offending substances, such as toxic airborne pollutants, is the first line of management and can significantly decrease the disease process. For instance, interventions may include the use of personal protective equipment (PPE) in the workplace, improved ventilation systems, and adherence to safety standards, which all reduce the risk for respiratory complications. Employee education and training on potential hazards, along with early reporting of respiratory symptoms, are also important. These interventions also support patients and promote a safety culture and health awareness within the workplace, ultimately translating to better health outcomes among workers in hazardous occupations (Hirsch et al., 2024). Pharmacological treatment is another cornerstone in the management of occupational and environmental lung diseases. Maintenance therapies, including corticosteroids and bronchodilators, will alleviate symptoms of diseases such as COPD and occupational asthma. These medications enhance airflow and reduce airway inflammation, improving the patient's quality of life. On top of this, supplemental oxygen therapy must be applied to patients with severe respiratory impairment to maintain adequate oxygenation and overall pulmonary function. Rehabilitation treatments, including pulmonary rehabilitation, are also helpful as they allow patients to regain strength and functional reserve through exercise, education, and support, thereby aiding in the recovery and management of occupational exposure-related chronic symptoms (Bray et al., 2024). Occupational and environmental causes of chronic lung diseases require lifelong follow-up and regular assessment of pulmonary function. Regular follow-ups with health professionals allow timely modifications in treatment protocols tailored to the evolving status of patients. In addition to this, integration of prevention measures into public policy is important for reducing the incidence of these diseases. This includes lobbying for better control of industrial effluents and occupational safety practices, as well as raising awareness programs to educate employers and workers about the risks posed by toxic exposures. Research into new therapy options, as well as the implementation of wide-scale public health programs, will play a central role in minimizing the threat posed by occupational and environmental lung disease, with a healthier workforce for future generations (Hirsch et al., 2024) (Figure 7.17).

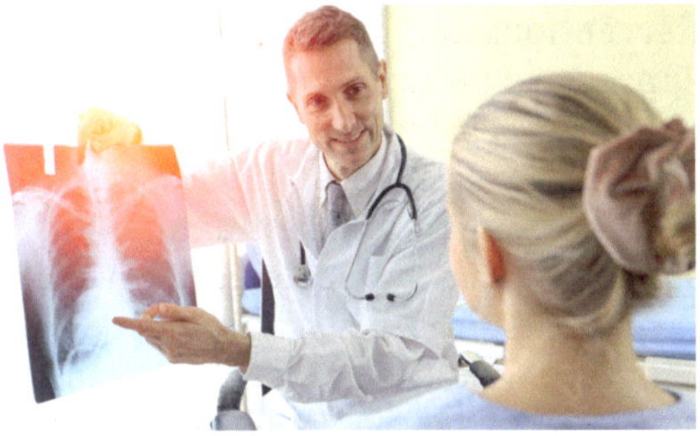

Figure 7.17. Effective treatment and management of occupational and environmental lung diseases.

Source: https://cdn.prod.website-files.com/647888ca92d03e3fca3f1ea0/647888ca92d03e3fca3f23dc_shutterstock_1667964562.jpg.

7.6.1. Medical Treatments Available

Medical treatments for occupational and environmental lung diseases encompass an array of therapies tailored for specific diseases and causative agents. The therapies can include pharmacologic treatments such as bronchodilators and corticosteroids, which are commonly used to provide relief and improve airflow in conditions like asthma and COPD. These medicines work by reducing inflammation in the airways and relaxing the surrounding muscles, thereby enhancing respiratory function. Other measures may involve giving antibiotics in cases where secondary bacterial infections have complicated the underlying lung conditions. Moreover, the importance of early diagnosis and continuous monitoring cannot be overestimated, as these elements significantly contribute to the effectiveness of treatment programs. Creation of a personalized treatment plan according to the requirements of each patient can significantly decrease the load of lung diseases on quality of life. In addition to pharmacotherapy, occupational and environmental lung diseases are also managed by non-pharmacological interventions to augment lung function and suppress exposure to noxious substances. Pulmonary rehabilitation programs are a part of this many-splendored treatment since they offer structured exercise training, nutritional counseling, and psychological counseling to the patients. The programs are designed to enhance physical tolerance and to instill self-management strategies that help patients control their conditions better. Environmental control measures, such as improvement in ventilation at the workplace and use of personal protective equipment, are also crucial in preventing further lung damage. The application of these measures not only aids in managing the existing disease but also significantly reduces the risk of further disease progression, ultimately leading to better long-term results for the patients concerned. New therapies also demonstrate promise for the treatment of occupational and environmental lung disease, particularly for those who will be resistant to conventional therapies. Research into targeted biologic treatments intended to manipulate the immune system is accelerating, especially for those diseases that have an inflammatory component, like asthma. These novel treatments could involve using monoclonal antibodies to prevent specific pathways involved in airway inflammation, thereby providing an added choice for severe patients. Further, innovations in gene therapy and stem cell technology may eventually provide new means of repairing or replacing lung tissue damaged by exposures at work. As studies and clinical trials progress, the status of medical therapy for lung diseases continually shifts and promises even better and more individualized treatment in the future (Figure 7.18).

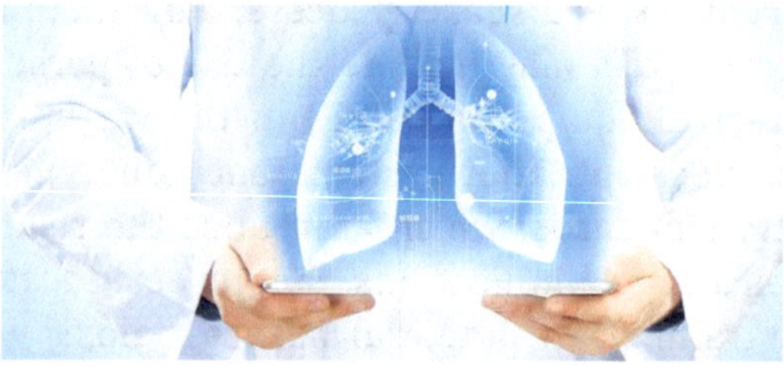

Figure 7.18. Medical treatments available of occupational and environmental lung diseases.

Source: https://careandcurehospital.co.in/wp-content/uploads/2025/05/Best-Respiratory-Medicine-Treatment-In-Chembur-800x350-1.jpg.

7.6.2. Lifestyle Changes and Preventive Measures

The significance of lifestyle changes in preventing occupational and environmental lung diseases cannot be overemphasized. A healthy lung strategy involves adopting habits that lower risk factors for lung disease, such as smoking, obesity, and exposure to pollution. Avoidance of smoking is the most crucial lifestyle change since smoking is the leading cause of lung cancer and respiratory illness. The facts reveal that nearly 49% of lung cancer cases are directly linked to smoking, indicating the urgency of public health initiatives for reducing tobacco consumption. Moreover, following a healthy nutrition plan and engaging in proper physical exercise can actually improve respiratory health by enhancing lung function as well as overall health. By targeting lifestyle modifications, individuals can reduce their risk for lung disease and promote a better quality of life (Bray et al., 2024). Apart from individual decisions, systemic preventive measures play a major role in reducing occupational and environmental lung disease. Exposure controls that limit exposure to poisonous chemicals in the workplace have been effective in reducing instances of diseases such as asbestosis and pneumoconiosis. Portfolio investments in improving air quality, combined with occupational safety interventions, can make a significant contribution to declining workers' risk of lung disease. Moreover, companies are quickly embracing the position of mental and emotional health in holistic lung health, given that stress management and mental health treatment can contribute to one's capacity to cope with occupational exposure. The development of supportive environments strengthens adherence to health-promoting habits, thereby confirming the significance of preventive interventions in reducing lung disease risk (Bray et al., 2018). Awareness and education are the pillars of effective lifestyle changes and preventive interventions for occupational and environmental lung diseases. Community outreach programs will raise awareness of the risks associated with exposure in some working environments, thereby empowering employees to voice their concerns for their own health and safety. Furthermore, incorporating respiratory health education into occupational training sessions makes the workers familiar with the knowledge of proper safety measures, including the utilization of personal protective equipment. Creation of a safe workplace culture encourages the prevention of lung health and prepares individuals to defend against harmful exposures. By raising awareness and educating about risk factors and prevention, society not only improves individual health but also helps reduce the burden of lung diseases on the healthcare system and economy (Bray et al., 2018, 2024) (Figure 7.19).

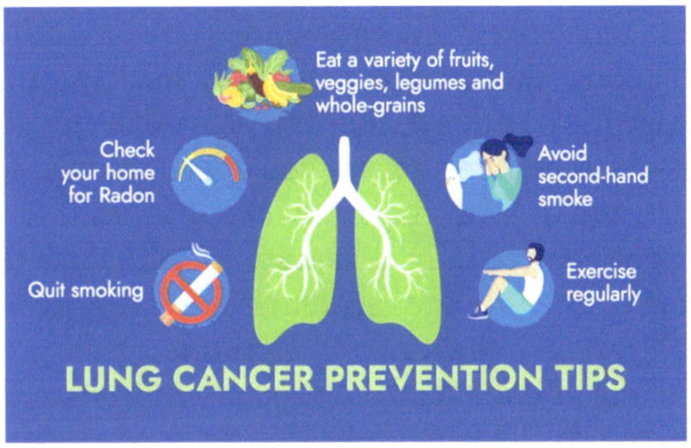

Figure 7.19. Lifestyle changes and preventive measures of occupational and environmental lung diseases.

Source: https://www.healzone.co.in/storage/app/public/blogs/December2024/Untitled%20design%20-%202024-12-18T123057.299.jpg.

7.6.3. Role of Rehabilitation Programs

The contribution of rehabilitation programs to managing occupational and environmental lung disease cannot be overemphasized, as they offer holistic interventions that address not only physical rehabilitation but also emphasize the psychological and social facets of well-being. Multidisciplinary interventions are often practiced in these programs, where healthcare providers, occupational therapists, and respiratory specialists collaborate to develop personalized rehabilitation plans tailored to the patients' needs. Patients usually find exercise training, disease management education, and strategies for improving lung function helpful. Focusing on these areas, rehabilitation programs are able to enhance patients quality of life and restrain symptom worsening characteristic in chronic lung diseases. The overall care model finally offers a clearer pathway towards recovery and accommodation across various settings, whether in the work environment or daily living. One of the most significant advantages of rehabilitation programs is that they emphasize informing patients about their illnesses, which renders patients active in their care and management. Education modules are likely to cover topics such as symptom recognition, environmental provocation, and self-management strategies, particularly for individuals with chronic occupational and environmental lung diseases. In addition, the programs motivate patients to bring about changes in behavior, for example, giving up smoking or enhancing workplace environments, which also helps prevent symptom worsening. Identifying patients' active participation in their own healthcare process not only leads to improved health outcomes but also fosters resilience. With greater knowledge and proficiency, patients can better overcome the challenge of their lung ailments, thus leading to improved occupational functioning and overall well-being in the long term. The inclusion of rehabilitation programs within treatment also reduces the broader psychosocial impact of occupational and environmental lung diseases. A number of patients are isolated, anxious, or depressed following the challenge posed by their conditions. Therapy sessions usually consist of counseling and support groups that facilitate emotional recovery and attachment with others under the same circumstances. These psychosocial supports are essential as they improve total mental well-being, boost motivation, and encourage adherence to treatment protocols. As highlighted in various public health initiatives, such as the Allergy Program of Finland, awareness of the psychosocial determinants of health results in enhanced management of chronic conditions such as asthma and allergy, and thus evincing the role of a rehabilitation program as a whole person in minimizing the impact of occupational and environmental lung diseases on the lives of individuals and national productivity (Haahtela et al., 2021; N/A, 2023) (Figure 7.20).

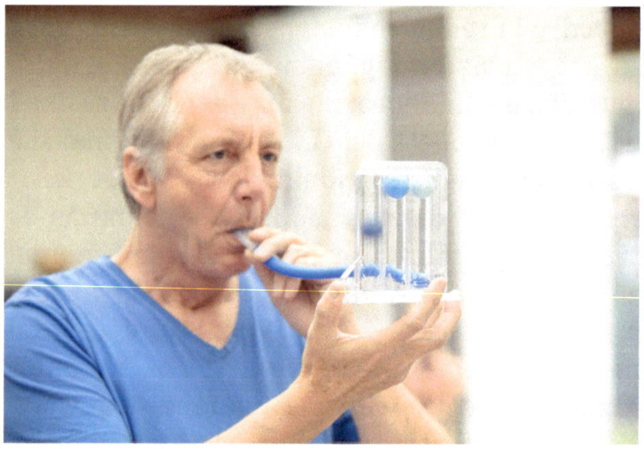

Figure 7.20. Pulmonary rehabilitation program.

Source: https://external-content.duckduckgo.com/iu/?u=https%3A%2F%2Fwww.nationalhealthexecutive.com%2Fwrite%2FMediaUploads%2FiStock-508011138.jpg&f=1&nofb=1&ipt=b11ae337d09aef56127c8bafac36d1d46148228c3065cfd3400b20b81665a3f0.

Test Your Knowledge

1. What are the lifestyle changes and preventive measures?
2. What is the role of rehabilitation programs?

SUMMARY

In the study of occupational and environmental lung diseases, it is clear that the diseases are a significant challenge not only to individual health but to public health systems as well. The intricacy of the diseases is brought out by their etiological associations with both work environments and overall environmental exposures. For instance, the longer time gap between symptom onset and referral to healthcare during crises such as the COVID-19 pandemic has exacerbated the diagnosis and management of many lung conditions, particularly lung cancer, which has increased referral times due to the strain on the healthcare system (Helsper et al., 2023). This waiting time illustrates the necessity of organized interventions to reduce such waiting times, thereby improving immediate access to care and eventually better health for those in question. In addition, the link between participation at work and occupational health remains recognized as an area of priority for intervention. As demonstrated by research showing improved work capacity after rehabilitation treatment, the significance of adequate respiratory health care cannot be overstated (Skinnes et al., 2023). Such programs are pivotal not only in ensuring recovery from lung disease but also in securing employment, which is crucial for economic and psychological stability in individuals. The findings also show that interventions in factors like comorbidities, pain severity, and general well-being can enhance one's ability to work following rehabilitation. This again highlights the need for comprehensive health interventions that consider both respiratory wellness and workplace support. Prevention of occupational and environmental lung diseases also involves an active approach that sets personal health against system policy changes. Regulations to manage exposure to harmful airborne particulates, setting work safety standards, and community awareness are essential in avoiding lung disease risks. It is also significant that health providers, policymakers, and industry join hands in developing targeted education programs, increasing awareness of the potential hazards of occupational and environmental exposure. By emphasizing prevention and early intervention, the stakeholders can best mitigate the prevalence of lung diseases and, in the process, contribute to healthier workplaces and communities for the coming generations.

Occupational and environmental lung diseases represent an important public health problem, which includes heterogeneous pathology due to inhalation of harmful agents. These diseases can be present as COPD, asthma, and pneumoconiosis, directly linked to exposure in occupational environments or polluted environments. Etiology and pathophysiology of these diseases should be identified in order to develop effective preventive strategies. As an illustration, mining, construction, and manufacturing sectors commonly expose employees to dangerous particles and gases that influence lung function in the long term. Knowledge regarding occupational exposures and respiratory health is significant at both a policy and an individual level for occupational health. Measurement of lung function is one of the most prominent features in diagnosing and tracking occupational and environmental lung diseases. The American Thoracic Society and European Respiratory Society's 2005 joint report on pulmonary function tests (PFTs) emphasizes the need for accurate interpretation of test results. By defining pulmonary function values as within or outside of normal limits, healthcare providers can become more informed about a patient's respiratory status and subsequent prognosis. The integration of clinical data and physiological determinants renders such tests more consistent, enabling interventions to be systematically crafted based on individual requirements. Stanojevic et al. (2021) ensure compliance with standards by keeping clinicians updated with current norms for the interpretation of PFTs, thereby improving patient care for occupational lung disease management. Prevention is paramount in minimizing the burden of occupational and environmental lung diseases. This also involves implementing strict safety measures and increasing awareness among the workforce about the risks involved in certain environments. For instance, the utilization of preventive measures such as proper ventilation, respirators, and continuous air quality monitoring can significantly reduce exposure to noxious fumes. Further, training in-house on the signs of respiratory issues can allow workers to receive medical care at an early stage. The ongoing process of updating guidelines, as encouraged by Vahanian et al. (2021), is crucial in establishing effective public health policy with regard to lung health. Through a concerted effort by employers, healthcare professionals, and regulators, we can encourage workplace safety and, in the long term, improve respiratory health outcomes across the affected populations.

KEY TERMS FROM THIS CHAPTER

- Asbestosis
- Bagassosis
- Berylliosis
- Black lung disease
- Bronchiolitis obliterans
- Byssinosis
- Caplan syndrome
- Chronic beryllium disease
- Hypersensitivity pneumonitis
- Lung fibrosis
- Occupational asthma
- Organic dust toxic syndrome (ODTS)
- Pneumoconiosis
- Pulmonary alveolar proteinosis
- Siderosis
- Silicosis
- Toxic inhalation injury

CRITICAL THINKING QUESTIONS

1. **Which of the following occupational exposures is classically associated with silicosis?**
   a. Coal dust
   b. Asbestos fibers
   c. Crystalline silica dust
   d. Cotton dust
2. **What is the most characteristic pathological feature of asbestosis?**
   a. Caseating granulomas
   b. Fibrosis with asbestos bodies
   c. Necrotizing vasculitis
   d. Non-caseating granulomas
3. **Byssinosis is a lung disease caused by exposure to:**
   a. Coal dust
   b. Cotton dust
   c. Silica dust
   d. Bird droppings
4. **Which occupational lung disease is associated with an increased risk of lung cancer and mesothelioma?**
   a. Silicosis
   b. Asbestosis
   c. Coal worker's pneumoconiosis
   d. Hypersensitivity pneumonitis
5. **Which hypersensitivity pneumonitis is associated with exposure to bird droppings?**
   a. Farmer's lung
   b. Bird fancier's lung
   c. Byssinosis
   d. Bagassosis

Short Answer Questions

1. What defines an occupational lung disease, and how are these diseases broadly classified?
2. Name three common types of pneumoconiosis and their causative agents.
3. What are the pulmonary diseases caused by asbestos exposure?
4. What is hypersensitivity pneumonitis, and what are some common occupational exposures causing it?
5. What are the typical clinical symptoms of occupational lung diseases?
6. What diagnostic tools are used to evaluate occupational lung diseases?

Answer to Critical Thinking Questions

1. (c); 2. (b); 3. (b); 4. (b); 5. (b)

References

1. Ahmad, M. M. (2024). Diffuse Parenchymal lung disease: An update, diagnosis & management. *Bangladesh Journal of Medicine*, 135. https://doi.org/10.3329/bjm.v35i20.73381Ali, H., Khan, E., & Ilahi, I. (2019). Environmental chemistry and ecotoxicology of hazardous heavy metals: Environmental persistence, toxicity, and bioaccumulation. *Journal of Chemistry, 2019*, 1–14. https://doi.org/10.1155/2019/6730305 (accessed on 30th June 2025).
2. Alzheimer's Association. (2023). 2023 Alzheimer's disease facts and figures. *Alzheimer's & Dementia, 19*, 1598–1695. https://doi.org/10.1002/alz.13016 (accessed on 30th June 2025).
3. Aziz, J., Shezali, H., Radzi, Z., Yahya, N. A., Kassim, N. H. A., Czernuszka, J. T., & Rahman, M. T. (2016). Molecular mechanisms of stress-responsive changes in collagen and elastin networks in skin. *Skin Pharmacology and Physiology, 29*, 190–203. https://doi.org/10.1159/000447017 (accessed on 30th June 2025).
4. Basanets, A., & Kurdil, N. (2022). Computed tomography densitometry of the lungs in the algorithm for the diagnosis of interstitial lung diseases, including occupational and ecological diseases. *Ukrainian Pulmonology Journal*. https://www.semanticscholar.org/paper/989009d33ac69ec685b5f6e512e3996000d1088a (accessed on 30th June 2025).
5. Bhakta, N. R., Kaminsky, D. A., Bime, C., Thakur, N., Hall, G. L., McCormack, M. C., & Stanojevic, S. (2021). Addressing race in pulmonary function testing by aligning intent and evidence with practice and perception. *CHEST Journal, 161*, 288–297. https://doi.org/10.1016/j.chest.2021.08.053 (accessed on 30th June 2025).
6. Blyth, K. G., Cherrie, J. W., & McElvenny, D. (2017). Estimating past inhalation exposure to asbestos: A tool for risk attribution and disease screening. https://core.ac.uk/download/111558060.pdf (accessed on 30th June 2025).
7. Bray, F., Ferlay, J., Soerjomataram, I., Siegel, R. L., Torre, L. A., & Jemal, A. (2018). Global cancer statistics 2018: GLOBOCAN estimates of incidence and mortality worldwide for 36 cancers in 185 countries. *CA: A Cancer Journal for Clinicians, 68*, 394–424. https://doi.org/10.3322/caac.21492 (accessed on 30th June 2025).
8. Bray, F., Laversanne, M., Sung, H., Ferlay, J., Siegel, R. L., Soerjomataram, I., & Jemal, A. (2024). Global cancer statistics 2022: GLOBOCAN estimates of incidence and mortality worldwide for 36 cancers in 185 countries. *CA: A Cancer Journal for Clinicians, 74*, 229–263. https://doi.org/10.3322/caac.21834 (accessed on 30th June 2025).
9. Cheng, E. S., Weber, M., Steinberg, J., & Yu, X. Q. (2021). Lung cancer risk in never-smokers: An overview of environmental and genetic factors. *Chinese Journal of Cancer Research, 33*, 548–562. https://doi.org/10.21147/j.issn.1000-9604.2021.05.02 (accessed on 30th June 2025).
10. Dharmage, S. C., Perret, J. L., & Ćustović, A. (2019). Epidemiology of asthma in children and adults. *Frontiers in Pediatrics, 7*. https://doi.org/10.3389/fped.2019.00246 (accessed on 30th June 2025).
11. El-Rahman, A., & Abd El-Hamid, S. M. (2018). Assessment of rehabilitation and smoking cessation strategies in patients with psychiatric disorders: Interventional study. *Journal of Environmental Sciences-China, 43*, 47–59. https://www.semanticscholar.org/paper/c143ce14dce05d6665ff19dacbf42764f27bbb02 (accessed on 30th June 2025).

12. Gardette, V., Sancey, L., Leprince, M., Gaté, L., Cosnier, F., Seidel, C., Valentino, S., et al. (2024). Quantifying titanium exposure in lung tissues: A novel laser-induced breakdown spectroscopy elemental imaging-based analytical framework for biomedical applications. *Small Science, 4*. https://www.semanticscholar.org/paper/e59f2d72a1a066ca928189b4dfd86428694051f9 (accessed on 30th June 2025).

13. Gauci, M., & Vella, N. (1997). Occupational screening. https://core.ac.uk/download/46601749.pdf (accessed on 30th June 2025).

14. Genchi, G., Sinicropi, M. S., Lauria, G., Carocci, A., & Catalano, A. (2020). The effects of cadmium toxicity. *International Journal of Environmental Research and Public Health, 17*, 3782. https://doi.org/10.3390/ijerph17113782 (accessed on 30th June 2025).

15. Haahtela, T., Valovirta, E., Saarinen, K., Jantunen, J., Lindström, I., Kauppi, P., Laatikainen, T., et al. (2021). The Finnish Allergy Program 2008–2018: Society-wide proactive program for change of management to mitigate allergy burden. *Journal of Allergy and Clinical Immunology, 148*, 319–326.e4. https://doi.org/10.1016/j.jaci.2021.03.037 (accessed on 30th June 2025).

16. Handra, C. M., Gurzu, I. L., Chirilă, M., & Ghiţă, I. (2023). Silicosis: New challenges from an old inflammatory and fibrotic disease. *Frontiers in Bioscience-Landmark, 28*, 96–96. https://doi.org/10.31083/j.fbl2805096 (accessed on 30th June 2025).

17. Helsper, C., van Gils, C. V., van Erp, N. F., Siepman van den Berg, M. F. R., Rogouti, O., van Asselt, K. V., Maarsingh, O., et al. (2023). Impact of the COVID-19 outbreak—Delayed referral of colorectal and lung cancer in primary care: A national retrospective cohort study. *Cancers, 15*. https://www.semanticscholar.org/paper/f4f6cd37db56a7143204dcd6e0abf3f470c31ede (accessed on 30th June 2025).

18. Hirsch, A., Goldberg, M., Martin, J. P., & Masse, R. (2024). *Prevention of Respiratory Diseases*. CRC Press eBooks. https://doi.org/10.1201/9781003573869 (accessed on 30th June 2025).

19. Knudsen, T. M., Rezwan, F. I., Jiang, Y., Karmaus, W., Svanes, C., & Holloway, J. W. (2018). Transgenerational and intergenerational epigenetic inheritance in allergic diseases. *Journal of Allergy and Clinical Immunology, 142*, 765–772. https://doi.org/10.1016/j.jaci.2018.07.007 (accessed on 30th June 2025).

20. Krefft, S., Wolff, J., Zell-Baran, L., Strand, M., Gottschall, E., Meehan, R., & Rose, C. (2020). Respiratory diseases in post-9/11 military personnel following Southwest Asia deployment. *Journal of Occupational & Environmental Medicine*. https://www.semanticscholar.org/paper/d99c71caf56277cd4e0bffed8be90e047bc7b18f (accessed on 30th June 2025).

21. Kriebel, D., Tickner, J., Jacobs, M., & Markkanen, P. (2011). Lessons learned: Solutions for workplace safety and health. https://core.ac.uk/download/71352756.pdf (accessed on 30th June 2025).

22. Labaki, W. W., & Han, M. K. (2020). Chronic respiratory diseases: A global view. *The Lancet Respiratory Medicine, 8*, 531–533. https://doi.org/10.1016/s2213-2600(20)30157-0 (accessed on 30th June 2025).

23. Liu, Y., Xu, Y., Li, Y., & Wei, H. (2023). Identifying the environmental determinants of lung cancer: A case study of Henan, China. *GeoHealth, 7*. https://www.semanticscholar.org/paper/fb86733d6c06e16346a195a2c41a68daf32b9785 (accessed on 30th June 2025).

24. Lloyd-Jones, D. M., Allen, N. B., Anderson, C. A. M., Black, T., Brewer, L. C., Foraker, R. E.,

Grandner, M. A., et al. (2022). Life's essential 8: Updating and enhancing the American Heart Association's construct of cardiovascular health: A presidential advisory from the American Heart Association. *Circulation, 146*. https://doi.org/10.1161/cir.0000000000001078 (accessed on 30th June 2025).

25. Mamyrbekova, S. A., Iskakova, G., Faizullina, K., Kuziyeva, G., Abilkaiyr, N., Daniyarova, A., Arynova, G., et al. (2022). The diagnostic accuracy of spirometry versus peak expiratory flow test for follow-up of adult asthma patients at primary care level. *Allergy and Asthma Proceedings, 43*(5), e58–e64. https://www.semanticscholar.org/paper/b1691edbf1eafc99a5cd7d14bd4fc831dd8a87ae (accessed on 30th June 2025).

26. Mkorombindo, T., Balmes, J., Custovic, A., & Dransfield, M. (2022). The air we breathe: Respiratory impact of indoor air quality in chronic obstructive pulmonary disease. *American Journal of Respiratory and Critical Care Medicine, 205*, 378–380. https://www.semanticscholar.org/paper/344e0b72257b7cb74ca4060eefc5fc073c3a657f (accessed on 30th June 2025).

27. Mocek, P. (2023). Mining dust as a health threat to employees of extraction departments of coal mines. *Scientific Papers of Silesian University of Technology. Organization and Management Series*. https://www.semanticscholar.org/paper/bd36e2a9d780e6e2f5d4b88dc6028b0b83077c1b (accessed on 30th June 2025).

28. Moretta, P., Cavallo, N. D., Candia, C., Lanzillo, A., Marcuccio, G., Santangelo, G., Marcuccio, L., et al. (2024). Psychiatric disorders in patients with chronic obstructive pulmonary disease: Clinical significance and treatment strategies. *Journal of Clinical Medicine, 13*. https://www.semanticscholar.org/paper/5b95391ecc29d1dcbf8b2424b80899fb9f63cc5c (accessed on 30th June 2025).

29. Nguyen, N. H. P. (2024). Pneumoconiosis and silicosis: Rising issues in developing countries. *Tạp chí Y học Việt Nam*. https://www.semanticscholar.org/paper/8a03d8910ab340efd05439e1cd709bc824df20cb (accessed on 30th June 2025).

30. Nishida, C., & Yatera, K. (2022). The impact of ambient environmental and occupational pollution on respiratory diseases. *International Journal of Environmental Research and Public Health, 19*. https://www.semanticscholar.org/paper/70072dfb08ee7a0574831007b1bd1e31d4277ab3 (accessed on 30th June 2025).

31. Partida-Zavala, N., Ponce-Gallegos, M. A., Buendía-Roldán, I., & Falfán-Valencia, R. (2018). Type 2 macrophages and Th2 CD4+ cells in interstitial lung diseases (ILDs): An overview. *Sarcoidosis, Vasculitis, and Diffuse Lung Diseases, 35*, 98–108. https://www.semanticscholar.org/paper/ac9f2861a409b4e5d60b033ba6002c641aa50cfc (accessed on 30th June 2025).

32. Siegel, D. A., Jatlaoui, T. C., Koumans, E. H., Kiernan, E., Layer, M., Cates, J., Kimball, A., et al. (2019). Update: Interim guidance for health care providers evaluating and caring for patients with suspected e-cigarette, or vaping, product use associated lung injury–United States, October 2019. *American Journal of Transplantation, 19*, 3420–3428. https://doi.org/10.1111/ajt.15690 (accessed on 30th June 2025).

33. Skinnes, M. N., Moe, R., Johansen, T., Lyby, P. S., Dahl, K., Eid, I., Fagertun, T., et al. (2023). Work ability in the year after rehabilitation—Results from the RehabNytte Cohort. *Journal of Clinical Medicine, 12*. https://www.semanticscholar.org/paper/e4a46c468f12ccc34ced60706ddf2bf550c939ac (accessed on 30th June 2025).

34. Stanojevic, S., Kaminsky, D. A., Miller, M. R., Thompson, B., Aliverti, A., Barjaktarević, I.,

Cooper, B., et al. (2021). ERS/ATS technical standard on interpretive strategies for routine lung function tests. *European Respiratory Journal, 60*, 2101499–2101499. https://doi.org/10.1183/13993003.01499-2021 (accessed on 30th June 2025).

35. Ta, R., Sen, P., Goswami, P., Gupta, L., Halder, I., Reddy, K. R. K., Pajanivel, R., et al. (2022). Sleep, occupational and environmental lung diseases. *Lung India: Official Organ of Indian Chest Society, 39*(S13), S13–S17. https://www.semanticscholar.org/paper/0647d8db5cc1b429c658d237f8ee53ef4dee8ced (accessed on 30th June 2025).

36. Thillai, M., Atkins, C., Crawshaw, A., Hart, S. P., Ho, L. P., Kouranos, V., Patterson, K., et al. (2020). BTS clinical statement on pulmonary sarcoidosis. *Thorax, 76*, 4–20. https://doi.org/10.1136/thoraxjnl-2019-214348 (accessed on 30th June 2025).

37. Vahanian, A., Beyersdorf, F., Praz, F., Milojevic, M., Baldus, S., Bauersachs, J., Capodanno, D., et al. (2021). 2021 ESC/EACTS guidelines for the management of valvular heart disease. *European Heart Journal, 43*, 561–632. https://doi.org/10.1093/eurheartj/ehab395 (accessed on 30th June 2025).

38. Vardoulakis, S., Jalaludin, B., Morgan, G., Hanigan, I., & Johnston, F. H. (2020). Bushfire smoke: Urgent need for a national health protection strategy. *The Medical Journal of Australia, 212*, 349–349. https://doi.org/10.5694/mja2.50511 (accessed on 30th June 2025).

39. Vos, T., Abajobir, A. A., Abate, K. H., Abbafati, C., Abbas, K., Abd-Allah, F., Abdulkader, R. S., et al. (2017). Global, regional, and national incidence, prevalence, and years lived with disability for 328 diseases and injuries for 195 countries, 1990–2016: A systematic analysis for the Global Burden of Disease Study 2016. *The Lancet, 390*, 1211–1259. https://doi.org/10.1016/s0140-6736(17)32154-2 (accessed on 30th June 2025).

40. Walters, G., Mokhlis, J., Moore, V., Burge, G., Robertson, A., & Burge, S. (2018). Profiling of hypersensitivity pneumonitis diagnosed at a UK specialist service for ILD and occupational lung diseases. *Occupational and Environmental Health*. https://www.semanticscholar.org/paper/f1ca552503c07bacf28ecae576aa670682fef765 (accessed on 30th June 2025).

41. Yatera, K., & Nishida, C. (2024). Contemporary concise review 2023: Environmental and occupational lung diseases. *Respirology, 29*, 574–587. https://www.semanticscholar.org/paper/f5cca9ac87fd49827e0ef34820f695ce3fc49589 (accessed on 30th June 2025).

42. Zekhnini, H., Mellouli, F., Salam, M., Bennis, F., & Chegdani, F. (2025). Evaluation of a commercial real-time polymerase chain reaction kit for the detection of *avian orthoavulavirus* type I. *Open Veterinary Journal, 15*, 1440–1445. https://www.semanticscholar.org/paper/02e8949ac79406915727eccd734d50711bed74e7 (accessed on 30th June 2025).

DISORDERS OF PLEURA AND MEDIASTINAL DISEASES

8

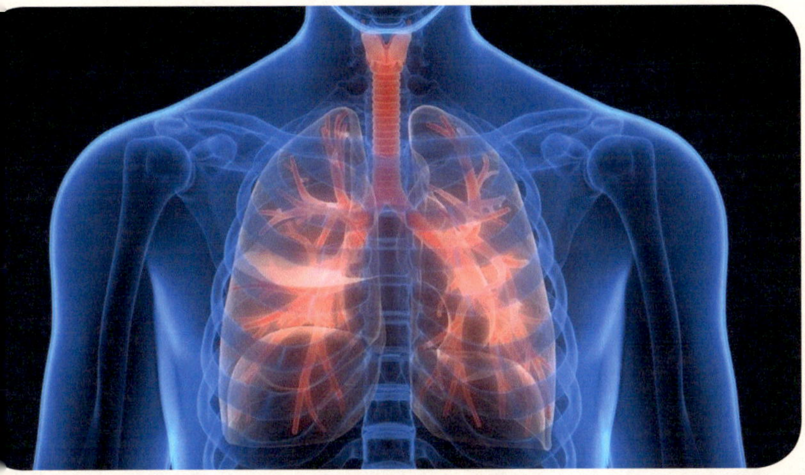

LEARNING OBJECTIVES

After studying this chapter, you will be able to:

1. Explain the anatomy of the pleura
2. List the common pleural disorders
3. Discuss mediastinal anatomy
4. Describe mediastinal diseases
5. Explore the diagnostic approaches
6. Illustrate the treatment options

Introduction

Pleura and mediastinum are significant structures of the respiratory system that play the roles of covering linings and compartments of essential organs. The pleura, consisting of a double layer of serous membrane, envelops the lungs and facilitates pleural fluid dynamics to support respiratory mechanics. Mediastinum, on the other hand, situated between the lungs, houses the significant components such as the heart, great vessels, esophagus, and trachea. These regions' disorders may result in serious morbidity and mortality, and knowledge of the pathophysiology is a necessity. Conditions such as mediastinal tumors, pneumothorax, and pleural effusions demonstrate the complexity of interactions within the thoracic cavity. With the higher incidence of respiratory disease and a better understanding of how systemic illness affects mediastinal and pleural disease, a distinct analysis of these diseases is warranted to inform clinical practice and improve patient outcomes. Comorbidities and effects of infectious disease have profoundly influenced the epidemiology of pleura and mediastinal disease. The COVID-19 pandemic illustrates how a respiratory virus can trigger a sequence of complications in these anatomical regions. There are signs that COVID-19 can lead to pleural effusion, respiratory distress, and even mediastinal lymphadenopathy due to massive inflammation and fluid accumulation in the thorax (Zhou et al., 2020). This has emphasized the importance of clinicians staying vigilant in diagnosing and managing pleural and mediastinal complications amid viral infections. This kind of evidence not only assists in the interpretation of acute presentation but also, even more so, supports the need for an integrated model of respiratory care amid a global health crisis. While therapists continue to enhance knowledge for better therapeutic outcomes, new treatments are being created for disorders of the mediastinum and pleura. For instance, developments in non-small-cell lung cancer (NSCLC) treatments have lessons about how targeted therapies may alter disease patterns in these regions. The addition of pemetrexed and carboplatin chemotherapy to first-line targeted therapies, such as EGFR tyrosine kinase inhibitors, has been found to augment overall survival and progression-free survival in NSCLC patients with specific mutations (Noronha et al., 2019). This guides the personalization of the treatment regimen for each patient based on their characteristics, particularly in complex cases involving pleural or mediastinal involvement. Understanding the evolving landscape in treatment modalities prepares practitioners to offer more ideal care, ultimately to better enhance patient quality of life and outcomes within the context of such challenging disorders (Figure 8.1).

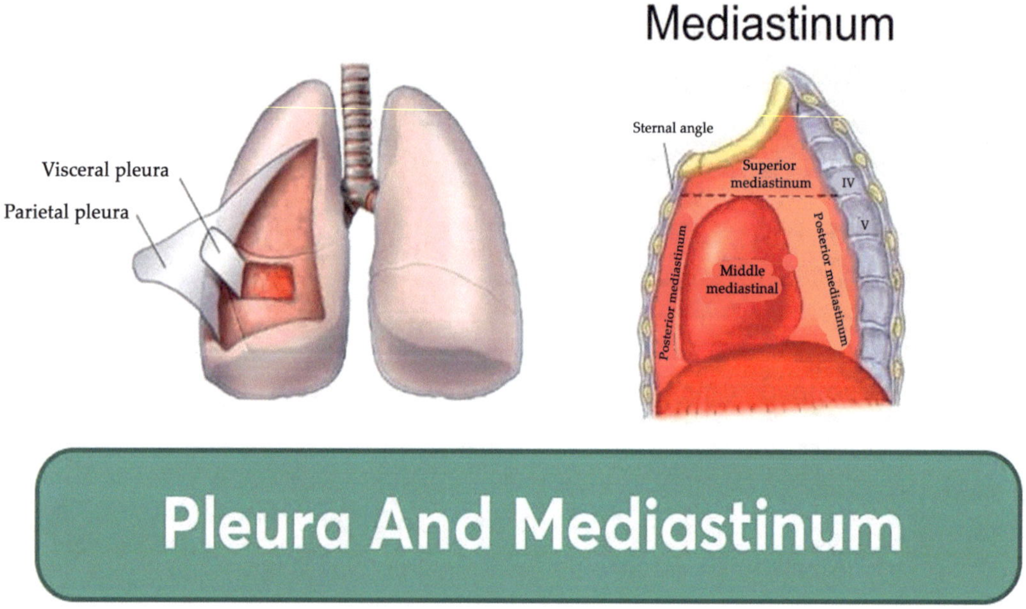

Figure 8.1. Pleura and mediastinum disorder.

Source: https://image.prepladder.com/prepladder/2024/04/26051141/Pleura-And-Mediastinum.webp.

Definition of Pleura and Mediastinum

The mediastinum and pleura are two crucial thoracic cavity anatomical structures, both playing an important role in respiratory and cardiac health. The parietal and visceral pleura are the two membranes that constitute the pleura, respectively lining the thoracic cavity and covering the lungs. This double-layered structure gives a pleural cavity containing serous fluid, which makes the gliding of the lungs during breathing easy while also providing surface tension in case of inflation of the lung. Any disruption to the pleura, such as in diseases like pleurisy or effusion of the pleura, can cause severe respiratory distress, illustrating its protective and functional position in thoracic anatomy. The mediastinum, between the lungs, serves as a corridor for vital structures such as the heart, great blood vessels, trachea, and esophagus. Sectioned into anterior, middle, and posterior divisions with distinct organs and tissue components vital to different body functions. For instance, the anterior mediastinal thymus gland plays a crucial role in developing the immune system. In contrast, the middle mediastinal heart and great vessels are crucial in ensuring proper blood circulation. The mediastinum is also implicated in various pathologies. For instance, mediastinal masses could be secondary to lymphadenopathy, tumors, or other systemic diseases, often indicating the need for extensive evaluation to facilitate successful diagnosis and treatment in a timely fashion. Understanding the pleura's relationship with the mediastinum is crucial to comprehending the disorders of these structures and the surrounding organs. As a clinical routine, extensive evaluation and imaging are conducted to diagnose diseases in these regions. Besides, recommendations such as those by the ESC emphasize the importance of diagnostic accuracy in the management of diseases of the pleura and mediastinum. This ensures that health professionals are in a better position to provide optimal patient care using the current scientific evidence, and thus highlights the importance of these anatomical regions within the grand framework of thoracic disease. Adherence to standard reporting practices, as emphasized by the ICCR within their cancer databases, enhances the capacity for proper diagnosis and treatment of thymic and other mediastinal tumors, eventually resulting in improved patient outcomes within thoracic medicine (Adler et al., 2015; Andrew et al., 2016).

Importance of Studying Pleural and Mediastinal Disorders

Pleural and mediastinal disease diagnosis is clinically significant due to its multifaceted associations with a range of respiratory diseases. The pleura, the two-layered membrane that encloses the lungs, can become inflamed or filled with fluid due to infections, malignancies, or extrapulmonary disease complications. Such alterations can profoundly influence respiratory physiology and lead to clinical manifestations of dyspnea, pain, and impaired exercise tolerance. Furthermore, mediastinal disease, e.g., infection or compressive lesions, may impinge on adjacent structures and thereby cause potential cardiovascular and neurologic morbidity. Thorough analysis and awareness of these illnesses enable clinicians to develop appropriate diagnostic and therapeutic plans, ultimately achieving improved outcomes for patients in numerous clinical situations. Reports also highlight the central role of pleural and mediastinal disease in life-threatening diseases, e.g., COVID-19. Autopsy results have shown that severe respiratory complications typically occur from pathologic alterations in the pleura and lung parenchyma during disease evolution. For example, the presence of diffuse alveolar damage and thrombosis can clarify the pathogenesis of acute respiratory distress syndrome (ARDS) in patients suffering. Pathophysiology of these complications needs to be understood for treating them with targeted therapies and optimizing management protocols. As global health patterns evolve, continued research on pleural and mediastinal diseases will provide insights into treating not only emerging infectious diseases but also chronic respiratory diseases, thereby enhancing public health overall. Additionally, advances in the therapy of thoracic cancers serve to illustrate the need to study pleural and mediastinal disease. As more advanced treatments for cancer, such as the treatment of non-small-cell lung cancer with targeted therapy, are developed, a working understanding of the interaction between the disease and the pleura is necessary. The combination of therapies, such as chemotherapy and tyrosine kinase inhibitors, can increase the patient's survival, but at the same time poses a risk of pleural effusion or other treatment- and disease-related complications. Thus, a clear understanding of pleural and mediastinal diseases enables medical professionals to anticipate and prevent these risks, ensuring that patients receive the optimum treatment. Such an interdisciplinary process not only enhances the quality of treatment but also brings in a better realization of the interdependent nature of several thoracic diseases (Figure 8.2).

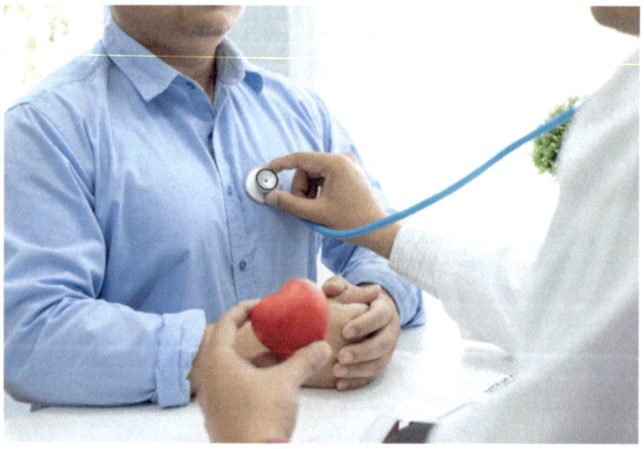

Figure 8.2. Mediastinal disease and its impact on pulmonary health.

Source: https://schmetterermd.com/wp-content/uploads/2023/11/4-1024x680.png.

Overview of Common Diseases Affecting These Areas

The mediastinum and the pleura are significant areas of the thoracic cavity that may be involved in an array of diseases and consequently manifest with a wide range of clinical symptoms. The most frequent conditions involving the pleura include pleuritis, pleural effusion, and pleural empyema, which is a result of an inflammatory response of the pleural space. Pleuritis, or inflammation of the pleura, usually manifests as stabbing chest pain that worsens with coughing or deep breathing. Pleural effusion is the accumulation of too much pleural fluid, which may be due to heart failure, pneumonia, or cancer. Pleural empyema, a more serious condition, arises when the pleural space becomes infected, typically by pneumonia, and requires drainage and antibiotics for effective control. It is essential to diagnose these frequent pleural disorders early in clinical settings. The mediastinum, the central compartment of the thoracic cavity, is also a site for various pathological conditions, among which are mediastinal tumors, both benign and malignant. Benign tumors in the region are usually of thymic tissue origin and may include thymic cysts and hyperplasia, which is an overgrowth due to inflammatory or autoimmune responses. Other nonmalignant masses can include mature teratomas or parathyroid glands and usually have a good prognosis if they are diagnosed early. However, malignant tumors such as lymphomas and primary mediastinal germ cell tumors can be special problems since they can spread and invade surrounding tissues. Identification of these tumors and their discrimination by imaging modalities relies on a solid understanding of the anatomical mediastinal divisions, which can offer vital information toward effective treatment approaches, as emphasized in recent publications (Gerber et al., 2023). The occurrence of high-attenuation pulmonary abnormalities is yet another critical problem in mediastinal disease evaluation. These abnormalities are commonly encountered on CT scanning and are signs of several underlying conditions, both benign as well as malignant. For instance, infectious granulomatous diseases like tuberculosis or sarcoidosis can have high-attenuation areas that mandate full workup. The diagnostic challenge that accompanies such abnormalities underscores the importance of a structured assessment, which involves screening for associated lesions and determining their morphological characteristics as established by existing research (Fukuda et al., 2023). This allows medical professionals to effectively differentiate between various conditions and administer appropriate therapeutic interventions. Hence, understanding these common diseases affecting the pleura and mediastinal regions is crucial for optimal clinical management.

8.1. Anatomy of the Pleura

Learning Outcome

1. Structure and function of the pleura
2. Types of pleura: visceral and parietal
3. Role of pleura in respiratory mechanics

The pleura is a critical component of the thoracic cavity that consists of two components: the visceral pleura, which covers the lung's surface in a close fit, and the parietal pleura, which covers the thoracic wall and the diaphragm. The serous membrane serves several important functions: it facilitates smooth respiration, aids in the movement of the lungs, and has an elastic recoil mechanism. The space between these layers is filled with a thin layer of pleural fluid that allows frictionless movement and also facilitates proper intrapleural pressure, upon which maximum expansion and contraction of the lungs depend. Abnormalities in this anatomical structure may result in pleural disorders like pleuritis and pleural effusion, which can significantly hinder respiratory and overall pulmonary efficiency. Several pathological abnormalities may result from changes in pleural anatomy, highlighting the importance of understanding these structures for diagnosing and treating pleural disease. Among the several potential complications, malignant pleural neoplasias can vary in their morphology and present as mesothelial, mesenchymal, or lymphoproliferative tumors. Malignant mesothelioma is the best-known of these tumors. However, other less common neoplasms may also be misdiagnosed due to a variety of reasons, including their closely related histological features. These neoplasms are diagnosed using a comprehensive clinical approach that incorporates imaging, pathology, and patient history to achieve accurate diagnosis and treatment, as highlighted by studies describing the clinical and pathological characteristics of these tumors (Maria et al., 2015). Apart from neoplastic disorders, the intrinsic anatomical associations of the pleura with mediastinal structures can lead to a disorder known as air leak syndrome (ALS). ALS involves a syndrome characterized by clinical manifestations such as pneumothorax, pneumomediastinum, and subcutaneous emphysema due to disruption in the thoracic cavity.

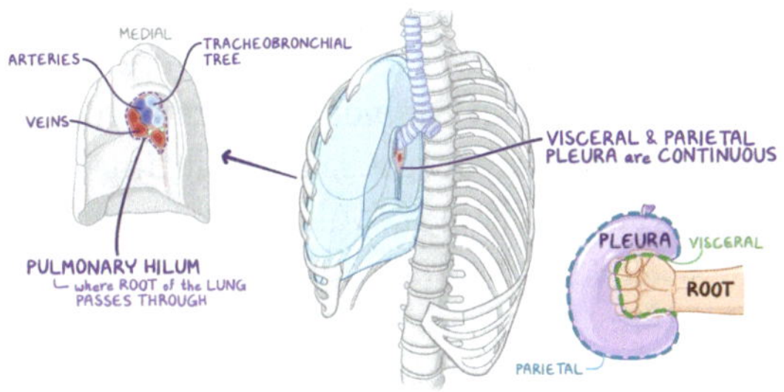

Figure 8.3. Anatomy of the pleura.

Source: https://www.osmosis.org/_next/image?url=https%3A%2F%2Fd16qt3wv6xm098.cloudfront.net%2FEEGu0wD_R4OP5mlNYHxBcYpKSN6_R1yr%2F_.jpg&w=3840&q=75.

The pathogenesis mechanism of ALS is based directly upon the unique anatomical characteristics of the mediastinum, which allow air leakage from the pulmonary cavity into adjacent spaces. The awareness of causative ALS factors, such as iatrogenic or secondary trauma, is necessary for effective management of the disease. Physicians need to be keen enough to identify these symptoms, bearing in mind that ALS can happen spontaneously or as a result of an underlying condition (Cuvertoret-Sanz et al., 2024) (Figure 8.3).

8.1.1. Structure and Function of the Pleura

The pleura is a significant anatomical structure enveloping the lungs. It is comprised of two membranes: the visceral pleura, which closely molds the lung surface, and the parietal pleura, which covers the thoracic cavity. The double-layered pleura serves a variety of functions critical to respiratory mechanics. The pleural membranes, primarily, secrete pleural fluid, which facilitates free movement of the lungs during inhalation and exhalation, reducing the friction between the lung surface and thoracic wall. Moreover, the negative pressure created in the pleural cavity helps to expand the lungs, which facilitates proper gas exchange. Interestingly, the pleura is not only a barrier to infection but also an enabler of the redistribution of inflammatory processes, highlighting its role in both ventilatory and pulmonary health and homeostasis functions. Pleural pathology can substantially compromise respiratory function, with attendant varied clinical presentations. For instance, pleural effusions, which are an excess of pleural fluid, can result from numerous etiologies including heart failure, infection, or malignancy. Accumulation of fluid can compress the lung and cause decreased lung volumes and impaired gas exchange, thus causing dyspnea and chest pain. The same applies to pleuritis, or inflammation of the pleura, which is usually described with stabbing, costal pain on breathing and pleuritic rub sounds on auscultation. The above diseases are typical manifestations of structural pleural changes, which are reflected as functional impairments, thus demonstrating the direct relationship between the pleura's anatomical integrity and its physiological functions. Equally important is knowledge of the pleura's structure and its functional significance, particularly in relation to mediastinal diseases. Mediastinal illness, be it a tumor or lymphadenopathy, can compress the pleura and impact pleural dynamics as well as lead to secondary pleural disease. Malignancies, for example, can produce pleural effusion secondary to inflammatory mediators or obstructive mechanisms and can result in significant morbidity. The presence of such illnesses as gout and its capability to produce unusual localizations of disease has also been reported to involve the pleura. In a fascinating report, monosodium urate crystal deposition was found in the pleural effusion of a gout patient, demonstrating the connection between metabolic illness and pleural disease (Kuzmina et al., 2023). Such a case speaks to the significance of holistic analysis of pleural structure and function in diagnosis-making and the treatment of pleural and mediastinal disease, reinforcing the pleura's fundamental involvement in respiratory health (Figure 8.4).

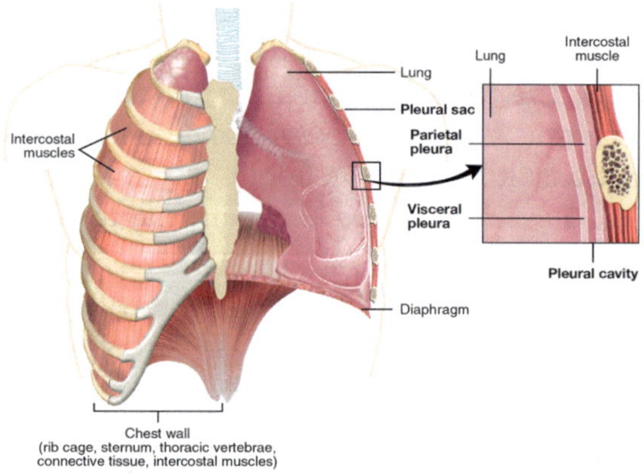

Figure 8.4. Structure and function of the pleura.

Source: https://upload.wikimedia.org/wikipedia/commons/0/0d/2313_The_Lung_Pleurea.jpg.

8.1.2. Types of Pleura: Visceral and Parietal

The human pleura is made up of two separate

layers: the visceral and parietal pleura, both having essential functions in respiratory physiology and disease pathology. The visceral pleura covers the lungs, resting directly on their surface and facilitating respiration by providing gas exchange. This layer is crucial not only for preserving lung structural integrity but also as an infection barrier that does not readily filter through the lung tissue. Pleural fluid between the two pleura acts as a lubricant, allowing the lungs to enter and leave the thoracic cavity with ease. The characteristics and functions of the visceral pleura must be understood, especially when assessing diseases such as malignant mesothelioma and other neoplastic pleural tumors, where alterations in this membrane can significantly affect breathing function and clinical outcomes (Maria et al., 2015). It is in contrast to the parietal pleura, which lines the thoracic cavity and is attached to the mediastinum, diaphragm, and chest wall. It is denser and more fibrous, providing protective support and housing sensory nerves that may be the source of pain in pleural disorders. The parietal pleura plays a vital role in the respiratory mechanics in general, since its movement is vital in forming the negative pressure needed for lung inflation. Diseases like pleuritis can result in inflammation of this layer, which may cause stinging pain in the chest and restrict respiratory ability. Additionally, since the parietal pleura comes into contact with several mediastinal disorders, one should have knowledge of its possible pathological reactions like pleural effusion. The pathophysiology of pleural effusions emphasizes the necessity of distinguishing between various etiologies, with the parietal pleura typically serving as a site of effusion accumulation in conditions like malignancy and tuberculosis (Baburaj et al., 2006). The relationship between the visceral and parietal pleura is significant in the diagnosis and management of various pleural and mediastinal disease conditions. Conditions affecting these layers can lead to significant clinical presentations, such as pleural effusion, caused by various factors, including infections, malignancy, and cardiac illness. The severity of pleural disease could influence therapeutic intervention, including the need for procedures like thoracentesis or pleural biopsy to determine the etiology of effusions. Precise identification of whether an effusion is visceral or parietal pleura, and what type, can direct appropriate interventions and improve patient outcomes. As more is learned about the subtleties of pleural disease, precise knowledge of the kinds of pleura will remain essential to helping develop pulmonology and oncology practice (Baburaj et al., 2006; Maria et al., 2015) (Figure 8.5).

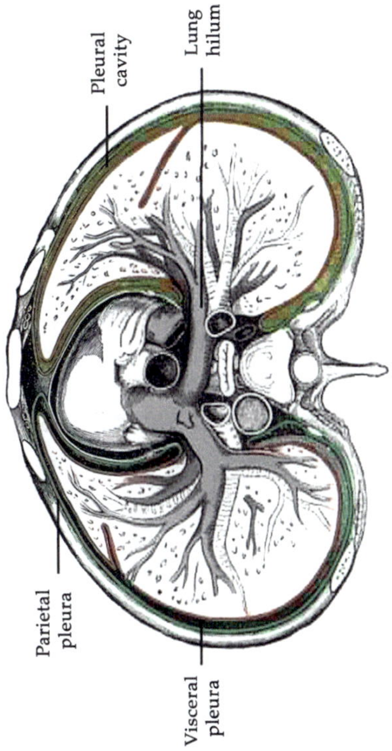

Figure 8.5. Types of pleura: visceral and parietal.

Source: https://teachmeanatomy.info/wp-content/uploads/The-Parietal-and-Visceral-Pleura-and-Pleural-Cavity.jpg.

8.1.3. Role of Pleura in Respiratory Mechanics

The pleura, a double membrane surrounding

the lungs, also plays a vital role in respiratory mechanics by facilitating effortless expansion and contraction of the lungs with every inhalation and exhalation. The visceral pleura adheres to the lung's surface, while the parietal pleura lines the thoracic cavity. This anatomical configuration creates a pleural cavity filled with pleural fluid, which reduces friction when the lungs expand and contract. The pressure gradient between the intrapleural space and the surrounding air is crucial for lung inflation; negative intrapleural pressure aids in drawing air into the lungs. Diseases that arise in the pleura, such as pleuritis or pleural effusion, may disrupt this delicate balance, leading to decreased lung volumes and compromised gas exchange. This ultimately impairs respiration and can result in conditions such as pneumonia or atelectasis, where segments of the lung collapse. The pleura also has a critical role in the mechanical functions of breathing by its influence on lung compliance and airway resistance. Pleura creates a coupling mechanism between the lung and the chest wall for force transmission generated during respiration. With expansion of the chest wall, negative intrapleural pressure enables the lung to expand, causing a rise in tidal volumes. Trauma or diseases like pneumothorax or hemothorax introduce air or blood into the pleural cavity, thereby creating the shifts in equilibrium, hindering lung expansion. The inability to create adequate negative pressure affects inspiratory capacity and necessitates immediate medical intervention to restore pleural integrity and return the respiratory device to normal mechanical operation. Otherwise, additional issues may develop, exemplifying the pleura's role in promoting respiratory health (Petrola et al., 2022). In addition to its mechanical purposes, the pleura is also vitally involved in mediastinal diseases, where pathological processes are responsible for compression of surrounding tissues and affecting overall respiration. Pleural tumors or significant pleural effusions can cause mediastinal shift, altering the position of the airway and prejudicing lung function. Because the volume within the pleura is limited, excess fluid or tumor bulk will compress lung tissue, reduce effective lung capacity, and produce dyspnea or pain in the chest. Successful diagnosis and management of the conditions depend on a thorough knowledge of pleural anatomy and pathology. The consequences of pleural dysfunction reflect the critical importance of early recognition of pleural-related conditions, focusing on the integrated function of global lung and respiratory mechanics within the context of pleura and mediastinal diseases (N/A, 2021) (Figure 8.6).

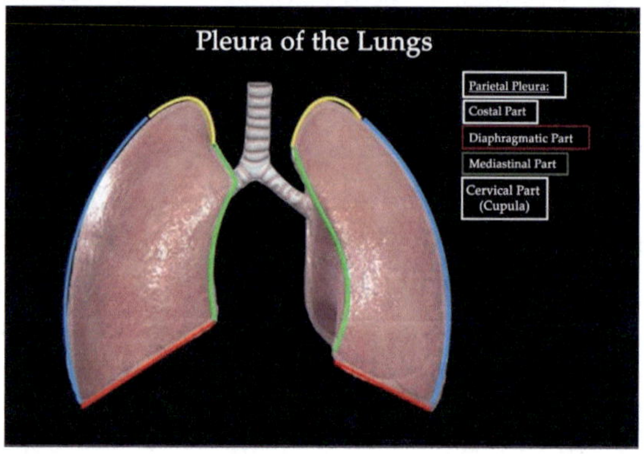

Figure 8.6. Role of pleura in respiratory mechanics.

Source: https://i.ytimg.com/vi/7va5QtWKLFk/hq720.jpg?sqp=-oaymwEhCK4FEIIDSFryq4qpAxMIARUAAAAAGAElAADIQj0AgKJD&rs=AOn4CLD945M9WYFAntaNfv6dlaRIPFxTEA.

Test Your Knowledge

1. What are the types of pleura?
2. What is the role of the pleura in respiratory mechanics?

8.2. Common Pleural Disorders

Learning Outcome

1. Pleural effusion: causes and symptoms
2. Pneumothorax: types and treatment options
3. Pleural fibrosis: implications and management

The pleura, a serous covering surrounding the lungs, participates in respiratory mechanics, and its pathology has significant implications in pulmonary function. Pleural effusion, a most common pleural pathology, is the condition of excess fluid within the pleural space. It may result from a variety of causes, including cardiac failure, infections, malignancies, and inflammation. In particular, congestive heart failure (CHF) is a recognized cause of pleural effusions, where fluid overload due to ineffective cardiac function leads to extravasation of fluid into the pleural spaces. As documented in studies, patients suffering from CHF are commonly observed to demonstrate adventitious signs, including jugular engorgement and pleural effusion, indicating a significant correlation between cardiac status and pleural disease. Comprehensive clinical evaluation and imaging studies, like ultrasonography, enable the detection of such underlying causes and thus proper treatment. Pneumothorax, another significant rib pleura condition, is the introduction of air into the interpleural space, leading to lung collapse. Spontaneous or traumatic, it is often seen in younger, thin males. The initial presentation may be acute dyspnea and chest pain, which need to be diagnosed and managed immediately to prevent respiratory distress. Treatment varies from observation alone if the condition is mild to interventions like chest tube insertion, depending upon the severity. An interesting overlap of systemic disease and pleural conditions is exemplified by Kikuchi-Fujimoto disease, a benign lymphohistiocytic condition associated with bilateral pleural effusions and mediastinal lymphadenopathies. This underlines the necessity of considering a broad differential diagnosis when evaluating patients with pleural disease, as systemic disease may manifest as a pleural abnormality. The impact of pleural disease extends beyond direct respiratory symptoms and may predate underlying systemic diseases. Pleuritis, inflammation of the pleura, can be secondary to infection, autoimmune disorders, or cancer. In extreme cases, pleuritis may lead to serious complications such as pleural fibrosis or trapped lung, which may cause restriction in lung expansion and exacerbate respiratory status. The association between pleural pathology and malignancy is of concern in the sense that pleural effusions may sometimes be the presenting feature of a primary or metastatic tumor. This organization highlights the importance of placing a high index of suspicion for cancer in patients presenting with new-onset pleural effusions. Successful therapy of such pleural diseases usually requires a multidisciplinary strategy, integrating clinical assessment, imaging studies, and potential invasive procedures to optimize patient outcomes (Figure 8.7).

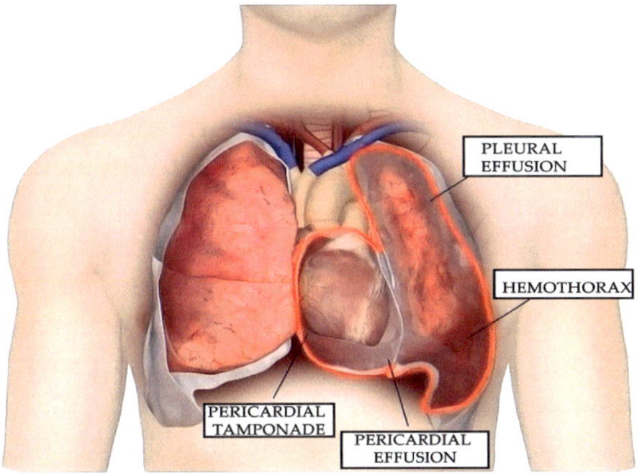

Figure 8.7. Common pleural disorders.

Source: https://cdn.storymd.com/optimized/OoY1l4fMoG/original.jpg.

8.2.1. Pleural Effusion: Causes and Symptoms

Pleural effusion refers to the buildup of fluid in the pleural space that can occur secondary to several underlying etiologies. Pleural effusion etiology is typically characterized as either transudative or exudative. Transudative effusions normally result from systemic diseases like CHF or cirrhosis, where fluid leaks into the pleural space secondary to elevated hydrostatic pressures or low oncotic pressures. Alternatively, exudative effusions are due to local processes, such as infections, malignancies, or inflammatory conditions, leading to increased vascular permeability. This is important in deciding on appropriate clinical management since management options vary significantly between the two. For instance, while diuretics may be of value in the treatment of transudative effusions due to heart failure, exudative effusions often need treatment of the underlying disease causing the accumulation of fluid. Pleural effusion symptoms can be diverse, usually being nonspecific or minor in character. Dyspnea or shortness of breath is a potential presentation that develops due to the limited lung expansion because of fluid accumulation. This can be supplemented by concomitant medical illnesses such as pneumonia or neoplasms that similarly produce pleural effusion. Patients can also present with dry cough or pleuritic chest pain, the latter of which is particularly accentuated on inhalation or cough. With gross accumulation, dullness to percussion or decreased breath sounds can be found on the affected side on exam. Diagnostic tests, such as thoracentesis, not only improve symptoms but also provide valuable information about the nature of the effusion, as seen in one case of multiple myeloma where pleural fluid examination confirmed malignancy-associated effusion (لدری‌ش et al., 1386). Presentation and meaning in some populations, such as those with CKD, may be especially challenging. In CKD patients, pleural effusion typically indicates complicating renal function-related aggravating complications such as infection or fluid overload to complicate the clinical picture. From research, it is clear that the incidence of exudative effusions is profoundly elevated among this population, mainly due to opportunistic infections such as tuberculosis, which remains an endemic problem in most regions (Muralitharan et al., 2017). The immunocompromise underlying CKD can potentially lead to practitioner challenges in differentiating the causes of pleural effusion, indicating the need for sophisticated diagnostic methods. Practitioners, therefore, have to exercise vigilance in assessing patients with CKD for potential pleural effusion in order to perform early interventions for the effusion as well as its etiologic causes (Figure 8.8).

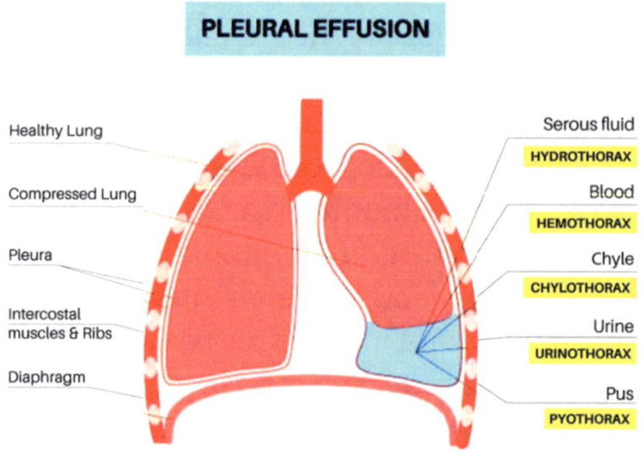

Figure 8.8. Pleural effusion.

Source: https://www.carehospitals.com/ckfinder/userfiles/images/pleural_effusion.webp.

8.2.2. Pneumothorax: Types and Treatment Options

The differentiation of pneumothorax is critical to determining its importance and consequent treatment plans. Pneumothorax is initially broadly classified into spontaneous and traumatic types. Spontaneous pneumothorax, one occurring without any external trauma, is further subdivided into primary and secondary pneumothorax. Primary spontaneous pneumothorax in young, tall men without a pre-existing lung disease may result from the rupture of tiny blebs on the lung surface. Secondary spontaneous pneumothorax is seen in patients with established pulmonary disease, like COPD or cystic fibrosis. Traumatic pneumothorax occurs after penetrating or blunt thoracic trauma and usually needs exceptional management based on the location and severity of trauma. An understanding of these distinctions is crucial for practitioners, as they determine subsequent management options and influence outcomes in pleural and mediastinal disease patients. Treatment of pneumothorax varies broadly based on the size and severity of the condition. Small, asymptomatic spontaneous pneumothoraxes may be treated conservatively by physicians with observation and follow-up imaging to ensure resolution. However, larger pneumothoraces or those accompanied by severe respiratory distress require more invasive procedures. These procedures include needle decompression for immediate relief of pressure, followed by the insertion of a chest tube for continued drainage of air from the pleural space. Operations, such as video-assisted thoracoscopic surgery (VATS), may be warranted in the case of recurrent pneumothorax or the failure of initial management. The management of choice ultimately rests on the clinical condition of the patient, the cause of the pneumothorax, and the presence of any co-morbid lung disease, highlighting the role of individualized therapeutic methods in managing pleural conditions. The newer imaging and therapeutic techniques have made a major contribution to the treatment of pneumothorax. The application of newer imaging modalities, as reported in recent literature, provides physicians with critical diagnostic information on the size and character of the pneumothorax. Developments such as ultrasound and CT scans allow pleural pathology to be accurately visualized, enabling effective planning of interventions (N/A, 2021). Moreover, progress in minimally invasive therapy has revolutionized management, improving outcomes while minimizing complications associated with traditional surgical procedures. The ongoing research into the pathophysiologic mechanisms of pneumothorax is likely to create novel treatment protocols, potentially addressing underlying etiologies and enhancing preventive strategies. As knowledge of pleural diseases advances, clinicians should stay abreast of the most current information to optimize treatment modalities and maximize overall patient care within the scope of mediastinal disease (N/A, 2025) (Figure 8.9).

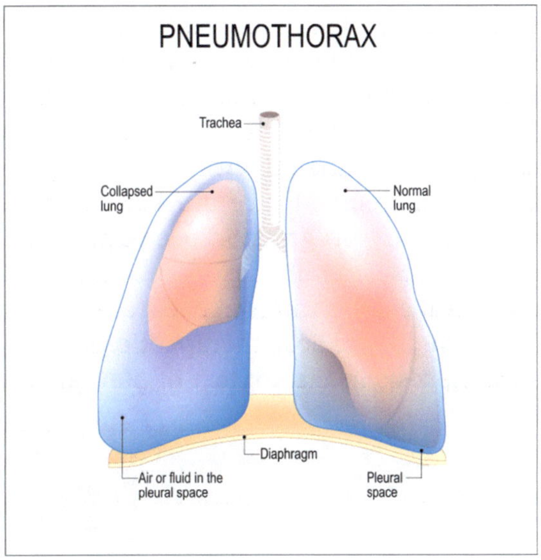

Figure 8.9. Pneumothorax.

Source: https://www.netmeds.com/images/cms/wysiwyg/blog/2019/08/Pneumothorax_Causes_big_898.jpg.

8.2.3. Pleural Fibrosis: Implications and Management

Pleural fibrosis, i.e., scarring and thickening of the pleural tissue, is a complex respiratory medicine condition. Most commonly, it is a chronic inflammatory process due to various etiologies, such as environmental exposures, infections, or systemic diseases that involve the entire body. The inductive and progressive form of pleural fibrosis can lead to compromised lung function as the fibrous tissue prevents the normal pleural expansion during respiration. In this context, effective management is the key to counteract both the underlying causes and symptomatic presentations of the condition. Diagnosis usually involves imaging modalities like chest X-ray or CT scans to establish the extent of fibrosis and associated complications, like pleural effusion or breathlessness, which have the potential to impact a patient's quality of life drastically. Management of pleural fibrosis needs to be addressed in a multidimensional way, the needs of the patient, and the specific causative factors involved. Therapeutic management can include pharmacologic interventions for anti-inflammatory and lung function improvement, complemented by pulmonary rehabilitation programs that seek to enhance respiratory mechanics via physical conditioning. Where the fibrosis is linked with occupational exposure, as noted in current research, correct diagnosis becomes crucial both for treatment and for applying preventive measures to limit further exposure and resulting harm (Calabrese et al., 2024). Multidisciplinary communication among pulmonologists, pathologists, and occupational health workers is central to formulating a comprehensive management plan that considers the complexities of pleural fibrosis and its relation to patient management. In advanced pleural fibrosis, surgery can be scheduled when conservative management is ineffective. Pleurodesis, a procedure that adheres the pleura to the thoracic wall to seal off recurrent pleural effusions, can benefit certain patients, particularly those with malignant pleural disease. Additionally, lung transplantation also is an option in patients with end-stage pulmonary pathology due to extensive fibrosis. Watchful follow-up and surveillance are key components of the treatment regimen, given the probability of the disease's progression over time. Moreover, awareness of the thoracic imaging features of pleural diseases, as discussed in contemporary literature, also adds validity to the application of radiological examinations in decision-making (Ilieva et al., 2022). This multi-disciplinary approach, which includes medical, therapeutic, and surgical therapy, emphasizes the complexity of managing pleural fibrosis in the context of pleural and mediastinal disease disorders (Figure 8.10).

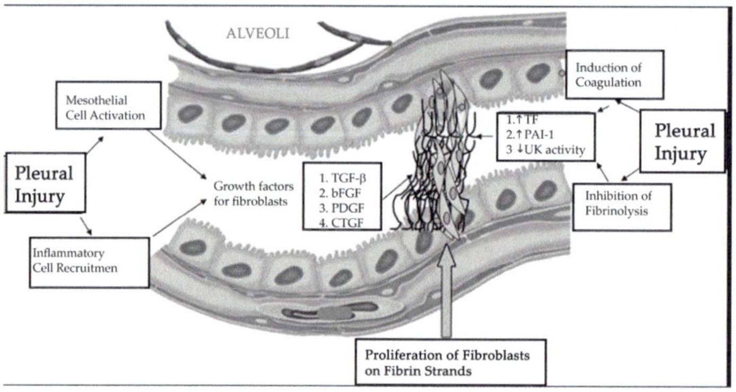

Figure 8.10. Pleural fibrosis.

Source: https://www.chestmed.theclinics.com/cms/10.1016/j.ccm.2005.12.003/asset/41f6fde5-1209-4024-8c21-c0494830f63a/main.assets/gr1.jpg.

Test Your Knowledge

1. What is pleural effusion?
2. What are the types of pneumothorax?

8.3. Mediastinal Anatomy

Learning Outcome

1. Divisions of the mediastinum
2. Key structures within the mediastinum
3. Importance of mediastinal anatomy in disease diagnosis

The mediastinum, an intermediate compartment of the thoracic cavity, is a pivotal area for numerous anatomical structures like the heart, great vessels, trachea, and esophagus. Anatomically, the superior and inferior mediastina split the latter into the anterior, middle, and posterior mediastina. An understanding of the complex arrangement and interactions between these structures is necessary to diagnose mediastinal disease. For instance, mediastinal masses or lymphadenopathy can hide vital anatomical landmarks and complicate assessment and treatment. Thus, clear knowledge of mediastinal anatomy not only allows for the diagnosis of disorders but also results in appropriate interventions and therapeutic regimes, especially in the case of tumors or inflammatory diseases where precise surgical planning or radiologic intervention is needed. The primary function of the mediastinal anatomy is blood supply, particularly concerning pulmonary and bronchial arteries. The pulmonary arteries carry deoxygenated blood from the heart to the lungs, while the bronchial arteries supply systemic blood to the lung tissues. Even if bronchial arteries constitute only 1% of cardiac output, they do directly impact pathological diseases concerning the lungs. Their anatomical variation and potential anomalies, e.g., dilatation of the bronchial artery, are indicators of specific obstructive respiratory conditions or developmental defects. Their recognition enhances the diagnostic knowledge of clinicians, particularly in evaluating diseases like chronic thromboembolic disease or infections that alter normal bronchial circulation pathways (Christopher et al., 2015). Thus, knowledge of mediastinal vascular anatomy is essential for the diagnosis and management of thoracic disease. For proper diagnosis of mediastinal disorders, sophisticated imaging plays an increasingly significant role in careful anatomical examination and pathology detection.

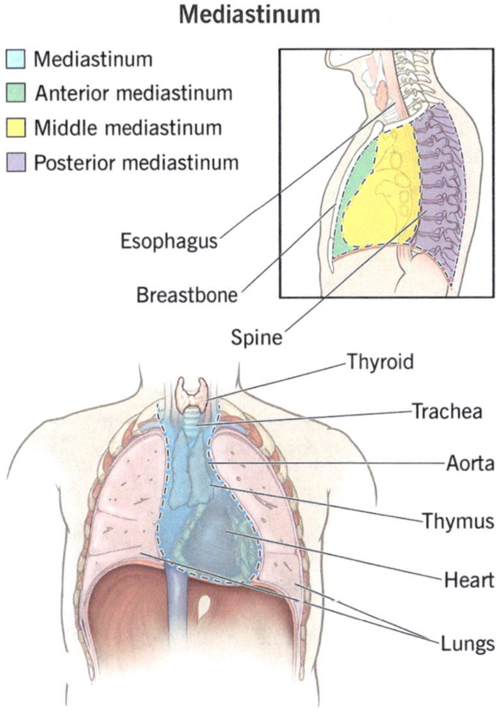

Figure 8.11. Mediastinal anatomy.

Source: https://my.clevelandclinic.org/-/scassets/images/org/health/articles/13792-mediastinal-tumors.

Blending imaging modalities such as multidetector computed tomography and ventilation/perfusion single photon emission computed tomography (V/PSPECT) enhances the structural evaluation of the mediastinum, along with related vascular anatomy. V/PSPECT, in particular, has been demonstrated to be highly sensitive and specific for detection of pulmonary embolism even in patients with intrinsic lung diseases such as COPD or heart failure, showing its potential in mediastinal disease diagnosis (Bajc et al., 2019). Furthermore, these imaging technologies allow accurate visualization of mediastinal masses and differential diagnosis between neoplastic and infectious etiologies. Therefore, engagement between mediastinal anatomy and newer imaging modalities is at the forefront to enhance diagnostic accuracy, ultimately improving patient care in patients suffering from pleural and mediastinal disease (Figure 8.11).

8.3.1. Divisions of the Mediastinum

The mediastinum is a critical compartment of the thoracic cavity, functioning to separate the contents of the thorax into individual anatomical spaces. It is crucial in both clinical evaluation and intervention, as it provides a means for diagnosing various mediastinal disorders, particularly those revealed by imaging modalities. With advancing medical imaging tools, particularly through the deployment of multidetector computed tomography (CT), a more precise division of mediastinal compartments has been created.

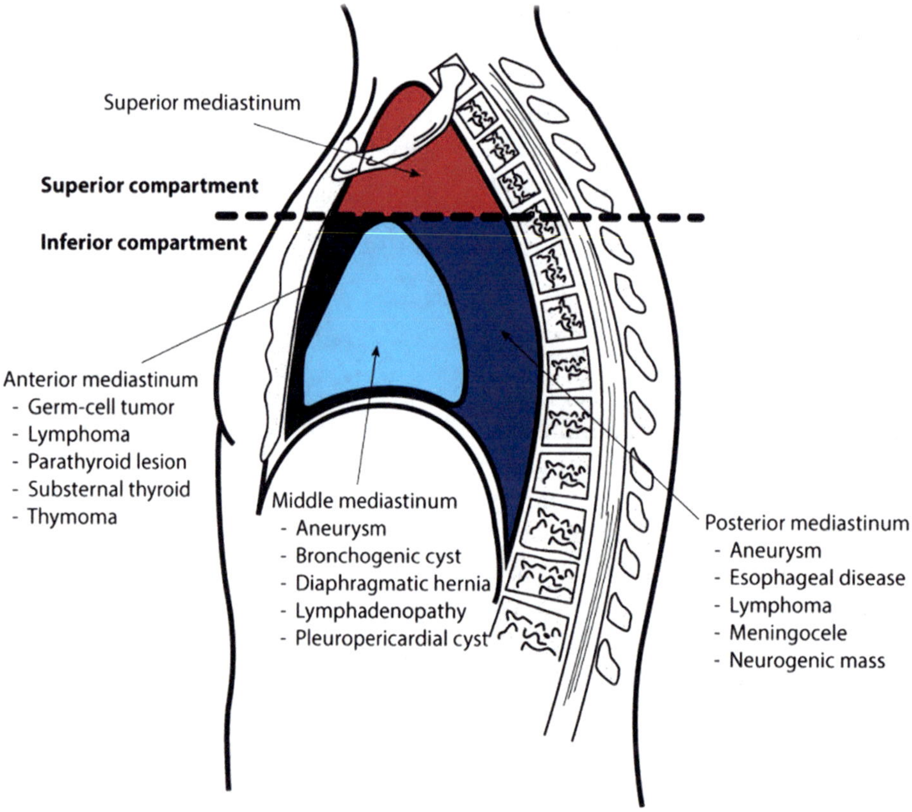

Figure 8.12. Divisions of the mediastinum.

Source: https://www.ncbi.nlm.nih.gov/books/NBK539819/bin/Mediastinum_Compartments.jpg.

The International Thymic Malignancy Interest Group (ITMIG) advocated for a new standard demarcating the mediastinum into prevascular, visceral, and paravertebral compartments, offering greater clarity for clinicians treating mediastinal illnesses. This division not only facilitates effective communication among multidisciplinary teams but also streamlines the process of diagnosis, allowing clinicians to formulate specific differential diagnoses based on the location of anomalies revealed during patient imaging studies (Brett et al., 2017). The role of these divisions even exceeds the management of specific diseases, including benign and malignant tumors that could occur within the mediastinal spaces. Tumors in this region may range from primary lesions, such as thymomas and lymphomas, to secondary metastatic deposits, specifically those related to ectopic disorders or other malignant processes. Ectopic thyroid tissue is particularly rare, as it may occur due to developmental anomalies during thyroid gland migration. The ectopic thyroid may complicate diagnosis, and it must be differentiated from metastatic masses of the orthotopic gland (Noussios et al., 2011). Therefore, anatomical mediastinal divisions are essential for proper diagnostic imaging and further treatment planning. At an anatomical level, this information helps in the correct localization of pathology, which may assist in planning surgery and therapy. In clinical practice, structural mediastinal organization is a framework for assessing and interpreting various mediastinal diseases. By encouraging a systematized methodology of imaging and diagnosis, the mediastinal division assists clinicians in ordering their differential diagnoses. For example, abnormalities in the anterior compartment would more likely point to other pathologies like thymic hyperplasia or germ cell tumors, whereas abnormalities in the posterior compartment are likely to signify neurogenic tumors or paravertebral masses. The evolving medical landscape demands clinicians become adept at identifying nuances in these compartments in a timely and appropriate manner. Therefore, the standardized division of the mediastinum, particularly by means of advanced imaging modalities, facilitates improved patient outcomes in the management of mediastinal disease (Brett et al., 2017) (Figure 8.12).

8.3.2. Key Structures Within the Mediastinum

The mediastinum, a middle space of the thorax, is characterized by its boundaries, which are the sternum anteriorly, the vertebral column posteriorly, and the lungs laterally. It is a necessary anatomical space that holds several vital structures important to systemic and respiratory functions. Among these structures are the heart, major blood vessels, and esophagus, all of which are enveloped by connective tissue that provides them with support and organization. The central location of these principal elements within the mediastinum accentuates the role of this compartment in the maintenance of physiological homeostasis. When disease arises in this region, it has the potential to generate severe clinical symptomatology, again underscoring the necessity of a thorough understanding of mediastinal anatomy to diagnose and manage disease efficiently. The heart and the major vessels of the mediastinum are focal to circulatory function. The pericardium encloses the heart and is an essential in protecting this organ while lubricating it in order to facilitate movement during cardiac cycles. The aorta, pulmonary trunk, and great veins encase the heart and serve as conduits through which oxygenated and deoxygenated blood move through the body. Trachea and main bronchi also extend from the mediastinum, dividing into the lungs, and facilitating air passage. Dysfunctions of the elements in this region—e.g., mediastinal tumors or vascular issues—may gravely impair these functions, leading to respiratory or cardiac problems. The mutual dependence of these anatomical structures highlights the importance of careful examinations when addressing mediastinal diseases and pleural conditions. Significance goes beyond anatomy; there is also an awareness of potential pathologies that are most apt to develop in this region. Disorders such as mediastinitis, malignancies, or tumors may cause obstructive symptoms affecting both the respiratory and cardiovascular systems. Moreover, the location of the lymphatic system within the mediastinum, specifically the lymph nodes, which are traditionally used as primary markers in the staging of thoracic cancers, underscores the role of this anatomical space. The combination of different systems makes the mediastinum a pivotal site for diagnosing thoracic diseases. The intricacies of such interactions are of paramount significance to health professionals, as the ESC Guidelines suggest, emphasizing the importance of good clinical judgment in determining treatment strategies and interventions for mediastinal conditions and pleural disorders (Adler et al., 2015; Members et al., 2014).

8.3.3. Importance of Mediastinal Anatomy in Disease Diagnosis

Knowledge of mediastinal anatomy is essential in accurately diagnosing pleural and mediastinal illness. The mediastinum, that area between the lungs, harbors vital structures such as the heart, trachea, esophagus, and large vessels, and thus can potentially need differentiation on an anatomical basis in different pathologies. Pathology within the compartment can yield diverse clinical presentations. For instance, a pathology of an abnormal mass within the mediastinum may be a sign of lymphoma or other tumors. Clear imaging of the mediastinal structures by imaging modalities like CT scans or MRIs allows the clinicians to establish an accurate diagnosis and subsequently guide treatment strategies, which accentuates the mediastinum's contribution to effective disease management.

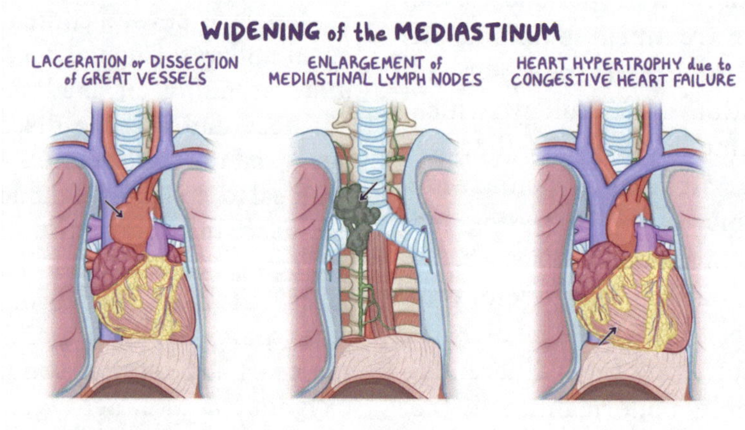

Figure 8.13. Mediastinal anatomy in disease diagnosis.

Source: https://www.osmosis.org/_next/image?url=https%3A%2F%2Fd16qt3wv6xm098.cloudfront.net%2Fu7SAJNL0SpOxEy_A2Lh0O3LQ4SZsZ4_%2F_.jpg&w=3840&q=75.

Advanced imaging techniques play a significant role in delineating mediastinal anatomy and its association with pleural diseases. For example, the integration of ventilation/perfusion (V/Q) scanning and volumetric CT imaging enhances the diagnostic sensitivity for conditions such as pulmonary embolism (PE) and heart failure, which can have overlapping clinical signs and symptoms. V/Q scans, when positive with specific patterns, can provide clinicians with information about likely underlying disorders, which then necessitate early interventions. The ability to perform tomographic imaging allows for a more precise understanding of how pleural diseases relate to mediastinal structures, with an emphasis on the interconnectedness of such anatomical regions in disease manifestation and diagnosis (Bajc et al., 2019). Thus, the application of sophisticated imaging modalities is paramount in optimizing diagnostic outcomes in patients with suspected mediastinal pathology. Moreover, the inclusion of ultrasound techniques for evaluating mediastinal and pleural illnesses has redesigned diagnostic approaches to the anatomic area. Previously underutilized, ultrasound provides a non-invasive alternative for analyzing the pleura and surrounding structures and can be applied in real-time imaging for diagnostic and therapeutic procedures. Ultrasound scanning, with its increased resolution, facilitates the visualization of fluid collections, masses, and other disease processes that are not characteristically apparent on usual imaging modalities. It is also significantly useful in the follow-up of chronic diseases, indicating changes of mediastinal anatomy that can be indicative of disease evolution. This use highlights the importance of understanding mediastinal anatomy in optimizing disease diagnosis and management, further confirming the correlation between these two fields of anatomy (Christoph et al., 2015) (Figure 8.13).

Test Your Knowledge

1. What are the divisions of the mediastinum?
2. What are the importance of mediastinal anatomy in disease diagnosis?

8.4. Mediastinal Diseases

Learning Outcome

1. Mediastinal tumors: types and characteristics
2. Mediastinitis: causes and clinical presentation
3. Lymphadenopathy in the mediastinum: diagnostic challenges

Mediastinal disease is a heterogeneous group of conditions of the central compartment of the thoracic cavity, between the lungs. It is a vital location for the housing of important structures such as the heart, great arteries and veins, esophagus, trachea, and lymph nodes, and therefore mediastinal pathology is relevant in clinical practice. Pathological mediastinal conditions can arise due to infection, tumors, autoimmune disorders, or congenital abnormalities. Significantly, the clinical presentation of mediastinal illness could be insidious and nonspecific, making timely diagnosis and treatment challenging. Symptoms often overlap with other thoracic diseases, even leading to confusion among healthcare providers and thus potentially delaying proper management. Therefore, knowledge of the pathogenesis of such diseases is crucial in bridging the gap to devise effective care strategies. Of the more frequent forms of mediastinal disease, anterior mediastinal tumors are noteworthy because of the degree of their malignancy and clinical impact. Thymomas, lymphomas, and germ cell tumors constitute the significant tumors in this group, with varying degrees of malignancy and challenges in diagnosis and treatment. Thymomas, for instance, may be associated with myasthenia gravis and may present in the form of encapsulated masses or invasive tumors. Their identification is generally based on imaging studies such as chest X-rays, CT scans, or magnetic resonance imaging (MRI), which help define their size and location. Furthermore, treatment of these disorders relies on a multidisciplinary approach consisting of surgery, chemotherapy, and radiation therapy, based on the type and stage of the tumor. Precise knowledge of the tumors enables healthcare professionals to optimize patient results through tailored treatment modalities. The importance of early diagnosis of mediastinal disorders cannot be overstressed, especially given their complex presentations. The use of advanced imaging and histopathologic examination is crucial in establishing a conclusive diagnosis, which directly influences therapies and prognoses in turn. Mediastinal lymphadenopathy, for instance, tends to manifest as an imitator of other disorders, and a clinico-workup becomes indispensable in ruling out malignancies. New technologies such as endobronchial ultrasound (EBUS) are increasingly credible in the acquisition of biopsies from mediastinal lymph nodes, enhancing diagnostic yield and facilitating timely intervention. With new research, additional information on the biological behavior of mediastinal diseases, combined with successful therapeutic measures, remains essential. In the final analysis, promotion of early diagnosis and individually tailored management will remain paramount to survival outcomes and quality of life in patients with these complex disorders.

8.4.1. Mediastinal Tumors: Types and Characteristics

Mediastinal tumors represent a heterogeneous group of neoplasms located within the mediastinal cavity, the space between the lungs that houses critical structures such as the heart, great vessels, trachea, and esophagus. Mediastinal tumors can be broadly categorized into three types: anterior, middle, and posterior mediastinal tumors, each with its own specific features and varying clinical implications for diagnosis and treatment. Anterior mediastinal tumors consist mainly of thymomas and germ cell tumors, which are often found with some clinical syndromes, like myasthenia gravis. Middle mediastinal tumors are most likely to consist of lymphadenopathy and bronchogenic cysts, while posterior mediastinal tumors are neurogenic in nature, such as schwannomas or neuroblastomas. Recognizing these divisions guides the appropriate clinical management and patient care algorithms for those suffering from these potentially complex syndromes. Diagnosis of mediastinal tumors typically depends on a combination of imaging studies and histological analysis. Chest X-ray and CT scan are valuable tools for identifying the mass effect of tumors and demarcating their anatomical locations. MRI can also delineate the relationship between the tumors and surrounding structures, an issue of paramount significance in determining the need for surgery. After being identified, biopsy continues to be a part of the diagnostic workup, enabling specific histopathological identification of tumor type and behavior. This data is pivotal not only in determining prognosis but also in designing treatment regimens that can include surgical resection, radiation therapy, or chemotherapeutic drugs, such as the association of pemetrexed and carboplatin, where indicated in certain types of tumors, producing favorable outcomes in local disease advancement (Noronha et al., 2019). The therapeutic approach to mediastinal tumors is evolving, driven by advances in medical therapy and a better understanding of tumor biology. For instance, specific molecular characteristics in tumors, for instance, those carrying epidermal growth factor receptor (EGFR) mutations, can be treated using targeted treatments such as tyrosine kinase inhibitors. The inclusion of such therapies introduces a new level of sophistication in the management of mediastinal tumors, as they can potentially offer superior progression-free and overall survival in certain cohorts, despite an incremental rise in toxicity (Noronha et al., 2019). Additionally, policies sanctioned by health authorities emphasize the imperative of individualized treatment modalities, with interventions tailored based on patient-specific elements and tumor characteristics. This individualized care paradigm is increasingly critical in the management of mediastinal tumors, as physicians balance the complex interaction between disease characteristics and treatment modalities to achieve the best patient outcomes (Figure 8.14).

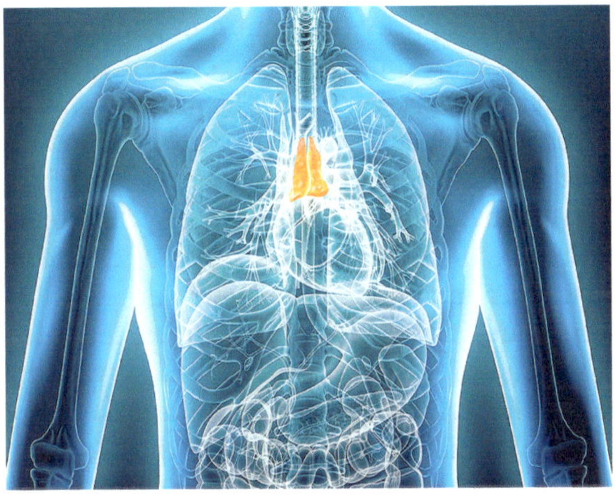

Figure 8.14. Mediastinal tumor.

Source: https://www.saintjohnscancer.org/thoracic/wp-content/uploads/sites/5/2023/06/thymoma-tumor-anterior-mediastinum.jpg.

8.4.2. Mediastinitis: Causes and Clinical Presentation

Mediastinitis is defined as an acute inflammatory process of the mediastinum, typically categorized as acute or chronic based on its duration and cause. The cause can be broadly divided into infectious and non-infectious etiology. Most frequently, acute mediastinitis is caused by postoperative complications of cardiac or thoracic surgery, esophageal perforation, or contiguous spread from adjacent infectious sites. Of interest, odontogenic infections and retropharyngeal abscesses are major sources of mediastinitis by direct extension. Immunocompromise or foreign bodies further predispose individuals to the disease and increase their vulnerability, significantly impacting its clinical presentation. While the management of the patient relies on early diagnosis, recognizing these diverse causative factors is a prerequisite for medical practitioners to diagnose the disease and implement proper interventions. The course of mediastinitis can be highly unpredictable, but it will typically present with evidence of systemic infection, such as fever, chills, and malaise. Localized chest pain, dyspnea, and dysphagia can also present, particularly when the process is complicated by esophageal perforation. Physical examination can produce differential signs such as decreased breath sounds or wheezing, depending on the mediastinal structures involved. Imaging diagnosis, primarily CT, is important for making the diagnosis and assessing the severity of the illness. One severe challenge lies in the early detection of acute mediastinitis, as imaging findings can mimic normal postoperative results, interfering with accurate diagnosis and early treatment (Tabotta et al., 2020). Therefore, there is a need for collaborative efforts involving clinical suspicion and high-technology imaging modalities to achieve proper management. Under treatment, early therapy is necessary to prevent fatal complications of mediastinitis. The treatment cornerstones typically involve broad-spectrum intravenous antibiotics, followed by the use of a specific antibiotic regimen based on culture data and sensitivity. Surgical intervention may be necessary, particularly in those caused by esophageal perforation or abscess formation, to permit drainage and debridement. According to current clinical observations, managing the underlying condition or risk factors is also important to prevent recurrences. Of interest is the emphasis on immunoglobulin G4-related disease (IgG4-RD) as a potential etiology of chronic mediastinal disease through fibrosing mediastinitis. Knowledge of association points towards proper evaluation and treatment in patients with chronic symptoms or refractory conditions in conventional management practices (Katz et al., 2021). Knowledge of the vast variety of mediastinitis assists the clinician to deal with complexities associated with diagnosis and therapeutic practice (Figure 8.15).

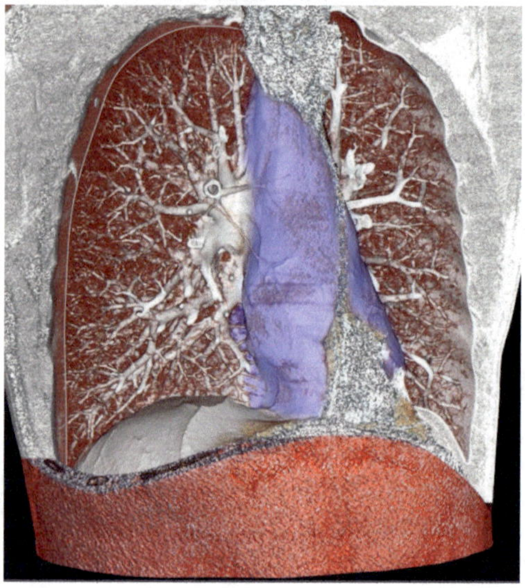

Figure 8.15. Mediastinitis.

Source: https://upload.wikimedia.org/wikipedia/commons/8/82/Mediastinum.jpg.

8.4.3. Lymphadenopathy in the Mediastinum: Diagnostic Challenges

Mediastinal lymphadenopathy is a difficult diagnosis to establish since it encompasses such a broad range of conditions, from infection to malignancy. The mediastinum is an intricate region of anatomy containing vital structures such as the trachea, esophagus, significant vascular elements, and expansile lymphadenopathy. Expansile lymphadenopathy within this region has the potential to generate compressive syndromes, creating a complicated clinical picture. A thorough understanding of the potential etiologies and their clinical features is essential to a proper diagnosis. Diagnostic testing in the form of imaging studies, such as CT or positron emission tomography (PET), is generally employed; yet sensitivity and specificity are not always assured. Consequently, clinicians can become frustrated when trying to differentiate between benign and malignant mediastinal lymphadenopathy, often delaying optimal treatment and impacting patient outcomes. In the management of the diagnostic challenge of mediastinal lymphadenopathy, it is critical to be aware of rare but life-threatening disorders such as POEMS syndrome, which characterizes the issue in clinical practice. This rare multisystem disease has the association of polyneuropathy and monoclonal plasma cell dyscrasia and typically presents with a masquerading presentation. The presentation of a 61-year-old male patient with lymphadenopathy as an indication necessitates extensive testing to avoid overlooking underlying pathologies, for instance, malignancy or systemic disease. Diagnostic imaging tests, alongside extensive clinical evaluation, are needed to make the diagnosis. Here, determining high vascular endothelial growth factor (VEGF) levels or other laboratory markers becomes critical for such conditions, illustrating the significant interaction between clinical symptoms and the subclinical biochemical processes that regulate diagnosis and management plans (Kumar et al., 2025). Lymphadenopathy in the mediastinum may also occur alongside infectious causes, again making it difficult to diagnose. A disease such as tuberculosis or bronchial anthracofibrosis could share radiological appearances and presentations, making meticulous distinction for non-missing a prerequisite. An example is the association of bronchial anthracofibrosis with anthracotic pigments together with respiratory signs, which emphasizes the need for high-tech imaging diagnostic procedures and bronchoscopy to establish the etiological cause correctly. With the dynamic pattern of mediastinal diseases, the inclusion of state-of-the-art diagnostic techniques becomes a necessity. Better imaging techniques, combined with judicious clinical assessment, play a crucial role in distinguishing benign from malignant processes, thus enabling timely and appropriate interventions for affected patients (Louis et al., 2024) (Figure 8.16).

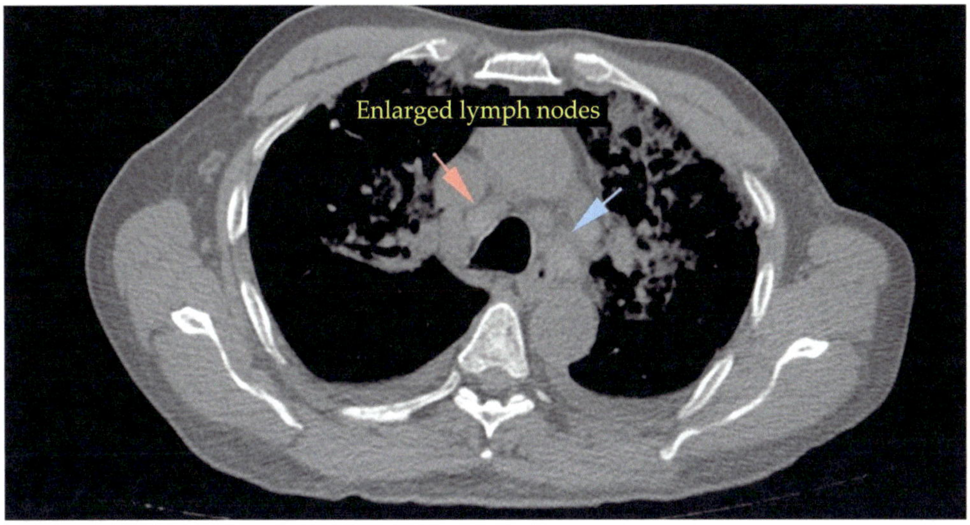

Figure 8.16. Lymphadenopathy in the mediastinum.

Source: https://external-content.duckduckgo.com/iu/?u=https%3A%2F%2Fwww.medrxiv.org%2Fcontent%2Fmedrxiv%2Fearly%2F2022%2F03%2F14%2F2022.03.10.22272193%2FF2.large.jpg%3Fdownload%3Dtrue&f=1&nofb=1&ipt=0a973e46e4574d500507fa023ae114c3942c1fed9298511da1d678d0e2c1ed40.

Test Your Knowledge

1. What are the types of mediastinal tumors?
2. What are the causes of mediastinitis?

8.5. Diagnostic Approaches

Learning Outcome

1. Imaging techniques: X-ray, CT, and MRI
2. Role of thoracentesis in pleural disease diagnosis
3. Biopsy methods for mediastinal lesions

Diagnostic approaches to pleural conditions and mediastinal disease are critical in managing treatment and maximizing patient outcomes. The complexity of the diseases requires that one have a masterful overview of diagnostic modalities. Endoscopic bronchial ultrasound (EBUS) is now a valuable modality for examining mediastinal lymph nodes, especially with suspected lung cancer. Through the provision of ultrasound-guided transbronchial needle aspiration, EBUS provides a less invasive method of acquiring tissue samples from intrathoracic lymph nodes, minimizing the dependency on more invasive surgery. With its high specificity and sensitivity, the application of EBUS is an essential component in lung cancer staging, and its role significantly contributes to accurate diagnosis and patient management of patients with mediastinal involvement and other cancers of the intrathoracic region (Bilocca et al., 2016). Another key diagnostic method is the application of low-dose helical CT, an innovation that has revolutionized lung cancer screening. Evidence has shown that low-dose CT detects more nodules and lung cancers, particularly in their early stages, compared with traditional chest radiography. The outcome of the National Lung Cancer Screening Trial highlights the efficiency of this modality, revealing the dramatic reduction in lung cancer mortality rates with aggressive screening practices. Further, guidelines by the National Comprehensive Cancer Network also urge lung cancer screening, citing early detection as an important component of improving survival. Screening tests therefore require a meticulous patient history and physical exam to direct further diagnostic strategies such that those who are going to present with lung cancer are adequately assessed and managed (Ferreira et al., 2012). The use of all these diagnostic techniques demonstrates the necessity of a multi-disciplinary management of pleural and mediastinal diseases. Tissue sampling remains a key component in diagnosing, and determining whether non-surgical or surgical means are to be used can have profound effects on patient outcomes. The careful analysis of mediastinal lymph nodes is particularly pertinent because it dictates the staging of lung cancer based on the tumor-node-metastasis (TNM) system. This staging provides important prognostic information and directs therapeutic management. Continuous advances in imaging technology and biopsy techniques promise to make differential diagnoses more precise, ultimately leading to better management of pleural and mediastinal diseases, as well as continued research aimed at refining current guidelines and practices within the specialty. The establishment of these diagnostic techniques underscores the importance of early intervention for improving patient survival and quality of life (Bilocca et al., 2016).

8.5.1. Imaging Techniques: X-Ray, CT, and MRI

Imaging tests are critical in the diagnosis as well as treatment of mediastinal and pleural disorders. X-ray imaging constitutes the initial non-invasive test, giving a general impression of the thoracic cavity. X-rays can easily identify gross abnormalities such as pleural effusion or huge masses in the mediastinal cavity. They often lack sensitivity to subtle changes, necessitating the use of more advanced imaging modalities like CT and MRI. These are more detailed and specific, allowing for better differentiation among various pathologies. For example, while an ordinary chest X-ray may identify a pleural thickening, CT and MRI can define the extent of infiltration and associated structures, thereby directing the diagnostic and treatment process more specifically. Computed tomography is a beneficial imaging modality with high-resolution cross-sectional information of the thorax, which is critical in the evaluation of mediastinal disease and pleural disease. In comparison with standard X-rays, CT scans can demonstrate sophisticated relationships between anatomy and pathologic change with excellent clarity. They are particularly valuable in assessing the extent of disease, guiding biopsies, and monitoring response to treatment. In the wide range of mediastinal disorders, including tumors and lymphadenopathy, CT yields subtle information that informs clinical decisions. In addition, its ability to image in more than one plane makes it more useful for diagnosis, revealing fine details valuable for effective treatment planning. In the words of the literature, improving technology in CT continues to augment diagnostic confidence and efficiency, ensuring thorough patient care in diagnosing pleural and mediastinal disease (N/A, 2021). Magnetic resonance imaging has emerged as an important modality in the evaluation of pleural and mediastinal illness, particularly where the major priority is soft tissue contrast. MRI is optimal in assessing complex diseases of the pleura, such as mesothelioma, and provides exquisite images of the mediastinal organs without the use of ionizing radiation. This advantage is particularly helpful in certain patient populations, e.g., in pediatric patients and patients who must have repeated imaging examinations. In addition, MRIs ability to perform functional imaging through diffusion-weighted imaging and dynamic contrast-enhanced sequences enables to better characterize tumors and evaluate vascular structures.

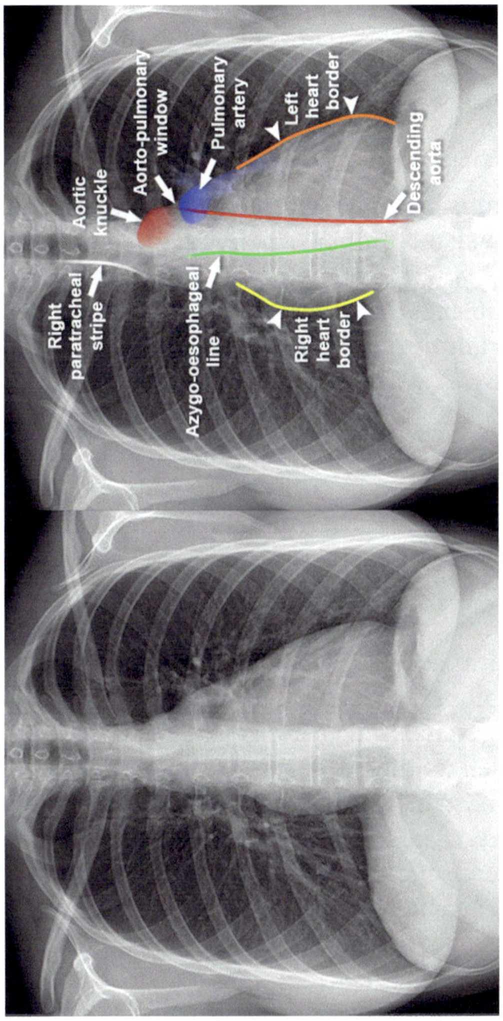

Figure 8.17. Mediastinum imaging techniques.

Source: https://external-content.duckduckgo.com/iu/?u=https%3A%2F%2Fwww.radiologymasterclass.co.uk%2Fimages%2Fchest-images%2Fgallery-mediastinum%2Fnormal.jpg%3Fmtime%3D20210304211316%26focal%3Dnone&f=1&nofb=1&ipt=5461cc89634ec257d03aa392b200b53d1803ea3c0cd8932575c6b79efef24d08.

As shown in current literature, complete imaging strategies with MRI, in combination with other modalities such as CT and X-ray, are necessary for multi-faceted thoracic disorder evaluation (N/A, 2025). By integrating various imaging modalities, clinicians can enhance diagnostic accuracy and optimize treatment strategies for patients with mediastinal and pleural diseases (Figure 8.17).

8.5.2. Role of Thoracentesis in Pleural Disease Diagnosis

The role of thoracentesis in diagnosing pleural pathology is important, especially in differentiating the causes of pleural effusions. Thoracentesis grants access to drainage of pleural fluid, which, after examination by the clinician, can render it feasible to distinguish between transudative and exudative effusions. This has relevance because it guides further treatment and management. For instance, the transudative form of effusion typically represents systemic conditions such as CHF, while exudative forms normally arise from infectious etiologies, malignancy, or inflammatory disorders. The initial criteria proposed by Lights have been widely applied, providing a valid guide for interpretation. The results of thoracentesis inform sound clinical practice and can direct additional diagnostic testing, such as imaging, to determine the etiology of the underlying pleural condition (Cashen et al., 2017). Thoracentesis, in addition to being diagnostic, is therapeutic, particularly in symptomatic individuals with large effusions. By decreasing pressure from built-up fluid, thoracentesis can enhance respiratory status and improve the overall quality of life for patients. The method is particularly valuable in cases where effusions are huge and cause important respiratory distress. Use of ultrasound guidance during thoracentesis has been shown to increase procedural success and patient safety, avoiding complications such as pneumothorax or vascular penetration. The utilization of ultrasound may also make it easier to identify loculated or complex fluid collections, which may require more aggressive therapy. Thus, not only does thoracentesis facilitate diagnosis, but it may be a therapeutic aspect of symptomatic treatment for patients with pleural effusion (Daniel, 2014). Thoracentesis is also relevant in pediatric practice because diagnosing pleural disease is crucial. The pattern of pleural effusions and their causes differ from those in adults and are most frequently due to infectious diseases, such as pneumonia, which can complicate to parapneumonic effusion and empyema.

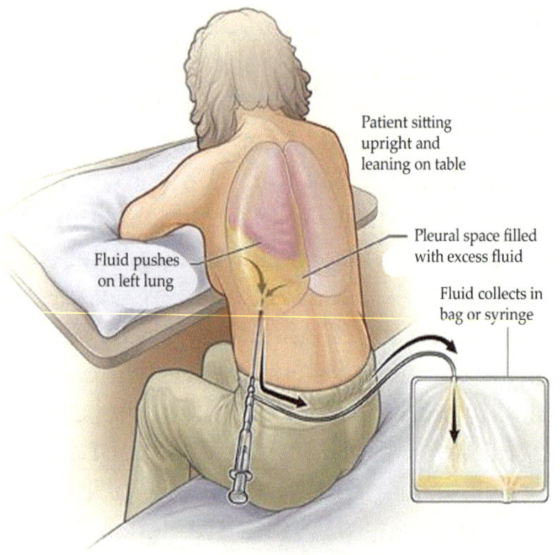

Figure 8.18. Role of thoracentesis in pleural disease diagnosis.

Source: https://external-content.duckduckgo.com/iu/?u=https%3A%2F%2Fwecaregolp.com%2Fwp-content%2Fuploads%2F2023%2F05%2FThoracocentesis-e1683455235198.jpg&f=1&nofb=1&ipt=06e4832d02f19a9e853cbeeea8a55eb77efdaddb9bc5e0c9d0d9d54c011fe308.

In this setting, diagnostic thoracentesis is particularly useful for establishing the fluid type, guiding the utilization of appropriate antibiotic therapy, and possibly preventing complications. Although pediatric patients may need to be anesthetized or sedated due to their age, advances in ultrasound technology have made the procedure safer and more effective. The pleural space can now be more thoroughly assessed by clinicians to avoid suboptimal management of pleural effusion-associated complications. Therefore, thoracentesis remains a cornerstone of treatment and diagnostic management of pleural disease across all ages (Cashen et al., 2017) (Figure 8.18).

8.5.3. Biopsy Methods for Mediastinal Lesions

Diagnosis of mediastinal lesions often requires the use of biopsy methods to obtain tissue samples for histopathologic examination. Two of the most utilized methods are fine needle aspiration biopsy (FNAB) and core needle biopsy (CNB). FNAB is most commonly utilized for its minimally invasive nature and is performed under ultrasound or CT guidance to precisely locate the lesion. This approach is particularly valuable to assess lymphadenopathy or masses that are not easily palpable. Alternatively, CNB provides larger tissue samples, which are vital for final diagnoses, especially in challenging situations such as lymphoma. The selection of the biopsy procedure is influenced by various factors, including the size and site of the lesion, as well as the patient's general condition, thus emphasizing the complexity in the management of these mediastinal conditions. Barring FNAB and CNB, mediastinoscopy offers a more invasive but extremely valuable means of performing a biopsy, particularly in cases involving suspicious anterior mediastinal masses or mediastinal lymphadenopathy. The surgical procedure allows for direct visualization and access to the mediastinal organs, with capabilities for extensive tissue sampling that would be difficult to achieve using percutaneous methods. Mediastinoscopy has been shown to have excellent diagnostic yields, particularly in malignancy, and may be of great value in cancer staging in thoracic malignancies. In any case, the invasiveness of the procedure and associated risks, such as anesthetic complications and bleeding, call for judicious patient selection. By considering both the probability of benefits and risks with mediastinoscopy, clinicians can determine optimal biopsies to use in cases, resulting in more accurate diagnoses and targeted treatment plans. Imaging also plays a critical role in the planning of mediastinal lesion biopsy, with the choice of modality directly impacting the success of the procedure. The developments in newer diagnostic imaging modalities such as CT and MRI over recent years have improved lesion characterization and localization, thereby improving the accuracy of biopsies. The addition of image-guided interventions, such as ultrasound- or CT-guided biopsies, is commonplace today, offering real-time imaging and reduced complications. The overview of imaging modalities discusses imaging-interventional synergy in the clinical setting. The recent past literature emphasizes that multimodal imaging enhances the diagnostic process with efficient decision support and improved patient outcomes in the context of mediastinal disorders (N/A, 2021, 2025).

Test Your Knowledge

1. What is the role of thoracentesis in pleural disease diagnosis?
2. What are the biopsy methods for mediastinal lesions?

8.6. Treatment Options

Learning Outcome

1. Medical management of pleural disorders
2. Surgical interventions for mediastinal diseases
3. Emerging therapies and research directions

The best management of mediastinal and pleural disease is multidisciplinary, and the choice of treatment varies greatly depending on the specific diagnosis and the patient's personal features. Pleural effusion, a persistent condition, can be managed with therapeutic thoracentesis, ie, removal of the excess fluid from the pleural space. It not only prevents the symptoms but is also helpful in diagnostic workup by analysis of pleural fluid. During infection, as in empyema, additional therapy with antibiotics and possibly surgical drainage can be required to manage loculated collections of fluid. Overall, a broad understanding of the individual patient's specific clinical presentation is crucial in determining the most appropriate initial treatment of pleural disease. For mediastinal disease, the treatment paradigm is also dependent on proper pathology determination. For instance, mediastinal tumors that are either benign or malignant may often demand combinations of surgical excision, chemotherapy, or radiation. Targeted agents have dramatically transformed therapy for chosen malignancies, most notably in non-small-cell lung cancer (NSCLC). A common first-line therapy for EGFR-mutant advanced NSCLC is an EGFR-targeted oral tyrosine kinase inhibitor. Adding pemetrexed and carboplatin chemotherapy with an oral tyrosine kinase inhibitor can improve outcomes (Noronha et al., 2019). Such a multidisciplinary approach ensures that each treatment is tailored to individual tumor characteristics and patient tolerance, maximizing patient outcomes and minimizing treatment-related morbidity. Finally, imaging and diagnostic technology have further refined treatment options in pleural and mediastinal disease. The introduction of minimally invasive surgery, such as video-assisted thoracoscopic surgery (VATS), has revolutionized the clinicians' approach to both diagnosis and treatment. VATS not only facilitates correct biopsy sampling for histological examination but also allows therapeutic interventions, such as pleurodesis, in cases of recurrent pleural effusion. Moreover, the use of molecular profiling in diseases such as lung cancer also assists in understanding targeted therapy and enhancing overall efficacy (Lax et al., 2020). A treatment plan that incorporates both the emerging trend of changing technology and patient-dependent values can significantly help in the treatment outcomes of pleural and mediastinal disorders.

8.6.1. Medical Management of Pleural Disorders

The treatment of pleural disease requires a complete understanding of the various etiologies of the pleural disorder and the associated pathophysiologies. Infectious, neoplastic, and cardiovascular illnesses cause pleural effusion and pneumothorax, each necessitating a specific treatment regimen. In children, parapneumonic effusions are common and typically secondary to pneumonia, whereas in adults, malignancy and CHF are frequent etiologies of pleural disease. Management is maximally effective when distinguishing between exudative and transudative effusions through the analysis of pleural fluid, which helps guide treatment strategies specific to the etiology. Supportive therapy with antibiotics and respiratory management tends to be preliminary, while the selection of a drainage modality becomes important for severe respiratory impairment or symptomatic pleural accumulation (Zhou et al., 2020; Cashen et al., 2017). After pleural effusions have been established to be infected, the initiation of empiric antibiotics promptly is necessary before identification of the causative organisms. Local resistance and the assumed pathogens should guide antibiotic choices, typically protecting against Streptococcus pneumoniae and Staphylococcus aureus, especially in those complicated by severe pneumonia or empyema. In the past, large thoracostomy tubes were used for draining complicated effusions, but the latest evidence supports the efficacy of minimally invasive procedures, such as small-bore catheters or VATS. These interventions reduce morbidity in addition to reducing recovery times by minimizing operative trauma (Zhou et al., 2020; Cashen et al., 2017).

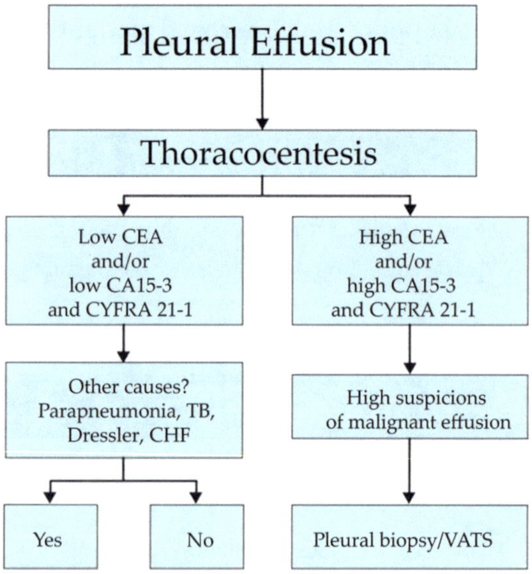

Figure 8.19. Management of pleural effusion.

Source/. https://www.researchgate.net/profile/Mordechai-Kramer-2/publication/7681338/figure/fig1/AS:280886550515715@1443979980327/Management-of-pleural-effusion-a-clinical-practice.png.

Where medical management and drainage fail to improve empyemas, additional intervention will be contemplated. Fibrinolytic therapy has also grown in use, offering a promising alternative aimed at lysing septations and allowing for reabsorption of the effusion. Studies indicate that fibrinolytics, i.e., intrapleural tissue plasminogen activator, are effective in producing significant reduction in empyema size compared to routine drainage alone and with improved functional outcome. Further, the applicability of early intervention cannot be downplayed since early treatment interventions are associated with lower hospital length of stay and morbidity. With innovations in the area, continuous monitoring of treatment patterns is crucial in order to agree with alterations in clinical practice as well as new evidence on best practice in the management of pleural disease (Cashen et al., 2017; Zhou et al., 2020) (Figure 8.19).

8.6.2. Surgical Interventions for Mediastinal Diseases

Surgical interventions are a key component of treating most mediastinal diseases, which encompass vital structures including the heart, lungs, and major blood vessels. Surgery is often required in the context of malignancy or congenital structural abnormalities that pose direct threats, such as airway compromise or vascular compromise. Surgical approaches can range from minimally invasive, such as thoracoscopic biopsies and resections, to more elaborate approaches such as median sternotomy and thoracotomy, depending on the nature and site of mediastinal illness. Evolution in surgical technologies and multidisciplinary approaches has enhanced patient outcomes in mediastinal illnesses. In particular, VATS has been revolutionary in allowing for less recovery time and shorter hospital stays, thereby significantly enhancing the candidacy of surgical patients in need of intervention for mediastinal masses or disease. The nature of mediastinal disease also necessitates having a proper appreciation of the possible emergencies that can arise. Surgical interventions, combined with careful preoperative assessment, can avoid potentially life-threatening complications such as massive hemoptysis or airway obstruction, which are the usual association of mediastinal malignancies and other conditions. For instance, bronchoscopic interventions allow direct intervention of central airway obstructions secondary to a tumor or a foreign body. Certain interventions entail the placement of stents to stabilize compromised airways and enhance airflow. The interaction between surgical care and intensive care is of utmost importance, as numerous patients are likely to need ICU placement for careful monitoring due to the high-risk status of their conditions. Therefore, proficiency in both surgical care and critical care becomes necessary in order to manage such cases properly, allowing for the best patient outcomes (Abramian et al., 2016).

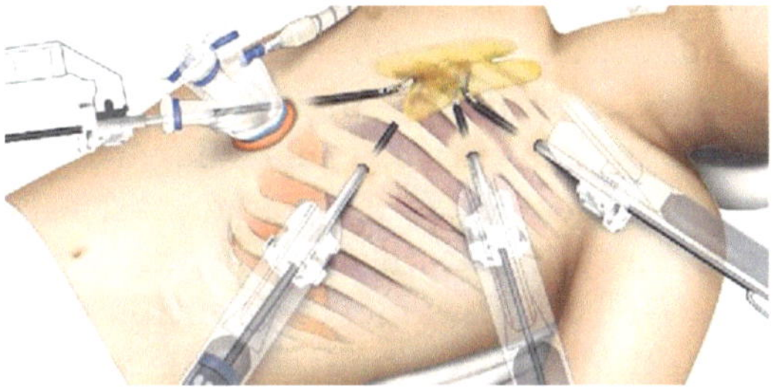

Figure 8.20. Mediastinal surgery.

Source: https://lirp.cdn-website.com/8d5123f4/dms3rep/multi/opt/fig3-640w.jpg.

Emergent and elective mediastinal disease surgery must be carried out with a well-defined treatment plan that considers individualized patient characteristics and disease presentation. Of note, conditions like Ortner's syndrome are a reminder of the need for correct diagnosis prior to surgery. Silent thoracic aortic aneurysm dissection can manifest as thoracic malignancy and lead to inappropriate invasive procedures like thoracentesis if it is not correctly diagnosed. The surgery must be accompanied by precise preoperative imaging, as in those cases which require CT scans before deciding on surgery (Ranasinghe et al., 2015). Management of mediastinal disease is often a multidisciplinary process involving intensivists, radiologists, and thoracic surgeons. Such consultation ensures that surgical interventions not only address the continuous immediate dangers of mediastinal illnesses but also align with total treatment protocols specific to each patient's unique clinical scenario (Figure 8.20).

8.6.3. Emerging Therapies and Research Directions

Research into the development of emerging therapies and avenues of research into pleural disorders and mediastinal diseases reflects heightened sensitivity to the necessity for new approaches to treatment. One advanced development is the increased use of point-of-care thoracic ultrasound (T-POCUS) in veterinary medicine as well as human medicine. This technology delivers real-time imaging of the thorax that facilitates immediate assessment of a variety of respiratory conditions. As noted, T-POCUS is able to identify pleural space abnormalities and diagnose several pulmonary conditions, enhancing clinical decision-making and patient outcomes in the emergency department. Increased use of T-POCUS does increase the demand for practice and terminology standardization to enable general clinical utility and effectiveness (Armenise, 2025). By refining and improving questionnaires, the field comes closer to the timely and precise questionnaires for patients with pleural and mediastinal diseases. Another new line of research involves exploring new therapeutic targets for the treatment of pleural mesothelioma, a highly malignant neoplasm and with serious therapeutic problems and poor prognosis. Current studies have focused on maximizing the efficacy of targeted therapy and immunotherapy, which hold promise for improving patient survival and quality of life. Of most interest are combination treatments that integrate conventional chemotherapy with biologic agents, holding promise for improved treatment. As has been clear in recent summaries, while advancements have been made with the biology and clinical presentation of pleural mesothelioma, there is still much to be done to maximize these treatments. Studies continue to emphasize not only the advancement in treatment but also the necessity to advance early diagnosis techniques to enhance patient outcomes and overall survival rates (Bertuccio et al., 2023). The shared evolution of imaging techniques and treatments highlights the inherent link between advanced medical technology and the evolving art of treating pleural and mediastinal diseases. Further studies will define genetic and molecular pathways of these diseases, creating opportunities for personalized medicine approaches tailored to unique patient profiles. A multidisciplinary research partnership can catalyze innovations in treatment approaches, paving the way for novel interventions that can revolutionize the management of pleura and mediastinum involved diseases. By networking of professionals from various fields and with the utilization of technological innovation in the implementation of such in clinical practice, the ability to revamp the treatment of patients in this such specialized field becomes increasingly realistic, a viable future for the management of pleural and mediastinal disease.

Test Your Knowledge

1. What are the medical management of pleural disorders?
2. What are the surgical interventions for mediastinal diseases?

Summary

Upon reviewing the pleural diseases and mediastinal diseases, it is clear that an integrated approach towards understanding these diseases is necessary for effective diagnosis and management. The interconnectedness of the pleura, lungs, and mediastinal tissues, which a patient relies on for the proper functioning of the respiratory system, makes interdisciplinary management of related diseases significant. From neoplastic disease processes to pleural effusions, practitioners must navigate a host of complications and symptoms in these regions. From considering clinical presentation and optimizing therapeutic interventions, practitioners are able to enhance outcomes for patients. This systems approach is essential because it supports the contribution of both clinical acumen and empirical evidence to guiding treatment regimens in patients with these diseases. Additionally, the growing importance of etiological factors such as COVID-19 and associated respiratory disorders emphasizes the dynamic nature of pleural and mediastinal diseases. Pandemic disruption has highlighted the importance of aggressive scientific research aimed at addressing the significant consequences of viral infections on the pleural apparatus and the mediastinum. For instance, COVID-19 has shown a propensity to lead to diffuse alveolar damage and venous thromboembolism, complicating traditional comprehension of respiratory conditions and treatment. Data-driven insights are more crucial than ever, particularly with the dynamic interaction between viral infections and chronic pulmonary diseases in the clinic. An investigation is called for to shed light on these subtleties and guide future treatment interventions aimed at avoiding danger, ultimately leading to optimal practice in this specialty medicine (Lax et al., 2020). Finally, ongoing research and trials, such as those on treating advanced non-small-cell lung cancer, indicate the need for creativity in treatment techniques. Of particular importance, the integration of targeted treatments such as tyrosine kinase inhibitors with traditional chemotherapy has yielded promising results toward improving survival in patients. Not only do such results and enhance understanding of individualized mediastinal conditions, but they also highlight the importance of tailoring treatment modalities based on patient profiles, particularly those with comorbidities. Through ongoing research, integrating new information into practice will play an important role in improving management strategies. Hence, collaboration between clinicians, researchers, and patients will be the solution to the complexities of mediastinal and pleural disease with the foundation for future advancements in respiratory medicine (Noronha et al., 2019).

Detection of pleural and mediastinal diseases is crucial for efficient clinical care, particularly since these conditions can markedly impair respiratory function and overall health. Pleura are two layers of tissue covering the lungs, and any disruption in the form of pleurisy, pleural effusion, or pneumothorax will lead to severe respiratory distress and pain. Furthermore, the mediastinum, where key structures such as the heart, trachea, and esophagus reside, is also susceptible to numerous diseases, including mediastinal tumors and infections. Not only are these diseases difficult to diagnose, but they must also be treated by personalized therapeutic strategies to correct symptoms and outcome in the patient, thus placing considerable emphasis on a thorough understanding of anatomical structures as well as their respective pathologies. Recent studies highlight gaps in knowledge regarding post-viral complications, such as those from COVID-19, and worsening pleural and mediastinal diseases. According to post COVID-19 condition systematic review, a notable proportion of patients experience long-lasting symptoms of fatigue, dyspnoea, and cognitive impairment far beyond their first diagnosis (Domingo et al., 2021). These findings thus indicate that associations between respiratory illness and post-viral syndromes need higher sensitization of health workers. Discovery of long-term effects is necessary, as it allows for early intervention and complete follow-up care, ultimately improving patients' lives and avoiding the dangers associated with uncontrolled respiratory complications. Moreover, pleural and mediastinal disease management typically involves multidisciplinary care in complicated presentations like acquired tracheoesophageal fistulas. The typical causes of the condition often arise from external injuries related to medical intervention, representing a significant area for improving procedure quality and patient safety. Efficient management involves preoperative assessment, precise surgical procedures, and follow-up monitoring in an effort to prevent complications (Santosham, 2018). Such a combined model enhances clinical outcomes and reduces the long-term morbidity commonly associated with these conditions. Therefore, creating standardized protocols and increasing awareness of such conditions are crucial for optimizing treatment in the context of pleural and mediastinal pathology.

KEY TERMS FROM THIS CHAPTER

- Bronchogenic cyst
- Chylothorax
- Empyema
- Fibrothorax
- Hemothorax
- Mediastinal fibrosis
- Mediastinal lymphoma
- Mediastinal mass
- Mediastinitis
- Mesothelioma
- Neurogenic tumors
- Parapneumonic effusion
- Pericardial cyst
- Pleural effusion
- Pleural plaques
- Pleural thickening
- Pneumothorax
- Teratoma
- Thymic cyst
- Thymoma

CRITICAL THINKING QUESTIONS

1. **Which of the following is the most common cause of a transudative pleural effusion?**
   a. Tuberculosis
   b. Congestive heart failure
   c. Malignancy
   d. Bacterial pneumonia
2. **Light's criteria are used to differentiate:**
   a. Exudative from transudative pleural effusions
   b. Empyema from hemothorax
   c. Malignant from benign pleural effusions
   d. Chylothorax from pseudochylothorax
3. **What is the most common primary tumor of the anterior mediastinum?**
   a. Thymoma
   b. Teratoma
   c. Lymphoma
   d. Neurogenic tumor
4. **Which type of pleural effusion is characterized by a milky appearance and elevated triglycerides?**
   a. Hemothorax
   b. Chylothorax
   c. Empyema
   d. Pseudochylothorax
5. **Which mediastinal mass is most commonly found in the middle mediastinum?**
   a. Thymoma
   b. Bronchogenic cyst
   c. Neurogenic tumor
   d. Teratoma

Short Answer Questions

1. What are the most common causes of a pleural effusion?
2. How do you differentiate between transudative and exudative pleural effusions based on pleural fluid analysis?
3. What clinical features are commonly seen in patients with spontaneous pneumothorax?
4. Describe the pathophysiology and clinical presentation of malignant pleural mesothelioma.
5. What are the main types of mediastinal masses, and how are they typically classified anatomically?

Answer to Critical Thinking Questions

1. (b); 2. (a); 3. (a); 4. (b); 5. (b)

References

1. Raouf, M. a. E., Elgioushy, M., & Ezzeldein, S. A. (2020). Congestive heart failure in cattle; etiology, clinical, and ultrasonographic findings in 67 cases. *Veterinary World, 13*(6), 1145–1152. https://doi.org/10.14202/vetworld.2020.1145-1152Abramian, E., Abramian, O., & Kolman, D. (2016). Oncological airway emergencies in the critical care unit. https://core.ac.uk/download/322428540.pdf (accessed on 30th June 2025).
2. Adler, Y., Charron, P., Imazio, M., Badano, L. P., Barón-Esquivias, G., Bogaert, J., Brucato, A., et al. (2015). 2015 ESC Guidelines for the diagnosis and management of pericardial diseases. *European Heart Journal, 36*, 2921–2964. https://doi.org/10.1093/eurheartj/ehv318 (accessed on 30th June 2025).
3. Armenise, A. (2025). Point-of-care lung ultrasound in small animal emergency and critical care medicine: A clinical review. *Animals, 15*, 106–106. https://doi.org/10.3390/ani15010106 (accessed on 30th June 2025).
4. Authors Task Force Members, Erbel, R., Aboyans, V., Boileau, C., Bossone, E., Di Bartolomeo, R., Eggebrecht, H., et al. (2014). 2014 ESC guidelines on the diagnosis and treatment of aortic diseases. *European Heart Journal, 35*, 2873–2926. https://doi.org/10.1093/eurheartj/ehu281 (accessed on 30th June 2025).
5. Baburaj, K. (2006). Etiological diagnosis of pleural effusion in hundred cases. https://core.ac.uk/download/235663749.pdf (accessed on 30th June 2025).
6. Bajc, M., Schümichen, C., Grüning, T., Lindqvist, A., Le Roux, P. Y., Alatri, A., Bauer, R. W., et al. (2019). EANM guideline for ventilation/perfusion single-photon emission computed tomography (SPECT) for diagnosis of pulmonary embolism and beyond. *European Journal of Nuclear Medicine and Molecular Imaging, 46*, 2429–2451. https://doi.org/10.1007/s00259-019-04450-0 (accessed on 30th June 2025).
7. Bertuccio, F., Agustoni, F., Galli, G., Bortolotto, C., Saddi, J., Baietto, G., Baio, N., et al. (2023). Pleural mesothelioma: Treatable traits of a heterogeneous disease. *Cancers, 15*, 5731–5731. https://doi.org/10.3390/cancers15245731 (accessed on 30th June 2025).
8. Bilocca, D., Montefort, S., & Vella, C. (2016). Endoscopic bronchial ultrasound in mediastinal staging of lung cancer. https://core.ac.uk/download/46604248.pdf (accessed on 30th June 2025).
9. Calabrese, F., Montero-Fernandez, M. A., Kern, I., Pezzuto, F., Lunardi, F., Hofman, P., Berezowska, S., et al. (2024). The role of pathologists in the diagnosis of occupational lung diseases: An expert opinion of the European Society of Pathology Pulmonary Pathology Working Group. *Virchows Archiv, 485*, 173–195. https://doi.org/10.1007/s00428-024-03845-1 (accessed on 30th June 2025).
10. Carter, B. W., Benveniste, M. F., Madan, R., Godoy, M. C. B., de Groot, P. M., Truong, M. T., Rosado-de-Christenson, M. L., et al. (2017). ITMIG classification of mediastinal compartments and multidisciplinary approach to mediastinal masses. *Radiographics, 37*, 413–436. https://doi.org/10.1148/rg.2017160095 (accessed on 30th June 2025).
11. Cashen, K., & Petersen, T. L. (2017). Pleural effusions and pneumothoraxes. *Pediatrics in Review, 38*, 170–181. https://doi.org/10.1542/pir.2016-0088 (accessed on 30th June 2025).
12. Clinical Practice and Cases in Emergency Medicine. (2021). *Clinical Practice and Cases in*

Emergency Medicine, 5. https://doi.org/10.5811/cpcem.2021.4.54351 (accessed on 30th June 2025).

13. Cova, M., Assunta, D. P., Gennari, L., Poillucci, A., et al. (2015). Imaging characteristics of pleural tumours. https://core.ac.uk/download/160651504.pdf (accessed on 30th June 2025).
14. Cuvertoret-Sanz, M., Domingo, M., Duignan, P. J., López-Figueroa, M., et al. (2024). Air leak syndrome in animals: Definition and pathogenesis. https://core.ac.uk/download/630817451.pdf (accessed on 30th June 2025).
15. Dietrich, C. F., Mathis, G., Cui, X. W., Ignee, A., Hocke, M., & Hirche, T. O. (2015). Ultrasound of the pleurae and lungs. *Ultrasound in Medicine & Biology, 41*, 351–365. https://doi.org/10.1016/j.ultrasmedbio.2014.10.002 (accessed on 30th June 2025).
16. Division of Genetics and Metabolomics Child Disease, Chen, X., Sun, Y., Yang, Y., Han, L., & Huang, X. (2021). [Consensus on screening, diagnosis and treatment of multiple acyl-CoA dehydrogenase deficiency]. *Zhonghua Yi Xue Yi Chuan Xue Za Zhi = Chinese Journal of Medical Genetics, 38*(5), 414–418. https://www.semanticscholar.org/paper/1ce57a8fdc80542e65879dd6c28841e7624f1623 (accessed on 30th June 2025).
17. Domingo, F. R., Waddell, L., Cheung, A. M., Cooper, C., Belcourt, V. J., Zuckermann, A. M. E., Corrin, T., et al. (2021). Prevalence of long-term effects in individuals diagnosed with COVID-19: An updated living systematic review. *medRxiv* (Cold Spring Harbor Laboratory). https://doi.org/10.1101/2021.06.03.21258317 (accessed on 30th June 2025).
18. Ferreira, J., Magalhães, M., Marques, F., Rocha, A., et al. (2012). Non-small cell lung cancer: Screening, diagnosis, and staging. https://core.ac.uk/download/71742541.pdf (accessed on 30th June 2025).
19. Fukuda, T., Egashira, R., Ueno, M., Hashisako, M., Sumikawa, H., Tominaga, J., Yamada, D., et al. (2023). Stepwise diagnostic algorithm for high-attenuation pulmonary abnormalities on CT. *Insights into Imaging, 14.* https://doi.org/10.1186/s13244-023-01501-x (accessed on 30th June 2025).
20. Gerber, T. S., & Porubský, Š. (2023). Benign lesions of the mediastinum. *Histopathology, 84*, 183–195. https://doi.org/10.1111/his.15088 (accessed on 30th June 2025).
21. Huang, C. (2020). The differential diagnosis of bilateral pleural effusion and multiple mediastinal lymphadenopathies includes Kikuchi-Fujimoto disease. *Journal of Investigative Medicine High Impact Case Reports, 8*, 232470962093342–232470962093342. https://doi.org/10.1177/2324709620933422 (accessed on 30th June 2025).
22. Ilieva, E., Kostadinova, V., Tzotcheva, I., Rimpova, N., Paskaleva, Y., & Lazova, S. (2022). Abdominal and thoracic imaging features in children with MIS-C. *Gastroenterology Insights, 13*, 313–325. https://doi.org/10.3390/gastroent13040032 (accessed on 30th June 2025).
23. Katz, G., & Stone, J. H. (2021). Clinical perspectives on IgG4-related disease and its classification. *Annual Review of Medicine, 73*, 545–562. https://doi.org/10.1146/annurev-med-050219-034449 (accessed on 30th June 2025).
24. Kumar, K., Daga, R., Singh, J., Kumar, N., & Dinkar, A. (2025). Diagnostic challenges of polyneuropathy, organomegaly, endocrinopathy, M-protein, and skin changes (POEMS) syndrome: A rare case report and review of the literature. *Cardiovascular & Hematological Disorders–Drug Targets.* https://www.semanticscholar.org/paper/1fae43e40d2a86ed03a5db3a1ae60e45b98923b5 (accessed on 30th June 2025).

25. Kuzmina, G. P., Lazarenko, O. M., & Markova, O. Y. (2023). Clinical case of severe visceral complications with atypical localization in a patient with gout. https://core.ac.uk/download/588445139.pdf (accessed on 30th June 2025).

26. Lax, S., Skok, K., Zechner, P., Kessler, H. H., Kaufmann, N., Koelblinger, C., Vander, K., et al. (2020). Pulmonary arterial thrombosis in COVID-19 with fatal outcome. *Annals of Internal Medicine, 173*, 350–361. https://doi.org/10.7326/m20-2566 (accessed on 30th June 2025).

27. Lichtenstein, D. A. (2014). Lung ultrasound in the critically ill. *Annals of Intensive Care, 4*, 1–1. https://doi.org/10.1186/2110-5820-4-1 (accessed on 30th June 2025).

28. Louis, B. S., Arshad, A., Muthu Raja, K., Ayub, I. I., & Dhanasekar, T. (2024). A report of two cases of tuberculosis with bronchial anthracofibrosis: Diagnostic challenges and therapeutic approaches. *Cureus, 16*. https://www.semanticscholar.org/paper/81b1cd73dbe8fc866ad8b17134a8b0d672e58892 (accessed on 30th June 2025).

29. Muralitharan, A. (2017). A study on exudative etiology of pleural effusion in chronic kidney disease in a tertiary care hospital. https://core.ac.uk/download/288215826.pdf (accessed on 30th June 2025).

30. Nicholson, A. G., Detterbeck, F., Marx, A., Roden, A. C., Marchevsky, A. M., Mukai, K., Chen, G., et al. (2016). Dataset for reporting of thymic epithelial tumours: Recommendations from the International Collaboration on Cancer Reporting (ICCR). *Histopathology, 70*, 522–538. https://doi.org/10.1111/his.13099 (accessed on 30th June 2025).

31. Noronha, V., Patil, V., Joshi, A., Menon, N., Chougule, A., Mahajan, A., Janu, A., et al. (2019). Gefitinib versus gefitinib plus pemetrexed and carboplatin chemotherapy in *EGFR*-mutated lung cancer. *Journal of Clinical Oncology, 38*, 124–136. https://doi.org/10.1200/jco.19.01154 (accessed on 30th June 2025).

32. Noussios, G., Anagnostis, P., Goulis, D. G., Lappas, D., & Natsis, K. (2011). Ectopic thyroid tissue: Anatomical, clinical, and surgical implications of a rare entity. *European Journal of Endocrinology, 165*, 375–382. https://doi.org/10.1530/eje-11-0461 (accessed on 30th June 2025).

33. Petrola, C., Castro, S., Rodríguez Conde, N., Gantxegi Madina, A., Jofra, M., Gil-Sala, D., & Armengol, M. (2022). Esophageal perforation due to acute esophageal necrosis: A case report and a comprehensive literature review. *Journal of Clinical and Investigative Surgery, 7*, 104–108. https://doi.org/10.25083/2559.5555/7.1.18 (accessed on 30th June 2025).

34. Ranasinghe, G., Samarasinghe, R., Kularatne, S., Handagala, S., & Pathirana, U. (2015). Ortner's syndrome presenting as thoracic aortic aneurysm mimicking thoracic malignancy: A case report. https://core.ac.uk/download/pdf/81194529.pdf (accessed on 30th June 2025).

35. Santosham, R. (2018). Management of acquired benign tracheoesophageal fistulae. *Deleted Journal, 28*, 385–392. https://doi.org/10.1016/j.thorsurg.2018.05.004 (accessed on 30th June 2025).

36. Tabotta, F., Ferretti, G., Prosch, H., Boussouar, S., Brun, A. L., Roos, J. E., Ebner, L., et al. (2020). Imaging features and differential diagnoses of non-neoplastic diffuse mediastinal diseases. *Insights into Imaging, 11*. https://doi.org/10.1186/s13244-020-00909-z (accessed on 30th June 2025).

37. Torres, T., Filipe, P., Menezes Brandão, F., Figueiredo, A., Pinto Soares, A., Sousa Basto, A.,

Rebelo, C., et al. (2023). Epidemiology of psoriasis in Portugal: A population-based study. *Acta Medica Portuguesa.* https://www.semanticscholar.org/paper/2212b929e6450009dba9de42612fb8b74f852eb1 (accessed on 30th June 2025).

38. Walker, C. M., Rosado-de-Christenson, M. L., Martínez-Jiménez, S., Kunin, J. R., & Wible, B. C. (2015). Bronchial arteries: Anatomy, function, hypertrophy, and anomalies. *Radiographic, 35*, 32–49. https://doi.org/10.1148/rg.351140089 (accessed on 30th June 2025).

39. Zhou, M., Zhang, X., & Qu, J. (2020). Coronavirus disease 2019 (COVID-19): A clinical update. *Frontiers of Medicine, 14*, 126–135. https://doi.org/10.1007/s11684-020-0767-8 (accessed on 30th June 2025).

DISORDERS OF THE DIAPHRAGM AND CHEST WALL

9

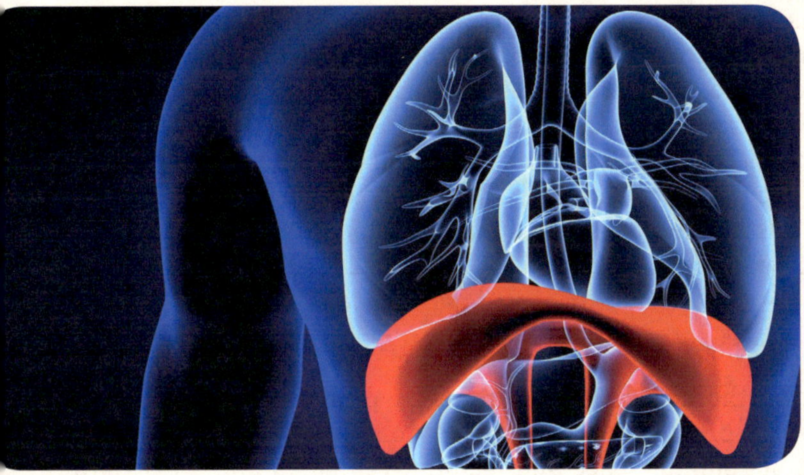

LEARNING OBJECTIVES

After studying this chapter, you will be able to:

1. Describe the diaphragm's anatomy;
2. Describe the chest wall's anatomy;
3. List the common diaphragmatic disorders;
4. Discuss the common chest wall disorders;
5. Understand the methods of diagnosis;
6. Highlight the treatment approaches.

Introduction

The diaphragm and chest wall play central roles in respiratory mechanics as key structures for effective ventilation. Complications of these structures result in serious respiratory dysfunction, which is characterized by compromised airflow and reduced efficiency of gas exchange. The recognition of these structural disorders necessitates a complex approach, integrating both the chest wall and diaphragm anatomy with the pathophysiological mechanisms underlying respiratory diseases. By exploring all these aspects in depth, it becomes clear that the interaction between muscle performance and structural integrity is critical for ensuring maximum respiratory performance. In addition, advances in the diagnostic technique illuminated the complexity of ascertaining diaphragm function, stimulating more studies along this line. The past two decades saw the clinical significance of diaphragm neuromechanical coupling (NMC) emerge as an area of priority research in respiratory medicine. NMC offers the efficiency of neural activation to transdiaphragmatic pressure conversion, which is significant in assessing diaphragm function, particularly in neuromuscular and cardiorespiratory diseases. Current gold standard methods for measuring NMC, such as invasive transdiaphragmatic pressure measurements and electromyography, have clinical drawbacks. Noninvasive techniques such as surface mechanomyography and surface electromyography are promising areas for the assessment of diaphragm function without invasive techniques. Through identifying a link between these methods, scientists are at the threshold of unlocking further knowledge regarding diaphragm mechanics and therefore more efficient treatment of patients with compromised respiratory function (Petrocelli et al., 2019). Further complicating the scenario regarding respiratory disease are the tasks performed by varying groups of inspiratory muscles, including the chest wall and diaphragm. New research on maximal inspiratory pressure has focused on the interdependency between these muscle groups and their relative contributions to respiratory efficacy. Interventions, such as inspiratory muscle training (IMT), have been discovered to increase maximal inspiratory pressure markedly, strengthening respiratory function. The relative contributions of diaphragm and chest wall muscles highlight the necessity of targeted rehabilitation interventions to optimize muscular coordination and strength in breathing. As treatment regimens improve, applying the outcomes of empirical studies will guide the formulation of customized treatment programs to address diaphragm and chest wall ailments, thereby improving patient outcomes (Brown et al., 2014).

Definition of Diaphragm and Chest Wall

The diaphragm is located at the base of the thoracic cavity, serving as the primary respiratory muscle and playing a very significant role in the breathing process. This dome-shaped muscular organ separates the thoracic space from the abdominal space and facilitates inhalation and exhalation. The diaphragm flattens and creates negative pressure in the thoracic space by contracting, hence pulling air into the lungs. The diaphragm relaxes to facilitate the expulsion of air during exhalation. Effective operation of the diaphragm is necessary for adequate oxygenation and carbon dioxide elimination, conditions closely correlated with the overall state of the respiratory system. The functional role of the diaphragm offers a basis for understanding many of the disorders subject to disturbing its function, which shall be discussed in the rest of this essay. Besides the diaphragm, the chest wall comprises ribs, intercostal muscles, and the rest of the thoracic cavity's supporting structures that facilitate respiration. Not only is the chest wall a protective shield over vital organs, but it is also a vital part that expands and collapses during breathing. Malformations or weakness in the chest wall can severely compromise respiratory mechanics. For example, diseases like scoliosis or kyphosis may restrict the expansion of the lungs and impair adequate ventilation. Besides, synergism between the chest wall and the diaphragm is critical; they cooperate to produce a harmonious respiratory effort. Compensation in one or other of these regions may lead to inefficient breath patterns, as well as to the onset of various respiratory disorders. Both components involve an appreciation of diagnosing and managing diaphragm and chest wall disorders. The co-operation between diaphragm function and chest wall integrity becomes even more relevant in diseases such as muscular dystrophy. These conditions lead to increasing weakness of respiratory muscles, including the diaphragm, significantly impacting respiration mechanics and gas exchange. Specifically, muscular dystrophy patients will be prone to both lung and pump origin respiratory failures, the function of the diaphragm being seriously impaired in advanced stages of the disease. This dual nature of effect emphasizes the importance of diaphragm function in respiratory disease, where alterations in thoracoabdominal patterns, hypoventilation, and increased airway resistance become evident. Furthermore, the interaction of the diaphragm with surgical procedures, such as lung transplant, adds complexity because the condition of the diaphragm significantly influences outcomes following these operations (Grasselli et al., 2024). Such interdependencies emphasize the necessity for incorporating both the chest wall and diaphragm in the assessment of respiratory illness (Aliverti et al., 2016) (Figure 9.1).

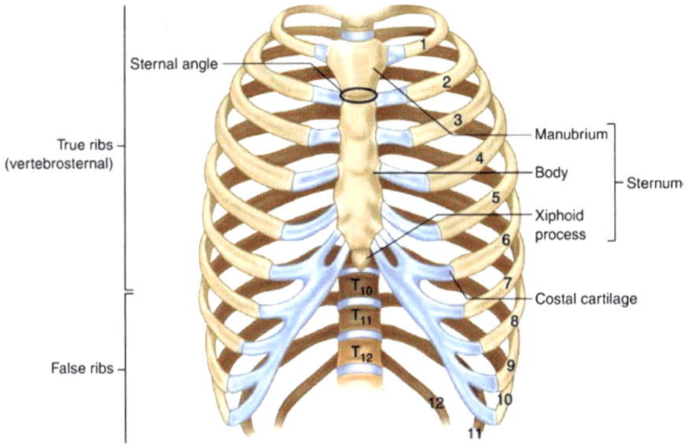

Figure 9.1. Chest wall and diaphragm.

Source: https://media.springernature.com/lw685/springer-static/image/chp%3A10.1007%2F978-3-030-31989-2_6/MediaObjects/469524_1_En_6_Fig4_HTML.png.

Significance of the Chest Wall and Diaphragm to Respiration

Both the chest wall and diaphragm are quite crucial in the mechanics of respiration, basically influencing the gas exchange process. The diaphragm, a dome-shaped muscle located beneath the lungs, contracts to create negative pressure during inspiration, enabling airflow into the thoracic cavity. This contraction increases the volume of the chest cavity, sucks air into the lungs, and provides oxygen entry with the removal of carbon dioxide. The chest wall, composed of rib cages, intercostal muscles, and associated structures, has structural support and helps with the expansion and contraction needed in breathing. This sophisticated coordination among the diaphragm and the chest wall is essential, as dysfunction in either can lead to serious respiratory comorbidities, highlighting their importance in facilitating proper respiratory function and overall wellness. In cases of respiratory disorders, the function of the diaphragm and chest wall becomes even more important. Conditions such as obesity, hypoventilation syndrome, or spinal cord injury can jeopardize the functioning of these tissues. As has been detailed in more recent studies, breathing disorders cannot just disrupt the mechanical process of respiration, but also affect physiological rhythms that foster cardiovascular health and overall health. For instance, dysregulation of the contraction of the diaphragm affects the equilibrium between oxygen and carbon dioxide levels in the body, leading to further complications such as respiratory failure or sleep hypoventilation. It is crucial to understand such dynamics in the development of effective intervention strategies, particularly in patients with varying degrees of respiratory dysfunction resulting from diaphragm and chest wall disorders (Barnes et al., 2014). Further, sleep-respiration interaction significantly emphasizes the diaphragm and chest wall mechanics, particularly in chronically respiratory-ill individuals. When resting, various nocturnal physiological changes influence ventilatory patterns, consequently affecting chest wall mechanics and the efficiency of gas exchange. Poor nocturnal ventilation can, therefore, lead to nocturnal hypoventilation and, in turn, complicate respiratory function and daytime quality of life. This condition emphasizes the role of therapeutic interventions like nocturnal nasal positive pressure ventilation (NIPPV), which is used to counteract the adverse effects of disrupted sleep breathing. Therapists must recognize, then, how respiratory events associated with sleep can have disastrous effects on daytime function. This recognition justifies the crucial role of the chest wall and diaphragm during both wakefulness and sleep and highlights their relevance to rehabilitative interventions (Piper et al., 1992).

Overview of Disorders Affecting These Structures

The chest wall and the diaphragm are integral components of the respiratory system, and disorders affecting these structures have the potential to produce serious respiratory dysfunction. Illnesses such as paralysis of the diaphragm due to neurological insult or mechanical compression prevent the diaphragm from contracting effectively. The defect leads to hypoventilation, reduced lung volume, and inefficient gas exchange. In addition, deformities of the chest wall, for example, scoliosis or pectus excavatum, may restrict the expansion of the thoracic cavity, further impairing ventilation. Such patients will report symptoms ranging from breathlessness to long-term respiratory failure, illustrating the impact of such disorders on overall well-being and quality of life. The relationship between obesity and respiratory function should also not be overlooked when evaluating diaphragmatic and chest wall disorders. Increased body fat, particularly within the thoracic region, can impede respiratory mechanics, leading to compromised lung function. A study examining the interrelation between percentage body fat and maximum expiratory flow strongly indicated that higher body fat does affect respiratory capacity, particularly in 10–12-year-old kids (Indahswari et al., 2019).

As excess weight exerts mechanical pressure on the diaphragm, it prevents movement, thus aggravating any concomitant respiratory disease and initiating a vicious cycle of declining pulmonary well-being. The therapy of obesity is therefore a vital component of the care of diaphragmatic and chest wall diseases. Along with that, sleep disorders have a profound influence on respiratory structure function, basically reorganizing gas exchange and overall health. Obstructive sleep apnea (OSA), for instance, may lead to nighttime hypoventilation and compromised gas exchange, ultimately manifesting as compromised daytime functioning and health. These are mainly induced by mechanical interruptions of the chest wall and diaphragm during sleep. NIPPV is an effective treatment strategy against such complications, helping to prevent worsening respiratory health at night (Piper et al., 1992). This technique not only alleviates nocturnal respiratory failure but also achieves maximum potential for rehabilitation in patients who are afflicted with underlying respiratory disease. Hence, integrating the best treatment for sleep-related respiratory disorders is essential in treating diaphragm and chest wall disorders (Figure 9.2).

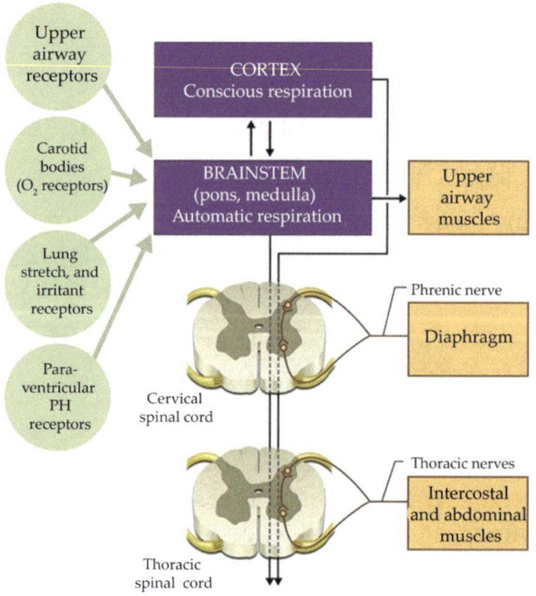

Figure 9.2. Disorders affecting the diaphragm and chest wall.

Source: https://thoracickey.com/wp-content/uploads/2016/06/B9780323082037000294_f029-001-9780323082037.jpg.

9.1. Anatomy of the Diaphragm

Learning Outcome

1. Structure and function of the diaphragm;
2. Innervation of the diaphragm;
3. Role of the diaphragm in breathing mechanics.

The diaphragm is the primary muscle of breathing, a dome-shaped membrane separating the thoracic cavity from the abdominal cavity. Its anatomy is important in that it has three primary components: the central tendon, muscle fibers, and lower rib and spinal attachments. The muscle fibers are both muscular and tendinous in character, originating from the xiphoid process, lower ribs, and lumbar vertebrae. When the diaphragm contracts, the central tendon flattens, tensing the thoracic cavity and facilitating inhalation. The action is vital to maintain gas exchange within the lungs, and limitation of diaphragm mobility can lead to serious respiratory ailments like hypoventilation and respiratory failure. Hence, comprehensive knowledge of diaphragm anatomy is essential in order to diagnose and manage associated pathologies that can be encountered in clinical practice. The function of the diaphragm is closely linked with respiratory mechanics and neuromuscular control. Innervation of the diaphragm is done by the phrenic nerve, which originates from cervical spinal roots C3 to C5. This nerve pathway is vital for coordinating the contraction of the diaphragm along with the respiratory cycle, which is primarily during inspiration. Disruptions of the signal of the phrenic nerve, either by injury, neurological disease, or systemic illness, could result in dysfunction of the diaphragm and produce respiratory problems. Diaphragmatic paralysis, for instance, can result from phrenic nerve damage, resulting in decreased lung volume and breathlessness. The chest wall can also have disorders such as scoliosis or muscular dystrophies, which restrict the movement of the diaphragm and hinder respiratory function. Hence, it is essential to have an association between neural control and diaphragm anatomy, which is most important in the diagnosis of respiratory disease. Awareness of anatomical variations in the diaphragm also improves discussion of pertinent clinical diseases.

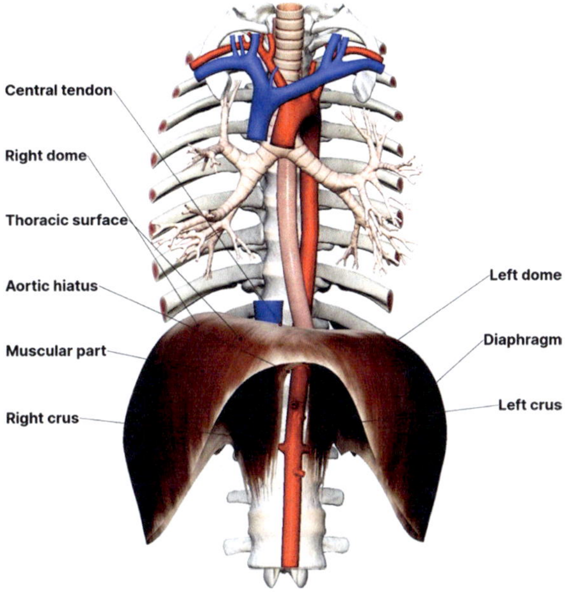

Figure 9.3. Anatomy of the diaphragm.

Source: https://anatomy.app/Media/slides/diaphragm-5-9477_medium.jpg.

The diaphragm can have anatomical faults, including congenital diaphragmatic hernias (CDHs), that can severely compromise respiratory function in neonates and require early surgical intervention. Also, dysfunctional mechanics of breathing because of diaphragm shapes and tones of abnormalities can potentially result in disorders such as obstructive sleep apnea, where the diaphragm fails to carry out effective ventilation when asleep. As respiratory physiology is dynamic in nature, alterations in diaphragm anatomy, like fibrosis or hypercurvature, may restrict effective tidal breathing patterns and sustain conditions like Parkinson's disease, where concomitant respiratory complications are common, including reduced lung capacity and abnormal breathing cycles. Therefore, an appreciation of the anatomical significance of the diaphragm for respiratory function capacity is essential for constructing purposeful therapeutic interventions against diaphragm and chest wall pathology (Arcieri et al., 2016; McGovern et al., 2020) (Figure 9.3).

9.1.1. Structure and Function of the Diaphragm

The diaphragm is a highly critical component of the respiratory system as the large muscle employed in inhalation and exhalation. Structurally, it is a dome-shaped sheet of muscle that separates the thoracic cavity from the abdominal cavity and consists of skeletal muscle fibers that facilitate both voluntary and involuntary movement. When the diaphragm contracts, it becomes flattened and descends, enlarging the volume of the thoracic cavity and generating a negative pressure that sucks air into the lungs. It is crucial not only for ventilation but also for ensuring proper gas exchange, as the movement of the diaphragms directly affects the influx of oxygen and the efflux of carbon dioxide. Diaphragmatic diseases, whether secondary to structural disease or muscular weakness, can tremendously impair this respiratory function and create significant clinical complications that underscore the diaphragm's critical position in respiratory physiology. The physiology of the diaphragm is inextricably bound to its anatomic structure and the muscle that envelops it. It is primarily innervated by the phrenic nerve, which is derived from the cervical spine (C3-C5) and has a vital role in motor control. Coordination of the diaphragm with accessory respiratory muscles such as the intercostals and the abdominal muscles is also crucial for effective breathing. The diaphragm's abnormal structure or neuromuscular function leads to ineffective ventilation and respiratory distress, particularly in conditions such as spinal muscular atrophy and amyotrophic lateral sclerosis. Davidescu et al. (2018) demonstrate that weakness of the respiratory muscles is a common cause of respiratory failure in neuromuscular diseases, which again highlights the significance of diaphragm integrity for optimal respiratory health. The recognition of these correlations highlights the diaphragm's significance not only in health but also in the pathophysiology of respiratory disease. In the examination of the clinical relevance of diaphragm dysfunction, several disorders can be identified that compromise its effectiveness. Disorders such as CDH, nerve injury-induced paralysis, or muscular dystrophies may lead to hypoventilation and impairment of gas exchange. Diaphragm dysfunction can present from exertional dyspnea to chronic exhaustion and reduced exercise tolerance.

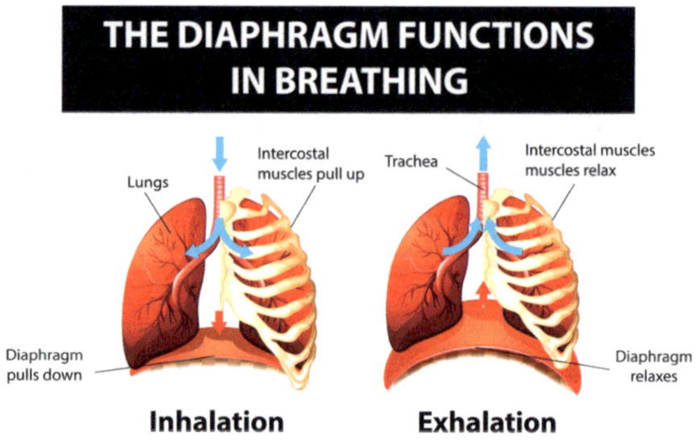

Figure 9.4. Structure and function of the diaphragm.

Source: https://img.freepik.com/free-vector/diaphragm-functions-breathing_1308-64803.jpg.

For patients with neuromuscular disease, as stated in Davidescu et al. (2018), respiratory muscle weakness may lead to chronic respiratory failure for which patients may need assistance through interventions such as noninvasive ventilation. Respiratory muscle function could be maximized by focused rehabilitation or surgery, leading to favorable effects on patient outcomes. Hence, understanding both the function and structure of the diaphragm becomes crucial when addressing the nuances of various respiratory ailments and creating effective treatment plans (Figure 9.4).

9.1.2. Innervation of the Diaphragm

The diaphragm, a muscular structure forming the base of the thoracic cavity, is extensively engaged in the act of respiration. Innervated primarily by the phrenic nerve, which originates from cervical spinal nerves C3 to C5, the diaphragm is responsible for the rhythm and volume of breathing. Disruptions in diaphragmatic innervation can cause respiratory disorders with a persistent effect on overall well-being. Spinal cord injury is but one disorder that can disrupt the neural flow of conducting respiratory impulses, leading to weakened or paralyzed diaphragm function. This disruption may lead to critical respiratory insufficiency, especially when injury occurs at more proximal cervical levels, which denervate not only the diaphragm but other significant respiratory muscles as well, thus complicating management of accompanying respiratory disorders. The coordination between diaphragm innervation and chest wall mechanics is a crucial element of respiratory function. Upon contraction of the diaphragm, negative intrathoracic pressure is created, thus allowing air to be inhaled into the lungs. Dysfunction of the diaphragm leads to ineffective ventilation patterns, with accessory muscles coming into action as a compensation mechanism, thus increasing the work of breathing. Neuromuscular patients, for instance, present with impaired respiratory function and trunk control due to deranged innervation, which further aggravates their breathing condition. Evidence of the interaction between trunk stability and diaphragmatic innervation suggests that any disruption in the optimal functioning of the diaphragm will have a cascading effect on respiratory health and postural control, as seen in spinal cord injury situations in children and adults (Singh et al., 2017). Recent evidence presents evidence of new interventions aimed at enhancing diaphragmatic function and overall respiratory capacity. Techniques such as abdominal binding have been attempted as mechanisms to optimize respiratory mechanics in patients with spinal cord injuries.

Research indicates that abdominal binding can maximize diaphragmatic movement by varying working lung volumes and elevating vital capacity, which are critical for effective breathing, especially with exercise (West et al., 2011). Such findings emphasize the importance of considering diaphragmatic innervation as a whole function rather than a single function, and as a component of a global respiratory strategy for the treatment of diaphragm and chest wall disorders. By considering the interdependence of innervation and mechanical function, medical professionals can develop targeted therapies to reverse the effects of respiratory loss in affected populations (Figure 9.5).

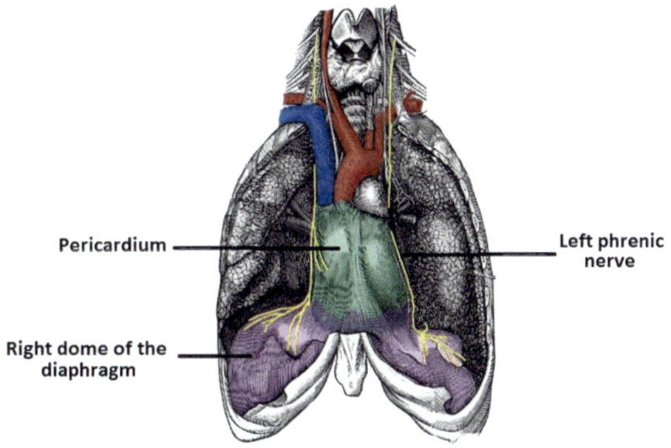

Figure 9.5. Innervation of the diaphragm.

Source: https://teachmeanatomy.info/wp-content/uploads/Phrenic-Nerve-Motor-Innervation-to-the-Diaphragm.jpg.

9.1.3. Role of the Diaphragm in Breathing Mechanics

The diaphragm is the primary breathing muscle and is significantly responsible for the mechanics of breathing. It takes the form of a dome-shaped structure positioned under the lungs and separating the thoracic cavity from the abdominal cavity. When it contracts, the diaphragm becomes flattened and the vertical height of the thoracic cavity increases, allowing air into the lungs. This negative pressure developed inside the thoracic compartment is essential for adequate ventilation. The diaphragm also assists by collaborating with accessory respiratory muscles, particularly during states of increased demand, such as exercise or respiratory distress. The diaphragm's maintenance of integrity is essential for effective ventilation and overall respiratory function, indicating its central role in the pathophysiology of most respiratory disorders. Diaphragmatic disorders can cause serious impairments in respiratory function.

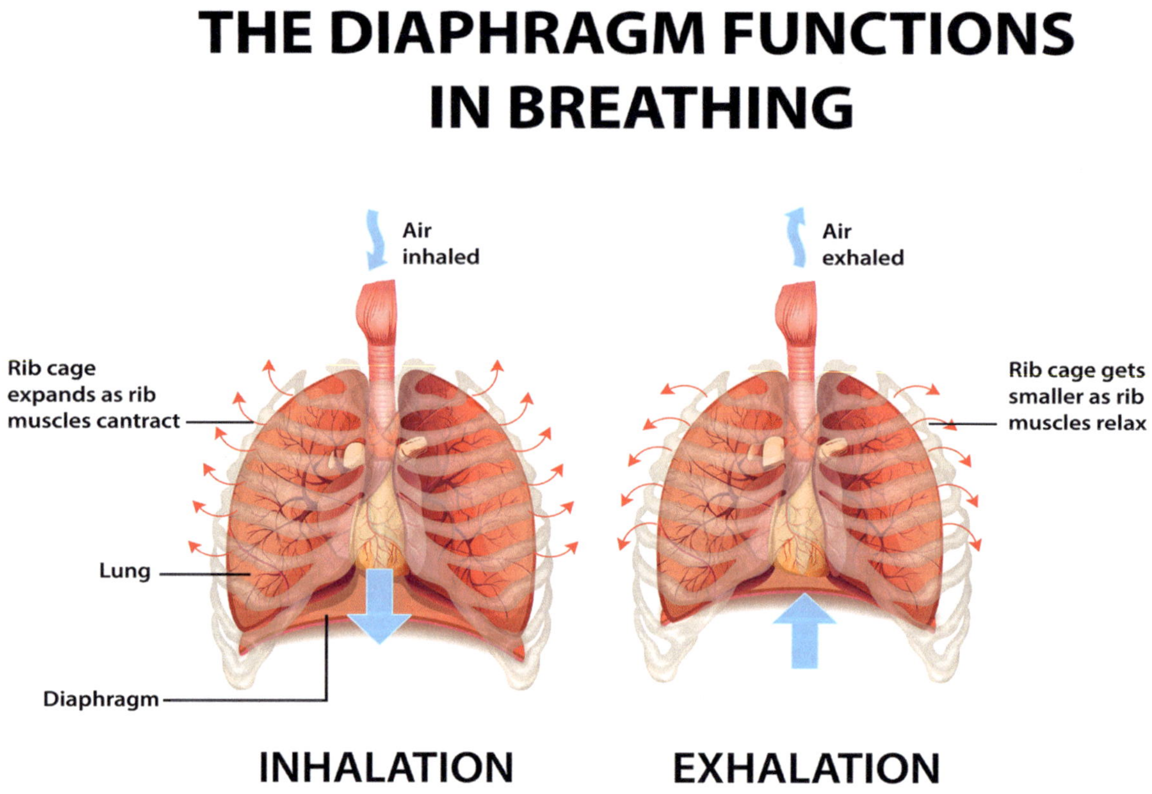

Figure 9.6. Role of the diaphragm in breathing mechanics.

Source: https://media.yogauonline.com/app/uploads/2023/02/27163516/2._the_diaphragm_functions_in_breathing_illustration_0.png.

Pathologies such as paralysis of the diaphragm can impair its contracting ability, which results in ineffective ventilation patterns. Ineffectiveness can cause hypercapnia and hypoxemia, also deteriorating the clinical condition of a patient. Moreover, the function of the diaphragm is of particular concern at night, when breathing mechanics can be altered due to changes in body position and muscle tone. Of particular interest is that sleep time is when the possibility of hypoventilation is high, as studies report a pivotal connection between nighttime respiratory disturbances and daytime functioning. Identification of such disruptions is crucial for medical workers because they significantly affect rehabilitation and the general well-being of patients (Piper et al., 1992). Additionally, the function of the accessory muscles enters the picture when the functioning of the diaphragm is impaired. Research has revealed that using respiratory accessory muscles can be beneficial for COPD patients. In a recent study, patients who received treatment aimed explicitly at stretching accessory muscles demonstrated increased chest expansion and decreased dyspnea (Anandh et al., 2016). This highlights the need for an integrated treatment approach, as improving respiratory muscle flexibility may alleviate some challenges presented by diaphragm disorders. Treatment of the groups of muscles together with the diaphragm can be best addressed by improving rehabilitation methods and exercise tolerance in cases of respiratory impairments, thus enhancing the quality of life (Figure 9.6).

Test Your Knowledge

1. Explain the structure and function of the diaphragm.
2. How does the diaphragm contribute to respiratory mechanics?

9.2. Anatomy of the Chest Wall

Learning Outcome

1. Structures of the chest wall;
2. Role of the chest wall in respiratory mechanics;
3. Interaction between the chest wall and diaphragm.

The chest wall is a protective shield that encloses significant thoracic organs, including the lungs and heart. Comprised primarily of ribs, intercostal muscles, and the sternum, this skeletal system is vital to breathing. The ribs, which attach both to the thoracic vertebrae and to the sternum, create a cage-like enclosure that not only supports the upper part of the body but also allows the lungs to expand and compress with each breath. Intercostal muscles, located between the ribs, contribute to the process of inhalation and exhalation through alteration in the volume of the thoracic space. Dysfunction or structural abnormality in this intricate anatomy can lead to severe respiratory impairment, highlighting the importance of understanding the chest wall in comparison to related disorders. Furthermore, the role of the diaphragm— a dome-shaped muscle at the bottom of the thoracic cavity— should not be overstressed in describing the mechanics of breathing and the pathophysiology of disorders of the same. As the master inspiration muscle, the diaphragm relaxes to increase the volume of the thoracic cavity, thereby lowering intrathoracic pressure to enable air to fill the lungs. Abnormalities in diaphragm function may lead to pathological conditions such as respiratory failure or chronic obstructive pulmonary disease (COPD), which drastically impair the mechanism of gas exchange. Research evidence supports diaphragm training and rehabilitation interventions in improving respiratory outcomes among specific populations, aligning with the need for targeted interventions to correct diaphragm activity dysfunction. These considerations demonstrate the interdependency between diaphragm health and overall pulmonary function. Lastly, the way anatomical structures interact with potential disorders validates the necessity for a comprehensive knowledge of the anatomy of the chest walls. Compression of the bronchi or pulmonary malformations may result from structural anomalies, with atelectasis or recurrent pneumonia ensuing. The relationship between elements of the chest wall and respiratory function validates the employment of the multidisciplinary approach in their management. Increased examination of diaphragm training and assessment strategies in athletic and rehabilitation settings, as presented through the experiences of sports medicine trainers, can yield valuable strategies in the treatment and rehabilitation of patients with chest wall disorders. Approaching these problems from a holistic perspective can lead to enhanced clinical outcomes, consistent with state-of-the-art practices in respiratory care (Arcieri et al., 2016; Foltz et al., 2016) (Figure 9.7).

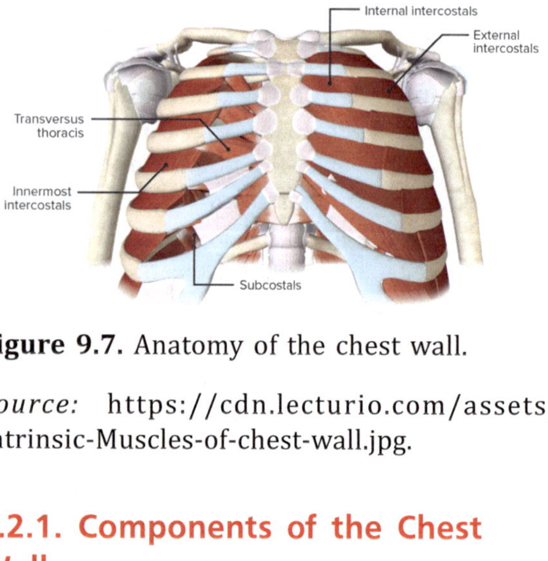

Figure 9.7. Anatomy of the chest wall.

Source: https://cdn.lecturio.com/assets/Intrinsic-Muscles-of-chest-wall.jpg.

9.2.1. Components of the Chest Wall

The chest wall is a significant body structure that plays a central role in respiratory mechanics, providing protective covering for the lungs and heart and enabling breathing. The chest wall, composed of bones, muscles, and connective tissue that form the rib cage, sternum, and diaphragm, acts together to offer effective pulmonary ventilation. The rib cage is composed of 12 pairs of posteriorly attached ribs to the thoracic vertebrae and arching around to the anterior. This allows for expansion and contraction of the rib cage with the respiratory cycle. The intercostal muscles between the ribs are also needed for breathing mechanics. During inhalation, they contract to elevate the rib cage, thereby increasing thoracic volume and lowering intrathoracic pressure. The diaphragm, situated at the base of the thoracic cavity, is the principal respiratory muscle, regulating the majority of inhalation. The bell-shaped muscle separates the thoracic cavity from the abdominal cavity and is under voluntary and automatic neural regulation. Diaphragmatic contraction flattens it and makes it move downward, creating an additional decrease in intrathoracic pressure and drawing in air into the lungs. Diaphragmatic dysfunction can lead to a variety of respiratory conditions, significantly impacting respiratory function. For instance, diaphragmatic paralysis can considerably hinder an individual's ability to breathe, leading to inadequate ventilation and thus respiratory distress. It is thus essential to appreciate the function of the diaphragm in relation to the chest wall so that one may diagnose and treat conditions arising from diaphragmatic dysfunction. Furthermore, the coordination of chest wall components and neuromuscular function underscores global assessment in clinical groups. Accompanying muscles, i.e., accessory abdominal and neck muscles, have the capacity to compensate in respiratory failure, a manifestation of the exquisite balance required to reach optimal breathing. Rehabilitation intervention may involve focused diaphragm training to optimize respiratory function and enhance overall pulmonary dynamics. There has been evidence of late from research that sporting trainers are increasingly cognizant of diaphragm training advantages in rehabilitation interventions for varied injuries and disorders, highlighting the muscle contribution to enhanced performance and recuperation (Foltz et al., 2016). As diaphragm and chest wall disorders continue to exist, for example, those noticed in neurological diseases like Parkinson's disease (McGovern et al., 2020), continuous research is needed to formulate the most effective treatment modalities for reclaiming normal respiratory function (Figure 9.8).

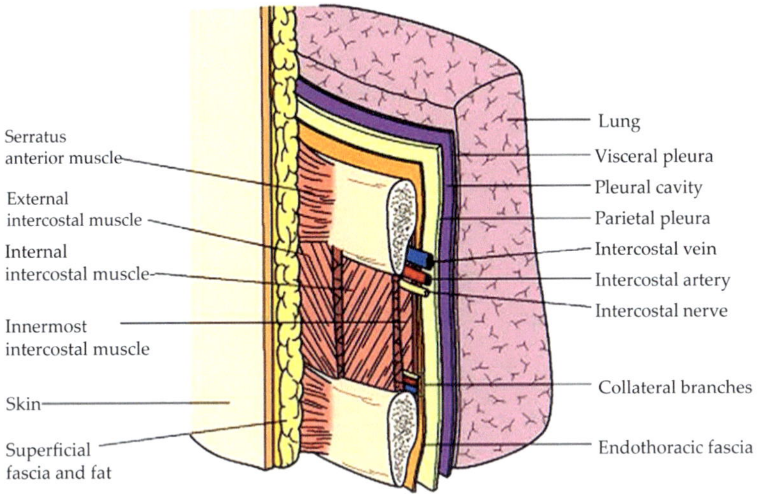

Figure 9.8. Components of the chest wall.

Source: https://radiologykey.com/wp-content/uploads/2018/10/C12-FF3-3.gif.

9.2.2. Function of the Chest Wall in Respiratory Mechanics

The chest wall has a significant role to play in the mechanics of breathing, allowing the expansion and contraction necessary for effective ventilation. Made up of the rib cage, sternum, and intercostal muscles, the chest wall acts as a protective framework and dynamic airflow regulator. During inspiration, the chest wall expands to allow the filling of the lungs with air. This reduction is enabled by synergistic action of the accessory muscles and diaphragm, which together decrease intrathoracic pressure to allow air entry into the lungs. The integrity of the chest wall is also basic to the best function of respiration, as disease of its structure or function will impair respiratory function severely. Coordination between the diaphragm and chest wall also contributes importantly to respiratory efficiency. The major muscle of respiration is the diaphragm, but it is assisted by the inspiratory chest wall muscles for its peak performance. Research has revealed that neuromechanical coupling (NMC) between muscle groups is essential for optimizing transdiaphragmatic pressure (Pdi) and respiratory mechanics in general. Enhanced function of the diaphragm measured both invasively and noninvasively can provide useful information about the respiratory health. As an example, noninvasive methods, such as sEMG, can provide information about the coordination of activity between the lower chest wall muscles and the diaphragm, helping to build insight into respiratory mechanics under conditions of loading (Petrocelli et al., 2019). Moreover, the proportional contributions of the chest wall and diaphragm to inspiratory pressures are significant in the evaluation of respiratory function, especially in disease states. Evidence is that maximal inspiratory pressure (PI,max) relies on the coordination between chest wall muscles and diaphragm. Inspiratory muscle training (IMT) has been shown to enhance PI,max, and thus targeted treatment could potentially contribute positively to respiratory strength and endurance. Importantly, a nuanced understanding of how chest wall mechanics affect diaphragm function can guide therapeutic approaches for respiratory disease. By addressing these interdependencies from a mechanical point of view, healthcare professionals can develop specific rehabilitation interventions to improve respiratory performance and improve patient outcomes (Brown et al., 2014) (Figure 9.9).

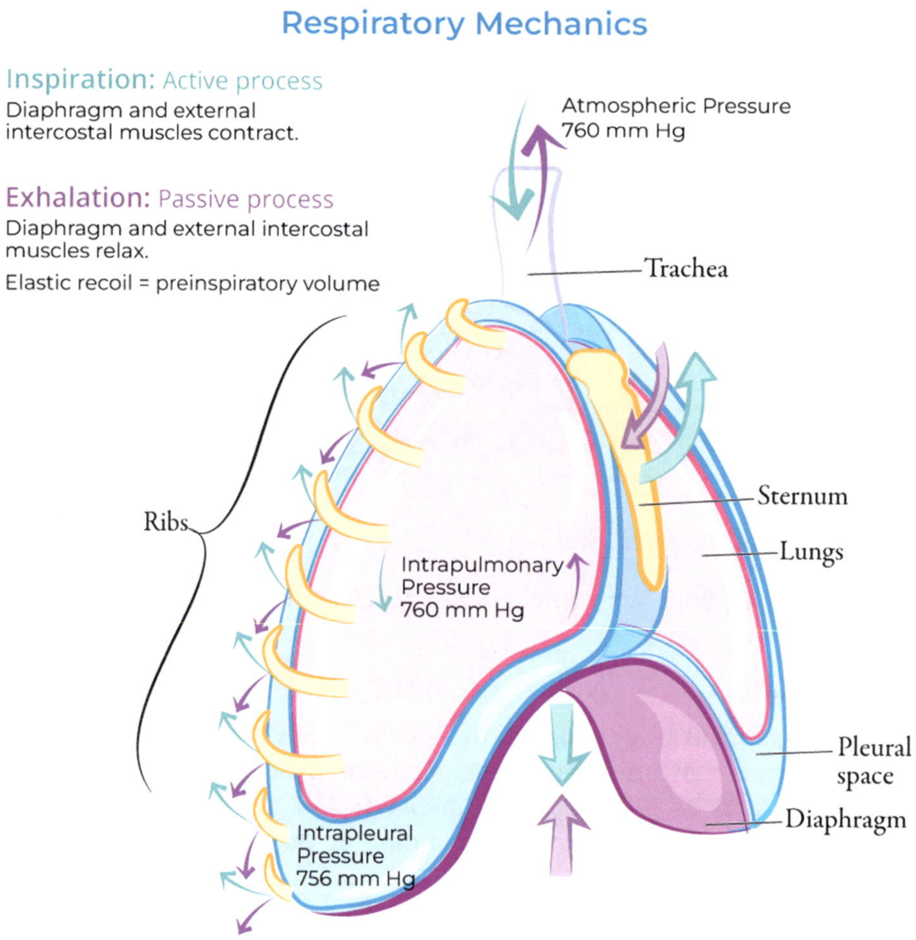

Figure 9.9. Function of the chest wall in respiratory mechanics.

Source: https://d1j63owfs0b5j3.cloudfront.net/term/images/respiratory-mechanics-1616.png.

9.2.3. Interaction Between the Chest Wall and Diaphragm

The intricate interaction of the chest wall and diaphragm is an elementary aspect of respiratory mechanics. The diaphragm, a dome-shaped muscle at the bottom of the thoracic cavity, plays a vital role in enabling inhalation through its contraction, which lowers pressure in the thoracic cavity and enables air to be drawn into the lungs. Together, the chest wall, which consists of ribs, intercostal muscles, and the sternum, provides structural support and protection to the thoracic cavity. Coordination between these two components is essential not only for respiration in a normal fashion but also for the best production of voice. For instance, alterations in chest wall motion can have a significant impact on diaphragmatic function and thereby predispose one to respiratory dysfunction. An understanding of how these interact is critical to the diagnosis and treatment of respiratory pathology, as deranged mechanics can exacerbate conditions such as diaphragmatic paralysis or restrictive lung disease. Furthermore, the interaction of the diaphragm, chest wall, and outcome with regard to performance cannot be overlooked, most particularly in applications such as speech and song. Diaphragm disorders can manifest as symptoms that affect effective communication, especially due to the crucial role the two segments play in developing adequate airflow. Empirical research has indicated that some therapeutic approaches aimed at promoting intercostal stretch and chest mobility have been found to yield positive outcomes in speech performance, particularly among the spastic cerebral palsy group, as demonstrated in improvements uncovered in sound pressure level and syllables per breath unit in a recent study (Varnado et al., 2015). This connection highlights the importance of understanding the biomechanical relationship between the diaphragm and chest wall, as therapy of these areas can lead to improved respiratory function and communicative abilities. Psychological factors, such as anxiety, may also have a substantial role in influencing the interaction of the diaphragm and chest wall, leading to constriction and dysfunction. For the performer, such as the singer and musician, the experience of Music Performance Anxiety can be the physical tension that disrupts breath control and vocal production. The subsequent chest constriction from anxiety restricts effective diaphragmatic movement, thereby ending the capacity to breathe deeply and phonate for an extended period. Identifying the role of anxiety in conjunction with breathing biomechanics highlights the importance of treating psychological and physiological factors when dealing with diaphragm and chest wall disorders. By highlighting growing awareness in breathing mechanics and relaxation, performers can rid themselves of the disabling symptoms attributed to anxiety, ultimately leading to improved performance outcomes in clinical and artistic contexts (Zecher et al., 2018).

Test Your Knowledge

1. What are the chest wall structures?
2. What are the functions of the chest wall in respiratory physiology?

9.3. Common Disorders of the Diaphragm

Learning Outcome

1. Diaphragmatic paralysis;
2. Diaphragmatic hernia;
3. Eventration of the diaphragm.

The diaphragm, an essential muscle involved in respiration, may be subject to a variety of disorders that lead to serious respiratory complications. The most common diaphragmatic disorder is muscular dystrophy, which is a collection of inherited myopathies with progressive muscle weakness, including respiratory muscles. Its impact on respiratory function is severe and results in respiratory failure, which ultimately becomes the most important cause of mortality in such patients. Diaphragmatic dysfunction contributes to the restrictive pulmonary pattern due to increased workload on the respiratory apparatus, decreased lung compliance, and diminished ventilatory drive, necessitating advanced management interventions. The nature and pattern of respiratory symptoms could vary significantly based on the type of muscular dystrophy involved, which emphasizes the use of tailored clinical strategies in management of these patients (Aliverti et al., 2016).

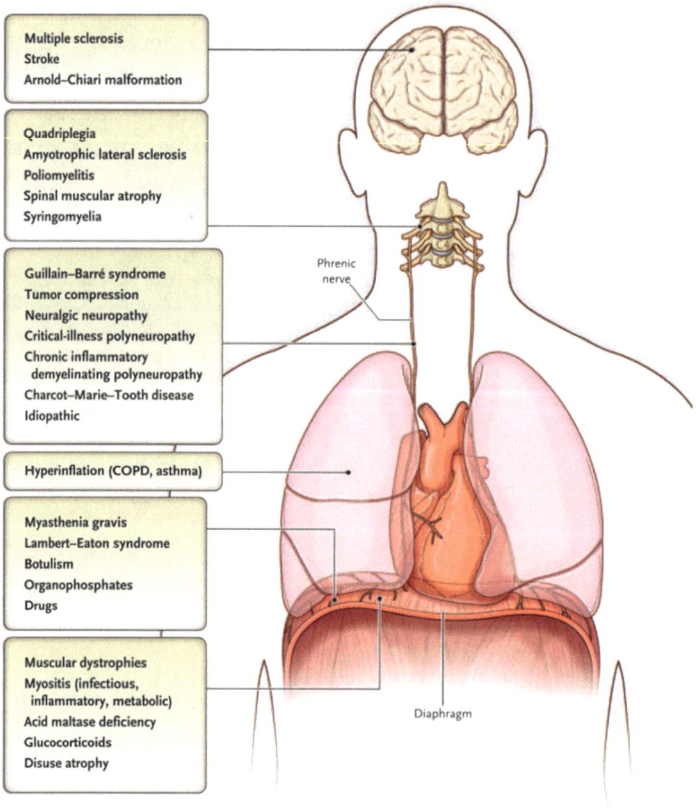

Figure 9.10. Name of the disorders of the diaphragm.

Source: https://www.nejm.org/cms/10.1056/NEJMra1007236/asset/1e4e3eff-55f1-48e8-96b4-5f97359c0d0e/assets/images/large/nejmra1007236_f3.jpg.

Another significant disorder that is associated with diaphragm dysfunction is diaphragmatic paralysis, which neurological illness, surgical complications, or trauma may cause. It is characterized by the inability to contract the diaphragm effectively during inhalation, leading to hypoventilation and eventual impairment of respiration. Patients with paralysis of the diaphragm generally have a characteristic pattern of breathing involving heavy use of the accessory respiratory muscles and reduced diaphragmatic movement. The assessment of diaphragm functioning has become more advanced, with added indices like diaphragm NMC providing insight into the efficiency of diaphragm activation as well as respiratory mechanics in general. The application of both invasive and non-invasive measurements has improved the interpretation of diaphragm functioning, particularly when handling neuromuscular diseases (Petrocelli et al., 2019). The effect of diaphragm disorders goes beyond respiratory function, significantly impacting the quality of life and overall health status. In patients with chronic respiratory issues secondary to diaphragm dysfunction, symptoms such as dyspnea, ineffective cough, and hypoventilation make daily living difficult. In addition, there is a present risk for sleep-disordered breathing too, which makes health issues more complicated. Effective management strategies demand multidisciplinary interventions, including respiratory therapy, drug therapy, and, in some cases, surgery such as diaphragmatic pacing or repair. Better comprehension of the pathophysiology of these diseases can lead to better clinical outcomes, emphasizing the importance of continued research and patient education to minimize the effect of diaphragm disorders on individual health and quality of life (Aliverti et al., 2016) (Figure 9.10).

9.3.1. Diaphragmatic Paralysis

Diaphragmatic paralysis, a significant disorder of respiratory mechanics, frequently occurs as a result of more than one etiology, including trauma, neurologic disease, or surgery. This presentation is defined by failure of the diaphragm to contract during inspiration adequately and will lead to compromised ventilation and resultant respiratory distress. As a result, patients may present with symptoms such as shortness of breath, particularly on exertion, and sleep disturbance secondary to apnea-related frequent wakefulness. The pathophysiology of diaphragmatic paralysis highlights the critical function of the diaphragm as a primary muscle of respiration, as its malfunction dramatically deforms airflow and gas exchange dynamics within the lung. This dysfunction can also cause the development of secondary complications, i.e., atelectasis and pulmonary infections, which further complicate the clinical situation and highlight the need for early diagnosis and intervention. Imaging modalities and pulmonary function tests are basically used for the detection and assessment of diaphragmatic paralysis. X-rays may reveal a paradoxical motion of the diaphragm with respiration, and more advanced imaging, such as ultrasound, can provide a real-time assessment of diaphragmatic function. Pulmonary function tests may measure the degree of respiratory impairment by measurement of vital capacity and flow rates. A polysomnography study is also often ordered to assess for secondary obstructive sleep apnea, which is often found in conjunction with diaphragmatic disease. Research establishes that postoperative care can be significantly enhanced by utilizing surgical procedures like diaphragmatic plication for individuals with accompanying sleep disorders. This illustrates how diaphragm functionality is linked to general respiratory well-being (Afsar et al., 2016). Management practices are essential in reducing respiratory complications and enhancing the ability of patients to conduct their daily activities. In addition, the effects of diaphragmatic paralysis extend beyond individual respiratory symptoms to impact global health and quality of life. The mutual interaction between the diaphragm and other chest structures, including lungs and chest wall, can lead to altered biomechanics to compromise pulmonary rehabilitation. For lung transplantation, for example, any preexisting diaphragmatic dysfunction will adversely influence surgical outcome by compromising graft performance and patient recovery (Grasselli et al., 2024). Increased understanding of the role of the diaphragm in the physiology of respiration and its relation to other systems offers possibilities for enhanced care and surgical management. Ultimately, treatment of paralysis of the diaphragm needs an integrated method involving immediate support for respiration through to long-term management as a way of maximizing lung function and enhancing the quality of life of the patient (Figure 9.11).

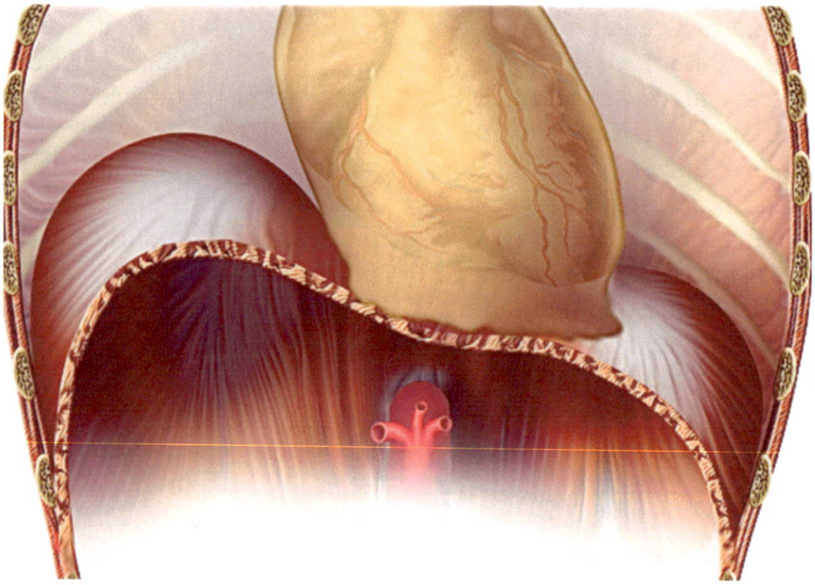

Figure 9.11. Diaphragmatic paralysis.

Source: https://middenrifcentrum.nl/wp-content/uploads/2022/04/middenrif-2.png.

9.3.2. Diaphragmatic Hernia

Diaphragmatic hernia is an anatomic fault with an abnormal opening of the diaphragm, through which abdominal visceral organs herniate into the thoracic cavity. Neonates have a high prevalence of this condition, in which CDH results from failure of the diaphragm to develop normally in embryonic life. These failures will have grave consequences for the respiratory system, most notably pulmonary hypoplasia, in which underdeveloped lungs limit oxygen intake and overall pulmonary function (N/A, 2021). The clinical presentation of diaphragmatic hernias will probably be in the form of respiratory distress shortly after birth and will require emergency treatment. Understanding the embryological pathogenesis of the condition is crucial for formulating treatment plans and appropriate antenatal management, which can subsequently have a significant prognostic effect on infants with this problem. The diagnosis of diaphragmatic hernia has evolved with advances in imaging technologies, particularly multi-detector computed tomography (MDCT). MDCT is an imaging modality that provides precise anatomical assessments and better demonstrates diaphragmatic defects and variations. By categorizing diaphragmatic appearances based not only on axial images but also sagittal reformatted images, MDCT provides critical information regarding the nature of defects (Elhamd et al., 2011). This enhanced visualization allows for hernia types to be differentiated and to identify their respective complications, hence enabling improved surgical planning. Also, the ability of MDCT in detecting and demonstrating structural variations of the diaphragm highlights its importance in delivering accurate diagnoses that are crucial for the treatment of such life-threatening conditions in clinical practice. Diaphragmatic hernia is treated primarily with surgery, with the ultimate goal of returning abdominal contents to normal anatomical positions and repairing the diaphragmatic lesion.

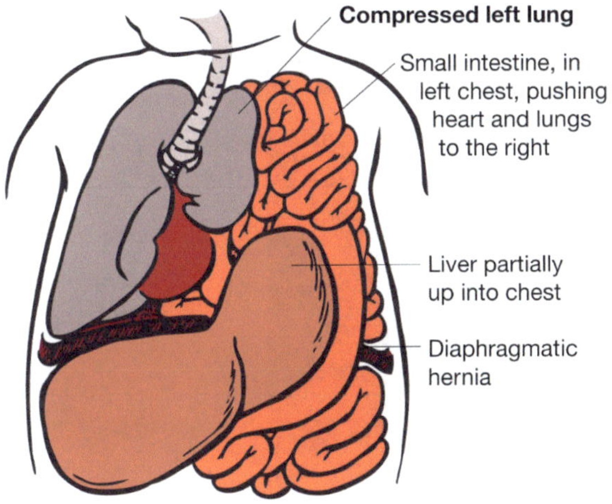

Figure 9.12. Diaphragmatic hernia.

Source: https://external-content.duckduckgo.com/iu/?u=https%3A%2F%2Ffetus.ucsf.edu%2Fuploads%2Fcdh.jpg&f=1&nofb=1&ipt=b25190cc857786761c151eaabaad289c21bfa7cca05274fb03414264246dc6e8.

Timing and type of corrective surgery are based on the status of the patients and degree of respiratory distress. Advances in minimally invasive surgical methods have shown promise to reduce postoperative complications, extend recovery periods, and improve overall outcomes in CDH patients (N/A, 2021). The complexities associated with this condition, however, extend far beyond surgical correction to include follow-up for an extended period to assess pulmonary function and monitor for potential complications. Due to the multifactorial etiology of diaphragmatic hernias, a multidisciplinary treatment involving pediatricians, surgeons, and respiratory medicine experts is essential to provide complete care to the affected patients throughout their lifespan (Figure 9.12).

9.3.3. Eventration of the Diaphragm

Eventration of the diaphragm is an underdiagnosed but clinically important disorder that impairs respiratory function. This condition occurs when the diaphragm, a muscle that aids in inhalation through contraction, is found to be abnormally positioned above instead of descending during respiration. This dislocation causes some significant clinical presentations such as dyspnea, fatigue, and compromised exercise tolerance. It is essential to be aware of the causative factors to ensure effective management. Eventration can occur due to several etiologies including neurological conditions, congenital malformations, and trauma. These are the causes of a dysbalance in muscle dynamics that disrupt regular thoracic mechanics, leading to compromised pulmonary functioning and the forced dislodgement of vital organs within the thoracic cavity. Clinical treatment of eventration of the diaphragm is most often a multidisciplinary approach, particularly when cases involving obstructive sleep apnea (OSA) are being weighed. It has been demonstrated in recent studies that the incidence of OSA in patients with diaphragmatic pathologies supports the interconnection of respiratory disease. It was quoted in one study that a significant percentage of patients presenting with diaphragmatic dysfunction also exhibited symptoms associated with sleep disorders, which required polysomnography before surgical intervention. Indeed, the linkage between sleep apnea and sustainable respiratory parameters indicates the broader implications of diaphragm disease on everyday quality of life. Treatment of these complications not only improves respiratory function but, more importantly, patient well-being overall by correcting concomitant conditions, making the clinical picture worse. Of course, accurate diagnosis of diaphragm eventration may be obscured by misinterpretation of imaging. For instance, a case report described how eventration may be localized and can create an imaging look of pleural effusion on chest radiographs. In this case, a patient with dyspnea and an initial clinical presentation of pleural effusion, according to preliminary imaging, was found to have diaphragm eventration through more intensive evaluation using spiral CT scans. These cases accentuate the necessity of thorough assessment and appropriate imaging techniques to avoid unwarranted interventions like thoracentesis, which can lead to complications when performed on a misdiagnosed effusion. Effective diagnosis and management are dependent on clinicians noticing subtleties of diaphragm pathology, applying targeted interventions that optimize respiratory function and avoid relapsing symptoms (Figure 9.13).

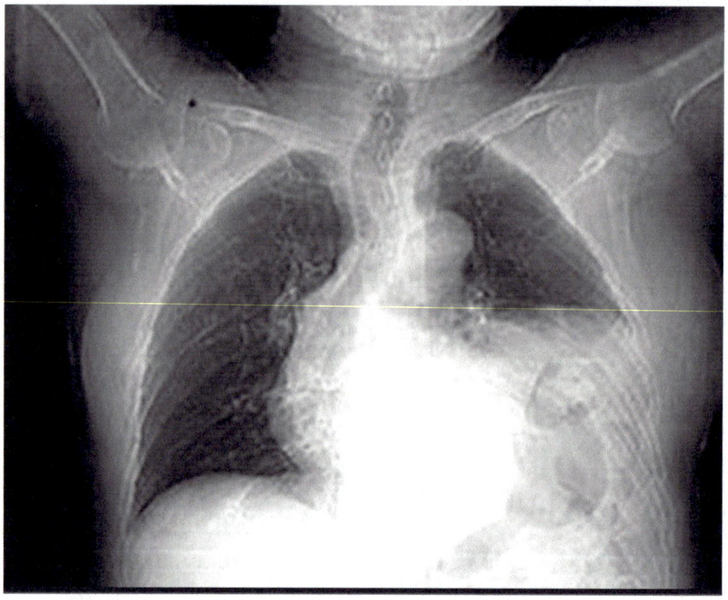

Figure 9.13. Eventration of the diaphragm.

Source: https://external-content.duckduckgo.com/iu/?u=https%3A%2F%2Fcasereports.bmj.com%2Fcontent%2Fcasereports%2F2013%2Fbcr-2013-008613%2FF1.large.jpg%3Fdownload%3Dtrue&f=1&nofb=1&ipt=d11733c39b4848e8635e88e3cdb9cb9ac7b447ec6464c2990a3ece6785c5492e.

Test Your Knowledge

1. What is diaphragmatic paralysis?
2. What is a diaphragmatic hernia?

9.4. Common Disorders of the Chest Wall

Learning Outcome

1. Pectus excavatum;
2. Pectus carinatum;
3. Rib fractures and their implications.

The chest wall is a vital component in respiratory function, and its disorder may significantly impair the mechanics of breathing. The most common chest wall disorders are scoliosis, kyphosis, and muscular dystrophies of various forms. Scoliosis, or a lateral abnormal thoracic spinal curvature, can compromise lung volume by restricting thoracic capacity, thereby affecting effective ventilation. In addition, kyphosis, in the form of a severe forward thoracic spinal curvature, can also impair respiratory mechanics. The structural abnormality often manifests as chest wall stiffness, affecting the positioning of respiratory muscles and resulting in ineffective respiratory patterns. All of these deformities combined can reduce oxygen uptake, leading to states of hypoxia, which immediately correlate with postural abnormality and respiratory dysfunction. Muscular dystrophies, a group of inherited disorders characterized by progressive muscle weakening and wasting, also bring their own complexities to normal function of the chest wall. In these conditions, respiratory muscles can be compromised, leading to reduced strength in the diaphragm and intercostal muscles. Therefore, individuals can experience respiratory failure due to a lack of muscle strength, rather than actual lung disease. Such an increase in load against which these muscles act can increase the work of breathing and lead to hypoventilation and impairment of gas exchange. Of specific interest is the impact of muscular dystrophy on respiratory function, which is multifaceted and manifests as a series of disorders that may impact restrictive pulmonary function, sleep-disordered breathing, and compromised cough reflexes, further complicating the clinical picture (Aliverti et al., 2016). Besides structural defects and muscle disease, the chest wall may be affected by traumatic injuries and inflammatory disorders. Rib fractures, for instance, not only lead to acute pain but also to altered respiration mechanics. The resulting respiratory distress is actually able to induce shallow breathing patterns, which compromise proper lung expansion, potentially leading to pneumonia and other respiratory complications. Inflammatory processes, such as pleuritis or costochondritis, can further produce pain and restricted movement, directly affecting respiratory dynamics. These conditions underscore the importance of recognizing the signs and implications of chest wall disorders in overall respiratory function. Thorough assessments and particularly targeted interventions, therefore, become crucial in managing these disorders to prevent long-term sequelae (Petrocelli et al., 2019).

9.4.1. Pectus Excavatum

Pectus excavatum, generally referred to as a concave deformity of the chest wall, is the most common congenital deformity of the chest wall, having a significant impact on both physical appearance and physiological functioning. The deformity results from abnormal growth of the rib cage, leading to depression of the sternum. Although most individuals have uncomplicated mild cases, moderate to severe types can present with significant cardiopulmonary hindrances. Symptoms typically include exercise intolerance, chest pain, and psychosocial issues as a result of the cosmetic impact of the deformity. Pectus excavatum has also been associated with other connective tissue diseases, which should be assessed to rule out underlying conditions that could complicate the treatment outcome and long-term prognosis (Messineo et al., 2013). Pectus excavatum is primarily treated using two kinds of therapy: non-surgical and surgical interventions. Non-operative techniques, such as the application of external vacuum-assisted devices or bracing, are typically indicated for mild cases, especially in children with developing skeletal systems. Surgical repair, frequently through the Nuss procedure or the Ravitch operation, then became the standard of care for more severe instances.

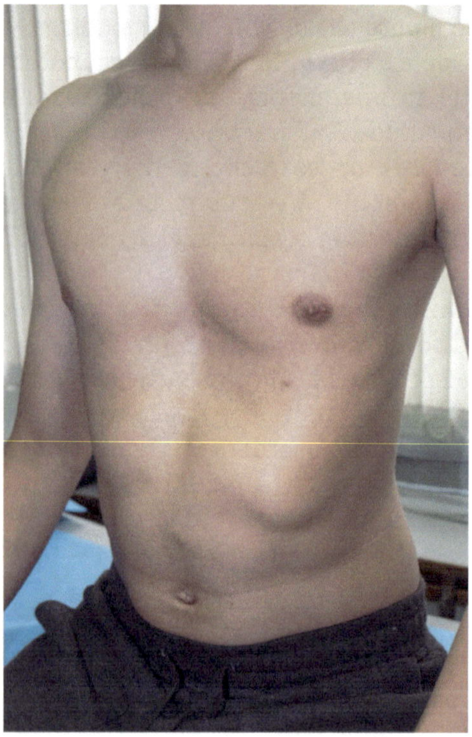

Figure 9.14. Pectus excavatum.

Source: https://external-content.duckduckgo.com/iu/?u=https%3A%2F%2Fwww.verywellhealth.com%2Fthmb%2FhGWBrD0OFilBm8Eqn3W9jLyuuUM%3D%2F1500x0%2Ffilters%3Ano_upscale()%3Amax_bytes(150000)%3Astrip_icc()%2FGettyImages-955109626-4b3292cc1af6404d8e85bd1145bd1193.jpg&f=1&nofb=1&ipt=56a669206170189b8fc4e6f8174e4d91bdd6b4625789888e3b6ff90cb297bc8f.

These treatments not only aim to enhance the cosmetic appearance of the chest walls but also to ensure improved respiratory function and quality of life. Despite the proven effectiveness of surgery, concerns regarding postoperative complications and psychological effects on the patient continue to affect debate on the most appropriate course of action in patients with pectus excavatum (Mompart et al., 2024). The relationship between pectus excavatum and associated disorders of the connective tissue contributes to the challenging nature of successfully treating the condition. Pectus excavatum patients may also have other disorders such as Marfan syndrome or Ehlers-Danlos syndrome that contribute to the complexity of their treatment. These comorbidities demand a multidisciplinary plan of management involving cardiology and genetic advice to assess for potential cardiovascular abnormalities and integrity of the connective tissue. As research continues, understanding the biological basis and implications of these correlations will be crucial for directing clinical management strategy. Treatment of pectus excavatum, in the end, not only improves physical deformity but also significantly affects overall health status and psychosocial functioning (Messineo et al., 2013) (Figure 9.14).

9.4.2. Pectus Carinatum

Pectus carinatum, or pigeon chest, is a classic chest wall deformity that consists of the abnormal forward protrusion of the sternum and the ribs. Pectus carinatum can have serious respiratory consequences and is often found to be associated with many genetic diseases, including Osteogenesis Imperfecta (OI). This underlying chest wall deformity due to the OI patient can result in functional impairments like decreased tidal volume and paradoxical rib cage motion during ventilation, which not only contaminates lung mechanics but also makes the patient susceptible to respiratory infections and overall cardiopulmonary insufficiency. Understanding the impact of pectus carinatum on integrated treatment planning is crucial, particularly for children whose chest wall deformities may be altered with time and influence their physical functioning and psychosocial adjustment. Pectus carinatum pathophysiology is multifactorial and an interaction of complex genetic susceptibility, biomechanical stress during growth and development, and alterations in collagen production. OI patients, especially those with a more severe type III, exhibit characteristic aspects of pectus carinatum, including accentuated thoraco-abdominal asynchrony and rib cage deformities. These structural changes have a considerable influence on the respiratory patterns and muscle coordination needed for effective ventilation. Studies have shown the need for cautious assessment and targeted interventions that encompass not only the physical deformity itself, but also the disabling breathing effects associated with such chest wall abnormalities. Therefore, identification and dissolution of pectus carinatum among chest wall deformities are of utmost importance to ensure optimal quality of life and to prevent other issues regarding respiratory health. Early identification and treatment of pectus carinatum are necessary, primarily due to its association with impaired respiratory function and psychosocial distress in patients, particularly children and adolescents. Although surgery is successful, it may not be appropriate for all patients, especially those with comorbidities of disease like OI, where perioperative morbidity can be considerable. Non-operative treatments, such as orthotic treatment and physical therapy, can be utilized as a first-line intervention to improve chest wall symmetry and function. Moreover, multidisciplinary management including orthopedists and pulmonologists is required in order to monitor cardiopulmonary status of the patients because those respiratory complications associated with pectus carinatum may have a significant role in long-term results in patients with disorders like OI. An appropriate understanding of the condition is necessary to provide proper management and rehabilitation plans to the concerned individuals (Figure 9.15).

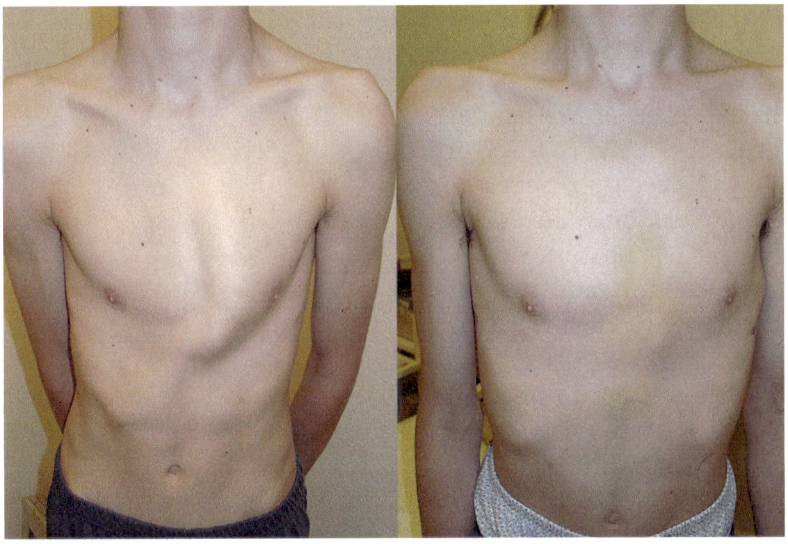

Figure 9.15. Pectus carinatum.

Source: https://external-content.duckduckgo.com/iu/?u=https%3A%2F%2Fels-jbs-prod-cdn.jbs.elsevierhealth.com%2Fcms%2Fattachment%2F7acbc5db-e8a1-4a4e-93e4-6624be5a2f41%2Fgr4_lrg.jpg&f=1&nofb=1&ipt=a3434c71ec27234637e78cfc360d0bd9608d91127b16e378fe9c0de6d0823729.

9.4.3. Rib Fractures and Their Implications

Rib fractures are one of the primary concerns in the case of chest wall disorders, as they can lead to a variety of acute and chronic respiratory function-related complications, as well as overall health problems. The most significant effects of rib fractures are their potential to compromise the integrity of the rib cage, which protects vulnerable organs such as the lungs and heart. Rib fractures may also lead to significant pain, which can discourage effective deep breathing and result in hypoventilation. This disrupted breathing pattern can then heighten the likelihood of respiratory complications such as pneumonia and atelectasis. Where there are several fractures or displaced fragments, the risk of progressing complications is heightened. It requires vigilance in assessment and, in certain instances, surgical intervention to stabilize the chest wall and restore optimal respiratory mechanics. Rib fractures have implications that extend beyond transient pain and distress and often impact long-term pulmonary function and rehabilitation outcomes. In some patients with existing conditions, such as OI, where the geometry of the rib cage is pre-existing, rib fractures aggravate such respiratory conditions. According to research, severe OI type III patients not only exhibit reduced tidal volumes but also present with paradoxical rib cage motion during respiration, and this may lead to disturbed ventilation patterns (Aliverti et al., 2012). Patients with severe OI type III are most susceptible to restrictive lung disease since having rib fractures and sternal abnormalities drastically impairs the respiratory muscle efficiency. Thus, rehabilitation in such patients ought to aim not only at the short-term effects of fractures but also at the long-term consequences on chest wall physiology. Moreover, diagnostic care of rib fractures requires interdisciplinary intervention to check chest wall complications. Advanced imaging techniques, such as computed tomography and ultrasound, allow for accurate determination of the extent of rib injury and identification of concomitant damage to surrounding tissue (N/A, 2021). These comprehensive assessments are required to develop individualized treatment programs that involve pain management, respiratory therapy, and surgery if needed. Compliance with an integrated system that accounts for both the structural and functional consequences of rib fractures enables practitioners to improve patient outcomes significantly. Preservation of lung function and volume following rib fractures is critical, particularly in the presence of pre-existing illness, thus highlighting the importance of effective interventional and diagnostic techniques in managing chest wall and diaphragmatic disorders (Figure 9.16).

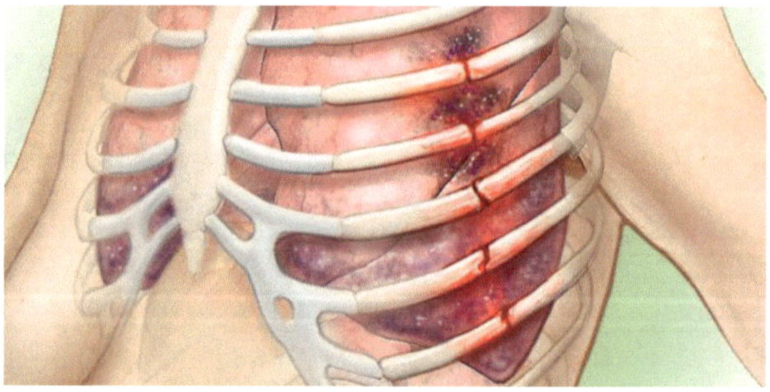

Figure 9.16. Rib fracture.

Source: https://external-content.duckduckgo.com/iu/?u=http%3A%2F%2Fiytmed.com%2Fwp-content%2Fuploads%2F2015%2F11%2F6_rib-fracture.jpg&f=1&nofb=1&ipt=e4e4499a0b86510106d340fc09c42aad73ebd96ec48fa9b34b169a64ed25789f.

Test Your Knowledge

1. What is pectus excavatum?
2. What are the rib fractures and their implications?

9.5. Diagnostic Approaches

Learning Outcome

1. Imaging modalities (X-ray, CT, MRI);
2. Pulmonary function tests;
3. Clinical assessment and history taking.

In diagnosing diaphragmatic and chest wall disorders, an accurate diagnostic workup is critical for adequately evaluating and treating these conditions. A clean history and physical are typically a part of the initial evaluation, used to provoke symptoms like dyspnea, pain, or abnormal respiratory patterns. Imaging modalities subsequently play a crucial role in outlining internal pathology. The application of standard modalities like CT scans and chest X-rays is prevalent; however, advancements in technology, particularly in magnetic resonance imaging (MRI), are revolutionizing diagnostic techniques. One of the benefits of MRI is that its technology is non-radiation, which is advantageous for vulnerable individuals such as children and pregnant women. As noted in various studies, MRI not only provides accurate morphological information but also quantifies functional respiratory mechanics, with the possibility of further information regarding disorders of the chest wall and diaphragmatic disease (Hebestreit et al., 2011). Aside from imaging tests, functional tests are essential in understanding diaphragm involvement in respiratory disease. Techniques such as ultrasound and electromyography can provide valuable information about diaphragmatic innervation and movement. Ultrasound, for instance, allows real-time visualization of diaphragm movement during breathing and can identify paralysis or dysfunction. Electromyography assists in the evaluation of neuromuscular function, an important consideration in suspected diaphragm dysfunction due to neurological disease or postoperative issues. Pulmonary function tests (PFTs) also determine the impact of diaphragm and chest wall dysfunction on overall lung capacity and efficacy in gas exchange. By integrating these unrelated diagnostic modalities, clinicians can formulate a clearer concept of disease process and devise a more effective treatment strategy for diaphragm and chest wall abnormalities. In addition, the interaction between diaphragmatic function and operative interventions, such as lung transplantation, underscores the need for more rigorous diagnostic criteria. The pre- and postoperative status of the diaphragm may influence outcomes dramatically, with surgical trauma and altered mechanics possibly influencing respiratory function. The lack of a standardized evaluation method makes it to assess diaphragmatic dysfunction in this context, and less-than-ideal management strategies may result. Current literature suggests that awareness of such complexities is needed to enhance patient care. With ongoing research, the integration of evolving multimodal diagnostic techniques will be crucial in resolving the multifaceted function of the diaphragm and its influence on respiratory disease pathophysiology, as well as outcomes following surgery (Grasselli et al., 2024).

9.5.1. Imaging Techniques (X-Ray, Computed Tomography (CT), Magnetic Resonance Imaging (MRI))

Imaging modalities are crucial for the diagnosis and treatment of diaphragmatic and chest wall diseases. X-ray imaging continues to be the modality of choice when imaging these regions because of its ubiquitous availability and expeditious performance. X-rays yield valuable structural information, including abnormalities such as elevation or paralysis of the diaphragm as a result of phrenic nerve trauma or hernia formation. Although X-rays can, however, serve to determine gross anatomical alterations, they are usually not satisfactory in assessing subtle pathologies such as minor disruption of muscle or incipient tumors. Thus, while X-ray imaging is a suitable screening method, it is often supplemented by more advanced techniques to yield the integral diagnostic data necessary for treating involved diaphragm and chest wall disorders. CT extends the imaging capability beyond the reach of X-rays, such as a three-dimensional perspective that significantly helps evaluate disorders of the diaphragm and associated chest wall abnormalities. CT scans provide accurate visualization of the diaphragm anatomy and enable the diagnosis of diaphragmatic hernias not visible on an X-ray. CT is also handy to define the extent of tumor or pathology that may involve the diaphragm and adjacent thoracic structures. Its high-resolution imaging quality allows it to be used for accurate lesion classification, which aids in surgical planning and intervention. CT has thereby emerged as the cornerstone of thoracic imaging, yielding valuable information required for the management of various respiratory and chest wall diseases. MRI is increasingly recognized as a valuable adjunct modality in diaphragm and chest wall pathology diagnosis, especially in patients who are at risk of radiation exposure, such as children and pregnant women. As illustrated in contemporary research, MRI offers unique advantages through the combination of morphological and functional assessments. For instance, it can measure congenital abnormalities, diaphragmatic function, and regional perfusion in conditions like cystic fibrosis or pulmonary embolism. The noninvasive nature and lack of ionizing radiation in MRIs make it possible to conduct repeated studies without risk using standard imaging techniques. The latest technology advancements in MRI, including motion-compensated imaging, merely add to its benefits. Therefore, with continued innovation in MRI, it is still a potential contender for diverse clinical uses in the diagnosis and management of chest wall and diaphragmatic disorders, complementing conventional imaging modalities appropriately (Hebestreit et al., 2011; N/A, 2021) (Figure 9.17).

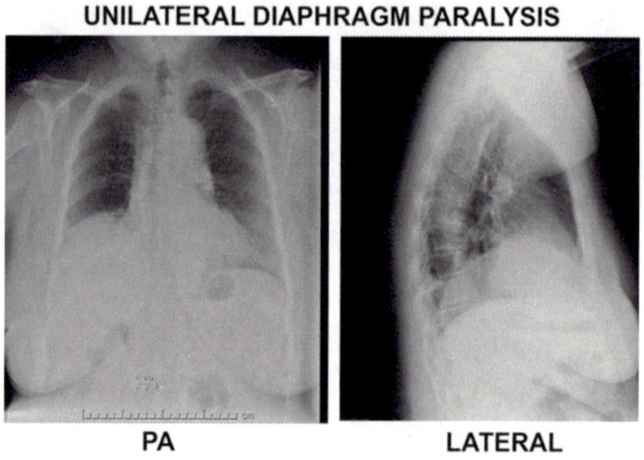

Figure 9.17. Imaging techniques disorders related to the diaphragm and chest wall.

Source: https://external-content.duckduckgo.com/iu/?u=https%3A%2F%2Fwww.chestmed.theclinics.com%2Fcms%2Fattachment%2Fdfbca058-d8af-4636-8533-550cc4f0788d%2Fgr3_lrg.jpg&f=1&nofb=1&ipt=480b27f57325c63759a58d65826ab105e7c1f08758f859a29c7c5a83120d6de0.

9.5.2. Pulmonary Function Tests (PFTs)

Measurement of pulmonary function is critical in the diagnosis and management of various diaphragmatic and chest wall conditions. PFTs are standardized measurements of the lungs' effectiveness, providing valuable information on lung volumes, capacities, and airflow rates. PFTs, consisting of spirometry, determination of lung volumes, and determination of diffusing capacity, are employed to distinguish obstructive and restrictive ventilatory patterns. For instance, spirometry quantifies airflow and will pick up on obstructive disease like asthma or COPD, but tests can quantify the effect of obesity or neuromuscular disease on pulmonary function. Thus, interpretation of PFT results is important to clinicians because they develop individualized treatment plans that address the specific challenges presented by chest wall and diaphragm disorders. Moreover, the contribution of the diaphragm to lung function must not be exaggerated, as it is the major respiratory muscle. Diaphragmatic neuromuscular disease due to muscle weakness, structural disease, or extrinsic compression can lead to severe impairment of the mechanics of breathing. The inter-relationship between diaphragm function and overall pulmonary function performance highlights the importance of specific evaluation methods. As indicated by studies, the influence of body fat percentage on peak expiratory flow rates suggests that changes in abdominal physiology affect respiratory mechanics, particularly in pediatric subjects. These correlations call for the incorporation of body composition testing alongside standard PFTs in the evaluation of patients with diaphragm disability disorders. These multidisciplinary approaches can assist in delineating the complexity of respiratory disease while guiding appropriate therapeutic interventions (Indahswari et al., 2019). In the case of lung transplant recipients, diaphragmatic and pulmonary interaction plays a greater role. It has been established that conditions like prior respiratory disease and surgery trauma can negatively affect post-transplant diaphragmatic function. Such a trend makes it more crucial to continue monitoring respiratory mechanics to ensure that the lung function in transplant recipients remains at its optimum level. The overall evaluation of the diaphragm during transplantation is still not fully investigated although its major role in defining both acute and long-term outcomes remains. The development of normative standards for diaphragmatic dysfunction can enable better management algorithms and provide a clear understanding of the interaction between diaphragmatic function and successful lung transplantation. Thus, a more in-depth review of diaphragm mechanics with PFTs could explain important components of care for patients with chest wall and diaphragm disorders (Grasselli et al., 2024) (Figure 9.18).

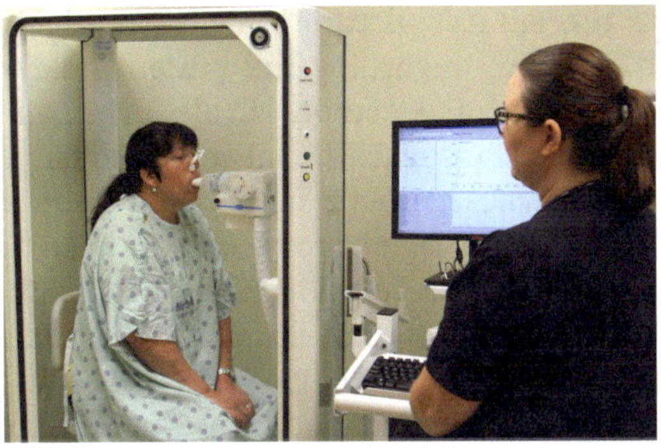

Figure 9.18. Pulmonary function test (PFT).

Source: https://external-content.duckduckgo.com/iu/?u=https%3A%2F%2Fwww.mercy.net%2Fcontent%2Fdam%2Fmercy%2Fen%2Fimages%2Fmercy_carthage_plethysmograph.jpg&f=1&nofb=1&ipt=5c65fa834826e4334a1b3cc7c5291511517e667194bbecb4ae2a581a31743371.

9.5.3. Clinical Evaluation and History Taking

History taking and clinical evaluation play a pivotal role in the diagnosis of diaphragm and chest wall disorders. A thorough patient history, detailing the onset and development of symptoms, provides a background for understanding the respiratory function and potential pathologies of these regions. The history of respiratory symptoms like dyspnea, cough, and intolerance to exercise needs to be noted by clinicians, as these presentations may indicate an underlying dysfunction in the respiratory muscles or chest wall mechanics. In addition, any previous history of neuromuscular diseases, previous respiratory diseases, or significant issues regarding lifestyle, such as smoking, should be recorded since these may tend to complicate the clinical profile and influence laboratory findings seriously. Detailed history taking can maximize the chances of obtaining relevant information and offer clues regarding the patient's overall respiratory status, and guide future clinical decision-making. Assessing respiratory muscle strength, particularly that of the diaphragm, involves not only familiarity with the clinical picture but also meticulous history-taking regarding the patient's day-to-day activities and activity level. For example, some conditions, such as muscular dystrophy, have been noted to be marked by profound impairment of respiratory muscle function, with consequent complications in the form of hypoventilation and ultimately respiratory failure (Aliverti et al., 2016). Therefore, patients can experience a gradual decline in respiratory function, identified by variability in respiratory mechanics and gas exchange. Clinicians are supposed to determine whether the patient's respiratory symptoms have improved over time, as this helps confirm the presence of underlying structural or muscular abnormalities. Variations in the severity of the symptoms should also be noted since this helps in prognosis and guiding rehabilitation design that addresses particular clinical requirements. On top of that, sleep-respiratory interaction cannot be overlooked in clinical evaluation, particularly in diaphragm and chest wall patients. Notably, sleep hypoventilation can exacerbate existing respiratory impairment and results in severe daytime functional disability and reduced quality of life. Appropriate evaluation would include inquiry about sleep habits, nighttime symptom history, and sleep's impact on daily function (Piper et al., 1992). Understanding these factors is important as they may reveal the necessity for nocturnal nasal positive pressure ventilation (NIPPV) to prevent the deterioration of nocturnal respiratory capacity. By examining the interaction between clinical symptoms and sleeping patterns, health care professionals can create comprehensive management strategies that optimize nocturnal and diurnal respiratory function and lead to better patient outcomes.

Test Your Knowledge

1. What are the imaging techniques?
2. What are the pulmonary function tests?

9.6. Treatment Options

Learning Outcome

1. Surgical interventions;
2. Physical therapy and rehabilitation;
3. Pharmacological treatments.

Treatment of disorders of the diaphragm and chest wall is multifaceted, involving a multidisciplinary intervention that addresses the underlying disease as well as enhancing respiratory mechanics. Application of respiratory therapy modalities, including physical rehabilitation and breathing exercises designed to maximize diaphragmatic function, is one of the most prominent avenues. These interventions aim to increase respiratory mechanical efficacy and may incorporate strategies such as incentive spirometry and diaphragmatic pacing to ensure maximum inflation of the lungs and oxygenation. Since recent studies suggest a physiological link between respiration and rhythm modulation, being aware of such relationships can further enhance the accuracy of therapeutic interventions and improve treatment modalities for various diseases (Barnes et al., 2014). Surgical interventions have become an indispensable therapeutic option, especially for diseases related to structural defects. In particular, new techniques for reconstructing diaphragmatic, pericardial, and thoracic wall defects hold promise. New surgical techniques paired with nickel-titanium implants, made possible by new computer technologies, have significantly enhanced surgical planning and execution. Clinical applications describe satisfactory and better functional results following surgery, with no severe pathology of respiratory function or rib cage instability revealed on later monitoring (Dambaev et al., 2017). These advancements are the promise of surgical treatment to reduce the incapacitating symptoms typically associated with diaphragmatic and chest wall pathology. Pharmacologic therapy complements non-invasive and surgical interventions by treating the pathophysiologic imbalances usually found in patients with diaphragm or chest wall disease. Medication treatment may include bronchodilators, steroids, and other medications intended to reduce inflammation or enhance airway mechanics. Further, an understanding of the precision of respiratory-induced changes in autonomic nervous system function could form the foundation for adjuvant treatment exploiting breathing's potential to influence cell and systemic functions (Barnes et al., 2014). By integrating pharmacological treatment with rehabilitative and surgical interventions, clinicians can design a management program specifically tailored to the needs and pathophysiology of each patient, thereby improving their quality of life.

9.6.1. Surgical Interventions

Surgical interventions play an essential part in the treatment of diaphragmatic and chest wall disorders, especially in cases where conservative interventions prove to be insufficient. Surgical treatment ranges from minimally invasive to more invasive reconstructive procedures, to maintain normal respiratory function and alleviate distress caused by structural abnormalities. For instance, in patients suffering from diseases such as Duchenne muscular dystrophy (DMD), life-threatening respiratory complications arise with the degeneration of respiratory muscles. Utilization of multidisciplinary approaches, including surgical treatment, extends lifespan and enhances quality of life through the direct management of respiratory complications. These interventions are essential not only to improve pulmonary function but also to help patients maintain independence for more extended periods, highlighting the significant interrelationship between surgical care and patient care overall in the context of diaphragm and chest wall disorders (Aliverti et al., 2015). Reconstructive surgery is particularly pertinent when treating defects caused by trauma or disease. Improvements in surgical techniques, such as the use of nickel-titanium implants, have demonstrated effective methods for repairing diaphragmatic and chest wall defects. These repairs allow precise restoration with reduced complications associated with standard techniques. Diaphragm defect conditions demonstrate this ability, wherein not only is anatomical continuity regained but respiratory function also becomes stable. Clinical experience has shown that such reconstructive patients have favorable outcomes, with few respiratory disorders of function following surgery. Such findings affirm the value of surgical treatment, opening the doors for the recovery and improved respiratory health of patients (Dambaev et al., 2017). Furthermore, surgical interventions play a critical role in the management of scoliosis and chest wall defects, which can lead to restrictive lung patterns. Corrective interventions typically involve manipulations such as realigning the chest wall, thereby allowing better lung capacity and function. For instance, patients with progressive scoliosis will have severe losses of pulmonary function due to thoracic instability. Corrective interventions for this malalignment not only halt the progression of decreased respiratory status but also provide psychological benefits through improved body mechanics and cosmetic appearance. The importance of integrating surgical techniques into treatment programs cannot be overstated, as these treatments are critical in achieving normalization of respiratory mechanics and a return of patients' quality of life despite chest wall and diaphragmatic disease (Aliverti et al., 2015) (Figure 9.19).

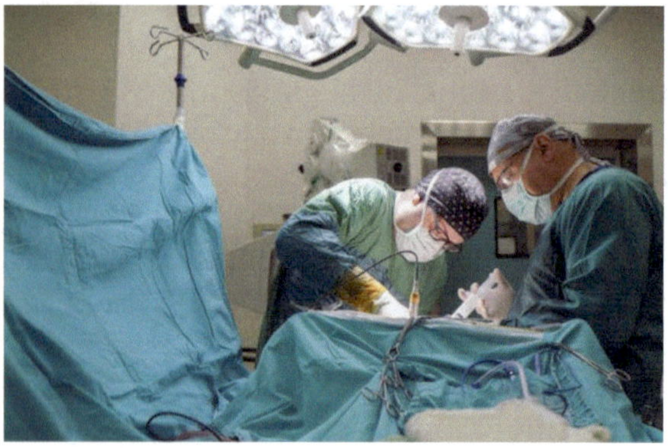

Figure 9.19. Surgical interventions of the diaphragm and chest wall.

Source: https://external-content.duckduckgo.com/iu/?u=http%3A%2F%2Fdrraveesh.com%2Fwp-content%2Fuploads%2F2023%2F12%2Fsurgical-intervention.jpg&f=1&nofb=1&ipt=ef70e8a762dad4b71f0bb29b7181d8fb2c99bd95f359bf8fbb5b47f71f024e84.

9.6.2. Physical Therapy and Rehabilitation

Physical therapy and rehabilitation for patients with diaphragm and chest wall diseases should be integrated to enhance respiratory function and quality of life. Rehabilitation training tends to restore strength and make respiratory muscles, particularly the diaphragm, more efficient. Therapists apply diaphragm training techniques, as noted by Foltz et al. (2016), to address disorders such as tension and disordered breathing that affect patients with respiratory distress. There are interrelated rehabilitation models that include observational approaches, palpation, and goniometry, allowing practitioners to tailor interventions based on the specific needs of patients. By utilizing these strategies, healthcare providers are not only able to improve performance but also allow patients to gain greater control of their diseases, ultimately leading to better therapeutic outcomes. Furthermore, intervention of the physiological intricacies of sleep breathing is also an important part of rehabilitation in patients suffering from chest wall and diaphragm disorders. Research emphasizes the adverse effects of nocturnal hypoventilation and fragmentation on daytime performance and quality of life, necessitating an integrative therapeutic approach.

As proposed in Piper et al. (1992), NIPPV is presently an established intervention for the prevention of respiratory complications via sleep. Physical therapists working in pulmonary rehabilitation must appreciate the significance of nocturnal respiratory events and the potential they have to detract from rehabilitation improvement. By incorporating procedures that maximize nocturnal respiratory function, rehabilitation therapists can optimize patients' daytime functions and rehabilitation potential. The development of evidence-based physical therapy practices is crucial for maximum management of diaphragm and chest wall disorders. Clinicians should keep looking for and implementing new rehabilitation approaches that reflect both the mechanical and functional modalities of respiratory well-being. The narratives of athletic trainers demonstrate a growing recognition of the diaphragm's function during performance and recovery, as seen in Foltz et al. (2016). Training methods, including biofeedback and manual interventions, are becoming powerful instructional tools that enhance patient engagement and sensitivity. By embracing a holistic approach that includes both physical and pedagogical interventions, physical therapy can significantly improve the quality of care for patients with respiratory conditions. Lastly, the commitment to developing new treatment approaches will foster better functional outcomes, securing long-term health and resiliency in this patient group (Figure 9.20).

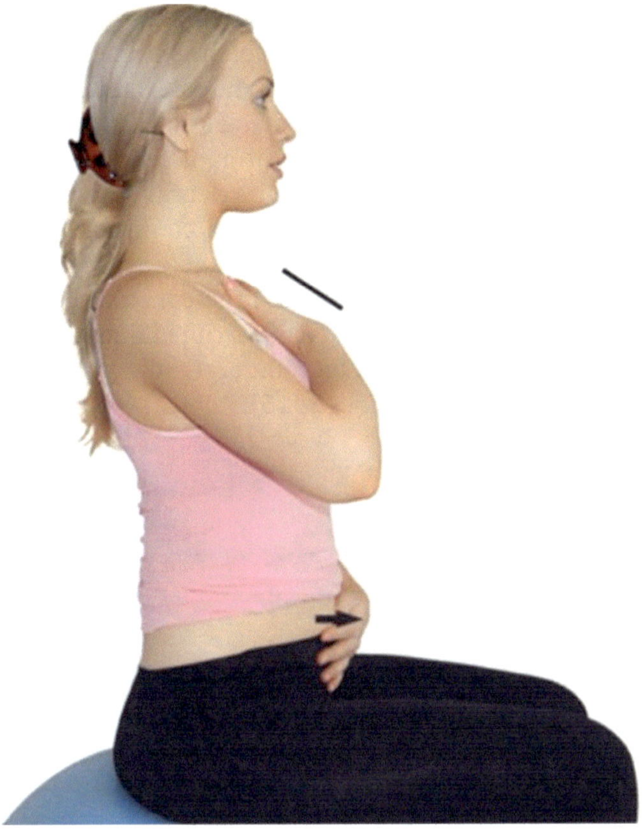

Figure 9.20. Physical therapy and rehabilitation of the diaphragm.

Source: https://external-content.duckduckgo.com/iu/?u=https%3A%2F%2Fwww.rehabmypatient.com%2Fmedia%2Fuploads%2Farticles%2FDiaphragmatic-breathing-sitting.jpg&f=1&nofb=1&ipt=21ab5d08047482a5cb41912a675cd56f2127560d6ef488ad4073751ee7840107.

9.6.3. Pharmacological Treatments

Pharmacological therapies are a primary means of treating diaphragmatic and chest wall disease, notably in conditions such as DMD, which involves the gradual weakening of respiratory muscles. Due to such complexities, there is usually a considerable loss of pulmonary function, and treatment interventions must keep changing. The new advancements in pharmacological treatments, including corticosteroids and idebenone, are significant since they have shown efficacy in slowing the deterioration of spirometric parameters. Not only do these enhance the quality of life, but they also increase the survival rate of patients by delaying respiratory failure, which is common in patients with DMD. Drug therapy is thus one component of comprehensive therapy to reduce pulmonary complications of chest wall and diaphragm disease (Aliverti et al., 2015). In addition to corticosteroids, comprehensive respiratory care also involves rehabilitative pharmacology as well as add-on therapies. Evidence has indicated that recruitment maneuvers in the lung can be effectively used with pharmacologic treatments to further increase pulmonary function. This synergistic approach works by excluding atelectasis—the lung tissue collapse, which can contribute to breath difficulty. Furthermore, the use of non-invasive mechanical ventilation plays a vital role in treating nocturnal hypoventilation, sleep-disordered breathing, and general respiratory support, highlighting the necessity for an integrated model of care. The model emphasizes individualized pharmacologic therapy taken alongside rehabilitative measures to strengthen respiratory outcomes and optimize patient survivability (Almendros et al., 2019). Moreover, the role of interdisciplinary treatment cannot be emphasized enough, as it addresses multiple aspects of patient care, including pharmacological and non-pharmacological interventions. By implementing a dual modality of steroid therapy and cough-amplified devices, physicians can improve airway clearance and reduce respiratory infection risk. Each intervention alone addresses the multifactorial condition of chest wall and diaphragm disorders. With the integration of new research findings and novel pharmacologic approaches, the dynamic nature of respiratory care is exemplified, and the constant spirit of innovation embodied within this medical specialty is highlighted. High-tech multimodal methods not only improve clinical outcomes but also revolutionize the treatment and understanding of respiratory disorders related to the diaphragm and chest wall (Aliverti et al., 2015).

Test Your Knowledge

1. What is the surgery of the diaphragm and chest wall?
2. What is the physical therapy and rehabilitation of the diaphragm and chest wall?

Summary

It is important to gain insight into chest wall and diaphragmatic diseases in clinical practice to ensure appropriate diagnosis and treatment. The disease significantly affects respiratory function and can lead to reduced quality of life and excessive healthcare spending. The diaphragm plays a role in ventilation, and its failure may be due to a variety of factors such as neuromuscular disease and mechanical loads. Progress in the past few years in assessing diaphragm function with invasive and noninvasive methods underscores the importance of accurate measurement of diaphragm performance to tailor treatment interventions accordingly. By integrating these methods into routine clinical practice, clinicians can more accurately identify the compromised issues in respiratory mechanics and diaphragm function, resulting in improved patient outcomes. Furthermore, it has been established in studies that IMT can enhance the function of the diaphragm, as evidenced by higher PI,max, and improved neuromechanical coupling. The research illustrates a robust correlation between baseline inspiratory capacity and the efficacy of IMT across various populations. Specifically, the interaction between the inspiratory chest wall and the diaphragm contributes to respiratory mechanics and plays a critical role in the creation of targeted treatment regimens. As elaborated in the findings, recognizing how different muscle groups contribute to breathing can aid healthcare professionals in formulating more effective rehabilitation schemes. Thus, a consideration of increasing diaphragm effectiveness through IMT can lead to considerable improvements in breathing function among patients with diaphragm and chest wall disorders. Finally, as we continue to move forward with understanding of diaphragm and chest wall disease, it becomes necessary to promote continuing study into new forms of assessment and training. The disparity discovered between invasive and noninvasive measurements provides insightful information regarding the heterogeneity of diaphragm function. It suggests that a multi-faceted approach will lead to optimal diagnostic and therapeutic outcomes. The integration of new technologies, such as surface mechanomyography and electromyography, may facilitate simpler assessment of diaphragmatic function and enhance clinical practicability. Finally, it is a multifaceted process with concerted advances in research, clinical assessment, and therapy that comes closer to knowing and effectively treating diaphragm and chest wall disorders. The aim is to optimize respiratory function in those with heterogeneous disease populations, delivering the optimal care possible.

By investigation into the diseases of the diaphragm and chest wall, a good appreciation of the pathophysiology behind them gives the necessary information to account for their clinical presentation. The diaphragm, being the large respiratory muscle, is the principal muscle responsible for the majority of the effort of ventilation. Dysfunction of this muscle can be brought about by a wide range of conditions, including neuromuscular disease affecting its coordination and strength. For example, in muscular dystrophy, respiratory failure is the major clinical problem, ultimately resulting in patient death. The combination of weak respiratory muscles and the high resistance they must overcome creates a spectrum of respiratory disturbances that can profoundly compromise gas exchange and overall pulmonary function. The need for early diagnosis and treatment of such respiratory complications is critical in optimizing patient results. The role of chest wall disorders is also important, with conditions such as kyphoscoliosis and obesity influencing respiratory mechanics. These structural abnormalities can lead to restrictive lung disease, limiting the lung capacity of inspiration and expiration. When the chest wall becomes stiff and deformed, even the elastic ability of the lungs is lost, leading to dyspnea and hypoxemia. Diseases like kyphoscoliosis, for example, specifically alter the effective volume for lung expansion, ultimately reducing the efficiency of gas exchange. This compromise in structure requires a multi-dimensional management approach that may include physical therapy, surgical intervention, and the use of non-invasive ventilation strategies to provide optimal respiratory function and quality of life. The interlink between respiratory muscle involvement and systemic effects also highlights the complexity of managing chest wall and diaphragmatic disorders. In muscular dystrophy, respiratory issues may vary depending on the type and progression of the disease, leading to differences in the onset and severity of hypoventilation and sleep-disordered breathing. These disturbances in respiration are secondary to alterations in thoracoabdominal dynamics and the failure to generate effective inspiratory pressures. Hence, complete knowledge of these main points is key to developing effective care strategies that address not only respiratory conditions but also the systemic consequences associated with diaphragm and chest wall disorders, thereby improving patient prognosis and quality of life (Aliverti et al., 2016; Cheung et al., 2017).

KEY TERMS FROM THIS CHAPTER

- Chest wall deformity
- Costochondritis
- Diaphragmatic hernia
- Diaphragmatic rupture
- Flail chest
- Pectus carinatum
- Phrenic nerve injury
- Respiratory muscle weakness
- Thoracic cage rigidity
- Tietze syndrome
- Chest wall tumor
- Diaphragmatic eventration
- Diaphragmatic paralysis
- Eventration of diaphragm
- Hypoventilation syndrome
- Pectus excavatum
- Poland syndrome
- Scoliosis (affecting chest wall)
- Thoracic outlet syndrome

Critical Thinking Questions

1. **Which of the following is the most common cause of diaphragmatic paralysis?**
   a. Trauma to the phrenic nerve
   b. Myasthenia gravis
   c. Spinal cord injury above C5
   d. Multiple sclerosis
2. **What is the typical chest X-ray appearance in unilateral diaphragmatic paralysis?**
   a. Elevated hemidiaphragm on the affected side
   b. Bilaterally flattened diaphragm
   c. Bilateral pleural effusions
   d. Pneumothorax
3. **Which disorder is characterized by inappropriate chest wall movement during respiration, typically secondary to flail chest?**
   a. Pectus excavatum
   b. Paradoxical chest wall movement
   c. Kyphoscoliosis
   d. Platypnea
4. **Which congenital deformity leads to sunken appearance of the anterior chest wall?**
   a. Pectus carinatum
   b. Pectus excavatum
   c. Poland syndrome
   d. Klippel-Feil syndrome
5. **Which of the following is NOT a common cause of restrictive lung disease secondary to chest wall disorders?**
   a. Kyphoscoliosis
   b. Ankylosing spondylitis
   c. Obesity
   d. Asthma

Short Answer Questions

1. What are the common causes of diaphragmatic paralysis?
2. Describe the clinical features and diagnosis of a diaphragmatic hernia.
3. What is the pathophysiology of flail chest, and how does it affect respiration?
4. How is diaphragmatic rupture diagnosed following blunt trauma?
5. What is the distinction between congenital and acquired diaphragmatic hernia?

Answer to Critical Thinking Questions

1. (a); 2. (a); 3. (b); 4. (b); 5. (d)

References

1. Oruc, O., Sarac, S., Afsar, G. C., Topcuoglu, O. B., Kanbur, S., Yalcinkaya, I., Tepetam, F. M., & Kirbas, G. (2016). Is polysomnographic examination necessary for subjects with diaphragm pathologies? *Clinics*, *71*(9), 506–510. https://doi.org/10.6061/clinics/2016(09)04Agin, K. H., Khoshkar, A., & MoinAzad Tehrani, M. (2013). Eventration of diaphragm or pseudo pleural effusion? https://core.ac.uk/download/483635408.pdf (accessed on 30th June 2025).
2. Aliverti, A., & Lo Mauro, M. A. (2016). Physiology of respiratory disturbances in muscular dystrophies. https://core.ac.uk/download/80335401.pdf (accessed on 30th June 2025).
3. Aliverti, A., D'Angelo, M. G., & Lo Mauro, M. A. (2015). Assessment and management of respiratory function in patients with Duchenne muscular dystrophy: Current and emerging options. https://core.ac.uk/download/55257285.pdf (accessed on 30th June 2025).
4. Aliverti, A., De Troyer, A., Lo Mauro, A., Aliverti, A., Turconi, A. C., LoMauro, A., et al. (2012). Rib cage deformities alter respiratory muscle action and chest wall function in patients with severe osteogenesis imperfecta. https://core.ac.uk/download/pdf/8718939.pdf (accessed on 30th June 2025).
5. Almendros, I., Baillieul, S., Caballero, C., Degani-Costa, L., et al. (2019). Highlights from the 2018 European Respiratory Society International Congress: Sleep and clinical physiology. https://core.ac.uk/download/226984864.pdf (accessed on 30th June 2025).
6. Anandh, V., Samuel Sundar Doss, D., Rekha, R., Rai, R., et al. (2016). Effect of stretching respiratory accessory muscles in chronic obstructive pulmonary disease. https://core.ac.uk/download/477852018.pdf (accessed on 30th June 2025).
7. Arcieri, L., Assanta, N., Baggi, R., Di Maurizio, M., et al. (2016). The role of posterior aortopexy in the treatment of left mainstem bronchus compression. https://core.ac.uk/download/74319435.pdf (accessed on 30th June 2025).
8. Barnes, V. A., Crawford, M. W., Harden, K., Ravinder, K., et al. (2014). Widespread depolarization during expiration: A source of respiratory drive? https://core.ac.uk/download/131210052.pdf (accessed on 30th June 2025).
9. Brown, P. I., Johnson, M. A., & Sharpe, G. R. (2014). Determinants of inspiratory muscle strength in healthy humans. https://core.ac.uk/download/30635175.pdf (accessed on 30th June 2025).
10. Cheung, J. P. Y., Cheung, K. M. C., Luk, K. D. K., Wong, K. W., et al. (2017). A rare postoperative complication of anterior lower thoracic instrumentation: Diaphragmatic laceration with hemothorax. https://core.ac.uk/download/95561003.pdf (accessed on 30th June 2025).
11. Clos Mompart, M. (2024). 3D-printed bracing system for female pectus carinatum treatment. https://core.ac.uk/download/613973071.pdf (accessed on 30th June 2025).
12. Dambaev, G. T., Gunther, V. E., Hodorenko, V. N., Shchadenko, I., et al. (2017). Reconstruction of thoracic postresection defects by TiNi-based implant. https://core.ac.uk/download/417409049.pdf (accessed on 30th June 2025).
13. Davidescu, L., Manolescu, D., Oancea, C., Ulmeanu, R., et al. (2018). Noninvasive ventilation in neuromuscular diseases. https://core.ac.uk/download/322437445.pdf (accessed on 30th June 2025).

14. Elhamd, E. A., & Seifeldein, G. S. (2011). Multidetector computed tomography of diaphragm: Anatomic variants and diagnostic problems in adult population. https://core.ac.uk/download/pdf/81121157.pdf (accessed on 30th June 2025).
15. Foltz, M. R. (2016). Diaphragm training and evaluation as a therapeutic tool by athletic trainers in orthopedic rehabilitation. https://core.ac.uk/download/233949873.pdf (accessed on 30th June 2025).
16. Grasselli, G., Lo Mauro, A., Mattioni, G., Morlacchi, L., Musso, V., Palleschi, A., Privitera, E., et al. (2024). Diaphragm and lung transplantation. https://core.ac.uk/download/638781948.pdf (accessed on 30th June 2025).
17. Hebestreit, A., Kluge, A., Kluge, A., Kluge, A., Bankier, A. A., Henderson, A. C., Brody, A. S., et al. (2011). MRI of the lung (3/3)—Current applications and future perspectives. https://core.ac.uk/download/28969132.pdf (accessed on 30th June 2025).
18. Indahswari, N. W. (Ni), Indrayani, A. W. (Agung), Thanaya, S. A. (Sayu), Wibawa, I. D. N., et al. (2019). The correlation between body fat percentage and peak expiratory flow in children aged 10–12 years at SD Negeri 8 Dauh Puri. https://core.ac.uk/download/234033578.pdf (accessed on 30th June 2025).
19. McGovern, K. (2020). Acoustic intensity and speech breathing kinematics in a patient with Parkinson's disease. https://core.ac.uk/download/328827036.pdf (accessed on 30th June 2025).
20. Messineo, A., Tocchioni, F., Ghionzoli, M., & Romagnoli, P. (2013). Pectus excavatum and heritable disorders of the connective tissue. https://core.ac.uk/download/26474530.pdf (accessed on 30th June 2025).
21. Petrocelli, L. C. E., Campos, R. J., Jolley, J., Lozano García, C., et al. (2019). Noninvasive assessment of inspiratory muscle neuromechanical coupling during inspiratory threshold loading. https://core.ac.uk/download/294829794.pdf (accessed on 30th June 2025).
22. Piper, A. J. (1992). Sleep and respiration: Implications for pulmonary rehabilitation. https://core.ac.uk/download/pdf/82529960.pdf (accessed on 30th June 2025).
23. Primorac, D., Turkalj, M., Lulić-Jurjević, R., Gjergja Juraški, R., & Miranović, V. (2017). Kardiorespiracijske komplikacije u bolesnika s *osteogenesis imperfecta*. https://core.ac.uk/download/212469295.pdf (accessed on 30th June 2025).
24. Singh, G. (2017). Trunk and respiratory motor control in typically developing children and its implications in children with chronic spinal cord injury. https://core.ac.uk/download/143835340.pdf (accessed on 30th June 2025).
25. Varnado, C. B. (2015). Treatment efficacy of manual therapy on speech outcomes in children with spastic cerebral palsy: A single-subject experimental design. https://core.ac.uk/download/217392798.pdf (accessed on 30th June 2025).
26. West, C. (2011). Effect of abdominal binding on cardiorespiratory function in Paralympic athletes with cervical spinal cord injury. https://core.ac.uk/download/9633120.pdf (accessed on 30th June 2025).
27. Zecher, K. (2018). Performance anxiety and the benefits of proper breathing for singing. https://core.ac.uk/download/236388320.pdf (accessed on 30th June 2025).

CONGENITAL ANOMALIES OF THE RESPIRATORY SYSTEM

10

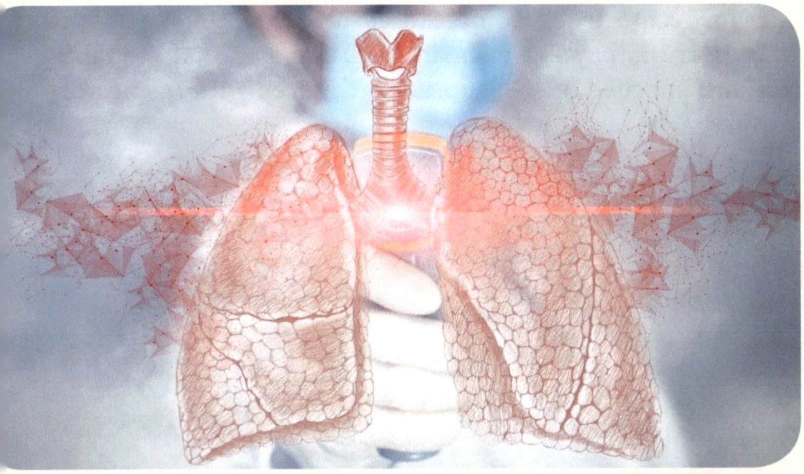

Introduction

Congenital respiratory abnormalities are a heterogeneous collection of fetal diseases that produce structural or functional defect of the respiratory apparatus. They have significant implications for the health of the neonate and are generally marked by various clinical expressions of different severities. Early diagnosis is bolstered by the potential early medical therapy has to rectify respiratory function as well as general quality of life in patients. Etiologic determinants for the development of such anomalies could include genetic predispositions, environmental causes, and maternal conditions during pregnancy. Prevention and clinical practice management of such high-risk groups are dependent on the identification of such etiologic factors. The interplay of systemic disease considerations with congenital anomalies highlights the necessity for multidisciplinary management. For instance, there have been reported cases of some congenital conditions affecting normal respiratory development in infants and therefore more complexity in the treatment and diagnostic process for doctors.

LEARNING OBJECTIVES

After studying this chapter, you will be able to:

1. Describe the types of congenital anomalies;
2. List the causes and risk factors;
3. Understand the diagnosis of congenital anomalies;
4. Discuss clinical manifestations;
5. Explain treatment options;
6. Explore the prognosis and outcomes.

The interesting part of this argument is the fact that the mother's well-being can be a causative factor in causing respiratory abnormalities in infants. Maternal diabetes could lead to an array of complications including respiratory defects, e.g., infants with congenital malformations like arthrogryposis, who have resultant attendant respiratory complications (Kumar et al., 2009). The intersection of maternal and fetal health warrants specific research so as to direct prevention measures and therapeutic interventions. Further, medical advances have elucidated the genetic and immunologic determinants in the expression of congenital respiratory disease. The more that has been realized concerning the interplay between genetics and the disorders, the wider the horizon of possible treatments grows. The International Union of Immunological Societies has facilitated the clarification of the complexity involved in the inborn errors of immunity, which can manifest as respiratory complications (Ailal et al., 2020). This involves conducting extensive research in both genetic and environmental settings to decipher the complexities of congenital anomalies in an integrated manner. These recognitions are important to healthcare professionals, enabling them to provide personalized patient care and improve the prognosis for children with respiratory congenital anomalies (Figure 10.1).

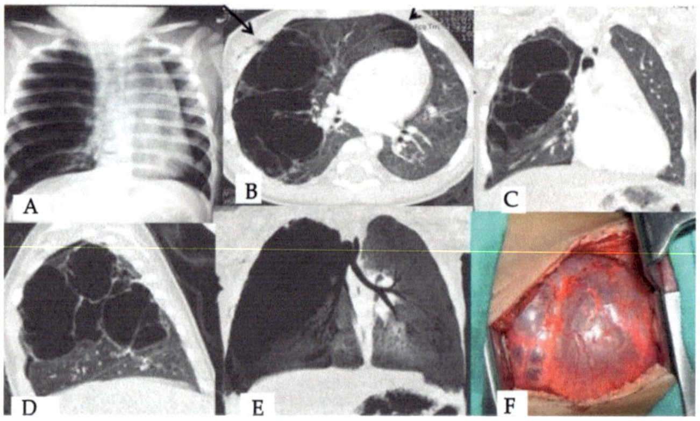

Figure 10.1. Congenital anomalies of the respiratory system.

Source: https://media.springernature.com/lw685/springer-static/image/art%3A10.1007%2Fs40134-014-0071-y/MediaObjects/40134_2014_71_Fig3_HTML.jpg.

Definition of Congenital Anomalies

Congenital anomalies or birth defects are structural or functional prenatal developmental defects that may affect the impairment of a variety of organ systems, including the respiratory system. Congenital anomalies result from a multifactorial etiology of environmental, genetic, and socioeconomic factors, which lead to aberrations in normal fetal development. Although some congenital anomalies occur as physical deformities, others can impair organ function without any visible external characteristics. As far as the respiratory system is concerned, tracheoesophageal fistula and congenital diaphragmatic hernia (CDH) highlight the critical need for awareness of these abnormalities. Implications are significant when detected early and treated early, and therefore enhanced awareness and screening of at-risk populations should be guaranteed in the process of prenatal diagnosis. The term congenital anomalies is also quite broad in application, and the disorders may vary in severity and impact on the health of an individual. Congenital respiratory system anomalies, for example, may vary from benign anatomical variation to life-threatening disorders requiring emergent operation. Their classification is typically complex, typically separated by the type of anomaly—structural or functional—or involved system. Some environmental exposures that are teratogenic in nature have been defined to cause some congenital anomalies, and, therefore, public health policy guidelines have been established for the avoidance of such exposure during pregnancy. Understanding these complications is critical for health care professionals to provide appropriate care and support to families affected by these disorders, ensuring they can be treated and managed accordingly. Also, the lifelong implications of congenital defects go beyond physical health and tend to affect psychological and social health. Infants born with respiratory system defects may experience impaired body development, respiratory performance, and quality of life. The evidence suggests that supportive care through early intervention programs and family therapy is the cornerstone in effective management of these disorders. For instance, treatment is typically applied with a general strategy that takes into account a multidisciplinary group of individuals to address the numerous problems that children such as these will have throughout their lifetime. The demand for interventions aimed at the condition highlights the importance of informing parents and communities about congenital anomalies and available resources, thereby contributing to the improved health status and quality of life of the afflicted individual and their family.

Importance of Studying Respiratory System Anomalies

Anomalies of the respiratory system are significant to research given their far-reaching impact on health outcomes, particularly in neonates. Congenital conditions of this system have the potential to cause serious consequences, such as respiratory distress and long-term morbidity, which greatly influence quality of life. The realization of such conditions highlights prospects of prenatally diagnosing and treating them, which can limit infant mortality from respiratory failures. Applicable literature highlights the importance of measuring health outcomes in the context of delivery and labor procedures, describing the connection between increased maternal health and decreased instances of respiratory system failure among children (Nizalova et al., 2025). By studying these anomalies, medical practitioners can design better treatment and screening protocols tailored to the individual's specific needs of having such anomalies, resulting in better practice of care and management in neonatal care. Respiratory system anomaly studies are also crucial for developing public health policy and practice recommendations. It supports the creation of comprehensive prenatal care packages that emphasize early detection and prevention of congenital malformations. Improving healthcare practice based on evidence has the potential to generate standardized birth and delivery procedures that can ultimately enhance infant and maternal well-being outcomes. For example, early antenatal care interventions can lead to significant improvements in health profiles, as demonstrated by the Mother and Infant Health Project, which reported declining infant mortality rates due to respiratory complications (Vyshnya et al., 2025). Investment in the care and study of these anomalies enables health systems to optimize resources and allocate care more equally among at-risk populations, thus meeting the twin goals of saving lives and eradicating health disparities. In addition, the importance of respiratory system anomalies extends beyond clinical practice, as it advances our basic scientific understanding of developmental biology and genetics. Research into etiologic mechanisms and causes of congenital malformations has the potential to yield significant insight into how environmental, genetic, and pathologic factors interact during fetal life. In addition to adding to the literature, this study has implications for family planning recommendations and clinical genetic counseling in risk groups. Data derived from the study of anomalies of the respiratory system can chart the path of upcoming medical research and discovery, with improved health outcomes for the patients suffering from these debilitating diseases. The accurate understanding of respiratory system congenital anomalies remains fundamental in the quest for better healthcare and scientific discovery, leading to improved public health interventions (Figure 10.2).

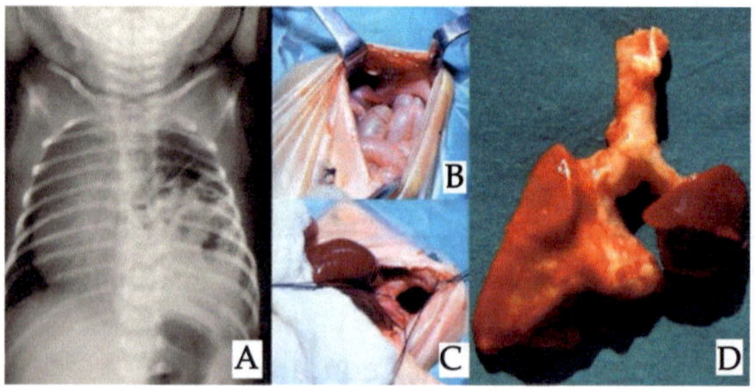

Figure 10.2. Respiratory system anomalies.

Source: https://embryology.med.unsw.edu.au/embryology/images/thumb/6/66/Congenital_diaphragmatic_hernia_01.jpg/600px-Congenital_diaphragmatic_hernia_01.jpg.

10.1. Types of Congenital Anomalies

Learning Outcome

1. Tracheoesophageal fistula;
2. Congenital diaphragmatic hernia;
3. Pulmonary agenesis.

Anomalies of the congenital respiratory system are categorized into different groups according to their pathological and clinical characteristics. Structural anomalies include tracheoesophageal fistula and congenital diaphragmatic hernia (CDH). These presentations reflect the heterogeneity of abnormalities of the congenital respiratory tract. They are caused by both environmental factors and genetic influences or even a combination of the two. Early diagnosis of these anomalies is significant as they significantly affect the development and functioning of the infant's lungs. For instance, CDH is likely to result in pulmonary hypoplasia, leading to lethal respiratory distress at birth. An understanding of the various categories of congenital anomalies is vital for healthcare providers to initiate appropriate management methods and improve outcomes for affected infants. Another critical category of congenital anomalies are malformations of the airway, which can lead to profound compromise of respiratory function. Laryngomalacia and congenital vocal cord paralysis are two examples of how structural issues within the airway can disrupt normal respiratory function. Laryngomalacia, or softening of the laryngeal tissues, is most frequent in infants presenting with stridor and generally improves over time as the infant grows. On a separate note, congenital vocal cord paralysis may cause acute airway obstruction, requiring closer observation and potentially surgical intervention. The complexity of these defects only emphasizes the need for ongoing study and observation, since advancements in diagnostic techniques and therapies can result in improved patient care. An understanding of the pathophysiology and clinical importance of these respiratory defects is essential for providing optimal care to affected patients. Finally, syndromic conditions are also present in congenital respiratory abnormalities, hence making them harder to treat and diagnose. For example, Pierre Robin sequence and certain craniosynostosis syndromes are often coupled with intrinsic congenital respiratory issues, including obstructive sleep apnea and airway patency difficulty. The complexity of the syndromic presentations requires a multidisciplinary intervention involving pediatricians, pulmonologists, and geneticists to address the varied challenges posed by the anomalies. Comprehensive management plans, like ongoing monitoring and teamwork, are essential to improve respiratory outcomes among affected subjects. The combination of large population-based studies is important, as demonstrated by the Hungarian Congenital Abnormality Registry, which highlights the occurrence and relationship between respiratory anomalies and other congenital conditions, eventually allowing us to gain a better understanding of their etiology and treatment (Czeizel et al., 2005).

10.1.1. Tracheoesophageal Fistula (TEF)

The existence of a TEF is a severe congenital anomaly in the range of respiratory system diseases. This malformation is caused by an abnormal connection between the trachea and esophagus that jeopardizes life. Diagnosed classically at birth, TEF often coexists with esophageal atresia, where the formation of the esophagus is halted, leaving a gap that compromises normal respiration and feeding. This route can lead to severe respiratory compromise, aspiration pneumonia, and failure to thrive, and requires immediate detection and treatment. As the severity of these conditions suggests, successful management generally requires a multidisciplinary treatment plan. This anomaly impinges not only upon respiratory function but also upon gastrointestinal well-being, contributing to the issues faced by involved infants and families. Clinical presentations of TEF may vary considerably, contributing to the challenge of diagnosis and management. In some instances, symptoms need not become apparent at initial presentation, with consequent misdiagnosis or delayed intervention. For instance, recurrent pneumonia can be the presenting feature of an underlying fistula, whereby saliva and food enter the trachea via the abnormal pathway. Ishibashi et al. (2022) describe a stunning case of a patient with CHARGE syndrome, with recurrent hospitalizations for respiratory issues culminating in the diagnosis of a TEF causing ventilatory insufficiency. This highlights the life-threatening significance of intimate monitoring in infants presenting with respiratory and feeding distress, since unrecognized TEF can lead to serious respiratory complications and needs surgery to minimize risk. Tracheoesophageal fistula treatment is a blend of medical and surgical treatment based on individual needs. Initial management is usually focused on the preservation of respiratory stability and the correction of nutritional deficiency brought about by feeding problems. Repair by operation typically includes fistula closure and, when necessary, concomitant esophageal atresia repair. In cases where tracheomalacia is among the clinical features, innovative approaches, such as the cervical approach to tracheopexy, may be applied to enhance airway stability, as discussed in Bjornson et al. (2014). This multi-disciplinary treatment philosophy not only addresses the anatomical condition of the fistula but also seeks to improve overall respiratory well-being, allowing for improved quality of life in affected patients (Figure 10.3).

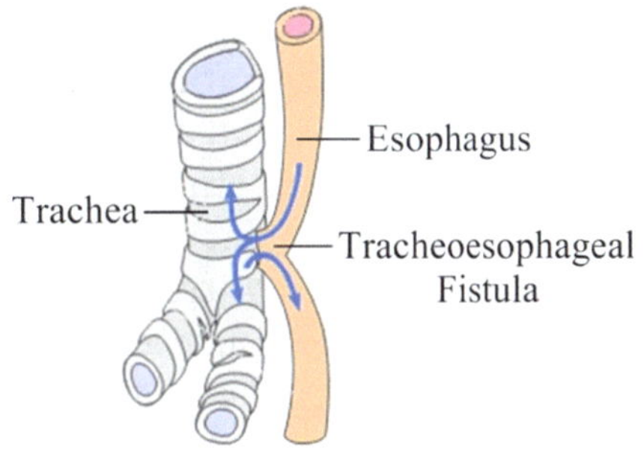

Figure 10.3. Tracheoesophageal fistula (TEF).

Source: https://external-content.duckduckgo.com/iu/?u=http%3A%2F%2F4.bp.blogspot.com%2F-419DWhikru4%2FT3cA8bHFErI%2FAAAAAAAABXs%2F-gWOvI4yaeM%2Fs1600%2FTracheosphageal%252BFistula.png&f=1&nofb=1&ipt=1f0477d944a366d65776f1d95ea4580dba7139d9740aca67f6f6e13fd5e7d4c3.

10.1.2. Congenital Diaphragmatic Hernia (CDH)

CDH is a life-threatening respiratory malformation characterized by an abnormal development of the diaphragm such that there is a defect through which abdominal contents can enter the thorax. This condition can significantly impair lung growth and function because the herniated organs restrict the space available for lung growth. It should be noted that the two common types of CDH are distinguished by their presentation. There are Bochdalek hernias, which are seen posteriorly, and Morgagni hernias, typically anterior in site. The impact of CDH is severe, normally resulting in high morbidity and mortality among affected neonates. Early detection, through methods primarily of prenatal screening such as ultrasound, is instrumental in improving outcomes by allowing for planned postnatal care to address respiratory assistance and surgery, to enhance the recovery and quality of life probability for infants with this defect. The effect of CDH isn't just an acute respiratory impact since infants with this diagnosis are at higher risk of developing long-term sequelae. Studies have indicated that patients with congenital malformations like CDH may create a cascade of respiratory afflictions during childhood and need ongoing medical monitoring. In agreement with clinical findings, most of these children incur frequent hospitalizations due to lower respiratory tract infections, expanding the importance of an extensive follow-up program for their individual healthcare requirements (Mussi et al., 2024). It demands a multidisciplinary approach that involves pediatric pulmonologists, neonatologists, and surgeons to detect and manage these risks effectively. By ensuring interprofessional collaboration among care providers, treatment for CDH should encompass not only surgery but also preventive respiratory therapy, specific nutrition management, pulmonary rehabilitation, and an all-inclusive model of patient care. Treatment of CDH varies with the severity of the anomaly and the overall clinical condition of the patient. Surgical repair is the treatment of choice, with techniques varying based on the size and site of hernias and patients' individual needs. Of specific note, peritoneopericardial diaphragmatic hernia, although less common, also falls into this class of congenital defects and has been successfully treated with median celiotomy for herniorrhaphy (García et al., 2024). Recovery following surgery is good in the majority of cases, with most patients showing significant improvement in respiratory function and overall condition. Research underscores the importance of routine follow-up and vigilance after surgery for several years, as early detection of any problem can lead to practical measures that ensure the best possible outcomes for the patient. Ultimately, treatment of CDH with a well-planned approach not only alleviates acute respiratory problems but also maximizes the long-term health trajectory of affected individuals (Figure 10.4).

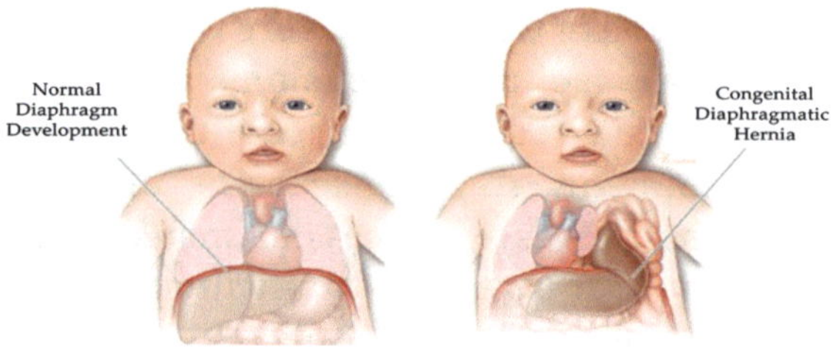

Figure 10.4. Congenital diaphragmatic hernia (CDH).

Source: https://external-content.duckduckgo.com/iu/?u=https%3A%2F%2Fwww.choc.org%2Fwp%2Fwp-content%2Fuploads%2F2023%2F07%2FCDH-normal-vs-not.png&f=1&nofb=1&ipt=87e3319fc7d2676befe02f84b2cc39619fa77ad0f73a608a2b68f77b9e1243b4.

10.1.3. Pulmonary Agenesis

Pulmonary agenesis is one of the most severe congenital anomalies within the category of respiratory system anomalies. Pulmonary agenesis is characterized by the absence of lung parenchyma, bronchial tree, and associated vasculature, and also tends to present in early childhood. Pulmonary agenesis severely cripples patients since it may present with other congenital anomalies that complicate diagnosis and management. The most common cause of this anomaly is identified by a chest X-ray, which shows the etiology through the presence of homogeneous opacities that may then be confirmed by a computed tomography of the thorax. Early and accurate diagnosis is thus crucial in the management of pulmonary agenesis with resultant early therapeutic maneuvers aimed at preventing potential complications and improving the quality of life of the patients as discerned in relevant clinical observations. Pulmonary agenesis is managed clinically through a multidisciplinary approach based on the complexity and variability of concomitant congenital anomalies. Evaluation is often extended to echocardiogram and ultrasonography of the abdomen to rule out other developmental abnormalities that may increase the risk of respiratory failure or other complications. For instance, a recent case report reported a one-month-old male with pulmonary agenesis who presented with cough and dyspnea, where imaging modalities supported the diagnosis and revealed associated situs solitus and dextroposition of the heart (Das et al., 2022). These associations necessitate careful planning of care that addresses the broad spectrum of potential complications, emphasizing the need for close observation and intervention to optimally manage symptoms and enhance respiratory function. Although the prognosis in pulmonary agenesis patients largely depends on the occurrence of associated anomalies and the availability of early intervention, advances in treatment modalities have been encouraging. Some control actions may include intravenous antibiotics, oxygen therapy, and bronchodilation nebulization to reduce respiratory symptoms and health effects. Unfortunately, as reported in research, such children have a risk of recurrence of respiratory infections in the future, thus requiring regular follow-up and a potential surgical intervention for severe cases (Das et al., 2022). Comprehension of pulmonary agenesis within the broader context of congenital respiratory abnormalities allows healthcare professionals to enhance diagnostic performance, facilitate early intervention, and eventually reduce childhood mortality from the disorder (Figure 10.5).

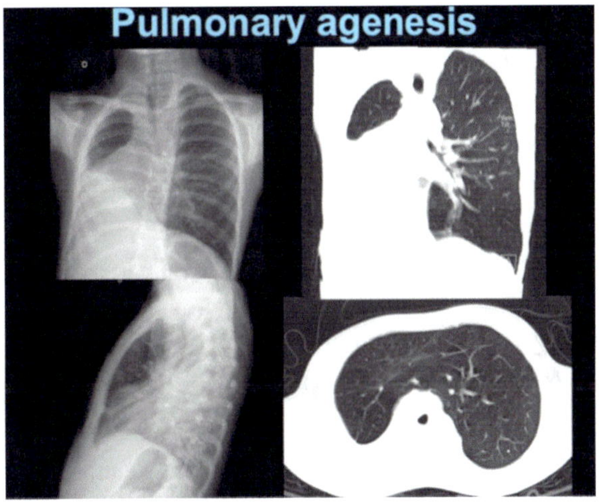

Figure 10.5. Pulmonary agenesis.

Source: https://www.researchgate.net/profile/Maria-Serrado/publication/343239798/figure/fig1/AS:917991977914368@1595877751408/Pulmonary-agenesis-Frontal-and-lateral-chest-radiograph-present-a-small-radio-opaque.jpg.

Test Your Knowledge

1. What is a tracheoesophageal fistula?
2. What is a congenital diaphragmatic hernia?

10.2. Causes and Risk Factors

Learning Outcome

1. Genetic factors;
2. Environmental influences;
3. Maternal health and lifestyle.

Congenital respiratory defects occur due to a complex interaction between environmental and genetic factors. Genetic predisposition plays a crucial role, with various studies confirming the presence of specific genetic mutations in the formation of structural malformations of the respiratory system. For instance, chromosomal abnormalities like trisomy 21 have been related to an enhanced incidence of congenital respiratory malformations, suggesting the contribution of hereditary factors to the anomalies. Moreover, disruption of the genetic regulatory pathways during embryogenesis may lead to abnormal respiratory structure development and, consequently, to congenital anomalies.

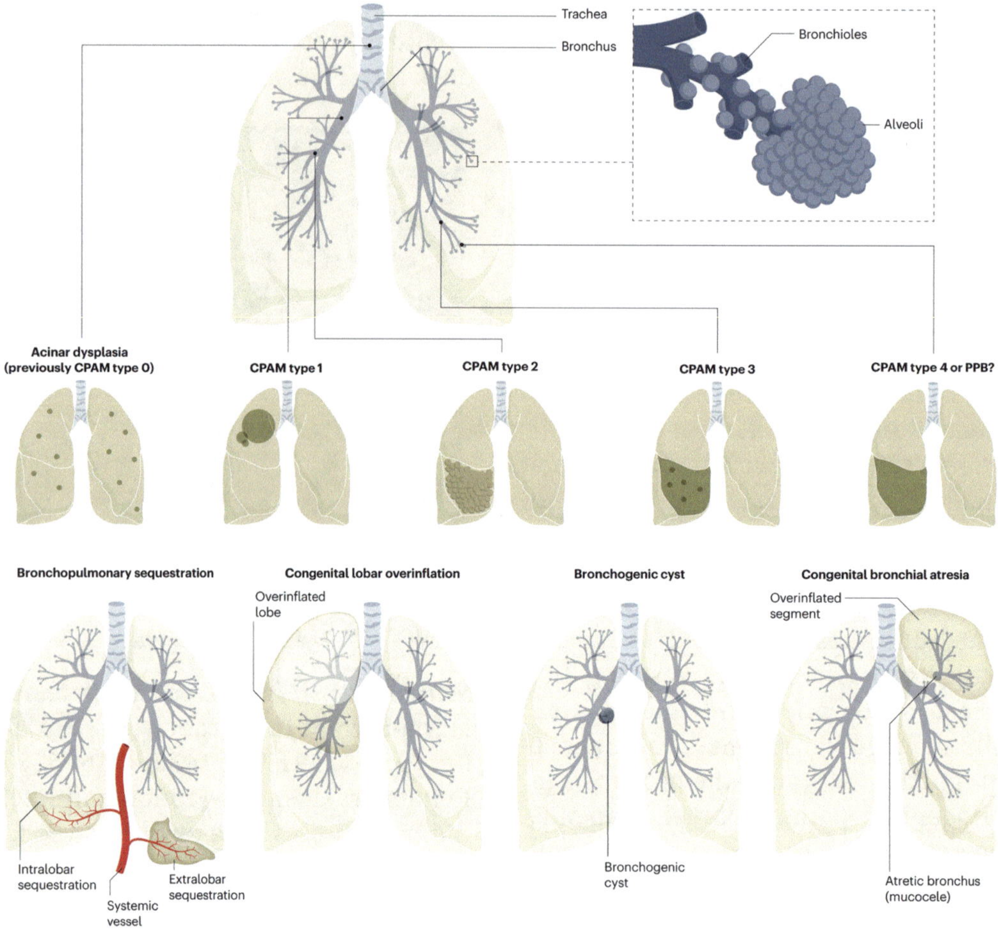

Figure 10.6. Causes and Risk Factors for the congenital anomalies of the respiratory system.

Source: https://media.springernature.com/full/springer-static/image/art%3A10.1038%2Fs41572-023-00470-1/MediaObjects/41572_2023_470_Fig1_HTML.png.

An understanding of these underlying gene factors is essential to early diagnosis and treatment, which in turn can maximize the outcome for the affected population. Environmental factors during pregnancy also play a role in the risk of congenital respiratory anomalies. Maternal health, including underlying conditions and lifestyle habits, may significantly affect fetal development. For instance, maternal exposure to harmful chemicals such as tobacco smoke and certain drugs can lead to the risk of respiratory defects at birth. Infections during pregnancy, particularly those caused by organisms such as the flu virus, are known risk factors that can lead to abnormal development of the respiratory system. Understanding such environmental risks can lead to the formulation of guidelines for pregnant women, emphasizing the importance of prenatal checkups and lifestyle changes that can neutralize such impacts. Socioeconomic status is also an important risk determinant associated with congenital respiratory anomalies. Mothers belonging to lower education groups are often faced with delays or challenges in accessing good-quality healthcare, leading to underlying medical conditions going unattended and putting pregnant women at greater risk of congenital anomalies. In a study, it was discovered that inadequate prenatal care has been linked to more instances of complications, such as maternal infection, each with the potential to cause respiratory defects during birth (Ornaghi et al., 2022). Also, there is the prevalent rate of cesarean delivery in certain regions, where the baby can be subjected to the lack of exposure to the mother's vaginal flora, essential for the development of healthy microbiota, which can affect respiratory health (Executive Board of IJMS, 2022). Resolution of such inequalities through targeted interventions can decrease the incidence of congenital anomalies and improve maternal and infant health status (Figure 10.6).

10.2.1. Genetic Factors

Genetic factors play a crucial role in the research regarding congenital anomalies of the respiratory system since certain hereditary disorders directly cause malformations. Genetic vulnerabilities are responsible for susceptibility to the development of a number of respiratory anomalies, such as CDH or tracheoesophageal fistula. These are caused by disruptions during embryogenesis, regulated by inherited gene mutations or chromosomal abnormalities. For example, specific gene mutations affect normal development of the thoracic cavity, which subsequently leads to structural defects. Transparency of genetic contributions not only explains the etiology of anomalies but also helps identify populations at risk, enabling early interventions to prevent or minimize congenital disorders. In addition to individual genetic mutations, the interaction between genes and the environment is paramount to understanding the subtleties of congenital respiratory anomalies. Family histories tend to show patterns implying a genetic component; these aberrations can also occur due to teratogenic exposures during pregnancy. For example, maternal smoking or the intake of certain drugs may interact with genetic vulnerabilities to render an individual more susceptible to developing congenital respiratory defects. It is thus possible to explain the multifactorial etiology of such conditions by identifying these gene-environment interactions, and this serves to emphasize the importance of thorough genetic counseling. Health practitioners need to be aware of these interactions during assessing patients with congenital anomalies in order to make informed decisions regarding management and therapy as well as preventive care planning in future pregnancies that can be at risk. Additionally, advancements in genetic screening technology have significantly enhanced our knowledge of the hereditary elements involved in congenital respiratory system anomalies. Techniques such as next-generation sequencing (NGS) have made it possible to identify extensive panels of genetic variation associated with respiratory malformations. By discovering specific genetic markers, physicians can better predict outcomes and create personalized treatment plans based on an individual's own genetic profile. Additionally, research still highlights discrepancies in the frequency of such anomalies among various populations, hinting at a probable relationship with genetic disorders alongside socio-environmental issues. As suggested in recent research, increasing awareness regarding genetic testing and its effects can empower families with knowledge, inspiring proactive control over their health in accordance with their genetic compositions, considering the broader demographic factors involved (Baumgartner et al., 2020; Siegel et al., 2024).

10.2.2. Environmental Influences

Environmental factors play an important role in the pathogenesis of congenital anomalies of the respiratory system. Various factors, ranging from air quality to exposure to toxic agents, significantly influence fetal development. Air pollution, particularly particulate matter and noxious fumes from industrial processes, has been associated with adverse pregnancy outcomes. Those women who live near highways or industrial sites are potentially at a greater risk of the infant suffering from respiratory abnormalities. The most important aspect of exposure to the environment is the chemical composition of pollutants, which, through abnormal fetal development, can result in lung structural abnormalities (Bruen et al., 2004). Furthermore, such an environmental hazard can complicate what has already occurred, with a compounding factor that maximizes the risk of a congenital defect. Climate is also an environmental influence that can initiate congenital anomalies of the respiratory tract. Extreme weather conditions, such as extreme heat waves or unexpected cold snaps, can influence maternal health and, hence, fetal development. High and low temperatures have been known to elevate the risk of ischemic heart disease, suggesting that environmental temperature could be exerting the same influence on congenital health outcomes (Armstrong et al., 2012). These temperature fluctuations could be stressing the maternal body, leading to compromised blood supply and oxygenation of the fetus, hence affecting the development of respiratory system. This underscores the need to attain a good understanding of how local climatic conditions and weather extremes might influence maternal and child health, particularly concerning respiratory anomalies. Waste management operations and landfilling also contribute to environmental hazards associated with congenital anomalies. Uncontrolled landfills emit toxic gases, including landfill gas and leachate, both of which can contaminate local air as well as water sources (Bruen et al., 2004). Exposure to these toxic conditions during pregnancy has been observed to increase the risk of congenital respiratory abnormalities due to exposure to unknown or poisonous chemicals found in the waste. The connection between living near unregulated landfills and adverse birth outcomes has been documented, but ultimate causal links to specific anomalies remain under investigation. This relationship underscores the need for strict waste management policies and comprehensive environmental studies to contain hazards and ensure healthier outcomes for developing fetuses. It also stresses the necessity of ongoing study into the environmental determinants of congenital malformations (Figure 10.7).

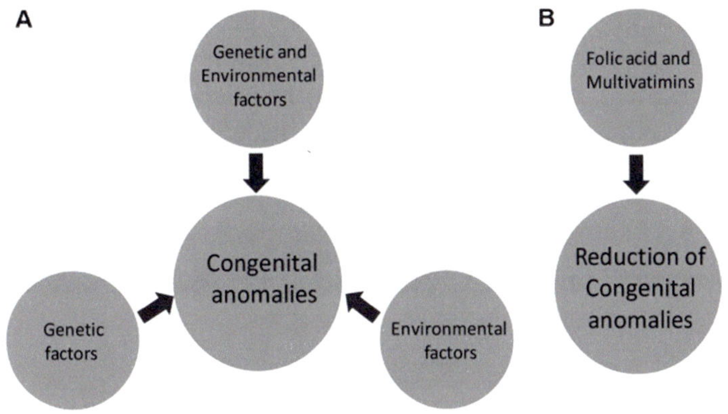

Figure 10.7. Common congenital anomalies: Environmental causes and prevention with folic acid containing multivitamins.

Source: https://onlinelibrary.wiley.com/cms/asset/79572e8c-a57a-4c5f-ba08-b0da0db42568/bdrc21138-fig-0002-m.jpg.

10.2.3. Maternal Health and Lifestyle

The diet and maternal health during pregnancy play crucial roles in the etiology of congenital anomalies, particularly respiratory anomalies. Diet, smoking, and exposure to environmental toxins among maternal factors play a significant role in fetal growth. Maternal undernutrition, for instance, may result in growth restriction in the fetus, making the newborn susceptible to respiratory problems at birth. Additionally, maternal smoking of cigarettes is an established risk factor found to be associated with higher incidences of congenital anomalies, including respiratory system anomalies. Public health initiatives promoting healthy lifestyle choices during pregnancy are paramount in reducing incidences of such congenital abnormalities. As research offers proof that some 70% of all infant deaths are linked with preterm birth or major congenital malformations, it is imperative to learn about the impact of maternal health in addressing these astronomical figures (Adamkin et al., 2016). Socioeconomic factors might also complicate outcomes of maternal health and influence both life decisions and healthcare access among pregnant women. Research has shown that the disparity in deprivation has increased with time as far as neonatal mortality is concerned, so that women in lower socioeconomic groups have a heavier burden as far as health experiences of their children are concerned. Women in lower socioeconomic groups are more likely not to receive adequate prenatal care, which could lead to uncorrected medical conditions that could lead to congenital respiratory system abnormalities. Maternal health professionals, therefore, have to consider such social determinants when they develop programs and strategies meant to promote maternal and child well-being. Closing prenatal care disparities can effectively counteract the risks associated with both congenital anomalies and adverse neonatal outcomes, consequently leading to healthier babies and families (Adamkin et al., 2016). The use of pharmacological treatments, including metformin in pregnancy, demonstrates the intricacy of mother health and the impact on fetal outcome. Metformin has been used for more than 40 years, primarily in gestational diabetes and maternal obesity, two conditions that are risk factors for neonatal respiratory abnormalities. More recent randomized controlled trials (RCTs) have assessed the safety and efficacy of this drug, showing both its possible benefits and potential long-term effects on fetal growth. While metformin does pass through the placenta, long-term programming concerns necessitate that careful consideration must be exercised prior to prescribing it to pregnant women. As public health messages change to facilitate a healthier life for the mother, there is a requirement to examine existing drugs' safety and efficacy so that they are in line with the overall aim of minimizing risks for congenital abnormalities, particularly respiratory-related ones.

Test Your Knowledge

1. What are the genetic factors of congenital anomalies?
2. What is the maternal health and lifestyle of congenital anomalies?

10.3. Diagnosis of Congenital Anomalies

Learning Outcome

1. Prenatal imaging techniques;
2. Postnatal diagnostic methods;
3. Role of genetic testing.

Accurate diagnosis of congenital abnormalities, particularly in the respiratory tract, is vital in enabling proper management and intervention strategies. The anomalies, including the CDH, not only affect the respiratory status but also the overall health of affected infants. Diagnostic techniques have evolved in prenatal care, allowing early identification of these abnormalities. The use of diagnostic imaging such as ultrasound combined with biochemical markers makes it possible to detect anatomical abnormalities and associated anomalies. Prenatal detection of the defects may prepare the medical teams for instant interventions at birth, which is crucial in cases of high rates of pulmonary hypoplasia for conditions such as CDH (Campo et al., 2018). The early diagnoses also emphasize that there should be a multidisciplinary team composed of obstetricians, pediatricians, and genetic counselors to optimize care. In the recent past, the inclusion of genetic testing has been an integral part of diagnosing respiratory system congenital anomalies. Rapid whole-genome sequencing (rWGS) has improved the diagnostic accuracy significantly, particularly in complex congenital disorders. Genetic information not only directs treatment options but also facilitates understanding of the risk of recurrence in families. For example, in CDH patients with congenital heart disease, genetic mutation explains the etiologic cause and directs appropriate medical care. Besides that, educating the parents on the genetic significance and potential requirement for surgery of the child can mitigate anxiety and improve decision-making processes at this critical moment (Helner et al., 2019). Lastly, the integration of genetics into routine diagnostic protocols represents a significant advancement in the treatment of congenital respiratory abnormalities. Moreover, the role of maternal health in the diagnosis and management of congenital defects cannot be overlooked. Research indicates that maternal conditions, e.g., respiratory disease and other somatic conditions, are linked with greater risks for congenital abnormalities, including anomalies of the respiratory system (Helner et al., 2019). Intensive maternal history screenings for medical conditions must thus become standard in prenatal care. Knowledge of the variety of potential risk factors enables healthcare providers to do the proper prenatal screening and diagnostic measures. Additionally, this data informs prevention interventions aimed at curtail infections-related risks during pregnancy, such as acute respiratory viral infections, which have been identified to affect fetal growth. Thus, developing comprehensive prenatal care regimens integrating maternal health is imperative in restricting the occurrence of these anomalies and promoting neonatal outcome in neonates with congenital anomalies of the respiratory system (Figure 10.8).

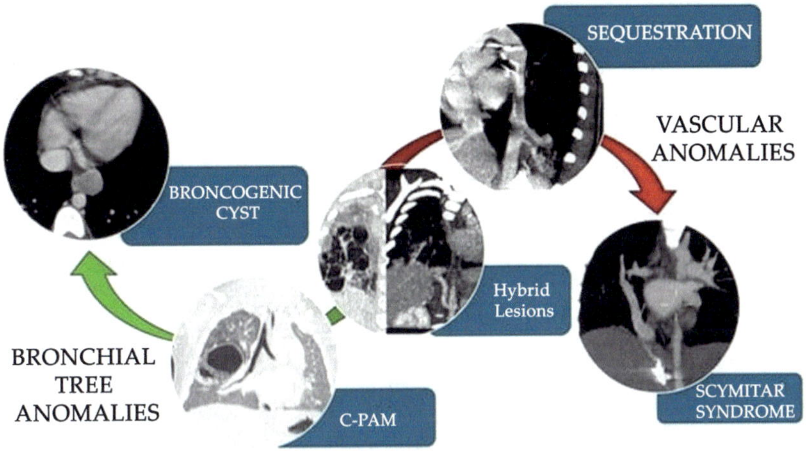

Figure 10.8. Diagnosis of congenital anomalies of the respiratory system.

Source: https://pub.mdpi-res.com/children/children-11-00638/article_deploy/html/images/children-11-00638-ag-550.jpg?1716629046.

10.3.1. Prenatal Imaging Techniques

The advent of prenatal imaging technologies has revolutionized early congenital anomaly diagnosis, particularly conditions related to the respiratory system. Ultrasound remains the most common modality used in prenatal scans, enabling clinicians to recognize anatomical features and monitor fetal development. While ultrasound provides valuable early information, the inability to resolve complex conditions necessitates the use of more advanced imaging technologies. Fetal MRI, for instance, has become an important adjunct, yielding additional information that ultrasound cannot provide by itself. Studies in the clinical literature indicate that MRI can clarify previously indeterminate findings and thus enhance diagnoses and risk assessments for a range of respiratory disorders. As documented in the literature, such universal knowledge allows for more effective parental counseling and management strategies, particularly in the case of congenital respiratory anomalies that may impact the infants' current and long-term health (Baldacchino et al., 2016). In addition, the application of advanced genetic testing has also complemented prenatal imaging techniques in identifying potential congenital anomalies. With the advancement of genetic diagnostics, early detection of various genetic illnesses that cannot be visually discerned through imaging alone is possible. The use of both imaging and genetic screening together offers a more insightful understanding of potential respiratory abnormalities. Genetic testing, for instance, can identify cystic fibrosis or CDH, often followed by imaging evidence of abnormal development. Additionally, the reality that existing genetic screening techniques are innocuous, including the analysis of cell-free fetal nucleic acids in maternal blood, has paved the way for a safer method of obtaining critical prenatal data. Consequently, the integrative methodology fortifies clinical management and decision-making options, emphasizing the importance of prenatal care in maintaining fetal and maternal well-being (Uzak et al., 2011). With improvements in the technology of prenatal imaging, the possibilities for the management of congenital respiratory tract anomalies are profound. Improvements in imaging tools, such as three-dimensional ultrasound and advanced MRI, have made visualization of complex fetal anatomy much easier. With these advancements, the detection of developmental abnormalities is more precise and occurs at an earlier stage, which can have a profound impact on prenatal and postnatal management strategies. Furthermore, utilizing multi-disciplinary approaches involving neonatologists, maternal-fetal medicine specialists, and genetic counselors ensures properly planned care. By permitting timely intervention and customized management plans, prenatal imaging techniques not only promote the outcome for infant respiratory anomalies but also give parents access to information to make an informed decision regarding their pregnancy. Finally, such collaborative works resulting from these imaging technologies reinforce the necessity of continuous adaptation of clinical practice in response to accruing evidence (Baldacchino et al., 2016) (Figure 10.9).

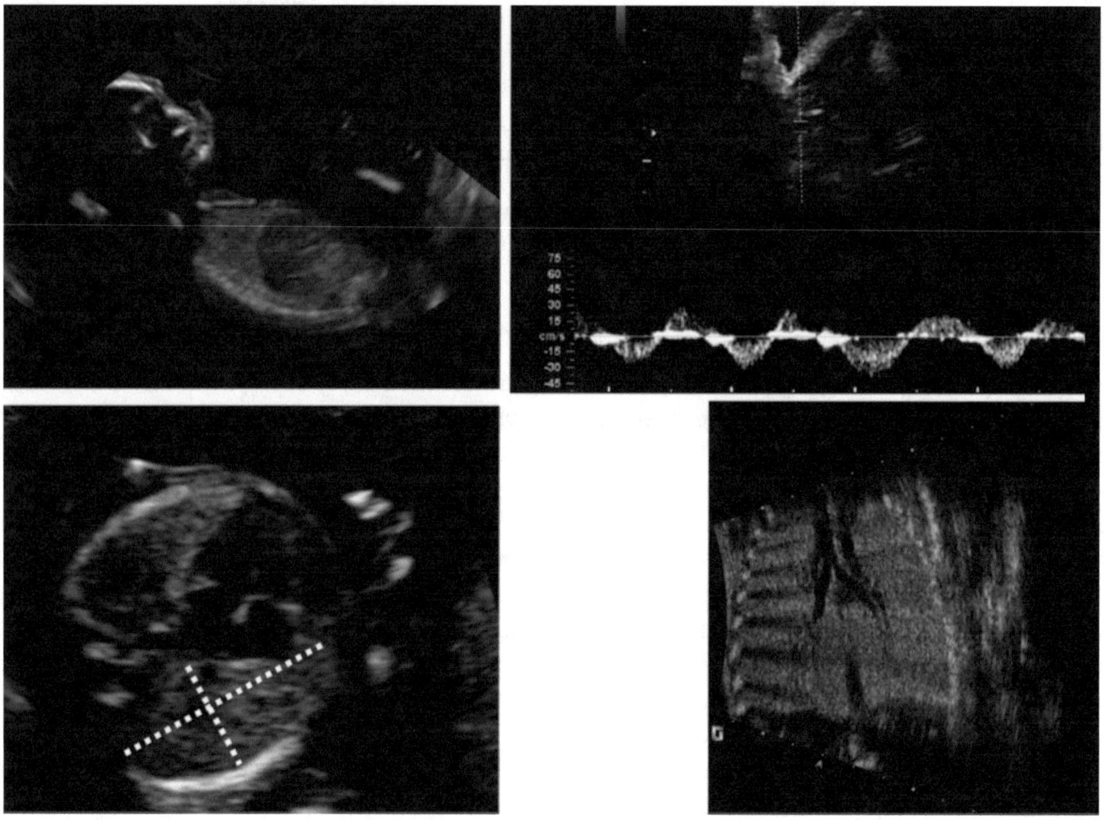

Figure 10.9. Prenatal imaging techniques of the respiratory system.

Source: https://www.researchgate.net/profile/Roland-Devlieger-2/publication/261772832/figure/fig1/AS:601690176761879@1520465525383/Normal-lungs-airways-and-diaphragm-a-Prenatal-ultrasound-of-the-normal-diaphragm-at.png.

10.3.2. Postnatal Diagnostic Methods

Postnatal diagnostic methods are also critically vital for early detection and management of congenital anomalies of the respiratory system. Following delivery, a full evaluation is needed to identify any structural or functional defects that may affect a newborn's respiratory health. Techniques such as chest X-rays, ultrasound scanning, and specialty imaging devices such as computed tomography (CT) scans are utilized to identify malformations such as CDH or tracheoesophageal fistula. Such imaging techniques assist healthcare providers in identifying anatomical structures and examining airflow patterns, facilitating early treatment. The integration of these diagnostic tests not only enhances the understanding of respiratory disease but also informs treatment approaches down the line, ultimately leading to improved patient outcomes. As part of imaging protocols, clinical assessment and laboratory investigation are the fundamental components of postnatal diagnostic protocols. Respiratory distress testing and genetic testing to identify syndromic associations with respiratory disease could be included in newborn screening programs. Such programs are vital for early intervention and can potentially reduce morbidity and mortality from congenital disorders. For instance, information on the genetics obtained from high-level screening programs can identify familial patterns of respiratory disorders, facilitating risk stratification and counseling for these families. Such multi-disciplinary approaches underscore the necessity of considering the genetic and environmental origins in the management of congenital anomalies, opening up possibilities for innovations in personalized medicine. Moreover, new developments in molecular diagnostics are transforming the practice of postnatal examinations. Techniques such as NGS enable rapid identification of genes associated with congenital respiratory diseases. This evolution not only brings about clearness in the diagnosis of complex conditions but also allows focused therapeutic interventions, furthering the overall care of affected newborns. With research ongoing, findings concerning the genetic basis of congenital anomalies should only further enhance clinical practice. Discussion of the genetic cause of congenital anomalies emphasizes integration across disciplines, validating cooperation between specialties to ensure adequate care, as outlined in recent studies on congenital heart disease and syndromes (Pierpont et al., 2018). Similarly, updated clinical practice guidelines reflect a commitment to optimizing the treatment of congenital disease, with patient-centered care (Speiser et al., 2018) (Figure 10.10).

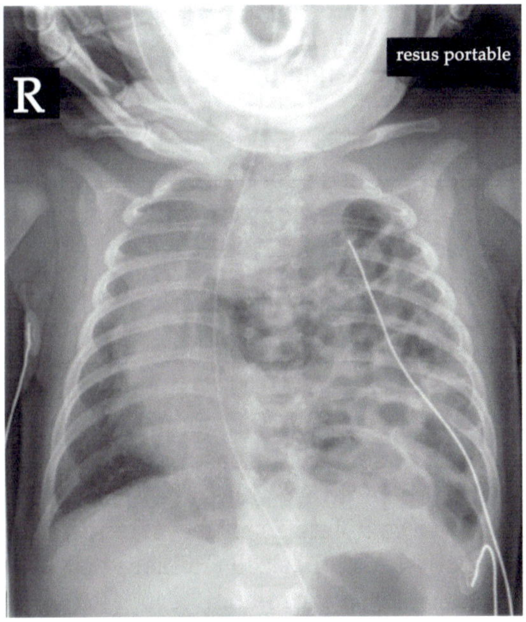

Figure 10.10. Postnatal diagnosis of congenital diaphragmatic hernia.

Source: https://external-content.duckduckgo.com/iu/?u=https%3A%2F%2Fprod-images-static.radiopaedia.org%2Fimages%2F65738723%2Fb043bbe3c18e9714d229fbed8b0c100863d52fc684b42c048b2321fef3050da5_gallery.jpeg&f=1&nofb=1&ipt=33cf23c7f67f0fdc987f7db195c89bd7caa0e8453a3d764960ee0781a3a28102.

10.3.3. Role of Genetic Testing

The significance of genetic testing in congenital anomalies of the respiratory system is increasingly central. Genetic testing offers an important means of identifying chromosomal abnormalities and genetic syndromes that may predispose the individual to congenital disease. For instance, specific genetic markers can determine the probability of respiratory anomalies, enabling clinicians to formulate individualized management strategies for affected neonates. The identification of such markers not only enables early intervention but also directs parental counseling for potential outcomes. Inclusion of genetic testing in prenatal care, especially when used in conjunction with imaging modalities, enhances fetal development and related risk perception, thereby influencing clinical decision-making appropriately. This preventive approach has been especially important as medical professionals attempt to minimize the occurrence of the impacts of congenital conditions on infant morbidity. In addition, the efficacy of genetic testing is further augmented by recent data illustrating its application in detecting congenital heart malformations, which are often co-associated with respiratory anomalies. In one study, a population of 67 pregnant women, some of the challenges of somatic diseases were observed, including respiratory abnormalities, and the necessity of complete genetic evaluation during pregnancy was emphasized (Helner et al., 2019). Using non-invasive prenatal tests (NIPT) and other genetic markers, healthcare providers can more accurately assess the risk of congenital heart disease that can further interfere with respiratory function. This dualism not only strengthens the process of diagnosis but also fine-tunes the management strategies by ensuring that high-risk pregnancies are subjected to targeted surveillance and interventions. Genetic testing, in this way, is a cornerstone in the complete strategy for the management of congenital anomalies of the respiratory system. In addition to its diagnostic benefits, genetic testing in congenital anomalies affects family planning and genetic counseling. Knowledge of the inheritance pattern of respiratory anomalies facilitates families to make decisions regarding future pregnancy and the likelihood of the need for pre-implantation genetic diagnosis. This aspect of genetic counseling serves to reduce the emotional burden on families who otherwise may have to live with the uncertainty of congenital disease among their children. The complexities of congenital muscular dystrophies and respiratory disease-associated disorders indicate the necessity of ongoing research and improved classification systems to prevent misdiagnosis and family counseling (Corsello et al., 2016). Last but not least, genetic testing not only aids in the identification of currently occurring anomalies but also paves the way for future medical advancements focused on prevention and treatment of congenital diseases of the respiratory tract.

Test Your Knowledge

1. What are prenatal imaging methods?
2. What are the postnatal diagnostic techniques?

10.4. Clinical Manifestations

Learning Outcome

1. Symptoms of respiratory distress;
2. Systemic complications associated with them;
3. Health implications in the long term.

Clinical presentations of congenital respiratory tract anomalies are highly diverse and are contingent upon the nature and severity of the defect. The most commonly observed symptoms include respiratory distress manifested as dyspnea, tachypnea, or gasping. Infants with such anomalies typically have cyanosis, a blue discoloration of the skin due to oxygen-poor blood. Tracheoesophageal fistula or CDH also disrupts the normal function of the airway. Early identification is critical because these findings lead to significant morbidity unless treated soon. The heterogeneity of clinical presentation requires a fine appreciation of the underlying pathophysiology, which can ultimately guide therapeutic approaches to improve such presentations and enhance the quality of life for affected individuals. The clinical presentation includes potential concomitant systemic abnormalities that further exacerbate respiratory impairment. For instance, hypotonia may occur in infant congenital muscular dystrophy patients, and thus, compromised respiratory muscle function and secondary hypoventilation can ensue, raising the risk for respiratory failure. The variability of symptoms in those with the condition makes it particularly challenging to diagnose, sometimes requiring the intervention of a multidisciplinary team of pediatricians, neonatologists, and pulmonologists to facilitate proper assessment. Early interventionary measures, depending on the accurate clinical features reported, are vital. These may include the use of ventilatory support and surgery for structural anomalies. Monitoring respiratory function and overall growth remains integral to managing the long-term status of these patients, highlighting the need for ongoing surveillance in clinical practice. Furthermore, congenital conditions like arthrogryposis multiplex congenita present with respiratory issues as a result of involvement in the musculoskeletal system, leading to impaired ventilation; therefore, it is important to assess every patient on a holistic basis. Arthrogryposis may impair diaphragmatic mobility through contractures of joints, which compromise the expansion of lungs and impair the effectiveness of ventilation. These structural abnormalities not only impact the respiratory dynamics but also compromise the infants' clearance of pulmonary secretions, predisposing them to frequent respiratory infections. The interplay between various organ systems necessitates multifaceted modes of care tailored to the unique clinical presentation. Therefore, clinicians should be alert to the risk of respiratory complications from congenital anomalies and refer the patient early to expert services for their effective management (Kumar et al., 2009; Corsello et al., 2016).

10.4.1. Respiratory Distress Symptoms

Clinical presentation of respiratory distress is a point of serious concern in congenital anomalies of the respiratory system. They represent a group of clinical signs that consist of increased respiratory effort, productive cough, wheeze, and cyanosis. In preschool-age and infant children, these symptoms are threatening and often require urgent medical attention to avoid severe complications. For instance, illness conditions such as bronchopulmonary sequestration can lead to chronic respiratory infections, which subsequently might aggravate predisposing respiratory distress symptoms. It is essential to note the above signs early since delayed treatment will cause severe morbidity and mortality. Thus, caregivers and healthcare workers must be on the lookout for respiratory distress, as it is usually a sign of serious underlying pathology that requires intense investigation and early intervention. Clinical presentation of congenital anomalies such as laryngeal and tracheal ones is usually by the presence of obvious respiratory distress symptoms. These can manifest as an obstructive airway leading to stridor or noisy respiration, repeated respiratory infections, and feeding difficulty that can impair growth and development. Of particular note are the variable symptoms seen among affected individuals, with some reporting more pronounced manifestations than others. For example, infants who have complete tracheal ring deformities can present with severe respiratory distress because of impaired patency of the airway. This presentation highlights the intricacy of treating congenital respiratory anomalies, as clinicians must address not only the immediate respiratory issue but also the potential long-term effects on the child's well-being. Correspondingly, a sensitive understanding of the etiology and treatment options is necessary for clinicians who treat affected populations (Fockens et al., 2024). Second, a respect for the symptoms of respiratory distress goes beyond having immediate clinical relevance; it also has significant psychosocial implications for families. Parents dealing with a child's respiratory distress due to congenital anomalies usually experience higher stress and anxiety, thereby complicating the whole caregiving process. The symptoms of respiratory distress can result in frequent hospital admissions, leading to stress and economic expenditure. Hence, it is the duty of medical practitioners to offer holistic care by addressing the child's medical requirements along with the emotional needs of the family. Knowledge regarding the symptoms, management, and prognosis of some of the congenital anomalies may enable the families to promote coping mechanisms. Through developing a spirit of collaboration, healthcare professionals can genuinely improve the quality of care, which finally guides the family through the complexities of congenital respiratory abnormalities (DeGiovanni et al., 2016) (Figure 10.11).

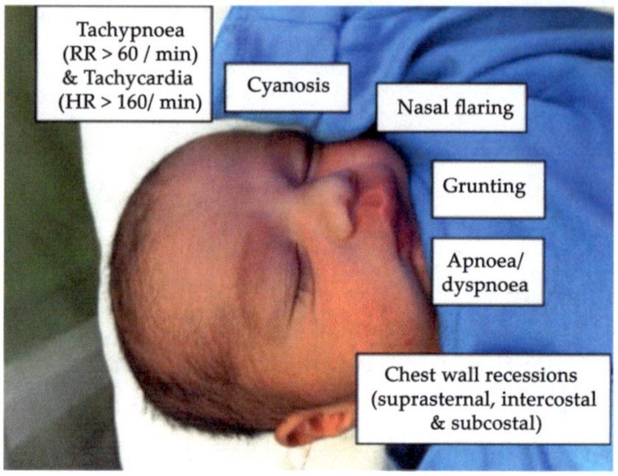

Figure 10.11. Respiratory distress symptoms.

Source: https://ars.els-cdn.com/content/image/1-s2.0-S1526054212000073-gr1.jpg.

10.4.2. Associated Systemic Complications

Congenital anomalies in the respiratory system may cause severe systemic complications affecting not just the immediate health but also future outcomes in the affected individuals. Notably, malformations such as CDH and TEF often impair pulmonary function. In children with CDH, for instance, the hypoplastic lungs can result in pulmonary hypoplasia, thus causing chronic respiratory compromise. This compromised respiratory status may set a cascade of complications like compromised gas exchange, recurrent respiratory infection, and risk for pulmonary hypertension. Moreover, systemic effects of such respiratory complications might be seen in enhanced use of medical care, longer hospital stays, and greater need for intensive medical management, as research on patients with craniofacial abnormalities who undergo complicated surgery has reported higher rates of infectious complications and longer recovery times (Allareddy et al., 2018). Beyond pulmonary complications, congenital anomalies may place patients at risk for overall systemic illness. For example, congenital respiratory abnormalities in infants can be accompanied by gastrointestinal difficulties, such as the extremely high incidence of feeding disorders in tracheoesophageal malformations. Assistance with feeding not only complicates nutrition but also increases the risk of malnutrition and resultant growth deficits. In addition, the chronic disease nature of respiratory disease also often leads to repeated cycles of hospitalization and medication requirements, as with findings in populations with other congenital conditions, where health consumption increases markedly following diagnosis (Canova et al., 2016). Such interaction between respiratory well-being and overall health necessitates the multidisciplinary nature of treating congenital anomalies, requiring a multi-factorial approach to address both respiratory and overall health in conjunction. Finally, the broader implications of this associated systemic complication extend beyond individual health to impact familial and societal issues as well. Families of children with respiratory impairment at birth will most often experience a financial and emotional burden, along with the need for long-term care planning and potential special education services. The economic cost arises not only from higher hospital visits and treatments but also from the loss of parental work hours from caregiving obligations. Therefore, knowledge of the system implications of congenital respiratory abnormalities is crucial for healthcare professionals, policymakers, and care organizations. Increased awareness and early intervention strategies will significantly improve individual health outcomes and reduce the socioeconomic costs of such congenital anomalies en masse, thereby providing a healthier tomorrow for patients afflicted by them.

10.4.3. Long-Term Health Implications

Long-term health implications of congenital anomalies of the respiratory system are vast and extensive, especially in disorders like CDH. While survival rates have been improved by medical technology to 80%–90% or more, such individuals often have some degree of functional impairment as they grow older. They can experience respiratory disease, delay in developmental processes, and increased vulnerabilities to chronic diseases and are seriously compromised in quality of life. Notably, the association of CDH with other severe conditions like congenital heart disease and pulmonary hypertension adds to the complexity of long-term prognosis and treatment. The financial burden of maintaining CDH, as indicated, may require up to $250 million annually, pointing to the need for effective follow-up treatment and intervention strategies in a timely manner to manage complications that could arise due to this disorder in the future (Campo et al., 2018). The second critical area of concern involves psychosocial complications faced by children with congenital respiratory abnormalities. Longitudinal studies have documented that such children are more likely to develop mental illness, including anxiety and depression, because of their long-term medical treatment and hospitalization. Furthermore, the social stigma associated with visible disabilities or chronic conditions may cause social isolation, further exacerbating mental illness. For instance, the experience of having had multiple surgical interventions, while necessary to stay alive, could make them feel more vulnerable and not quite "normal" for their age group. Addressing the psychosocial and mental health of these children is no less critical than curing their physical conditions and needs a multidisciplinary approach combining medical and psychological expertise (Doughty et al., 2014). In addition, long-term health outcomes influence the families of these children with congenital respiratory abnormalities. Psychological and economic stress on parents and caregivers is profound and impacts their overall well-being. Particularly in situations involving significant medical intervention, families go through a drastic alteration in daily routines, which typically means high caregiver strain and even burnout. The prevalence of related health issues, such as depression and obesity, highlights the importance of adequate support systems and mental health care access for such families. Counseling about long-term care needs of children with congenital malformations is instrumental in instructing families on the parameters required to sustain them through this arduous process. Ensuring that they are aware of their child's health needs and are part of the long-term care plan enhances the family's coping capacity and survival (Campo et al., 2018) (Figure 10.12).

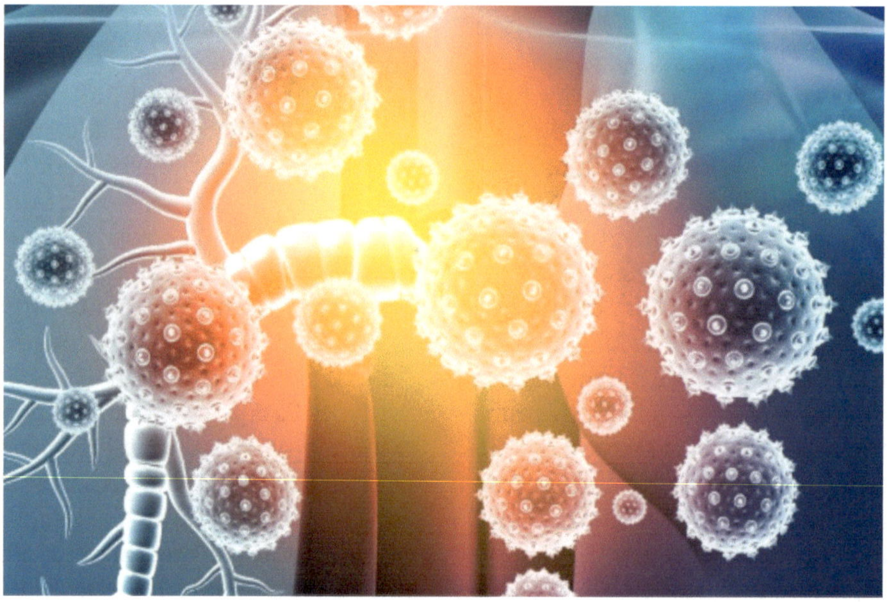

Figure 10.12. The long-term health implications of congenital anomalies of the respiratory system.

Source: https://external-content.duckduckgo.com/iu/?u=https%3A%2F%2Fd2jx2rerrg6sh3.cloudfront.net%2Fimages%2Fnews%2FImageForNews_734648_16723203205328165.jpg&f=1&nofb=1&ipt=1e05eaf77cd263bbb7f19d9f997839b2f79ef8ef47f56a1cd39ca651fc0ff397.

Test Your Knowledge

1. What is the respiratory distress syndrome?
2. What are the complications related to the system?

10.5. Treatment Options

Learning Outcome

1. Surgical management;
2. Medical management;
3. Supportive care and rehabilitation.

Management of congenital respiratory system anomalies is a complicated process, considering the nature and severity of the anomaly. The initial treatment in the majority of conditions, e.g., tracheal stenosis or congenital hernia of the diaphragm, is surgical intervention. In the majority of cases, the surgery can restore normal respiratory function and improve the quality of the patient's life. It is important that timing and surgical technique are proper; for instance, early surgery is usually able to overcome the complications due to a delay in treatment, such as pulmonary hypertension and chronic respiratory distress. Accurate preoperative assessment and planning are essential to obtain optimum results, as highlighted by various studies showing improved survival following early surgical correction of such anomalies. In addition to surgery, supportive management is an important factor in treating respiratory anomalies. These include respiratory therapy, which may consist of mechanical ventilation or oxygen therapy to facilitate patients with severe hypoxemia or respiratory failure. Besides, medications such as bronchodilators and corticosteroids may be used to manage associated airway inflammation and increase respiratory efficacy. Such intervention methods are increasingly relevant to present-day clinical practice, as evident from present guidelines illustrating the necessity of multidimensional treatment using both surgical and nonsurgical interventions to address the diverse presentation of respiratory abnormalities (Roth et al., 2020). Furthermore, customized treatment plans, tailored to the specific presentation and needs of each patient, are required for maximum therapeutic benefit and patient safety. Advanced technology and surgical technique further expand the scope for the surgical correction of congenital respiratory system deformities. Minimally invasive surgery, such as video-assisted thoracoscopic surgery, has evolved as a less disruptive alternative to open surgery, with the benefits of earlier discharge and reduced postoperative morbidity. Moreover, ongoing research in regenerative medicine and the development of biocompatible materials could possibly provide future alternatives for anatomical malformation repair with safety. Practitioners must remain current with new treatment approaches and guidelines to ensure optimal care for these complex conditions (Baumgartner et al., 2020). Finally, a multidisciplinary collaboration of pediatric experts, like pulmonologists, surgeons, and primary care doctors, views treatment options grounded in contemporary evidence, thereby yielding the best outcomes for concerned individuals (Figure 10.13).

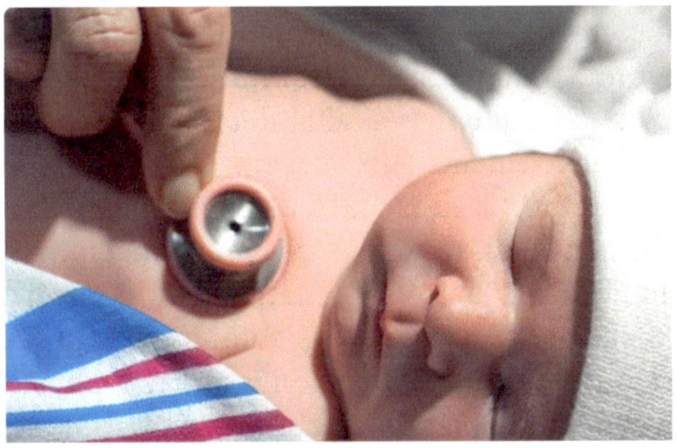

Figure 10.13. The management of congenital anomalies of the respiratory system.

Source: https://www.news-medical.net/image-handler/picture/Newborn%20medical%20exam%20-%20Susan%20McAnnally_thumb.jpg.

10.5.1. Surgical Interventions

The nature of congenital anomalies of the respiratory system typically necessitates surgical interventions for the best outcomes for patients. Surgical procedures are aimed at repairing the specific anatomical deformation and functional impairment of these malformations. Anomalies such as tracheoesophageal fistula or CDH, for instance, require urgent surgical repair to restore normal respiratory function and prevent severe morbidity. Such modalities of treatment can involve correction of abnormal connections between the trachea and esophagus or reconstruction of the diaphragm to ensure adequate ventilation. Without timely and effective surgical interventions, such infants are at greater risk of respiratory distress, failure to thrive, and prolonged hospital stay, underlining once again the crucial role to be played by surgery in the management of congenital respiratory malformations. Even beyond mere initial surgical correction, too, lies multidisciplinary patient management of individuals with congenital malformations. Long-term follow-up care is essential to monitor respiratory performance and manage resultant sequelae arising after the operation. For example, kids who have surgical intervention for congenital lung abnormalities may require ongoing pulmonary rehabilitation, nutritional care, and frequent re-evaluation to assess growth and development. This surgery is not limited to acute repair but is part of a comprehensive treatment plan that requires multi-disciplinary collaboration among pediatrics, pulmonology, and surgical services. This combined approach to care ensures that not only are the physical aspects of the anomaly addressed, but also the psychological and developmental needs of the child and family are considered, thus enhancing the overall quality of care. The intricacies in congenital anomalies, such as Apert syndrome, further adequately justify the necessity for meaningful surgical interventions. Interrelated anatomical defects can have multiple detrimental effects on different body systems, such as the respiratory system. Since the conditions are very complex, their control demands a multi-disciplinary approach. Surgical professionals often work along with respiratory therapists, pediatricians, and other health professionals to create treatment modalities that produce maximum functional outcomes. Treatment possibilities through surgery could range from craniofacial reconstruction to airway management surgeries, aiming to improve both breathing capacity and aesthetics. By establishing coherent care plans that take into account possible reduced intellectual functioning and cumulative anesthetic effects, practitioners can streamline treatment for patients while easing some of the distress for their families, highlighting the central position of surgical interventions in the treatment of congenital respiratory system malformations (Doughty et al., 2014; Caporlingua et al., 2015) (Figure 10.14).

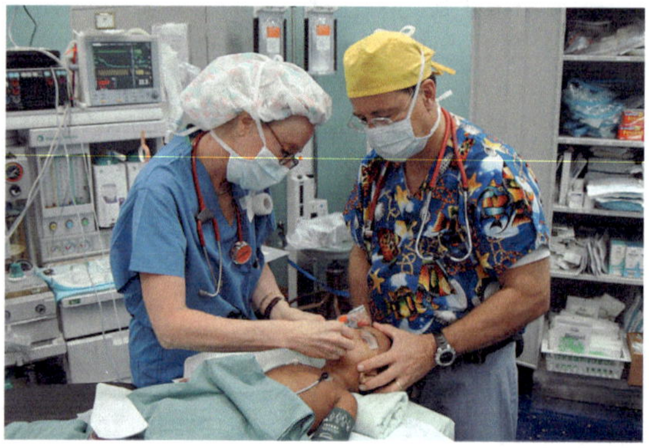

Figure 10.14. Surgical interventions of congenital anomalies of the respiratory system.

Source: https://external-content.duckduckgo.com/iu/?u=https%3A%2F%2Fwww.childheartspecialist.com%2Fwp-content%2Fuploads%2F2016%2F03%2Fchildren-heart-disease-non-cardiac-surgery.jpg&f=1&nofb=1&ipt=013333fcec7c6873fe3349e2075e6673ff562a795b26391bc0f393a7020f70c2.

10.5.2. Medical Management

Effective medical management of congenital anomalies of the respiratory system is critical in order to improve patient outcomes and the ideal quality of life. Early diagnosis and intervention are an integral part of such management. Advanced prenatal diagnostics, such as ultrasound and NIPT, play a significant role in the diagnosis of congenital heart and respiratory malformations during pregnancy. For instance, CDH abnormalities are usually diagnosed on routine prenatal ultrasounds to enable particular medical treatment plans at birth. Early detection makes it possible to plan for interventions that might be necessary, such as the immediate provision of respiratory support or surgical correction, which improves survival and reduces morbidity among affected infants. Furthermore, multidisciplinary management teams play an important role in treating complex cases of congenital respiratory anomalies. These teams include neonatologists, pediatric surgeons, pulmonologists, and geneticists who collaborate in formulating specialized treatment plans for the individual condition of each patient. In disorders like CDH, where pulmonary hypoplasia is a feature with the anomaly, other treatments like extracorporeal membrane oxygenation (ECMO) will be needed to support the infant's respiratory activity in vulnerable periods. This combined strategy not only addresses the surgical and medical needs of the patient but also familiarizes the family with the challenges involved with it, both hospitalization and the long-term care of their child's well-being, with the concern of delayed development and long-term medical care, as highlighted in previous studies (Campo et al., 2018). Genetic counseling's contribution cannot be ignored in the management of congenital respiratory malformations. The majority of such conditions are genetically caused, and therefore, there is a need for a comprehensive medical-genetic assessment of affected families. For example, knowledge of the genetic substrates of defects such as pulmonary agenesis or broncho-pulmonary dysplasia can assist in making more informed treatment choices and family consequences. In addition, gene-directed therapy from genetic diagnosis will enhance care of patients and direct steps for future pregnancy prevention. Recognition of the genetic contribution to respiratory malformations also changes paradigms in medical management because the addition of genetic counseling into standard care protocols has been proven to enhance education and assistance to families managing such complex conditions (Helner et al., 2019) (Figure 10.15).

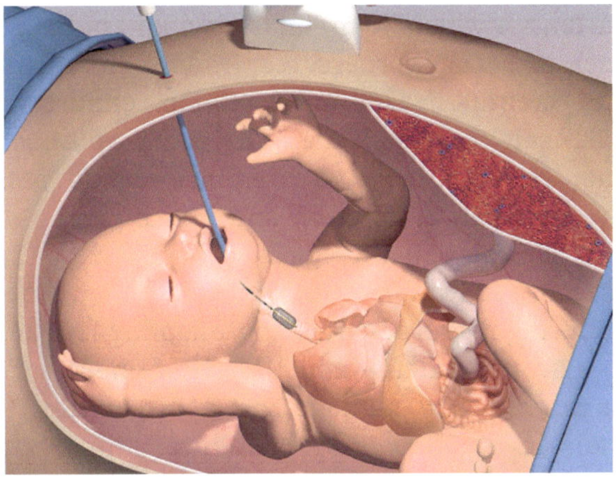

Figure 10.15. Medical management of congenital anomalies.

Source: https://www.bmj.com/content/bmj/370/bmj.m1624/F2.medium.jpg.

10.5.3. Rehabilitation and Supportive Care

Treatment of congenital respiratory system anomalies involves multidisciplinary management consisting of extensive rehabilitation and supportive care. They are crucial in optimizing respiratory function and improving the global quality of life in affected individuals. These programs are also important in this matter since they enable healthcare professionals to personalize therapy to suit the specific needs of every patient. Through continuous assessment and adjustment of therapeutic interventions, such as physical therapy and breathing training, recovery is able to contribute to lung function and capacity significantly. Rehabilitation not only takes into account the physiological but also the psychosocial well-being of patients, promoting resilience and adaptive coping as they deal with the complexities of disease. Supportive care, an integral component of rehabilitation, transcends the delivery of physical health treatments. It encompasses a wide range of interventions to address the emotional, social, and practical needs of congenital respiratory anomaly patients. Availability of multidisciplinary teams such as social workers, respiratory therapists, and mental health professionals ensures a balanced care approach. The team approach enables comprehensive care plans that address the medical, emotional, and social needs of families and patients. Further, emphasizing the care and education of caregivers creates a more enduring model of caregiving, enabling families to gain the training and experience necessary to successfully manage the complexities of their loved ones daily. Evidence supporting the effectiveness of these rehabilitative and supportive care practices favors their necessity in the management of congenital respiratory system defects. Evidence showed that proper coordination of care not only improves health outcomes but also reduces long-term costs in recurrent hospitalization and emergency admission. Investigating patient populations with successful integrated support systems reveals informative details about best practices that lead to successful rehabilitation outcomes. This corroborates the necessity for extensive rehabilitation interventions and supportive care integration, lastly advocating for policies that promote increased access to such vital services among patients diagnosed with congenital anomalies of the respiratory system, as indicated in articles on broad population health trends (Kitsiou et al., 2013) and assessing systemic health-related costs within various settings (Flaming et al., 2015) (Figure 10.16).

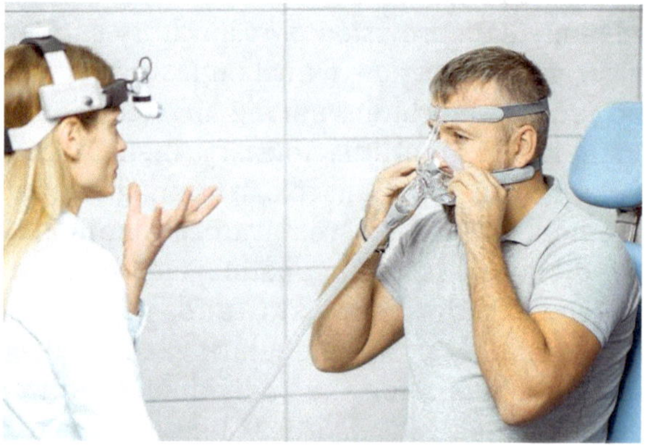

Figure 10.16. Rehabilitation of congenital anomalies of the respiratory system.

Source: https://external-content.duckduckgo.com/iu/?u=https%3A%2F%2Fblog.rehabselect.net%2Fhubfs%2Frespiratory-rehab.jpg&f=1&nofb=1&ipt=429a8b6d51f31c53e310c9b07a0af4168a793b58b439ac215e80997c4561ef0a.

Test Your Knowledge

1. What is the medical management of congenital anomalies of the respiratory system?
2. What is the rehabilitation and supportive care of congenital anomalies?

10.6. Prognosis and Outcomes

Learning Outcome

1. Factors influencing prognosis;
2. Quality of life consideration;
3. Long-term follow-up care.

The character and extent of the specific anomaly largely determines prognosis in a newborn with congenital anomalies of the respiratory system. Disorders like CDH have the potential to cause acute life-threatening complications, primarily respiratory distress as a consequence of lung hypoplasia. Early diagnosis through prenatal imaging modalities, such as ultrasound and fetal MRI, is of utmost importance in determining outcomes. A study found that not only does fetal MRI increase the accuracy of anomaly diagnosisbut , but it also aids in parental counseling and delivery planning, thereby improving overall management strategies (Helner et al., 2019). The most important determinant, however, is the timing of intervention; early surgical intervention can significantly improve survival rates and long-term health outcomes, justifying the necessity of ongoing surveillance and clinical assessment from the prenatal state to neonatal intensive care admission. The prognostic expectation of congenital anomalies also largely relies on the syndromic or non-syndromic conditions related to them. Those with single respiratory malformations may have better outcomes than individuals who have multiple congenital anomalies, for example, cardiovascular and neurological malformations. By evaluating the whole clinical record, healthcare providers may apply medical-genetic advice, as proposed in certain studies that point out family history and maternal health as predictors of the prognosis (Helner et al., 2019). For instance, the presence of comorbidities, such as maternal diabetes or high blood pressure, can have an adverse impact on both prenatal development and postnatal recuperation. Balancing findings from both genetic testing and advanced imaging can promote profound insights into challenges behind this disease so that special care plans can be created that meet the specific needs of each patient. Understanding the long-term prognosis for children with congenital respiratory malformations extends beyond initial survival; it includes assessing quality of life and functional status. Contemporary research indicates that most survivors will likely have chronic respiratory complications that necessitate long-term medical management and intervention for a lifetime. Gaining knowledge of the long-term effects allows for a proactive approach to treatment and rehabilitation, focusing on respiratory therapy, nutrition support, and mental health (Baldacchino et al., 2016).

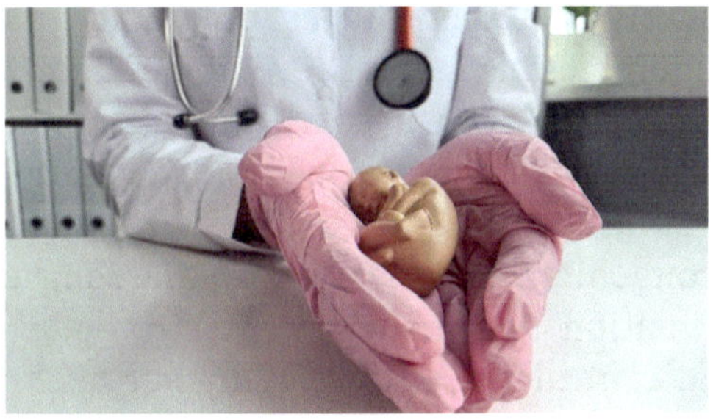

Figure 10.17. The prognosis for infants born with congenital anomalies of the respiratory system.

Source: https://images.onlymyhealth.com/imported/images/2023/June/09_Jun_2023/Main-congenital-anomalies.jpg.

Multidisciplinary treatment teams are highlighted by the need to address the children's overall needs, with appropriate follow-up and repeated reassessment. With an improvement in prognosis due to advancements in medical technology and surgical techniques, the emphasis is given to shared care and prolonged monitoring upon discharge so that the lives of affected individuals by congenital anomalies of the respiratory system are improved (Figure 10.17).

10.6.1. Factors Influencing Prognosis

The prognosis of congenital respiratory system defects is determined by a complex interplay of biological, environmental, and socio-economic factors. Among the biological determinants, the presence of coexisting associated congenital defects, particularly of other organ systems, significantly influences the prognosis. Certain evidence suggests that patients with underlying cardiovascular defects, for instance, have increased morbidity and mortality compared to those with isolated respiratory defects. It is important to understand these interactions since they can determine treatment strategy and outcome. Also, maternal clinical factors, including pre-existing medical conditions or infections occurring during pregnancy, play a considerable role in fetal development and later prognosis. In such a case, maternal medical history is a vital assessment instrument that may be used to predict the risk of individuals for congenital defects, thereby allowing early intervention and management strategies that play a central role in improving survival rates and quality of life for affected infants (Helner et al., 2019). The timeliness and efficacy of prenatal diagnosis are also other dimensions that significantly affect prognosis. Advances in imaging technology have enhanced the detection of congenital respiratory abnormalities in utero, enabling postnatal planning to be conducted in a hurry. Early diagnosis can lead to well-controlled deliveries and preparedness for instant medical intervention, which may enhance survival and outcome rates for affected newborns. Furthermore, prenatal genetic counseling is also essential, especially among families with a history of congenital malformations. The effectiveness of such counseling is likewise linked to the extent of maternal health screening, for example, measurement of genetic influences or chromosomal abnormalities that may put some pregnancies at risk for congenital disorders. Trimester-specific biomarkers of chromosomal disease follow the risk of fetal anomalies and therefore corroborate the predictive value of timely intervention procedures in establishing prognosis (Canova et al., 2016). Socio-economic determinants also contribute to the difficulty of the prognosis of congenital respiratory anomalies since they can influence access to care, environmental risk exposures, and overall health outcomes. Less socio-economically privileged families might be deterred from obtaining necessary prenatal care or treatment from decreased access to medical facilities and other amenities, further exacerbating the adverse effects of congenital conditions. Additionally, studies have shown that the extent of maternal education is related to better infant care methods and health outcomes for infants with congenital anomalies. The trend reveals that higher levels of maternal education regarding prenatal care can be a key method for alleviating the impacts of congenital respiratory anomalies. Thus, addressing socio-economic disparities is crucial for ensuring equal access to health care and improving the general prognosis for such infants, highlighting the importance of a comprehensive perspective when evaluating the factors influencing prognosis in congenital respiratory system anomalies (Canova et al., 2016).

10.6.2. Quality of Life Considerations

The quality of life for individuals with congenital anomalies of the respiratory system largely depends on the interaction between extensive care and medical treatment. These anomalies, from mild structural abnormalities to complicated, deadly conditions, are most likely to need complex treatments and long-term management solutions. The psychological and emotional dimensions of dealing with such illnesses contribute to the complexity of the general quality of life as individuals are bound to have chronic health problems, repeated hospitalizations, and the ongoing risk of respiratory distress. Such a burden does not only fall on the patients but also on their families, who need to find their way within the healthcare system and look after their relatives, very likely leading to increased stress and altered family structure. Moreover, the inclusion of effective health care programs is a significant determinant in assessing the overall standard of life for such individuals. For instance, programs like the Mother and Infant Health Project show how quality prenatal and postnatal care are essential parameters to improve infant as well as maternal health. By emphasizing early attendance at antenatal clinics and encouraging good delivery practices, such programs have the potential to minimize severe complications associated with congenital respiratory disease. The resulting increased healthcare use is typically expressed through better survival rates and a decreased incidence of respiratory failures, which in turn help maintain the quality of life for affected infants and their families. Moreover, the excellent return on investment in such ventures, as indicated by the cost-effectiveness ratio, highlights the immense benefits of guaranteeing quality over ensuring quantity in healthcare (Nizalova et al., 2025). Socioeconomic determinants of congenital anomalies also have a substantial impact on quality of life outcomes. Families that have difficulties with the respiratory illness of a child most often have burdensome financial demands, including healthcare payments, treatment methods, and potential loss of earnings due to caregiving responsibilities. These pressures can create limited accessibility to necessary services, including transport to hospitals, dietary requirements, and educational opportunities, which in total affect the health of the child. By resolving such socioeconomic inequalities, health care organizations can enhance quality of life through integrated support systems that go beyond clinical intervention. Community health programs focusing on educational assistance, logistics support, and economic assistance can strengthen families, thereby increasing their capacity to manage the complexities of respiratory irregularities. Therefore, a study of quality of life concerns in this case illustrates a complicated system to promote improvement for those concerned (Vyshnya et al., 2025) (Figure 10.18).

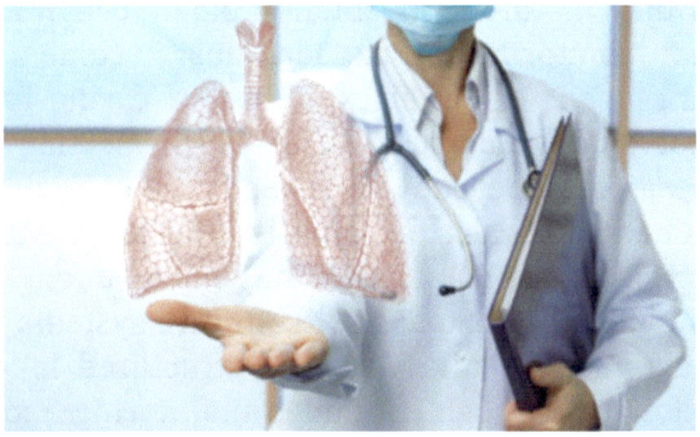

Figure 10.18. The quality of life for individuals with congenital anomalies of the respiratory system.

Source: https://admin.sarojhospital.com/storage/images/Respiratory-Disorders-in-the-Young-Population.png.

10.6.3. Long-term Follow-up Care

The relative complexity and challenge of these conditions necessitates long-term follow-up care for congenital anomalies of the respiratory system. Kids who are diagnosed with diseases such as CDH don't simply require emergency surgery; they're likely to have a whole range of health issues that extend into their early years. Campo et al. (2018) inform that even the kids who survive the initial neonatal period tend to have long-term functional disabilities, for which such children require comprehensive post-operative care. Such ongoing assessment is important to monitor pulmonary function, airway patency, and resolution of secondary pulmonary complications. Pediatric pulmonologists and other specialized medical professionals are inclined to use multidisciplinary approaches, in conjunction with other healthcare providers, to deliver complete follow-up care that encompasses physical and psychosocial aspects. Additionally, the impact of congenital anomalies on the child's neurodevelopment cannot be overstated, highlighting the importance of individualized long-term follow-up care. The chronic problems of the patients, such as developmental delay and recurrent respiratory infections, must be monitored regularly, with many of them involving screening for developmental issues and rehabilitation therapy. Correct comprehension of the patients' changing needs requires regular contact with all types of specialists, from speech therapists to occupational therapists. Such intensive care is designed to optimize each child's developmental trajectory, providing healthcare professionals with the information necessary to apply proper interventions as they mature. Congenital anomaly centers that focus on congenital anomalies increasingly see that monitoring and support must become an integral part of the very fabric of long-term health care. While financial expenses for caring for congenital respiratory abnormalities are high, as described in Campo et al. (2018), neglecting proper long-term follow-up care can further escalate these costs. Beyond the expenditure of prolonged hospital stays, it places a heavy emotional and monetary burden on families. The most expensive noncardiac congenital defect, as mentioned, highlights the implication that effective long-term care strategies may counteract both healthcare complications and costs. Healthcare systems can improve outcomes and quality of life for affected individuals by investing in a structured follow-up care regimen. The organization of long-term follow-up through continued monitoring and support finally aligns with the intention of holistic health, which is to allow for resilience and self-management capacity in patients as they traverse adulthood (Figure 10.19).

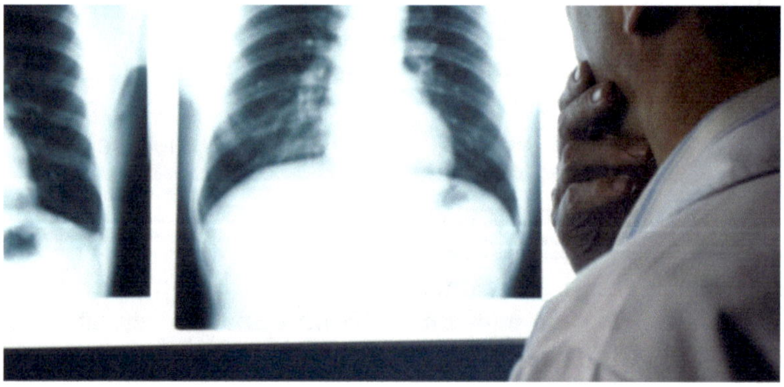

Figure 10.19. Long-term follow up of congenital lung abnormalities.

Source: https://external-content.duckduckgo.com/iu/?u=https%3A%2F%2Fwww.ersnet.org%2Fwp-content%2Fuploads%2F2022%2F09%2F16.png&f=1&nofb=1&ipt=06d5269892d2044dad03b7c14b5087092273d653cdce69690ff9b4222743ffac.

Test Your Knowledge

1. What are the factors influencing prognosis?
2. What is long-term follow-up care?

Summary

The research on congenital respiratory system abnormalities shows that such abnormalities have severe impacts on public and individual health as well as public health intervention. The abnormalities can occur in isolation or together with other congenital malformations, hence clinical assessment and intervention processes are complicated. Such an understanding of the complexity, particularly the association of socio-occupational status with these abnormalities, has to be ensured for the provision of widespread health equity interventions. Studies have established that low socio-occupational status is linked to increased prevalence of respiratory anomalies, hence the need for early screening, education, and dispensation of resources among marginalized groups (Llopis-Gonzalez et al., 2009). Secondly, the different patterns of congenital anomalies across disparate geographic and socio-economic settings prove that environmental and genetic determinants play a big role in their etiology. Research conducted in Dr. Sardjito General Hospital illustrates the prevalence of respiratory abnormalities among other prevalent conditions across various populations (Romi et al., 2015). This manifests as a general need for particular research work that addresses these inconsistencies, informing both clinical management and preventive intervention. By synthesizing outcomes across studies, healthcare systems can ultimately identify risk factors more accurately and implement specific preventive interventions in the expectation of minimizing the occurrence and outcome of such causally problematic conditions. Further, resolving congenital anomalies of the respiratory system entails the use of a multi-disciplinary approach by clinicians, researchers, and public health specialists. Coordination among these stakeholders will be essential for developing early diagnosis and intervention programs that can potentially lead to improved outcomes. Encouraging community awareness and education about potential risk factors associated with these abnormalities, such as maternal behaviors and socio-economic status, will also be key. Monitoring the incidence rate and clinical outcome will provide informative feedback for revising existing interventions as well as identifying successful ones. Such initiatives play an important role in reducing the burden of congenital respiratory malformations and providing improved health pathways for those affected (Llopis-Gonzalez et al., 2009; Romi et al., 2015).

It is considered to include many aspects of child health that are associated with early mortality rates with regard to congenital anomalies of the respiratory system. Recent findings have indicated that children who have congenital Zika syndrome (CZS) experience significantly larger mortality risks compared to their unaffected peers. In fact, the research reveals a staggering 13.10-fold increased risk of mortality among children less than five years of age with CZS. Importantly, cause-specific mortality due to respiratory illness is especially dramatic and suggests that congenital abnormalities are likely to seriously compromise respiratory function and general health status in impaired infants and toddlers. Thus, early diagnosis and targeted interventions are essential to avert these hazards and boost survival rates among this risk group (Cardim et al., 2025). Additionally, the complexity of diagnosing congenital respiratory anomalies in children underlines the necessity for elaborate health approaches. Practitioners must use a broad differential diagnosis whenever they present with respiratory signs in individuals with backgrounds of congenital conditions. For example, a patient presenting with respiratory distress may also have underlying cardiac defects, which complicate the clinical presentation. Understanding how the respiratory system behaves in the presence of other anatomical defects prevents children from experiencing delays in life-saving treatment due to misdiagnosis. Multidisciplinary care with the intervention of pediatrics, cardiology, and pulmonology specialists is essential in addressing such complexities and tailoring effective management protocols for these children (Ali et al., 2024). Lastly, a heightened awareness of the risks associated with congenital anomalies in the respiratory tract leads to an evaluation of public health policies. There is an immediate need to have more effective neonatal screening and community health campaigns to identify children at risk of respiratory issues secondary to congenital abnormalities. Furthermore, increased awareness among healthcare providers concerning the potential connections between the different congenital disorders can facilitate early intervention and coordinated care plans. With the evolution of research and clinical interventions related to congenital respiratory deformities, we can significantly improve the long-term well-being of affected children, reducing mortality chances and improving their quality of life (Ali et al., 2024; Cardim et al., 2025).

KEY TERMS FROM THIS CHAPTER

- Bronchial atresia
- Bronchogenic cyst
- Choanal atresia
- Congenital diaphragmatic hernia (CDH)
- Congenital lobar emphysema
- Esophageal atresia
- Laryngeal web
- Laryngomalacia
- Pharyngeal pouch
- Pulmonary agenesis
- Pulmonary hypoplasia
- Pulmonary sequestration
- Tracheal stenosis
- Tracheoesophageal fistula (TEF)
- Tracheomalacia
- Vascular rings

Critical Thinking Questions

1. **What is the most common congenital lung malformation?**
   a. Congenital pulmonary airway malformation (CPAM)
   b. Bronchogenic cyst
   c. Pulmonary sequestration
   d. Congenital diaphragmatic hernia
2. **Which congenital anomaly involves a nonfunctional mass of lung tissue with an abnormal blood supply?**
   a. CPAM
   b. Pulmonary sequestration
   c. Bronchogenic cyst
   d. Tracheoesophageal fistula
3. **A newborn with respiratory distress and scaphoid abdomen most likely has:**
   a. Bronchogenic cyst
   b. Congenital diaphragmatic hernia
   c. Tracheoesophageal fistula
   d. Laryngomalacia
4. **Which anomaly involves an abnormal connection between the trachea and esophagus?**
   a. Pulmonary sequestration
   b. Tracheoesophageal fistula (TEF)
   c. Bronchogenic cyst
   d. CPAM
5. **Which congenital respiratory anomaly is commonly associated with prenatal polyhydramnios?**
   a. Laryngomalacia
   b. Tracheoesophageal fistula
   c. Bronchogenic cyst
   d. Pulmonary hypoplasia

Short Answer Questions

1. What is tracheoesophageal fistula (TEF), and how does it typically present in newborns?
2. Describe the different types of congenital diaphragmatic hernias (CDHs) and their clinical significance.
3. What is congenital pulmonary airway malformation (CPAM), and how is it diagnosed?
4. Explain the pathophysiology and clinical features of bronchopulmonary sequestration.
5. How does congenital lobar emphysema present, and what are the typical radiologic findings?

Answer to Critical Thinking Questions

1. (a); 2. (b); 3. (b); 4. (b); 5. (b)

References

1. Field, D., Boyle, E., Draper, E., Evans, A., Johnson, S., Khan, K., Manktelow, B., Marlow, N., Petrou, S., Pritchard, C., Seaton, S., & Smith, L. (2016). Towards reducing variations in infant mortality and morbidity: a population-based approach. *Programme Grants for Applied Research*, *4*(1), 1–218. https://doi.org/10.3310/pgfar04010Aguilar García, D., & Jiménez Peláez, M. (2024). Use of autologous pericardial patch graft for treatment of large congenital peritoneopericardial diaphragmatic hernia in two cats. *Veterinary Record Case Reports*. https://www.semanticscholar.org/paper/767097147e58592f2dac8f3bd474d18304b06682 (accessed on 30th June 2025).
2. Ailal, F., Al-Herz, W., Bousfiha, A., Casanova, J. L., et al. (2020). Human inborn errors of immunity: 2019 update of the IUIS phenotypical classification. *Frontiers in Immunology*. https://core.ac.uk/download/323074666.pdf (accessed on 30th June 2025).
3. Allareddy, V., Fletcher, S., Metalwala, Z., Okunseri, C., et al. (2018). Orthognathic surgical outcomes in patients with and without craniofacial anomalies. *Journal of Oral and Maxillofacial Surgery*. https://core.ac.uk/download/213086834.pdf (accessed on 30th June 2025).
4. Armstrong, B., Guo, Y., Jaakkola, J. J. K., Li, S., et al. (2012). Extremely cold and hot temperatures increase the risk of ischemic heart disease mortality: Epidemiological evidence from China. *Environmental Health Perspectives*. [No URL provided].
5. Baldacchino, I., Gatt, A. S., & Saliba, I. (2016). Fetal MRI: An essential step in interpreting complex ultrasound findings. *Malta Medical Journal*. https://core.ac.uk/download/46604247.pdf (accessed on 30th June 2025).
6. Baumgartner, H., De Backer, J., Babu-Narayan, S. V., Budts, W., Chessa, M., Diller, G. P., Lung, B., et al. (2020). 2020 ESC guidelines for the management of adult congenital heart disease. *European Heart Journal, 42*, 563–645. https://doi.org/10.1093/eurheartj/ehaa554 (accessed on 30th June 2025).
7. Bjornson, C., Mitchell, I., Bailey, J. A., Brindle, M., & Soles, M. (2014). Delayed diagnosis of high proximal tracheoesophageal fistula in esophageal atresia and a novel approach to the treatment of tracheomalacia by sub manubrial tracheole. *Journal of Pediatric Surgery*. https://core.ac.uk/download/pdf/81737092.pdf (accessed on 30th June 2025).
8. Bruen, M., Crowley, D., O'Connor, P., & Staines, A., et al. (2004). Public health and landfill sites. *Environmental Health Review*. https://core.ac.uk/download/11309293.pdf (accessed on 30th June 2025).
9. Campo, M. D., Chowdhury, S., Dimmock, D. P., Jones, M. C., et al. (2018). The case for early use of rapid whole-genome sequencing in management of critically ill infants: Late diagnosis of Coffin-Siris syndrome in an infant with left congenital diaphragmatic hernia, congenital heart disease, and recurrent infections. *Genetics in Medicine*. https://core.ac.uk/download/323064060.pdf (accessed on 30th June 2025).
10. Canova, C., Ludvigsson, J. F., Pitter, G., Romor, P., et al. (2016). Risks of hospitalization and drug consumption in children and young adults with diagnosed celiac disease and the role of maternal education: A population-based matched birth cohort study. *Journal of Pediatric Gastroenterology and Nutrition*. https://core.ac.uk/download/53531106.pdf (accessed on 30th June 2025).

11. Caporlingua, A., Di Giorgio, G., Fadda, M. T., Ierardo, C., et al. (2015). Treatment timing and multidisciplinary approach in Apert syndrome. *Journal of Craniofacial Surgery*. https://core.ac.uk/download/54520953.pdf (accessed on 30th June 2025).
12. Cardim, L., Costa, M., Cunha Rodrigues, L., Carvalho-Sauer, R., Brickley, E., Arraes de Alencar Ximenes, R., Pescarini, J., et al. (2025). All-cause and cause-specific mortality in children with congenital Zika syndrome in Brazil. *JAMA Network Open, 8*. https://www.semanticscholar.org/paper/c6ae3d74d67a8b67c2353a9b258419f74215fb97 (accessed on 30th June 2025).
13. Corsello, G., Falsaperla, R., Parano, E., Pavone, P., Praticò, A. D., Rizzo, R., Ruggieri, M., et al. (2016). Congenital muscular dystrophy: From muscle to brain. *Italian Journal of Pediatrics*. https://core.ac.uk/download/286528712.pdf (accessed on 30th June 2025).
14. Creighton, E. K., Keating, M. K., Lyons, L. A., Sisó, S., et al. (2016). Characterization of an inherited neurologic syndrome in Toyger cats with forebrain commissural malformations, ventriculomegaly and interhemispheric cysts. *Veterinary Pathology*. https://core.ac.uk/download/323069548.pdf (accessed on 30th June 2025).
15. Czeizel, A. E., Sárközi, A., & Wyszynski, D. F. (2005). Oral clefts with associated anomalies: Findings in the Hungarian Congenital Abnormality Registry. *American Journal of Medical Genetics Part A*. https://core.ac.uk/download/142040219.pdf (accessed on 30th June 2025).
16. Das, R., & Roy, P. (2022). Unilateral pulmonary agenesis in a child with recurrent respiratory tract infections. https://core.ac.uk/download/539912931.pdf (accessed on 30th June 2025).
17. DeGiovanni, J. V., Grech, V. E., Micallef, S. P., Sammut, M., et al. (2016). 3-year-old with chronic wet cough: Interlobar bronchopulmonary sequestration. https://core.ac.uk/download/46604028.pdf (accessed on 30th June 2025).
18. Doughty, M. W. (2014). Determining the health problems of Alaska Military Youth Academy participants. https://core.ac.uk/download/162576817.pdf (accessed on 30th June 2025).
19. Elsayed Ali, R. H., Warrell, C., & Manson, J. (2024). P16 Concurrent sacroiliitis and infective endocarditis in a young male with congenital aortic stenosis: A diagnostic challenge and learning points. *Rheumatology Advances in Practice, 8*. https://www.semanticscholar.org/paper/cb19696b75a815a13dd3429da9549bf40468196b (accessed on 30th June 2025).
20. Executive Board of IJMS. (2022). Abstracts of the Medical University Congress of Mogi das Cruzes, COMUMC. *International Journal of Medical Students*. https://www.semanticscholar.org/paper/85408df6b2026213147cee7e5f22766ec456ebed (accessed on 30th June 2025).
21. Flaming, D., Toros, H., & Burns, P. (2015). Home not found: The cost of homelessness in Silicon Valley. https://core.ac.uk/download/75781793.pdf (accessed on 30th June 2025).
22. Fockens, M. M. (2024). Anomalies of the larynx and trachea: Developmental aspects and treatment considerations. https://core.ac.uk/download/604736713.pdf (accessed on 30th June 2025).
23. Helner, N., Makukh, H., Prokopchuk, N., Sharhorodska, O., et al. (2019). Medical genetic counseling of women with congenital heart diseases of fetus. https://core.ac.uk/download/301580705.pdf (accessed on 30th June 2025).
24. Ishibashi, H., Kitamura, A., Mori, H., Nakagawa, T., et al. (2022). Gross E esophageal atresia with unique course. https://core.ac.uk/download/521170966.pdf (accessed on 30th June 2025).

25. Kitsiou, A., Caforio, A. L. P., Porta-Sanchez, A., Vahanian, A., Iung, B., Carrera, C., Szymanski, C., et al. (2013). ESC core curriculum for the general cardiologist (2013). *European Heart Journal.* https://core.ac.uk/download/55756305.pdf (accessed on 30th June 2025).

26. Kumar, A., Taksande, A. M., & Vilhekar, K. Y. (2009). Arthrogryposis: A rare manifestation in infant of diabetic mother. https://core.ac.uk/download/pdf/87417.pdf (accessed on 30th June 2025).

27. Lindsay, R. S., & Loeken, M. R. (2017). Metformin use in pregnancy: Promises and uncertainties. https://core.ac.uk/download/84148422.pdf (accessed on 30th June 2025).

28. Llopis-Gonzalez, A., Andersen, A. M. N., Arntzen, A., Bille, C., Boeing, H., Borg, D., Carmichael, S., et al. (2009). Socio-occupational status and congenital anomalies. *Public Health.* https://core.ac.uk/download/pdf/8271647.pdf (accessed on 30th June 2025).

29. Mussi, N., Maugeri, E., Deolmi, M., Scarpa, A., Casolari, E., Pisi, G., Fainardi, V., et al. (2024). Respiratory follow-up in a cohort of children with congenital malformations affecting lung development: A cohort study. *International Journal of Pediatrics and Child Health.* https://www.semanticscholar.org/paper/5060a7c277720826d97026758a5942ba515dc45b (accessed on 30th June 2025).

30. Nizalova, O. Y., & Vyshnya, M. (2025). Evaluation of the impact of the Mother and Infant Health Project in Ukraine. https://core.ac.uk/download/pdf/6385781.pdf (accessed on 30th June 2025).

31. Ornaghi, S., Maraschini, A., Buoncristiano, M., Corsi Decenti, E., Colciago, E., Cetin, I., Donati, S., et al. (2022). Maternal sepsis in Italy: A prospective, population-based cohort and nested case-control study. *Microorganisms, 11.* https://www.semanticscholar.org/paper/3e8c017434af38361292748dabef8c7458ced7c0 (accessed on 30th June 2025).

32. Pierpont, M. E., Brueckner, M., Chung, W. K., Garg, V., Lacro, R. V., McGuire, A. L., Mital, S., et al. (2018). Genetic basis for congenital heart disease: Revisited: A scientific statement from the American Heart Association. *Circulation, 138.* https://doi.org/10.1161/cir.0000000000000606 (accessed on 30th June 2025).

33. Romi, M. M. (2015). Preliminary study on congenital anomaly in DR. Sardjito General Hospital Yogyakarta. https://core.ac.uk/download/297186891.pdf (accessed on 30th June 2025).

34. Roth, G. A., Mensah, G. A., Johnson, C. O., Addolorato, G., Ammirati, E., Baddour, L. M., Barengo, N. C., et al. (2020). Global burden of cardiovascular diseases and risk factors, 1990–2019. *Journal of the American College of Cardiology, 76*, 2982–3021. https://doi.org/10.1016/j.jacc.2020.11.010 (accessed on 30th June 2025).

35. Siegel, R. L., Giaquinto, A. N., & Jemal, A. (2024). Cancer statistics, 2024. *CA A Cancer Journal for Clinicians, 74*, 12–49. https://doi.org/10.3322/caac.21820 (accessed on 30th June 2025).

36. Speiser, P., Arlt, W., Auchus, R. J., Baskin, L. S., Conway, G. S., Merke, D. P., Meyer-Bahlburg, H. F. L., et al. (2018). Congenital adrenal hyperplasia due to steroid 21-hydroxylase deficiency: An Endocrine Society* clinical practice guideline. *The Journal of Clinical Endocrinology & Metabolism, 103*, 4043–4088. https://doi.org/10.1210/jc.2018-01865 (accessed on 30th June 2025).

LUNG TRANSPLANTATION

11

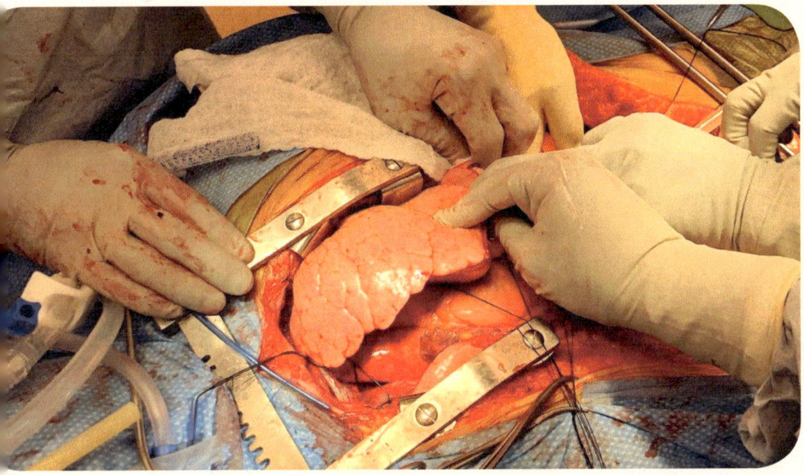

LEARNING OBJECTIVES

After studying this chapter, you will be able to:

1. Give a history of lung transplantation;
2. Describe indications for lung transplantation;
3. Explain the evaluation process for candidates;
4. Discuss the transplant procedure;
5. Understand the risks and complications;
6. Focus on the ethical considerations.

Introduction

The evolution of lung transplantation has undergone immense developments during the last decades to become a life-saving treatment for patients with advanced lung disorders. The principal cause of morbidity and mortality remains respiratory failure secondary to diseases like COPD, idiopathic pulmonary fibrosis, and cystic fibrosis, and thus, the demand for therapeutic interventions is raised. Lung transplantation is a practicable measure that not only gives patients a longer life, but also a better quality of life. However, the complex situation surrounding lung transplantation entails many medical, ethical, and logistics-related issues to be properly examined. Understanding these nuances is necessary for comprehending the profound meaning of this surgical procedure, as it requires a multidisciplinary approach from transplant surgeons, pulmonologists, immunologists, and ethicists working together to maximize recipient benefits. Recent technology has made lung transplants more effective by improving the precision of matching protocols between donor and recipient. Human leukocyte antigen (HLA) typing, for example, is among the important determinants in ensuring compatibility between recipient and donor. Serological approaches have hitherto relied on histocompatibility testing, which has its limitations in identifying certain HLA markers. The introduction of next-generation sequencing (NGS) technology has revolutionized HLA typing, and high-resolution two-field HLA typing (HR-2F) has been important in enhancing transplant success. Research has established that HR-2F typing has played a significant role in 41% of the analyzed cases, highlighting the importance of proper compatibility testing in reducing the risks of transplant rejection and improving post-operative patient care (Dinh et al., 2019). The use of such advanced methods not only increases the likelihood of higher success rates in lung transplants but also raises significant questions about resource allocation and ethical implications within the context. With the ongoing need for lung transplants outpacing the supply of organs for donation, the ethical foundations of allocation methods have come to play much greater significance. The issue of equitable allocation and prioritization in organ transplantation tends to raise considerations of access, equity, and fairness. With challenges of case-by-case scenarios and the finite supply of available organs, ethical considerations are essential in guiding transplant policy. Deliberative democracy offers itself as a probable solution to such ethical dilemmas, advocating for more sustained involvement of stakeholders in policy-making discourse. It favors multiple perspectives, allowing for a more nuanced consideration of the varied considerations in lung transplantation decisions (bosslet et al., 2019). Thus, addressing the ethical dilemmas of lung transplantation is more than a mere medical issue, needing the solid grounds of ethical concepts that guarantee social justice and patient care in transplant networks (Figure 11.1).

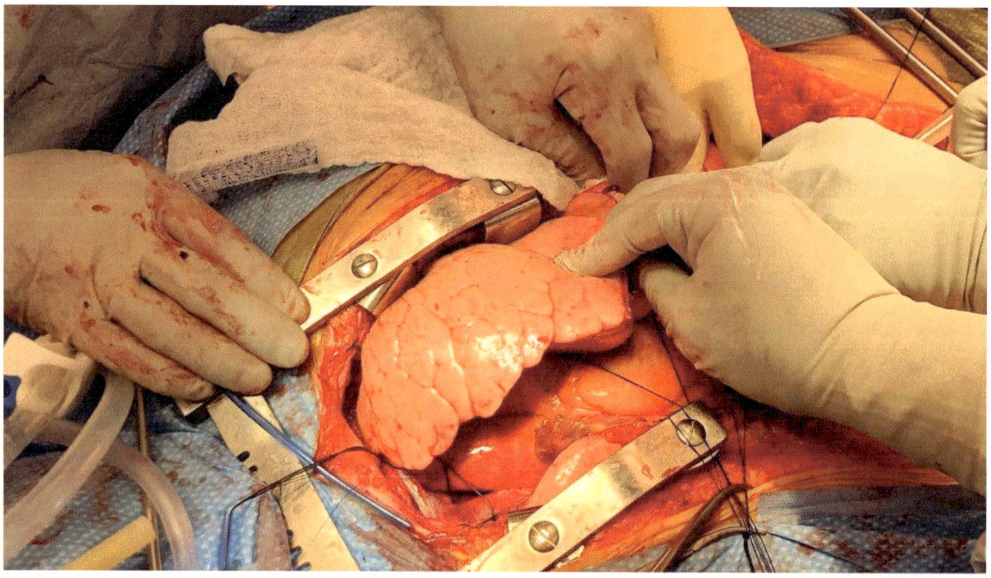

Figure 11.1. Lung transplantation.

Source: https://external-content.duckduckgo.com/iu/?u=https%3A%2F%2Faskthenurseexpert.com%2Fwp-content%2Fuploads%2F2023%2F09%2Fsuccessful-lung-transplantation-cases-4.jpg&f=1&nofb=1&ipt=645d7f9a9d866825e74ddc29ed1a144ef3b9a9ae438fc7364ef1cfd0ec8cc0c9.

Definition of Lung Transplantation

Lung transplantation is a surgical procedure meant to replace a dying or ruined lung with a donor lung from a deceased or living individual. This life-saving treatment is typically reserved for individuals with chronic pulmonary ailments, such as end-stage chronic obstructive pulmonary disease (COPD), pulmonary fibrosis, and cystic fibrosis, among others. The complexity of the procedure requires meticulous preoperative evaluations to determine organ compatibility and the suitability of the patient. The rationale for performing lung transplantation lies in the fact that, in selected patients, traditional medical management is no longer an option. Thus, lung transplantation not only represents a therapeutic form but also a critical chance for patients to regain valuable quality of life in the face of severe respiratory limitation. Lung transplantation entails a number of steps, including donor selection and organ procurement, surgical techniques, and postoperative care. To begin with, organ procurement can be from deceased donation, where lungs are acquired from an individual who has been declared brain dead, or from a living donor who can donate a portion of their lung tissue. According to Chapman (2024), successful procurement is dependent on the establishment of living and deceased donation programs that ensure an optimal supply of donor organs. Postoperative recipient care entails comprehensive management after surgery to avert rejection and infection. The use of immunosuppressive therapy is crucial in the prevention of rejection, thus necessitating ongoing medical attention in the life-long transplant recipients' process. Lung transplantation, even with potential benefit, also presents its challenges, particularly recovery after surgery and complications. Research, as characterized by Simanovski et al. (2022), indicates the state of poor quality sleep in lung transplant recipients exacerbated by age, gender, and psychological stressors. This helps to support the multidimensional nature of the experience of receiving a lung transplant, which transcends that of the surgical process itself. Regular follow-up of patients post-transplant is essential in identifying and addressing complications such as sleep abnormalities capable of compromising recovery. Besides this, scientists call for a more consistent approach in evaluating sleep quality and other postoperative outcomes. They also advocate for future research to establish clearer measurements and identify effective interventions to further enhance the transplant experience.

Significance of Lung Transplantation in Contemporary Medicine

Lung transplantation is a life-saving procedure in modern medicine, especially for patients with end-stage lung disease such as COPD, pulmonary fibrosis, and cystic fibrosis. Lung transplantation is not just survival; it enhances the quality of life significantly by providing the patient with a healthy and functioning lung. This surgical procedure not only alleviates symptoms, such as shortness of breath and weakness, but also allows patients to regain their independence and participate in daily activities that were once diminished by their illnesses. Further, with advancing technical innovation in surgery and postoperative care, results from transplant operations have become significantly improved, and lung transplantation can now be considered an option for more patients with severe pulmonary disease. Besides, lung transplantation is the epitome of sympathy and innovation in modern medicine. The expanding understanding of immunology, along with developing perioperative advancements, has been at the heart of reducing rejection rates and improving graft survival. Techniques such as immune modulation and personalized immunosuppressive treatments have helped break the formidable barriers in transplantation, including organ rejection and infection. Notably, the development of regenerative medicine, which involves approaches such as stem cell therapies and biomaterials, is providing a window of opportunity for better lung transplant integration with the tissues they replace to heal and function more efficiently. As defined in modern literature, multidisciplinary approaches in this field emphasize the ongoing evolution of lung transplantation and its fundamental role in managing complex pulmonary disease (Sarangi et al., 2024). Finally, as lung transplantation expands, it also holds fantastic implications for global healthcare systems. With the rising tide of lung disease, there are more donor organs needed than exist, and this forms a critical gap in public health provision. It is absolutely vital to promote awareness and advocacy of organ donation to fill this gap because each can significantly expand donor registries and ultimately lead to successful transplants. Additionally, the integration of conventional practices found in ancient medicine traditions, such as those documented in Persian medicine, could incite novel treatment methods that complement lung health together with transplant therapy (Akbari et al., 2024). The convergence of ancient and modern ways can create a society where alternative treatments flourish, leading to enhanced patient care and improved outcomes for lung transplantation as part of general healthcare practice (Figure 11.2).

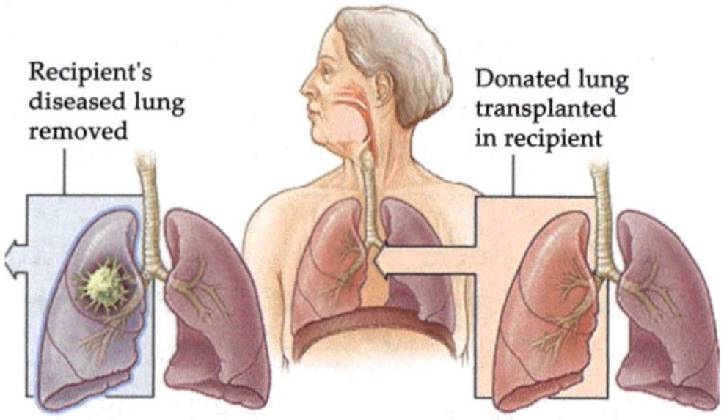

Figure 11.2. Lung transplantation in modern medicine.

Source: https://external-content.duckduckgo.com/iu/?u=https%3A%2F%2Fmodernclassics.info%2FMedical-Procedures%2Flung-transplant.jpg&f=1&nofb=1&ipt=8e89b25eeeadfeae45f6ef3988d2e773bfd7c72cec2187478381a6ef9d5fe76c.

11.1. History of Lung Transplantation

Learning Outcome

1. Early failures and challenges;
2. Landmarks in lung transplant techniques;
3. Evolution of surgical technique.

The history of lung transplantation began with significant developments in surgical skills and medical science in the mid-20th century. Initial organ transplantations were discouraging, particularly in terms of graft rejection and postoperative complications. But the initial pioneering efforts of surgeons such as Dr. James Hardy, who performed the first human lung transplant in 1963, were a turning point. In the early days, these procedures were the target of much criticism due to their high mortality rates and ethical issues regarding the distribution of donor organs. However, it was the persistence of researchers and clinicians that led to the establishment of improved methods and a better understanding of immunosuppressive therapy, which allowed subsequent developments in this area to progress. The introduction of cardiopulmonary bypass (CPB) technology was a key reason for advancing lung transplantation. CPB facilitated surgeons to offer circulatory and oxygenation support during lung and heart surgery. Not only did it simplify complex operations, but it also helped make operating rooms safer, thus enhancing lung transplantation viability. Other technological advancements, such as ECMO, came later, significantly enhancing lung transplant recipient postoperative care. The employment of imaging modalities, particularly computed tomography pulmonary angiography (CTPA), maximized the assessment of donors and recipients. Besides, improvements in pulmonary embolism treatment, including ex vivo lung perfusion (EVLP), have successfully expanded the donor base of lungs for transplantation, addressing the critical issue of organ supply in transplant practice (Russell et al., 2022). As lung transplantation advanced, the establishment of antibody-mediated rejection (AMR) brought an entirely new set of challenges. AMR, a leading etiology of acute allograft dysfunction, necessitated consensus diagnostic criteria to offer a uniform answer to this complex issue.

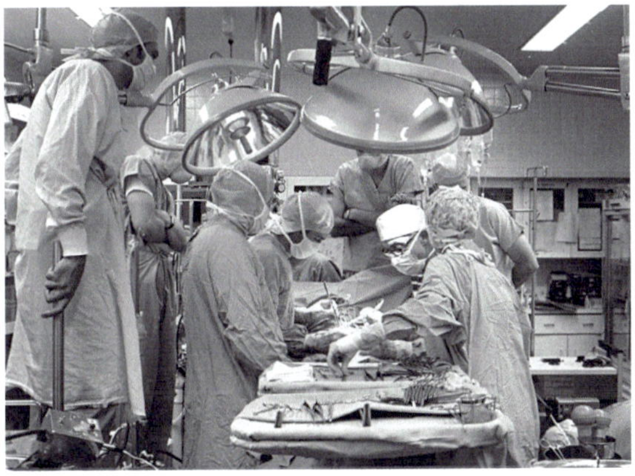

Figure 11.3. History of lung transplantation.

Source: https://external-content.duckduckgo.com/iu/?u=https%3A%2F%2Fwww.chestmed.theclinics.com%2Fcms%2Fattachment%2Fd3307352-33a9-4023-afd4-1d54d18a4b2a%2Fgr3_lrg.jpg&f=1&nofb=1&ipt=256478f4ec87d8612b25945a4ab0944a11f0907db42afafa7feab6db1b62b07f.

The limitations of the criteria recognized knowledge deficits in the mechanism and treatment methodology of AMRs. Currently employed therapies tend to borrow from other areas of medicine, illustrating the necessity for specialized therapies specific to lung transplant. Ongoing studies aim to bridge these knowledge gaps by researching new diagnostic technologies and effective treatment protocols. The ongoing nature of AMR complicates long-term prognosis; hence, researchers emphasize elucidating and controlling its role on chronic lung allograft dysfunction (CLAD) and survival rates in general (Bery et al., 2020) (Figure 11.3).

11.1.1. Early Attempts and Challenges

The early attempts at lung transplantation in the late 20th century were marked by immense optimism and daunting challenges that would shape the course of this medical innovation. Initial operations conducted in the 1960s and 1970s involved attempting to treat end-stage pulmonary conditions such as cystic fibrosis and COPD. But the initial phases of such pioneering operations were tainted with poor success rates due to the challenges of organ rejection and the body's immunological response. The surgeons found it impossible to create postoperative care strategies since the need for lifelong immunosuppression was realized. Then what resulted was a constant juggling of how to maximize the patients' quality of life and minimize the dangers of the anti-rejection medication, which came with unwanted side effects and complications. Thus, the early experiences of lung transplantation illustrated the need for a greater understanding of both transplant patient care and surgical techniques. Despite improvements in technologies and techniques, the inherent complexity of lung transplantation remained substantial, particularly in understanding the psychological management of transplants by medical doctors. The first studies found a high prevalence of depression in transplant patients, mirroring mental health issues previously overlooked through screening (Chernyak et al., 2020). The psychosocial impact of undergoing such a life-altering surgery necessitated exhaustive psychological assessments before surgery, since doctors recognized mental health could significantly influence adherence to treatment and outcomes. This interdisciplinary treatment aimed not only to bolster the physical healing but also to provide care that encompasses emotional equilibrium for patients which were essential in crafting an approach that was both medically feasible as well as psychologically rewarding to those undergoing life-threatening sickness. Ultimately, the initial difficulties with lung transplantation helped lay the groundwork for more recent advancements in the specialty, highlighting the necessity of enhancing surgical techniques and patient management strategies. Coordination among specialists in transplantation is also developing, as it addresses clinical issues and ethical dilemmas that arise in the care of complex cases, such as patients with concomitant disease or cancer (Burra et al., 2018). Besides, efforts to enhance organ preservation techniques and improve matching processes have joined the fray, further increasing the overall success rates of lung transplantations. The lessons learned from early trials and errors have established a more scientific approach, leading to thoughtful policies that focus on timely referrals and more comprehensive reviews of potential transplant candidates. With these developments, lung transplantation has become a complex but reliable form of treatment from a rudimentary one, offering new hope to patients with severe lung illness.

11.1.2. Milestones in Lung Transplant Procedures

Lung transplantation has radically improved since its initial phases, with a line of pivotal developments that have extended the procedure's effectiveness and scope. The initial successful lung transplant in the 1960s laid the foundations of a discipline that would flourish during the next few decades, marking a significant milestone in the history of surgery. With the introduction of technological as well as procedural advancements, the breakthrough of double lung transplantation in the late 1980s was a turning point, offering solace to patients with advanced pulmonary diseases. Furthermore, the application of immunosuppressive therapy improved the levels of transplant acceptance, tremendously reducing the risk of rejection. This advancement has made lung transplantation a viable therapeutic option for most respiratory ailments, significantly improving patient survival and prognosis, thus highlighting the ongoing need for development in this important field of medical science. Another turning point in lung transplant surgery was the development of formal criteria and guidelines for the choice of donor organs. Maximizing donor-recipient matching has been instrumental in enhancing short- and long-term success rates for transplants. The introduction of the lung allocation score (LAS) in the early 2000s transformed the process by ranking candidates according to clinical urgency and likely post-transplant survival. These advances have contributed to a more equitable distribution of donor organs, settling questions of access to transplantation on ethical bases. Concurrently, the addition of advances in surgical technology, such as VATS, has minimized postoperative complications, decreased recovery periods, and enhanced care for patients undergoing these taxing procedures. These landmarks are important because they improve the architecture of lung transplantation, evidencing the field's devotion to patient care and innovation. Advances in technology and surgery have been shaking the lung transplantation world in recent times, making way for future landmarks. Particularly, advances such as ECMO have been providing solutions to those patients with severe respiratory failure, maintaining them as potential candidates for transplantation. Further, the advent of robot-assisted surgery is now beginning to transform the mode of performing lung transplants to enhance surgical precision and minimize recovery. Spain's recent success with organ transplantation, as reflected in a donation rate of 52.6 per million population and dominance of lung transplant operations, underscores the importance of coordinated transplantation models, advanced practices, and commitment to sensitizing the public (Vispo, 2025). With ongoing development of lung transplantation, ongoing investigation, and ongoing refinement of surgery technique and patient management protocols will be essential to overcoming existing challenges of the field, ultimately broadening the horizon of what can be accomplished in the restoration of lung function and the improvement of quality of life in patients (Figure 11.4).

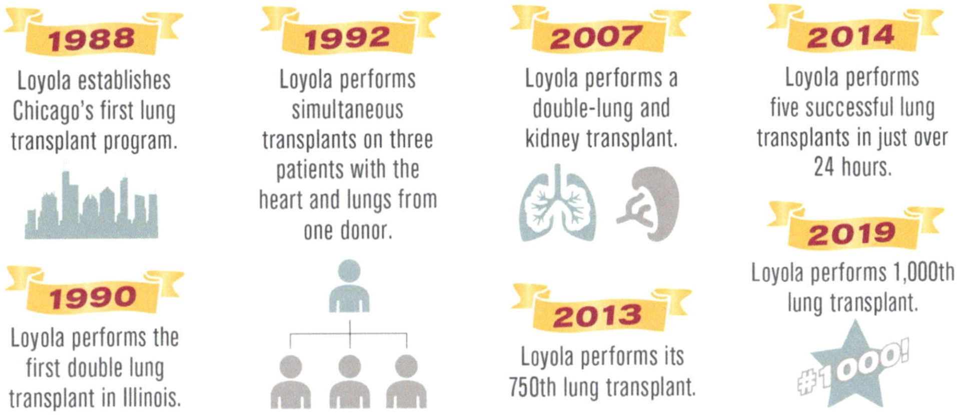

Figure 11.4. Milestones in lung transplant procedures.

Source: https://www.loyolamedicine.org/sites/default/files/hg_features/mercury_services/bde82229b54ef73adf48e9823db0ef10.jpg.

11.1.3. Evolution of Surgical Techniques

The history of surgical methods has played a critical role in the evolution of lung transplantation, transforming a once-standard procedure into a cutting-edge therapeutic intervention aimed at preserving life. Early transplantations were marred by a number of problems, with the fundamental surgical methods being rudimentary and prone to complications. Initial experimentation during the mid-20th century set fundamental principles for organ transplant, with experimental procedures by prominent players in the medical community. While researchers explored various surgical procedures, recognition of airway anastomotic complications was pivotal, ultimately leading to refined techniques that significantly improved outcomes for patients. An in-depth comprehension of these challenges enabled the creation of innovative methods that would appreciably enhance the success rates in lung transplantation, marking the beginning of a revolutionary phase in surgical technique evolution (Jacob et al., 2022). Building on these early innovations, subsequent innovations have centered on the importance of minimizing complications that are intrinsic to lung transplantation. The development of en bloc double lung transplantation was an innovation in this context. This technique offered an alternative to the traditional procedures and so reduced the frequency of airway complications (AC) usually encountered after single lung transplantations. In the recent past, the bilateral sequential technique was an even more advanced method, with improved results through enhanced healing of the airways after transplant. Furthermore, some surgical techniques have even gone so far as to include bronchial artery revascularization, which, while still in its limits, can minimize future complications and enhance long-term patient results. The significance of these innovative techniques cannot be overstated, for they represent continued striving for surgical excellence in the area of lung transplantation (Elgharably et al., 2021). With the progress in lung transplantation, the complexity of surgical methods has also evolved based on variable patient requirements and anatomical conditions. The introduction of more sophisticated surgical methods, including sternotomy and clamshell thoracotomy, has opened the doors for lung transplantations in patients with severe comorbidities. Furthermore, the application of intraoperative mechanical circulatory support (MCS) has enabled surgeons to surpass the particular challenges of fragile recipients. All of these advances necessitate a multidisciplinary approach in which careful planning and effective teamwork are fundamental to success. The evolution of surgical techniques in lung transplant techniques not only highlights the brilliance of modern medicine but also symbolizes the ongoing process of improving patient outcomes in the face of an ever-changing medical landscape, testifying to the complementary relationship between surgical development and patient care (Elgharably et al., 2021) (Figure 11.5).

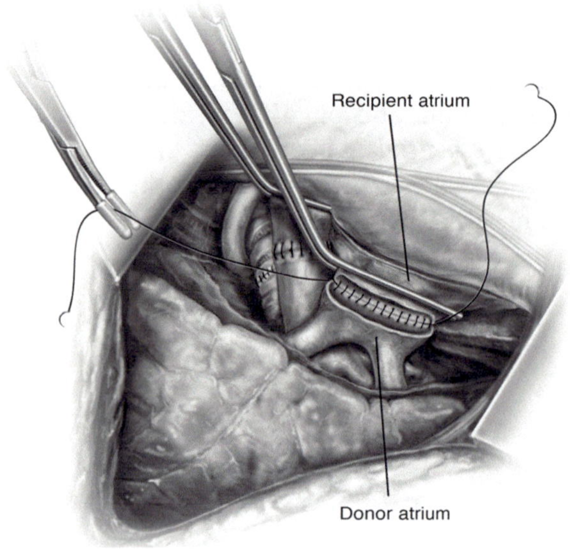

Figure 11.5. Evolution of surgical techniques in lung transplant procedures.

Source: https://cdn.amegroups.cn/journals/pbpc/files/journals/2/articles/2804/public/2804-PB9-R1.png/w300.

Test Your Knowledge

1. Allocate milestones in lung transplant procedures.
2. What are the evolution of surgical procedures?

11.2. Indications for Lung Transplantation

Learning Outcome

1. Chronic obstructive pulmonary disease (COPD);
2. Cystic fibrosis;
3. Pulmonary fibrosis.

Clinical indications for lung transplant are primarily concerning irreversible and end-stage lung diseases. COPD is one of the most common conditions that make an individual a candidate for this life-altering surgery, particularly where other treatments have failed. In patients with α-1 antitrypsin deficiency emphysema, a genetic form of COPD, patients are paradigm recipients for transplantation when other treatments—like oxygenation or lung reduction surgery—are lacking. While quality of life and life expectancy can both be significantly enhanced by transplantation, strict selection criteria ensure that only patients who are reaching certain medical and psychosocial milestones are considered. This prudent decision relieves the procedure's complications, such as CLAD, which complicates long-term outcomes by arising in as much as 50% of transplant recipients within five years (Verleden et al., 2023). In addition to COPD, the landscape of lung transplantation has evolved to encompass recipients with acute respiratory distress syndrome (ARDS), that is, secondary to viral infection such as COVID-19. A review of pathologic alterations in the lungs of COVID-19-infected patients has paralleled those for patients with other end-stage pulmonary diseases and has provided rationale for consideration for transplant in this population. Indications for lung transplant following respiratory failure resulting from COVID-19 must carefully consider the possibility of the patient recovering. Those that have no possibility of pulmonary function recovery, even with optimized therapy, are typically prioritized for transplant. This emerging evidence accentuates the adaptability of lung transplantation as a rescue procedure in response to emerging respiratory health crises. Importantly, survival rates among such patients have been reported to be commensurate with those of patients receiving a transplant for more traditional indications (Garza-Castillon et al., 2022). Other important indications for lung transplantation are those patients with interstitial lung disease (ILD), like idiopathic pulmonary fibrosis (IPF). These states typically lead to unresponsive progressive pulmonary dysfunction to normal medical intervention, and ultimately end with compromised life expectancy and quality.

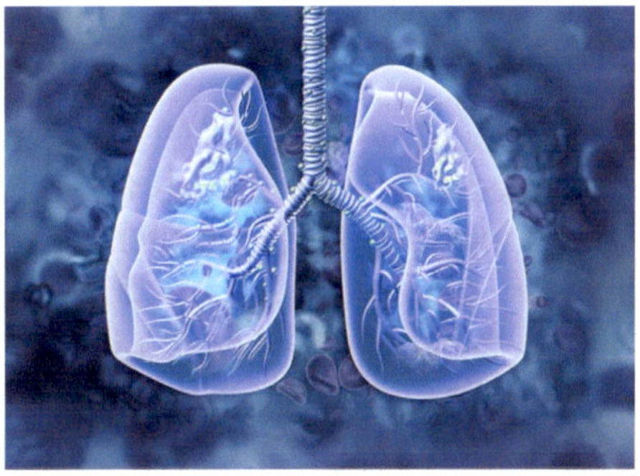

Figure 11.6. Indications for lung transplantation.

Source: https://www.mayoclinic.org/-/media/kcms/gbs/medical-professionals/images/2022/12/12/20/58/lung-transplant-767x535.jpg.

In this context, lung transplantation is a viable option when the disease has advanced to a stage where it becomes irreversible, as reflected by the fact that lung function dramatically deteriorates as assessed by pulmonary function tests. As with other indications, the transplantation process requires thorough evaluations to ensure that candidates are optimally matched for surgery, balancing potential benefits with inherent risks. Moreover, technical improvements in transplant and post-transplant management are increasingly improving outcomes, accounting for expanding demand for lung transplantation for a variety of chronic pulmonary conditions beyond COPD and ARDS (Verleden et al., 2023) (Figure 11.6).

11.2.1. Chronic Obstructive Pulmonary Disease (COPD)

COPD is a chronic respiratory illness that is defined by airflow limitation and persistent inflammation, caused mainly by long-term exposure to harmful particles such as cigarette smoke and atmospheric pollutants. The illness exists in various forms, such as chronic bronchitis and emphysema, leading to debilitating symptoms such as chronic cough, sputum production, and breathlessness. As COPD progresses, patients become more likely to develop severe deterioration of their quality of life and will likely become severely reliant on medical intervention. Even though improvement in drug therapy, such as the use of corticosteroids and bronchodilators, provides symptomatic management, the drugs fail to halt the disease's progression. For the majority of end-stage COPD patients, lung transplantation is a therapeutic option that holds the promise of restored pulmonary function and extended survival, despite the complexity present in donor matching and post-transplant care. Individualized care has been emphasized in current literature to be critical in choosing lung transplantation modalities for COPD patients. There are alternatives to bilateral and single lung transplantation, with new data suggesting that bilateral lung transplantation may yield more long-term survival benefits, particularly for younger patients with fewer comorbid diseases. There are many factors in the decision-making process, such as the patient's overall health, the severity of COPD, and the occurrence of other respiratory diseases like lung cancer, which is heavily impacted by COPD. Most significantly, there are differences by racial and ethnic group in outcomes, as highlighted by persistent research that has determined certain environmental and genetic factors contributing to the incidence and severity of COPD in Black/African American populations. Interplay among these factors necessitates continued efforts towards the understanding of underlying mechanisms that may contribute to health disparities in transplant outcomes (Thaiparambil et al., 2023).

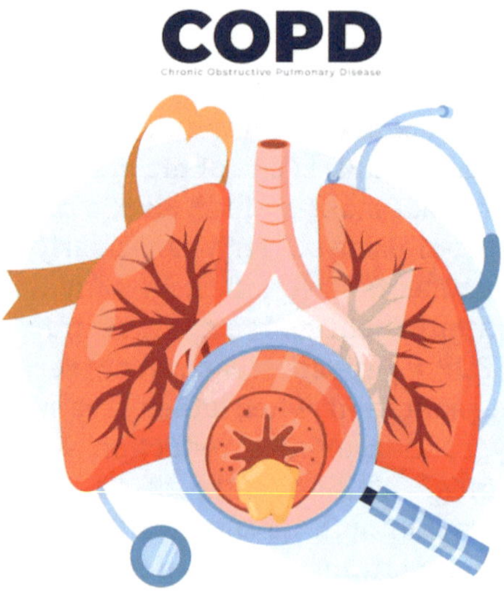

Figure 11.7. Lung transplant for chronic obstructive pulmonary disease (COPD).

Source: https://img.freepik.com/premium-vector/hand-drawn-flat-copd-illustration_23-2149101818.jpg?uid=R83560892&ga=GA1.1.1905821027.1699246592&semt=ais.

Moreover, post-transplant complications like CLAD further highlight the need for stringent monitoring and lengthy post-op treatment. While research has been optimistic with regard to quality of life and mid- to long-term survival rates for patients suffering from COPD undergoing lung transplant, the varying results are reflective of the complexity of the cases. Of particular note are patient age, co-existing medical conditions, and adherence to post-transplantation care as factors influencing survival rates. As emphasized in current narrative syntheses, the development of a culture for patient-centered care is essential to optimize outcomes maximally. In the evolving background of COPD lung transplantation, ongoing research remains a priority not only to optimize selection practices among bilateral and single-lung strategies but also to develop bespoke interventions to maximize care quality in this vulnerable population (Taghdiri, 2023) (Figure 11.7).

11.2.2. Cystic Fibrosis (CF)

CF is a genetic disorder that primarily affects the respiratory and gastrointestinal tracts, leading to the formation of thick, sticky mucus that interferes with normal lung function. As cystic fibrosis advances, patients experience recurrent pulmonary infections, inflammation, and extensive lung damage, and cystic fibrosis is a significant indication for lung transplantation.

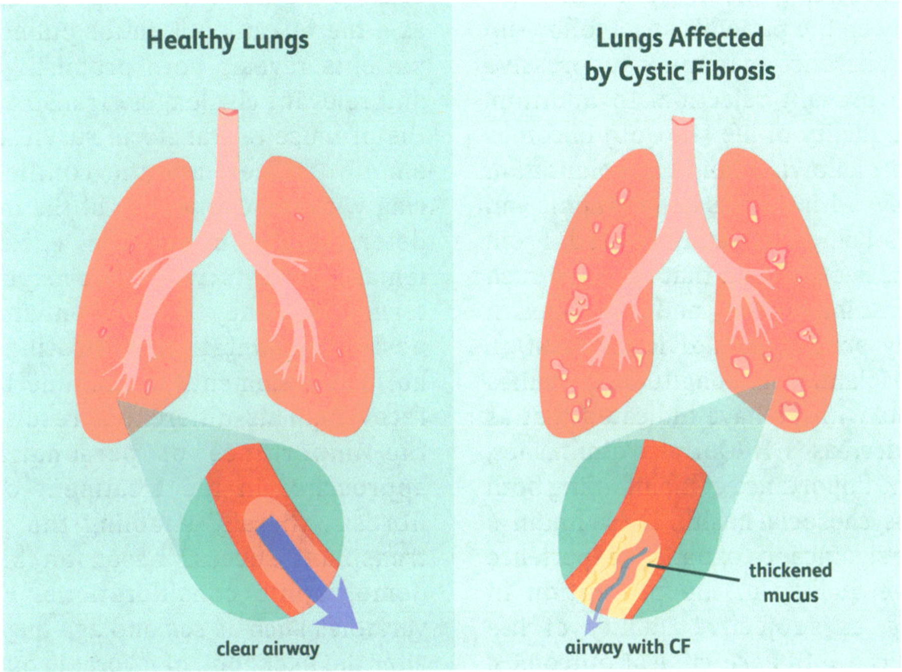

Figure 11.8. Cystic fibrosis (CF) for lung transplantation.

Source: https://www.verywellhealth.com/thmb/cD51qN450IpSwsPy7KgE_wBt2Q8=/1500x0/filters:no_upscale():max_bytes(150000):strip_icc()/understanding-cystic-fibrosis-998213_fin-f6b10f0a2a474ba08c40907fff1556dc.png.

The challenge of managing CF is that it is so multifaceted; not only will the patient have respiratory issues, but also nutritional challenges, diabetes secondary to the disease, and heightened psychological distress. Thus, lung transplantation often is the last resort when traditional therapy cannot offer sufficient lung function or quality of life. The surgical procedure is not only technically challenging but also requires careful patient selection to achieve optimal post-transplant results where chronic respiratory failure is a problem (Alves et al., 2024). The technical approach to lung transplantation in CF patients needs careful evaluation that takes into account the unique challenges presented by the disease. Notably, preoperative assessment must be a multidisciplinary effort where pulmonologists, transplant surgeons, dietitians, and psychiatrists collaborate to prepare the patient for the complex procedure. Postoperative management also requires close monitoring of potential complications such as graft rejection and infectious disease, given that the patients already have underlying diseases before the transplantation. This has been demonstrated in research, where lung transplant was found to significantly improve lung function and overall quality of life for CF patients, which is essential for managing the illness (Alves et al., 2024). Overall success with long-term outcomes relies primarily on the patient's strict follow-up regimen and adherence to immunosuppressive medication to prevent rejection. In addition, health-related quality of life (HRQoL) becomes a consideration following lung transplantation in cystic fibrosis, with various demographic and clinical factors being intricately related. From research, it has been proven that markers such as age, body mass index (BMI), and overall health status strongly predict an individual's HRQoL following transplantation. Longitudinal studies among patients with CF have indicated that as lung function decreases, HRQoL also diminishes, highlighting the importance of maintaining both physical and psychosocial health. These findings emphasize the significance of patient experience and subjective quality of life perception in care planning, as subjective quality of life measurement can influence clinical outcomes. By focusing on quality of life and functional status, health care practitioners can offer more total care for cystic fibrosis in the transplant setting (Figure 11.8).

11.2.3. Pulmonary Fibrosis

Pulmonary fibrosis is a serious clinical challenge in the lung transplant setting, primarily due to related morbidity and mortality. Characterized by progressive impairment of lung function because of excess scarring in the lungs, the condition poses challenging diagnostic and therapeutic issues. IPF, one of the most prevalent diseases with an etiology that is largely undefined, clearly shows the imperative need for efficient treatments. With a median survival rate of about 21.82 months after diagnosis, the condition is most dismal for the elderly, with males having 2.85 times the chance of death than females. Notwithstanding the progress made in elucidating the disease's pathophysiology, the unavailability of targeted therapies heightens the need to pay attention to lung transplantation as an available option for suitable patients with extensive pulmonary dysfunction (Creel et al., 2008). The landscape of lung transplant as a therapeutic option for pulmonary fibrosis patients reveals both promising possibilities and relevant challenges. Transplantation holds the promise to transform survival, particularly among females, but the conflicting findings ring with the complexity of the immunological determinants in question. Facts reveal that female patients who have experienced full-term pregnancy exhibit enhanced survival post-transplantation, indicating the role of hormonal elements in immune tolerance and recovery. This differential result underscores the importance of personalized medical approaches in the treatment of pulmonary fibrosis, thereby enabling the prediction of transplant success based on biological and demographic considerations. For instance, variables such as sex and age may significantly alter the likelihood of favorable outcomes. Thus, individualizing pre-transplant assessment to optimize patient prognosis is crucial (Creel et al., 2008). The impacts of ischemic circumstances on pulmonary fibrosis progression and exacerbation only further complicate the planning of lung transplant strategies. A report on bronchial artery blood flow and its influence on lung pathology, specifically in the case of bronchiolitis obliterans organizing pneumonia (BOOP), sheds light on the mechanisms of ischemic injury. The findings reveal that ischemia per se could trigger fibrotic transition and apoptosis of cells in distal airways that can potentially slow down healing post-transplant procedures. Elucidation of such ischemic events is necessary for the optimization of lung transplant results since effective treatment of ischemic damage may diminish the risk of sequelae such as BOOP. Emphasizing research studies that explore modes of ischemic signaling pathways could enhance future transplant strategies, with a focus on improving patient survival and quality of life upon transplantation (Figure 11.9).

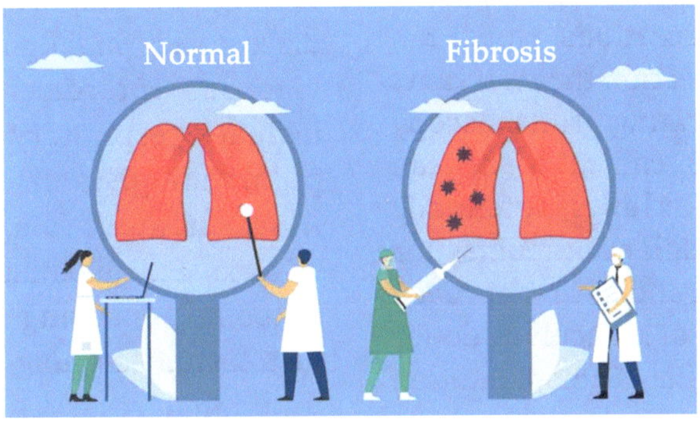

Figure 11.9. Pulmonary fibrosis.

Source:

Test Your Knowledge

1. What is cystic fibrosis?
2. What is pulmonary fibrosis?

11.3. Evaluation Process for Candidates

Learning Outcome

1. Medical evaluation and testing;
2. Psychiatric evaluation;
3. Determination of eligibility criteria.

The candidate's evaluation process of a lung transplant candidate includes a complicated and important process to ascertain the success of transplantation surgery. The evaluation process begins with the patient's strict scrutiny of their medical history, underlying respiratory disease, and functional status. Assessors consider some of the following parameters, including the patients' ages, comorbidities, and health status, which are powerful determinants of the chances of a successful transplant. Specific attention is paid to lung function dynamics, specifically the PaO2/FiO2 ratio, which is a critical determinant of respiratory effectiveness. Detailed examination may also include imaging tests that show structural and pathological changes in the lungs, establishing that potential candidates satisfy the rigorous criteria for transplantation. With the help of advanced evaluation devices, healthcare personnel have been able to determine a patient's candidacy better and make the process more efficient in the use of donor organs to their maximum potential (Çıtak, 2025). Another important aspect of candidate screening is the application of bronchoscopy in the assessment of donor lung quality. This procedure allows the doctor to look directly into the airways and identify problems such as airway secretions and infectious agents that could compromise lung function. For the lungs that are deemed acceptable for transplant, bronchoscopy is an excellent means of discriminating on vital details that are not included in imaging. One example is the finding of purulent secretions, which can represent a deep-seated infection that warrants organ rejection. In incorporating bronchoscopy into the evaluation process, clinical teams can more accurately assess donor lungs, potentially leading to better post-transplant outcomes for recipients. It is the comprehensive approach that reflects the importance of meticulous donor exams in managing risks in lung transplantation (Çıtak, 2025).

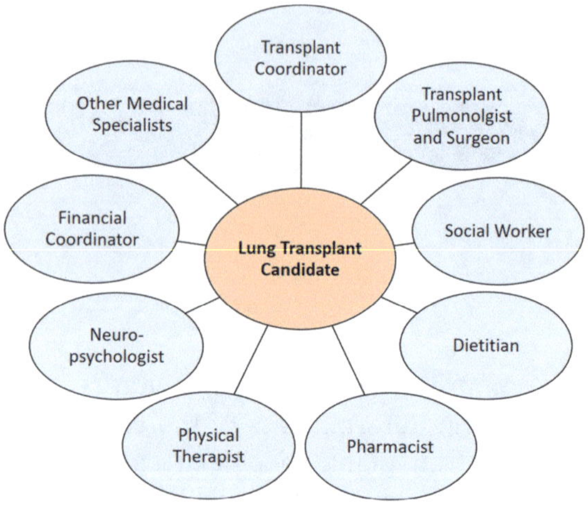

Figure 11.10. The lung transplant candidate.

Source: https://www.chestmed.theclinics.com/cms/10.1016/j.ccm.2022.10.001/asset/26e18551-bf28-4404-8579-296156fe352f/main.assets/gr2_lrg.jpg.

The candidate evaluation process must also assess the function of the diaphragm and its impact on outcomes following lung transplantation. Before the procedure, the patient's underlying respiratory illness and comorbid conditions affecting diaphragmatic function are thoroughly assessed. Post-transplantation, the procedure can alter the morphology and diaphragmatic functioning, which is of immense significance for respiratory function. Interestingly, despite the role played by the diaphragm in transplantation, no specific criteria have been established for testing for diaphragmatic dysfunction. This discrepancy highlights the necessity for more vigorous interdisciplinary assessment that includes respiratory therapists, surgeons, and pulmonologists in the evaluation process. Assessment of diaphragmatic performance criteria will maximize overall lung transplant outcome, ensuring that candidates are not just tested for lung function but also for the functional reserves necessary for long-term recovery and transplant success (Figure 11.10).

11.3.1. Medical Assessments and Tests

Clinical assessments and examinations play a significant role in the decision of patient suitability and transplant outcome for lung transplantation. Extensive assessment begins with a clinical evaluation through a thorough medical history, physical examination, and pulmonary function tests. The tests determine the extent of lung disease and comorbidities that affect the risk of surgery and recovery. Tests like forced expiratory volume in one second (FEV1) and lung diffusion capacity can account for the functional defect and guide interventions. Moreover, imaging tests such as chest X-rays and computed tomography (CT) scans provide valuable information on anatomy, enabling the transplantation team to assess lung morphology. Understanding these parameters is paramount because they inform not only clinical decision-making but also the broader prognostic evaluation necessary to triage candidates on the transplant list. *Ex vivo* lung perfusion (EVLP) is a new technology that has recently gained attention in the assessment of donor lungs, particularly those initially deemed unacceptable for transplant. The process involves perfusing and ventilating the lungs outside the body, allowing for an assessment of lung function and pathology that is not possible in standard donor evaluations. Research has demonstrated that up to 34% of lungs previously classified as unfit for transplant can be successfully reconditioned and utilized, underscoring the importance of incorporating EVLP into the organ transplant protocol. Nevertheless, while EVLP has the potential for greater donor availability, it introduces complexities regarding patient outcomes, as evidenced by lower survival rates at 12 months compared to conventional transplants. The studies indicate that there is a need for further examination to establish the long-term efficacy and safety of EVLP in improving transplantation practice (Andreasson et al., 2016).

Beyond patient selection and donor screening parameters, there is mounting evidence for the incorporation of patient-reported outcomes for lung transplantation. These range from survival to functional status, quality of life, and psychological well-being. Understanding the impact of interventions such as EVLP on these areas is relevant, as they ultimately dictate patient satisfaction and long-term adherence to post-transplant follow-up. Evaluation of these outcomes involves systematic questionnaires and graded scores that examine the patient's physical and psychological state before and after transplantation. Additionally, it has been noted that the costs of newly created technologies, such as EVLP, need to be balanced against their potential to achieve effective long-term outcomes, further complicating medical decision-making (Burra et al., 2018). Consequently, a multi-faceted assessment and test strategy becomes a necessity in the delivery of end-clinical effectiveness along with holistic patient management in lung transplantation (Figure 11.11).

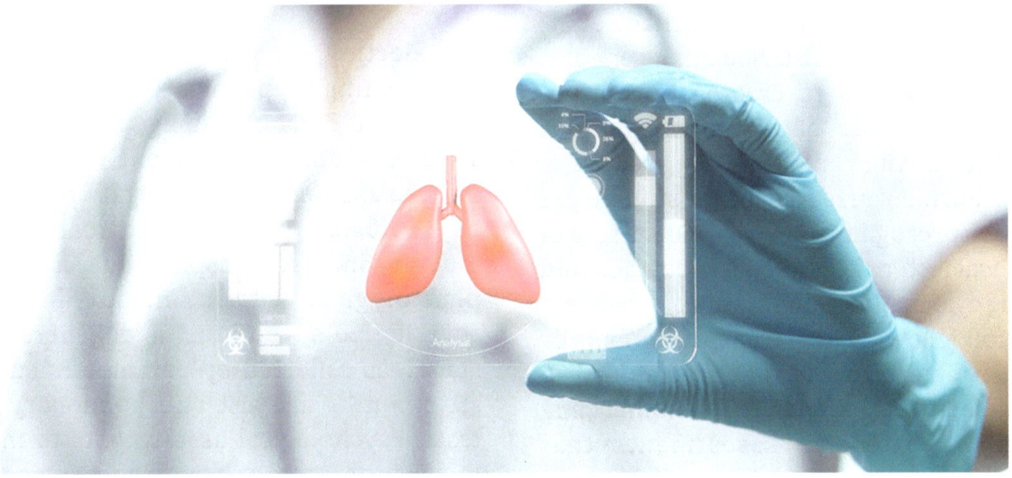

Figure 11.11. Pre-transplant evaluation for lung transplantation.

Source: https://www.kauveryhospital.com/blog/wp-content/uploads/2021/11/Lung-Transplant-Before-the-Procedure-1200x545_c.jpg.

11.3.2. Psychological Evaluations

Lung transplant is not merely a procedure encompassing the recipient's physical assessment but also psychological evaluations holistically. These evaluations are significant because they determine the psychological resilience, coping, and overall mental health of candidates prior to undergoing such an important surgery. Mental health has been well established as a significant predictor of post-transplant outcome and adherence to postoperative treatment plans. Candidates with evidence of psychological distress or those who cannot demonstrate adequate coping mechanisms can anticipate trouble with compliance in medication regimens, leading to poor outcomes. Therefore, psychological readiness must be assessed to determine if the candidates have the necessary tools to handle the challenge after the transplantation. Identifying probable personality traits and the influence of psychosocial aspects on patients' capacity to handle the stresses of lung transplantation is a crucial aspect of psychological evaluation. Social support networks, motivational scores, and awareness of their healthcare status are all being examined. In addition, research has documented that those with lower BMI may be at increased risk for postoperative complications, which necessitate psychological assessment to take into account the way in which mental health affects physical health outcomes (Atchade et al., 2024). Knowledge of these associations enables health care providers to create appropriate interventions capable of enhancing patient resilience and thus maximizing recovery processes. Further, research on postoperative complications recognizes the significant role of psychological factors in reducing aspiration and swallowing dysfunction complications, a frequent complication following lung transplantation. For instance, oropharyngeal dysphagia can lead to aspiration complications, thereby emphasizing the need for extensive assessments that include the measurement of physical status as well as psychological status (Graham et al., 2024). By embracing this integrated approach, not only a more holistic understanding of individual patients' risk but also of the ensuing interventions that are patient-specific can be achieved. Lastly, integrating psychological testing in the transplant process emphasizes the importance of combined patient care, improving short-term and long-term patient outcomes in lung transplantation (Figure 11.12).

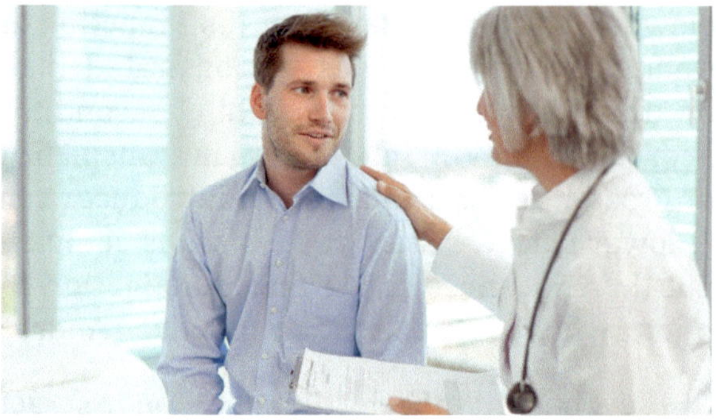

Figure 11.12. Psychological evaluations for Lung Transplantation.

Source: https://integrishealth.org/-/media/resources/articles/lung-transplant-patient-evaluation.ashx?as=1&mw=720&revision=89fd191e-bd1f-4591-ab62-dbeb24741aaf&hash=FEF5FA53D0D9B21D55B835793B2BA438.

11.3.3. Determining Eligibility Criteria

In selecting candidates for lung transplant, establishing appropriate eligibility criteria is crucial for optimizing patient outcomes. This evaluation frequently encompasses an assessment of several physiological, psychological, and sociological parameters that can impact transplant success. Important physiological factors include lung disease severity, comorbidities, and general physical status, as reflected by parameters such as the six-minute walk test and pulmonary function tests. Psychological assessments to measure a patient's ability to adhere to post-transplantation care, medication, and social support systems are also crucial. Ultimately, a multidisciplinary team, including pulmonologists, transplant surgeons, psychologists, and social workers, ensures that every aspect of a patient's health and circumstance is considered before listing for transplantation. Developments in medical technology have also informed the trajectory of eligibility criteria for lung transplantation. As a case in point, advances in ECMO have presented possibilities for those who might have been disqualified hitherto. ECMO is a life support technology for critically ill individuals, supporting them through to transplantation or facilitating the evaluation of potentially marginal donor lungs and thus redefining patient candidacy based on organ supply rather than traditional physiological criteria. Recent research indicates that ECMO therapy can improve the outcomes of otherwise complicated cases, supporting the revision of eligibility continually based on new medical knowledge and technology (Butt et al., 2024). Moreover, age is also a factor in deciding on eligibility, and research has indicated that recipient-donor age mismatch does not significantly impact late outcomes following transplantation. In a retrospective review of 409 patients, donor-recipient differences in age were not demonstrated to influence patient mortality, biopsy-proven rejection, or CLAD. Understanding the impact of age on success with transplantation will inform the use of older lung allografts and increase the donor pool without compromising patient outcomes. This evidence also supports expanding transplant programs' eligibility criteria, thereby fulfilling acute organ donor requirements and encouraging improved transplantation rates among various age groups (Franz et al., 2023).

Test Your Knowledge

1. What are the medical assessments and tests?
2. What are the psychological evaluations?

11.4. The Transplant Procedure

Learning Outcome

1. Pre-operative preparations;
2. Surgical techniques used in lung transplantation;
3. Post-operative care and recovery.

The transplant procedure for lung transplantation is a highly complex and specialized surgical intervention to provide a second lease on life to patients with end-stage pulmonary disease. The procedure usually starts with the choice of organ donors and recipients, which is paramount to the success of the transplantation. Patients undergo extensive evaluations to assess their candidacy, including medical history, lung function tests, and psychosocial assessments. The operating team utilizes sophisticated imaging modalities to ensure proper positioning of the donor lungs, which is an important determinant of optimal function following transplantation. With advances in surgical techniques, the coordination between transplant surgeons, anesthesiologists, and post-operative caregivers cannot be overstressed. These groups work together as a team to minimize post-operative and intraoperative complications, ensuring optimal patient outcomes. Following the surgical procedure, the patients undergo a severe post-operative period that requires careful attention and management to prevent complications. The most frequent complication is airway complication (AC), which can significantly influence short- and long-term outcomes. The incidence of AC may be as high as 15%–20%, thus making health teams vigilant against risks like airway stenosis or anastomotic leaks. Notably, most of these complications are seen in the first year following transplant and mandate close follow-up and management plans to preserve patient survival and quality of life. Technical nuances in managing these complications underscore the importance of specialized education and guidelines within transplant programs, as they remain a significant challenge in the current era of lung transplantation. In addition, the highly interdependent nature of the surgical technique, patient characteristics, and post-transplant management highlights the holistic approach required for effective lung transplantation. Aspects such as recipient age, surgeon experience in operating, and existing comorbidities all play crucial roles in dictating the outcome. As a case in point, older recipients often have a greater percentage of re-transplantation due to reduced regenerative capacity and heightened vulnerability to secondary medical complications (Hashemian et al., 2025). Furthermore, more recent studies emphasize the significance of standard diagnostic and therapeutic modalities to ensure proper management of AC. Consensus guidelines aim to standardize treatment protocols in airway management post-lung transplantation to ultimately enhance continuity of care for patients (N/A, 2025). By recognizing these challenges first and refining our methods, the science of lung transplantation continues to progress, bringing hope to all suffering from debilitating respiratory disease (Figure 11.13).

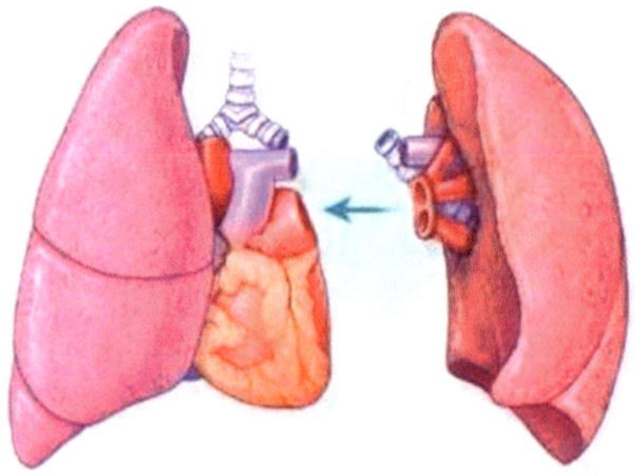

Figure 11.13. Lung transplant procedure.

Source: https://external-content.duckduckgo.com/iu/?u=https%3A%2F%2Fi.pinimg.com%2Foriginals%2Fa5%2F05%2Fa7%2Fa505a7d7cb680c2636a7da2183800276.jpg&f=1&nofb=1&ipt=465cb5ca9ccf33560a83239c113050e3faae57b3b996285e088e3131ff04ac9b.

11.4.1. Pre-Operative Preparations

Pre-operative preparations are a critical part of the process of lung transplantation, positioning patients appropriately for effective surgery. This phase involves comprehensive tests, which may include pulmonary function tests, imaging studies, and extensive medical evaluations. By taking a detailed look at a patient's clinical history and current state of health, transplant teams can ascertain candidacy for lung transplantation and create personalized treatment regimens. Pre-operative care, such as cessation of smoking, optimization of nutrition, and psychological evaluation, is also crucial in an attempt to maximize the condition of candidates. These preparations not only make the patients physically ready for the procedure but also address any emotional and psychological needs they may face during this complex and life-altering journey. With the assessments and lifestyle changes, multidisciplinary coordination is required for effective pre-operative preparations. Navigating the journey to lung transplantation often involves input from many healthcare professionals, including pulmonologists, surgeons, nutritionists, and mental health experts. This collaborative approach facilitates a comprehensive evaluation of the patients' fitness for surgery and helps establish whether there are any associated risks. For instance, the Canadian guidelines, developed based on interventions, demonstrated the merit of involving thoracic radiologists in the pre-operative process to ensure patient safety and optimal preparation. By ensuring that a patient's overall health is in good hands, transplant coordinators can create a well-defined plan that addresses both the surgical and post-operative needs, paving the way for successful lung transplantation. Pre-operative psychological preparation cannot be overemphasized in lung transplantation patients. Patients are usually paralyzed by fear, uncertainty, and anxiety, which seriously impair their readiness and recovery. Pre-operative information and advice are also important in this respect, giving patients the information they need about the operation, recovery, and long-term post-transplant changes to their health. There is evidence that physiotherapists' early intervention greatly enhances post-transplant outcome because it prepares the patient for the physical demands of the recovery process (Grehan et al., 2018). Moreover, therapy and support group sessions may provide emotional reassurance, allowing the patient to create a feeling of solidarity and share experiences. By providing equal emphasis on psychological welfare as physical readiness, the transplantation team enhances the prospect of improved post-operative results and successful recovery of the patient (Figure 11.14).

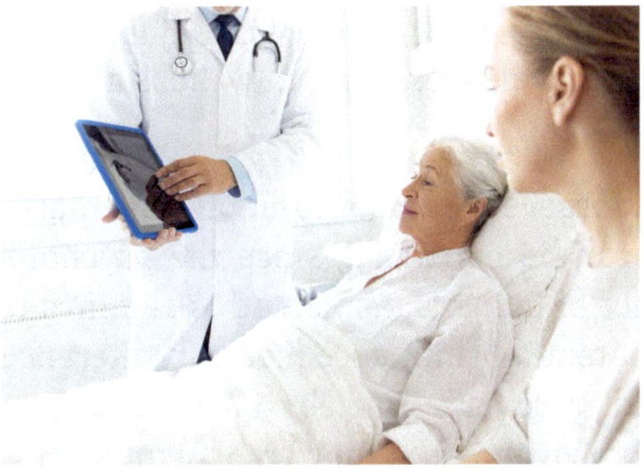

Figure 11.14. Pre-operative preparations.

Source: https://external-content.duckduckgo.com/iu/?u=https%3A%2F%2Fwww.dralinajafi.com%2Fwp-content%2Fuploads%2F2018%2F09%2Fpost-op.jpg&f=1&nofb=1&ipt=934c3ac84b0c027770c736742da3ae2ae77dd57309b794b53bda1b69b29c0a13.

11.4.2. Surgical Techniques Used in Lung Transplantation

The surgical procedures involved in lung transplantation have advanced significantly over the past decades, driven by improvements in medical technology and immunology. Conventional lung transplantation may be carried out through either the single or bilateral lung method, with the latter usually depending on the nature of the pathology. Bilateral transplant, or transplantation of both lungs or the left and right lung, has been associated with enhanced long-term survival, particularly for patients with specific diseases such as cystic fibrosis or pulmonary fibrosis. Precision of surgical technique is particularly important because technical errors can produce complications in the form of bronchial anastomotic failure, which is associated with significant morbidity and mortality for transplant recipients. With the introduction of minimally invasive techniques and better preoperative imaging, the viability of lung transplant has been made possible, which allows for more patients to be chosen for such intricate surgical operations (Cauchi et al., 1967). During the transplant, the surgeon typically employs techniques known as EVLP, which allows the examination of the donor lungs before their implantation in the recipient. This process enhances the selection of viable grafts, consequently reducing the incidence of primary graft dysfunction—a severe complication of lung transplantation. EVLP further provides a means for the direct administration of therapeutic agents to the lung graft, enhancing graft viability. In addition, the use of advanced techniques such as controlled donation after cardiac death has raised the number of donor organs, which is essential in view of the continued demand for lung transplantation. All these developments in surgery emphasize the dynamic aspect of lung transplantation and show that there is a demand for specialist surgical teams with current knowledge and equipment (Gardner et al., 2012). Postoperative surgical care and long-term patient management after lung transplantation also greatly contribute to the success of the surgery. Owing to the nature of lung transplantation, a team of surgeons, pulmonologists, and immunologists is required. Patients have to be regularly watched for the complications of organ rejection and infection, which are typical in the postoperative period. More sophisticated immunosuppression regimens are employed to lower the risk of rejection, but they present complications that need to be traded against avoiding rejection without lessening drug toxicity. Despite ongoing research into the mechanisms of graft rejection illuminating more of the process, technological advances in surgical techniques and postoperative care will likely yield improved outcomes and quality of life for lung transplant recipients (Cauchi et al., 1967) (Figure 11.15).

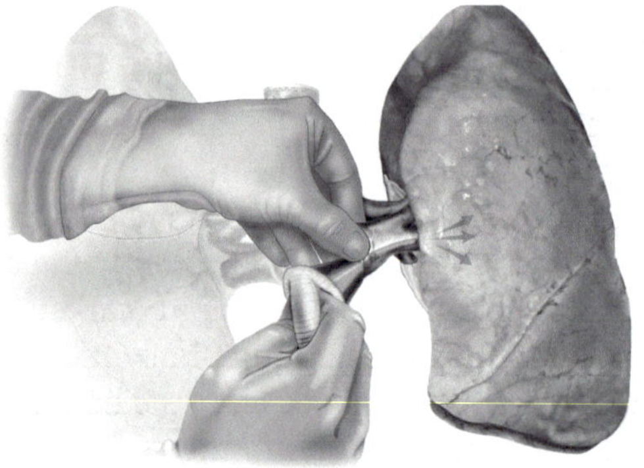

Figure 11.15. Surgical techniques used in lung transplantation.

Source: https://external-content.duckduckgo.com/iu/?u=https%3A%2F%2Fels-jbs-prod-cdn.jbs.elsevierhealth.com%2Fcms%2Fattachment%2F02de8abb-6f33-45d3-8e58-2ca008018283%2Fgr11_lrg.jpg&f=1&nofb=1&ipt=6540ba35f11195c8370bb75e0b731c7d88c530d6a6c6fa28417672b3656e156a.

11.4.3. Post-Operative Care and Recovery

Post-operative recovery and care following a lung transplant is a specific and very critical period that has a strong bearing on outcomes for the patient. The early post-operative period typically involves close monitoring to identify complications, such as rejection or infection, that may occur. Key signs, oxygen levels, lung function are closely monitored by medical staff to confirm that the transplanted organ is functioning correctly. Along with this comes the need to administer immunosuppressive drugs to prevent organ rejection, which in turn carries risks, such as increased susceptibility to infections. This fine balance of treatment necessitates a multi-disciplinary team of surgeons, physicians, nurses, and physical therapy/rehabilitation staff to ensure the optimum recovery and overall well-being of the patient (N/A, 2018). Patient education becomes important in the convalescent phase. Patients must be informed of the importance of adhering to medication regimens and post-operative instructions to minimize the risk of complications. Support programs like pulmonary rehabilitation are vital in helping patients restore their strength and activity levels after surgery. Multidisciplinary follow-up visits are an essential aspect of post-operative care, allowing healthcare providers to assess the patient's progress, adjust treatment plans, and address any new health problems that occur.

Moreover, the incorporation of mental health care can be beneficial, since the psychological impact of being transplanted is significant and can potentially influence medical adherence and overall recovery (Blazeby et al., 2009). Long-term recovery from lung transplantation is not limited to the immediate post-operative stage and entails extended care and surveillance. The patients are also monitored for chronic rejection, referred to as CLAD, which may occur months or years after the surgery. Regular checkup, such as imaging and functional tests, helps in the early identification of any complications. Proper nutrition is also crucial in the long-term recovery process, as it aids healing and overall health. Enabling lifestyle changes, such as smoking cessation and exercise, remains important to the preservation of lung function and improvement of quality of life. Proper incorporation of these factors within the domain of post-operative care can significantly contribute towards enhanced survival rates and results for lung transplant patients, and thus it remains a core element of transplantation programs (N/A, 2018) (Figure 11.16).

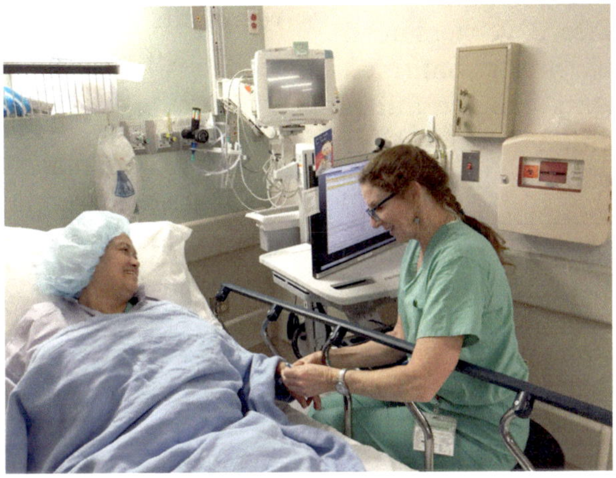

Figure 11.16. Post Op recovery care.

Source: https://external-content.duckduckgo.com/iu/?u=https%3A%2F%2Fhealth.ucdavis.edu%2Fsurgicalservices%2Fimages%2Fsame%2520day%2520surgery%2FPre-op-2-web.jpg&f=1&nofb=1&ipt=f008d4dcecc51aff52ebb2b262ee3c42faed777b224c95785fca7ae7a064374d.

Test Your Knowledge

1. What are the operative procedures for lung transplant?
2. What is post-operative care and convalescence?

11.5. Risks and Complications

Learning Outcome

1. Surgical risks of lung transplantation;
2. Long-term complications and rejection;
3. Risk of infection and management.

Lung transplantation is plagued by serious risks and complications that can impact patient outcomes considerably. Among the myriad of problems faced after the process of transplantation, the selection and use of extracorporeal life support (ECLS) techniques are particularly important determinants of patient safety. Cardiopulmonary bypass (CPB), off-pump techniques, and ECMO are some of the methods with varying degrees of efficacy and risk factors. In accordance with some recent studies, while off-pump techniques are now the order of the day, their increased use creates unique challenges. Even though it is thought to be a safer alternative to CPB, ECMO carries intrinsic risks and is more costly and necessitates stringent handling and monitoring to attain optimal patient outcomes. This delicate balance between the pros and cons attests to the complexity of lung transplantation and the absolute need for patient-specific care protocols (Yang et al., 2024). Post-transplantation complications are multifactorial and can impact long-term survival and quality of life. In particular, acute rejection, infection, and kidney complications are notable risks that healthcare workers need to expect and manage. Research has confirmed that preoperative assessments like the frailty index and nutritional condition are crucial in the prediction of complications. In a study with patients who have been undergoing lung transplantation, frailty indices were significantly correlated with postoperative mortality rates, thereby reaffirming the necessity of effective preoperative assessments. The data indicate that patients with high levels of frailty have worse postoperative results, highlighting the need for individualized strategies in patient handling and treatment. By designating those at risk in a timely fashion, healthcare teams can plan preventative interventions, thus improving survival rates and recovery profiles (Lee et al., 2024). Further, the emotional and psychological aspects of lung transplantation present an added risk for recipients. Patients often have comorbid depression and anxiety that complicates the recovery process and influences outcomes of surgery. The transplant procedure itself also results in dramatic quality-of-life alterations, provoking further emotional stressors. Screening for mental health and ongoing psychological treatment cannot be overstressed since these conditions directly impact compliance with post-transplant regimens and overall recovery. Incorporation of mental health evaluations in preoperative care can identify high-risk patients for adverse psychological consequences and allow early intervention practice, which can enhance the global success of the transplanting process. Troubleshooting the psychological component is important not only for short-term convalescence but also for long-term health and well-being among lung transplant recipients (Lee et al., 2024).

11.5.1. Surgical Risks Associated With Lung Transplantation

Lung transplantation, while lifesaving for recipients of end-stage lung disease, is also associated with a range of surgical risks that can have profound impacts on outcomes after surgery. These technical challenges are added to the need for advanced support modalities intraoperatively. ECLS and more familiar techniques like CPB or ECMO are often employed to offer circulation and oxygenation. Every procedure, however, carries inherent risks. As much as off-pump techniques have since become the technique of preference due to decreased complications, ECMO is now increasingly appreciated as a vital tool to bridge patients to transplantation. Although there are benefits to ECMO, its hidden hazards —such as bleeding, infection, and heavy healthcare expenditures —highlight the challenge for surgical teams to navigate maximally effective support approaches in lung transplantation (Yang et al., 2024). Along with the procedural urgency hazards, postoperative complications also become a determining factor in the success of lung transplantation. Surgical complications can include acute rejection, graft failure, and infection of various kinds, which are added to by the necessity of immunosuppressive treatment. The patient shares the risk of infection due to the requisite immunosuppression, which depresses their immunity to pathogens. Additionally, the complexity of treating graft rejection and infection necessitates rigorous attention during postoperative care. Investigation has demonstrated that careful monitoring and management can lead to positive outcomes, but these require significant resources and skilled clinical care. Awareness of these risks in the postoperative period is vital for optimizing treatment in lung transplant recipients and improving overall success in this risky field (Yang et al., 2024). Specific populations, such as pediatric recipients, bring additional risks in terms of surgery. It has been demonstrated in studies that concomitant cardiac surgery (CCS) is performed in a high percentage of pediatric candidates for lung transplant, and thus emphasis is placed on careful assessment and treatment of cardiovascular risk and lung risk. In a multicenter review, it was found that 15% of children undergoing lung transplant had CCS, and these were vastly less invasive repairs, such as closure of atrial septal defects. While these procedures have acceptable outcomes, they also contribute to the enhanced risk profile associated with lung transplant in children. Contributory factors, such as the prevalence of pulmonary hypertension as a primary diagnosis, necessitate comprehensive surgical planning and postoperative care across multiple dimensions (Figure 11.17).

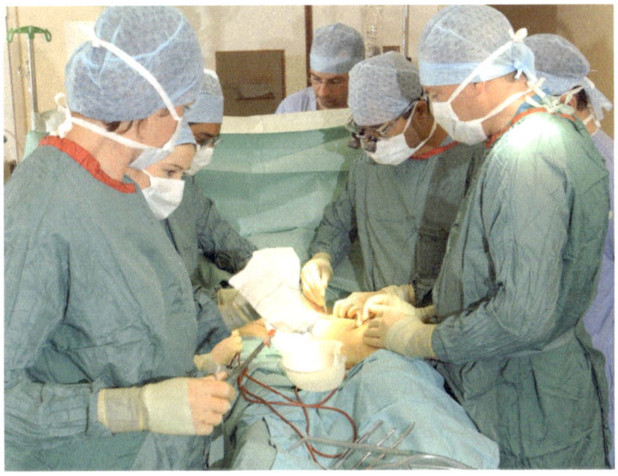

Figure 11.17. Surgical risks associated with lung transplantation.

Source: https://nhsbtdbe.blob.core.windows.net/umbraco-assets-corp/20205/2072212.jpg?width=310&height=235.

11.5.2. Long-term Complications and Rejection

The late transplant complications following lung transplantation present enormous challenges to patient management and survival. Acute cellular rejection (ACR), a frequent transplantation complication, is the result of the recipient's immune system perceiving the donor lung as foreign and mounting an immune attack against it. Most ACRs can be managed with immunosuppressive therapy, but refractory or recurrent ACR occurs in some patients, resulting in an accelerated decline in lung function. This loss can lead to CLAD, a syndrome that critically impairs long-term outcomes and is a primary cause of mortality in transplant recipients of the lung. It is crucial to understand ACR mechanisms and enhance early detection for intervention prior to damage becoming irreversible (Renaud-Picard et al., 2021). Aside from ACR, infectious complications also often result from the inevitable intensification of immunosuppressive treatment, adding further complexity to the postoperative situation. For most recipients of lung transplants, the level of immunosuppression to avoid rejection can be made at the expense of enhanced risk for opportunistic infection, which can negatively affect overall health as well as graft survival. Infections not only present immediate risks of morbidity but also give rise to longer-term complications that can inhibit recovery and reduce quality of life. Moreover, the link between infections and the development of CLAD identifies the interplay between rejection and infectious processes in this compromised population. Therefore, vigilant surveillance for infections and tailored immunosuppressive regimens are critical to improve patient outcomes without enhancing risks of rejection (McQuiston et al., 2021). Lastly, the role of pre-transplant autoantibodies in lung transplant illustrates the complex immune milieu that dictates long-term survival. These autoantibodies, if present before transplantation, have been implicated in graft injury and may augment the likelihood of acute as well as chronic rejection episodes following transplant. Research has identified a correlation of these antibodies with the development of primary graft dysfunction (PGD) and CLAD, and speculates that such autoantibodies will perpetuate autoimmune responses against the allograft. As science progresses, the place for application of biomarkers related to such autoantibodies is in the high promise category for both prediction and management of rejection. By highlighting the interaction between pre-transplant conditions and transplant outcomes, researchers can provide insights into individualized immunosuppression techniques and monitoring practices that can improve post-operative graft survival (McQuiston et al., 2021).

11.5.3. Infection Risks and Management

The lung transplant process is a collection of complexities, namely infection risk, that significantly jeopardize post-operative outcomes. Transplant recipients are also more prone to infections due to the nature of the potency of immunosuppressive therapy required to prevent organ rejection. This type of treatment, though vital to the survival of transplantation, blunts immune response function to eliminate infectious pathogens efficiently. This type of immunocompromised state increases the likelihood of acquiring multidrug-resistant pathogens, Cytomegalovirus, and fungi, which pose particular concern in the susceptible lung allograft setting. As evidenced by clinical studies, infection is the key cause of morbidity and mortality in the initial post-transplant period; thus, radical management measures are the most vital to avoid these risks and enhance patient survival after transplantation (Righi et al., 2024). Due to increased vulnerability to infection, a robust monitoring and management program must be instituted for lung transplant recipients. These include prophylactic administration of antibiotics, antiviral, and antifungal agents, tailored to each patient's specific risk factors. Close surveillance for the earliest signs of infection, such as fever or abnormal pulmonary function, is critical. In addition, advanced diagnostic techniques like bronchoscopy and culture techniques allow for prompt identification of pathogens so that prompt and specific treatment modalities can be initiated. Multidisciplinary teams, with infectious disease specialists and transplant surgeons, provide a comprehensive way to control infection. Teamwork can provide the fine balance between sufficient immunosuppression to maintain the allograft and sufficient immunity to combat infections (Righi et al., 2024).

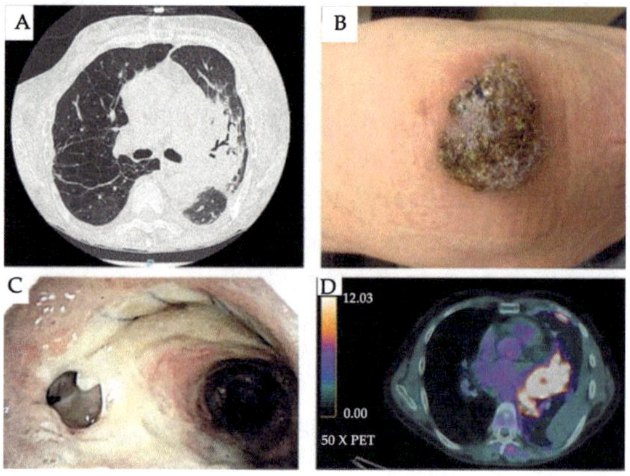

Figure 11.18. Infection risks and management with lung transplantation.

Source: https://www.tandfonline.com/cms/asset/fda231e5-0bd9-4f1d-8d97-62e091ee39bb/ierx_a_1843428_f0002_oc.jpg.

Central venous catheter insertion, in the form of totally implantable venous access devices (TIVADs), offers new options for the successful management of pulmonary infection and antibiotic treatment. Central venous catheters provide greater patient comfort and allow for extended intravenous infusion of antibiotics, which is crucial in clearing infections that may arise following lung transplantation. But their use is not without danger, as it predisposes to thrombosis and subsequent SVC obstruction, which is challenging to manage during transplantation. Case reports recognize successful management methods of SVC syndrome, noting the importance of meticulous planning and intervention during surgery. Overall, the integration of such advancements in infection management represents an improvement in the safe practice of lung transplantation, ultimately leading to improved patient outcomes and fewer complications during and after surgery (Figure 11.18).

Test Your Knowledge

1. What are the surgical risks involved with lung transplantation?
2. What are the long-term complications and rejection of lung transplantation?

11.6. Ethical Considerations

Learning Outcome

1. Organ allocation and donor shortages;
2. Ethical issues of transplant decision;
3. The issue of consent in organ donation.

The ethical issues involved in lung transplantation are multifaceted, highlighting the ethical issues that arise throughout the entire process, from the selection of the donor to the allocation of organs. The shortage of donor organs, relatively small compared to the number of patients actively listed for a transplant, makes it a pressing ethical issue. This shortage necessitates the implementation of allocation policies that prioritize patients based on criteria such as medical need and likelihood of transplant success. These policies, nevertheless, necessitate difficult decisions regarding who to give this lifesaving therapy to. Such choices affect not only those patients awaiting transplantation but also run counter to concerns about fairness and justice in healthcare, especially when socioeconomic factors that may affect access to transplantation services by patients are taken into account. The imperative of ensuring equal access while being subject to clinical guidelines remains a pressing issue in lung transplantation ethics. Additionally, ethical considerations are present in the effect of mental health on the success of lung transplantation. They can be depressed and anxious, and, therefore, can have a detrimental effect on their follow-up after surgery and recovery. Mental health is considered, as highlighted in allied research, when determining a patient's eligibility for transplantation. Preoperative detection of potential mental health issues is essential as failure to do so may result in a failure of compliance with medical treatment or advice post-transplant, and this ultimately puts the success of the surgery at risk. Therefore, adding comprehensive psychological evaluations and ongoing mental health services to the lung transplantation process is morally obligatory to provide for both the patients' well-being and fair allocation of resources in healthcare to provide all patients with the best outcomes following transplantation. Finally, retransplantation factors introduce still another ethical component to lung transplantation. Even as retransplantation can offer a second chance at life to recipients of a first transplant who have experienced chronic rejection or postoperative complications, ethical concerns are widespread in terms of resource use and the philosophy of pursuing additional life-sustaining therapies. The relative survival experience of retransplant candidates relative to primary transplant candidates would suggest potential worth; however, these decisions are confronted by the stigma of extending life at significant human and financial cost. As stated in recent literature, the ethical permissibility of retransplantation must be questioned, considering both patient quality of life and best use of limited healthcare resources. A clear understanding of these ethical components will ultimately guide the policies and procedures of lung transplantation and ensure that these life-and-death decisions reflect the values of justice, fairness, and compassion in health care (Maani et al., 2005; Chernyak et al., 2020).

11.6.1. Organ Allocation and Donor Shortages

Organ transplantation for transplant, particularly of the lungs, is a severe issue with a sensitive balance involving policy, ethics, and clinical need. Since the waiting list for lung transplants still exceeds the available supply, there is a need to allocate these limited resources equitably. Previous cases, such as those of Steve Jobs and Sarah Murnaghan, have established the occurrence of the urgent ethical concerns in organ allocation processes where medical personnel's decisions can be said to be unjust to the waiting list patients. Since these organs are in finite numbers, it is imperative to have fair and transparent policies of allocation so that confidence could be established among the masses and equal chance for life-saving treatment could be given to all the patients while creating a system of accountability within the medical community (Zarif et al., 2015). To offset the shortage of donors, the health sector is currently using new technologies such as Artificial Intelligence (AI) and Machine Learning (ML) to enhance organ allocation. These technologies revolutionize traditional practice by enhancing donor-recipient matching precision through analysis of large data pools of clinical, genetic, and demographic information. Hence, AI and ML technologies can potentially improve not only the rate of successful transplants but also the overall design of organ transplantation in many healthcare systems. With the prospect of predicting the outcome of surgery and adapting patient treatment regimens, such technological developments are a major breakthrough towards ending decades of shortages of donors for lung transplant (Marinze et al., 2025). With all the promise of technological advancements, there are also some challenges facing their large-scale implementation in organ allocation. All the key concerns such as data privacy concerns, regulatory requirements, and the integration of AI systems in current healthcare infrastructure must be addressed before they can be safely and ethically deployed. Apart from this, the rigorous clinical validation of AI techniques is a requirement for dependability in actual clinical applications. With coordination between medical professionals, researchers, and policymakers, the near future in these fields becomes crucial to maximize the effectiveness and productivity of organ transplantation through AI and ML. By overcoming these challenges, the science of transplantation can ride out the harsh realities of shortage donors and ultimately maximize patient benefits for lung transplantation (Marinze et al., 2025) (Figure 11.19).

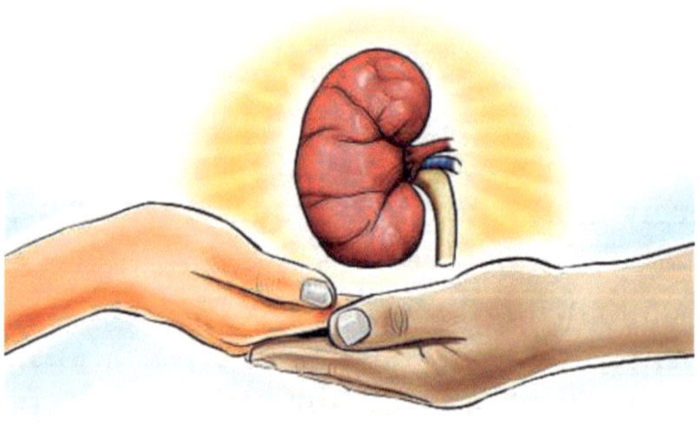

Figure 11.19. Organ allocation in lung transplantation.

Source: https://media.assettype.com/TNIE%2Fimport%2F2022%2F6%2F16%2Foriginal%2FCreating_awareness.jpg?w=480&auto=format%2Ccompress&fit=max.

11.6.2. Ethical Dilemmas in Transplant Decisions

Ethical issues in lung transplantation arise from

the immediate need to allocate scarce resources fairly to ensure optimal patient benefit. Principles of justice and beneficence inform the argument about organ allocation, in turn forcing health care providers to balance patient needs and donor shortages. With waiting lists growing, who gets a lung transplant is increasingly complex. Overall health of a patient, survival after the transplant, and socioeconomic status often complicate these decisions. Furthermore, the increasingly sophisticated technologies of organ preservation and transplantation raise ethical concerns. The questions need to rise above the personal needs of individual patients to consider the public social interests and how these choices can perpetuate and create inequities. Thus, the ethical context is a sensitive balance of moral obligation and pragmatism of convenience that needs equitable standards of transplant allocation (Wong et al., 2024). The cultural and religious factors also contribute to the ethical dilemma in lung transplantation. Beliefs of individuals influence organ donation and transplant choices. For instance, in those societies where familial and communal ties are most valued above everything else, the psychological stress of making decisions regarding organ donation will generate tensions that conflict with ethical norms. Findings in current studies show that personal characteristics, such as family size and cultural beliefs, shape organ donation attitudes, implying an interaction between the social environment and moral position (Aksoy et al., 2024). Cultural competence is significant to healthcare providers because, apart from educating patient care, it also promotes collaboration and rapport among families who choose organ donation. Experts need to address such tangled moral contexts by engaging with patients as human beings, considering individual and cultural values, and seeking the best outcomes. Finally, emerging organ transplant technologies like xenotransplantation and the utilization of AI raise ethical concerns that require serious consideration. They can potentially address the acute shortage of accessible organs but introduce new ethical concerns of consent, animal welfare, and long-term effects on human health. They also need strict regulatory frameworks to make sure that these technologies are used in a manner that upholds ethical standards and is in the interest of patients. The ethical subtlety of such developments highlights the dual responsibility of medical professionals: to remain adaptable in embracing advancements while upholding ethical standards. Bridging scientific progress with compassionate care is the answer to the very nature of the underlying lung transplant paradoxes, which demands prudent and ethical consideration not to allow ethical concerns to overshadow the life-saving nature of transplant interventions (Wong et al., 2024).

11.6.3. The Role of Consent in Organ Donation

Consent is a fundamental concern in organ donation, particularly in lung transplantation, where there is the most serious ethical concern. Organ donation is subsequently complicated by situational and emotional pressures on donor families. The dynamics of consent are therefore not legally rigid in form but can also encompass relational and contextual factors that influence decision-making. In the case of deceased donors, in fact, explicit expression of the deceased as well as of the survivors' will and best interests takes priority. If that is the situation, consent to organ donation is no longer routine but a nuanced interaction that requires tactfulness and subtlety, especially in terms of how medical professionals interact with families in such devastating loss (Cooper et al., 2020). Secondly, the moral implications of consent are evident in the controversy surrounding interventional donor studies, which aim to maximize the quality of transplant organs. While research is promising to offer more donor organs, the research is also contentious concerning who should do the consenting and what should constitute the content of the consent. The dual character of consent to dual uses like organ harvesting and medicine for what is called future research makes things even more complicated. Concerns about the sufficiency of information provided to relatives and possible misinterpretation necessitate reassessing consent practices to ensure openness and comprehension in relationships. If not carefully managed, the risk of erosion of public trust in organ donation programs looms, one that once more necessitates ongoing debate and policy revision (Cooper et al., 2020). Finally, consent issues should also consider evolving practice in organ donation, especially as practice adjusts to the utilization of donors with expanded criteria. For instance, donor use under support by mechanical circulatory assist is, as reported in existing experience, not only subject to strict clinical guidelines but also frank discussion of the impact of such technology on recipient and donor outcomes. Such innovation does necessitate informed consent, as an effort to bring home to the families the risks and complexities involved. Techniques like portable normothermic perfusion allow better evaluation of marginal donor organs, but such advances need to be accompanied by robust consent practice promoting the dignity of donors and relatives and enabling ethical transplantation practice (Figure 11.20).

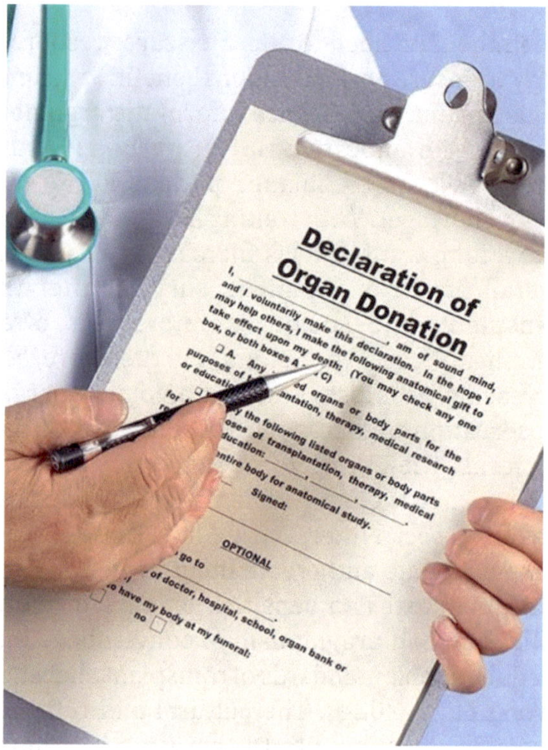

Figure 11.20. The role of consent in organ donation for lung transplantation.

Source: https://akm-img-a-in.tosshub.com/indiatoday/images/story/202505/organ-donation-200956975-3x4.jpg?VersionId=9oRGVvGqSfsrhjNx0VXRejiQKwSP8Gv7.

Test Your Knowledge

1. What are the ethical dilemmas with transplant decisions?
2. What is the importance of consent in organ donation?

Summary

Research on lung transplantation discovered that organ transplantation has both great promise and common issues associated with this form of medical treatment. Even while the technology continues to redefine the landscape of lung transplantation, and even more so with the application of technologies like ECMO in clinical practice, patients with end-stage lung disease increasingly have a living pathway to health recovery. ECMO has also emerged as a much-needed technology that provides vital support to seriously ill patients by stabilizing their pulmonary and circulatory systems, making them candidates for successful transplants. This capability is particularly important in the face of the widespread shortage of donor organs and the complexity of post-transplant care. Ultimately, these advances will certainly enhance patient outcomes and expand candidacy in patients otherwise transplant-ineligible (Butt et al., 2024). Aside from innovations in pre- and perioperative care, the future of lung transplantation is absolutely dependent on ongoing research into the prevention and comprehension of complications. Complications, such as post-transplant viral infection, including those caused by BK polyomavirus (BKPyV), still remain a significant danger to graft health. The recent findings on viral load monitoring have relevance that may be translational to enhanced control strategies and individualized immunosuppressive therapy. Enlightenment on successful biomarkers for BKPyV complication prediction highlights the role personalized medicine will have in improving transplant outcomes. With our knowledge in this area expanding, clinicians can better manage the nuanced interplay of infection and immunosuppression to achieve improved graft survival and patient health (Nourié et al., 2024). The future of optimal lung transplantation is one of collaboration that entails the combined action of investigators, caregivers, and patients. Future studies on long-term outcomes and complications will be of prime importance in defining practice and protocol in transplant centers globally. With continuing refinement of organ allocation strategies, surgical techniques, and post-transplant care, lung transplantation can meet the imperative needs of an aging population and the intricacy of chronic pulmonary disease. The integration of newer technology and treatment modes aims to build a stronger health system for lung transplantation, ultimately leading to improved survival and overall success of the life-saving operation. Emphasis on continued research and practice-related data will ensure that the future of lung transplantation is as bright as its promise (Butt et al., 2024; Nourié et al., 2024).

Lung transplantation is a landmark treatment for patients with end-stage lung disease. As demand for donor lungs is on the rise, complexity in candidate selection and meticulous candidate evaluation become critical. Specifically noteworthy is infectious complication management, which can have a profound influence on post-transplant outcome. Transplant teams should identify and treat pretransplant colonization or infection with multi-resistant bacteria, nontuberculous mycobacteria, and molds. All such information can serve to minimize risks and maximize the probability of a successful transplant, thereby improving the process of selection based on solid and improving data on the infectious milieu surrounding lung transplantation (as determined by new evidence of the role of these variables in graft survival and postoperative morbidity (Huang et al., 2025). Further, the late allograft complication of CLAD also highlights ongoing assessment of transplanted lungs. Advances in diagnostic methods have identified biomarkers such as matrix metalloproteinase 9 (MMP-9), which can provide indications of the potential risk of developing CLAD. Research has indicated that the elevated levels of MMP-9 after the second year following transplantation have been associated with higher risks of acquiring CLAD and, therefore, are a predictive factor for physicians as well. By monitoring these biomarkers, health care teams can respond early and individualize their management strategies to preserve graft function and improve patient outcomes. This can potentially redesign post-transplantation care and the success of lung transplants (Tissot et al., 2024). Generally, managing infectious diseases and using predictive biomarkers in lung transplantation are crucial to maximizing patient outcomes. As the field develops, it becomes increasingly clear that a multiaxial approach through careful selection, monitoring, and aggressive treatment of complications needs to be adopted. Enhancement in criteria for recipient suitability and donor lung allocation can be enabled by the progress in understanding infectious risk and the importance of biomarkers like MMP-9. It is for this reason that the present holistic approach aims not merely to maximize the rate of success in lung transplantation but to address the complex interplay of variables governing both graft survival and patient well-being in the long term (Tissot et al., 2024; Huang et al., 2025).

KEY TERMS FROM THIS CHAPTER

Acute rejection	Airway anastomosis
Bilateral lung transplant	Bronchiolitis obliterans syndrome (BOS)
Chronic rejection	Donor lung preservation
Donor matching	Graft-versus-host disease (GVHD)
HLA typing	Immunosuppressive therapy
Infectious complications	Ischemia-reperfusion injury
Lung allocation score (LAS)	Post-transplant surveillance
Pre-transplant evaluation	Primary graft dysfunction (PGD)
Pulmonary arterial hypertension (PAH)	Pulmonary function tests (PFTs)

Critical Thinking Questions

1. **What is the most common indication for lung transplantation?**
   a. Idiopathic pulmonary fibrosis
   b. Chronic obstructive pulmonary disease (COPD)
   c. Cystic fibrosis
   d. Pulmonary hypertension
2. **Which type of lung transplant involves transplanting both lungs simultaneously?**
   a. Single-lung transplant
   b. Bilateral lung transplant
   c. Heart-lung transplant
   d. Lobar transplant
3. **Which immunosuppressive drug is commonly used to prevent rejection after lung transplantation?**
   a. Methotrexate
   b. Cyclosporine
   c. Penicillin
   d. Aspirin
4. **What is the major cause of chronic lung allograft dysfunction (CLAD) after transplantation?**
   a. Acute infection
   b. Chronic rejection leading to bronchiolitis obliterans syndrome
   c. Pulmonary embolism
   d. Graft-versus-host disease
5. **Which infection is a common early post-transplant complication in lung transplant recipients?**
   a. Pneumocystis jirovecii pneumonia
   b. Tuberculosis
   c. Histoplasmosis
   d. Influenza

Short Answer Questions

1. What are the primary indications for lung transplantation?
2. Describe the contraindications for lung transplantation.
3. What types of lung transplantation procedures are commonly performed?
4. What immunosuppressive therapies are typically used after lung transplantation?
5. What are the major complications in the immediate postoperative period following lung transplantation?

Answer to Critical Thinking Questions

1. (b); 2. (b); 3. (b); 4. (b); 5. (a)

References

1. Akbari, F., Mollaei, M., Argani, P., Daneshfard, B., & Derakhshan, A. R. (2024). Spinacia oleracea: Exploring the therapeutic potential in Persian medicine and modern Pharmacology. *Current Drug Discovery Technologies, 21*(6). https://doi.org/10.2174/0115701638275971240201060710Aksoy, B., & Turker, E. K. (2024). Do ethical views of end-of-life patients' family members impact organ donation decisions? *Nursing Ethics, 32*, 530–542. https://www.semanticscholar.org/paper/d4c8b265d6348adeaeb00ddfdae9fd192236cb25 (accessed on 30th June 2025).
2. Alves, I. T., Alves, V. T., Rezende, E. H. M., Ribeiro, R. C. L., et al. (2024). Lung transplantation in cystic fibrosis patients: Clinical presentations and surgical considerations. https://core.ac.uk/download/617924771.pdf (accessed on 30th June 2025).
3. Andreasson, A., Anyanwu, A., Arcasoy, S., Avlonitis, V., Behrendt, C., et al. (2016). An observational study of donor *ex vivo* lung perfusion in UK lung transplantation: DEVELOP-UK. https://core.ac.uk/download/74230789.pdf (accessed on 30th June 2025).
4. A-Rahman, S., Abbott, J., Bradley, C., Arrington-Sanders, R., et al. (2015). Longitudinal impact of demographic and clinical variables on health-related quality of life in cystic fibrosis. https://core.ac.uk/download/42137142.pdf (accessed on 30th June 2025).
5. Atchade, E., de Tymowski, C., Lepitre, E., Zappella, N., Snauwaert, A., Jean-Baptiste, S., Tran-Dinh, A., et al. (2024). Impact of recipient and donor pretransplantation body mass index on early postoperative complications after lung transplantation. *BMC Pulmonary Medicine, 24*. https://www.semanticscholar.org/paper/d98591662c549bb0edd18e9ef21976082b144025 (accessed on 30th June 2025).
6. Bery, A., & Hachem, R. (2020). Antibody-mediated rejection after lung transplantation. *Annals of Translational Medicine, 8*. https://www.semanticscholar.org/paper/94c685c0103346eb2a84045bfce7ef63853b10ac (accessed on 30th June 2025).
7. Blazeby, J. M., Boutron, I., Clavein, P. A., Cook, J., et al. (2009). Challenges in evaluating surgical innovation. https://core.ac.uk/download/177132.pdf (accessed on 30th June 2025).
8. Bosslet, G. T., & Gutteridge, D. (2019). What should we learn from early hemodialysis allocation about how we should be using ECMO? https://core.ac.uk/download/322846895.pdf (accessed on 30th June 2025).
9. Burra, P., Caraceni, P., Ferri, F., Giannini, E., et al. (2018). Specific issues concerning the management of patients on the waiting list and after liver transplantation. https://core.ac.uk/download/159268374.pdf (accessed on 30th June 2025).
10. Butt, S. P., Kakar, V., Abdulaziz, S., Razzaq, N., Saleem, Y., Kumar, A., Ashiq, F., et al. (2024). Enhancing lung transplantation with ECMO: A comprehensive review of mechanisms, outcomes, and future considerations. *The Journal of Extracorporeal Technology, 56*, 191–202. https://www.semanticscholar.org/paper/e5ea9fdfc7a00b074a3fb82e04a81f290d9c0b30 (accessed on 30th June 2025).
11. Calabrese, F., Calabrese, F., Di Gregorio, G., Loy, M., et al. (2017). *Ex-vivo* recruitment and x-ray assessment of donor lungs in a challenging retrieval from a donor supported by LVAD using the portable normothermic perfusion system: A case report. https://core.ac.uk/download/84923815.pdf (accessed on 30th June 2025).

12. Cauchi, M. N. (1967). Organ and tissue transplantation. https://core.ac.uk/download/46604357.pdf (accessed on 30th June 2025).

13. Chapman, J. R. (2024). Moving boundaries for improving organ transplant availability. *Experimental and Clinical Transplantation, 22* (Suppl 4), 7–11. https://www.semanticscholar.org/paper/6f65de3a5b96caf9964f8881136c08108c114104 (accessed on 30th June 2025).

14. Chernyak, Y., Henderson, D. R., Patel, A., Teh, M., et al. (2020). Practice issues for evaluation and management of the suicidal left ventricular assist device patient. https://core.ac.uk/download/323269671.pdf (accessed on 30th June 2025).

15. Chinese Thoracic Society, Chinese Society of Organ Transplantation, & Guangdong Association of Primary Medicine. (2025). [Expert consensus on airway complications after lung transplantation]. *Zhonghua jie he he hu xi za zhi = Zhonghua jiehe he huxi zazhi = Chinese Journal of Tuberculosis and Respiratory Diseases, 48*(4), 318–328. https://www.semanticscholar.org/paper/075cb0de0087413bd18d3a11b0dcc4392fa394a1 (accessed on 30th June 2025).

16. Çıtak, S. (2025). Donor evaluation and the role of bronchoscopy in lung transplantation. *Laparoscopic Endoscopic Surgical Science*. https://www.semanticscholar.org/paper/febe17308718415319134 3ecf01e9738db82e3dd (accessed on 30th June 2025).

17. Clough, A. V., Cummens, B., Densmore, J. C., Jacobs, J., et al. (2013). Rattus model utilizing selective pulmonary ischemia induces bronchiolitis obliterans organizing pneumonia. https://core.ac.uk/download/213078972.pdf (accessed on 30th June 2025).

18. Cooper, J., Gardiner, D., & Harvey, D. (2020). Examining consent for interventional research in potential deceased organ donors: A narrative review. https://core.ac.uk/download/323306232.pdf (accessed on 30th June 2025).

19. Creel, M. E. (2008). Gender differences in survival in idiopathic pulmonary fibrosis and following lung transplant. https://core.ac.uk/download/12209464.pdf (accessed on 30th June 2025).

20. Dinh, A., Duke, J. L., Ferriola, D., Frackelton, E., et al. (2019). Assessing the utilization of high-resolution 2-field HLA typing in solid organ transplantation. https://core.ac.uk/download/213445234.pdf (accessed on 30th June 2025).

21. Elgharably, H., Javorski, M. J., & McCurry, K. (2021). Bilateral sequential lung transplantation: Technical aspects. *Journal of Thoracic Disease, 13*, 6564–6575. https://www.semanticscholar.org/paper/5a77cc2b76ac61be1b0b18af78e4ef9b89a9b929 (accessed on 30th June 2025).

22. Franz, M., Aburahma, K., Avşar, M., Boethig, D., Greer, M., Alhadidi, H., Sommer, W., et al. (2023). Does donor-recipient age mismatch have an influence on outcome after lung transplantation? A single-center experience. *European Journal of Cardio-Thoracic Surgery*. https://www.semanticscholar.org/paper/f6ad102dfde5ce9feb61b37f6ce3d38dae6dec10 (accessed on 30th June 2025).

23. Gardner, R. S., Haj-Yahia, S., Hawkins, N. M., Jhund, P. S., et al. (2012). How small is too small? A systematic review of center volume and outcome after cardiac transplantation. https://core.ac.uk/download/9652185.pdf (accessed on 30th June 2025).

24. Garza-Castillon, R., & Bharat, A. (2022). Lung transplantation for coronavirus disease 2019 associated severe acute respiratory distress syndrome. *Current Opinion in Anesthesiology, 36*, 11–19. https://www.semanticscholar.org/paper/ba7d831bd46052d820a6c8ae03023772baf56588 (accessed on 30th June 2025).

25. Graham, K., Kaiho, T., Thomae, B., Yagi, Y., Cerier, E., Martin-Harris, B., Bharat, A., et al. (2024). Risk factors and impact of swallowing impairment and aspiration after lung transplantation. *Journal of Thoracic Disease, 16*, 5755–5764. https://www.semanticscholar.org/paper/e53adc799c6e2e67160be0f397533e30c43b9b58 (accessed on 30th June 2025).
26. Grehan, P., Byrne, I., Egan, J., Danaher, D., & Heart and Lung Transplant Team. (2018). A review of lung transplantation for cystic fibrosis in Ireland in 2017. *Cystic Fibrosis*. https://www.semanticscholar.org/paper/882f52fdaafe981d45843a4b1935ed116ee72faa (accessed on 30th June 2025).
27. Hashemian, M., Zia, M. J., Khorrami-Nejad, M., Abed, Q. S., & Hashemian, H. (2025). Long-term outcomes of corneal transplantation: A review of 8,378 patients. *BMC Ophthalmology, 25*. https://www.semanticscholar.org/paper/289a26168d808d601212036318a8ec91b732eb7f (accessed on 30th June 2025).
28. Huang, J., Friedman-Moraco, R., & Pouch, S. (2025). Infections and lung transplantation: Key considerations for eligibility, management, and posttransplant care. *Current Opinion in Pulmonary Medicine*. https://www.semanticscholar.org/paper/a1154cb737d2db70bdb39f4615b4f7ea0d2c0412 (accessed on 30th June 2025).
29. Jacob, S., Pham, A. N., & Pham, S. M. (2022). Evolution of heart transplantation surgical techniques. In *Heart Transplantation [Working Title]*. https://www.semanticscholar.org/paper/6f91cfb185f3a1a8cd79bd3c77c44a2cc5623e5e (accessed on 30th June 2025).
30. Kang, M. W. (2025). Evolution of lung cancer surgery: Historical milestones, current strategy, and future innovations. *Journal of Chest Surgery, 58*, 79–84. https://www.semanticscholar.org/paper/5ba5ed79b7c56db9d4d1faf70427cf4d5d743672 (accessed on 30th June 2025).
31. Lee, S. W., Lee, D., & Choi, D. K. (2024). Comparison of the effects of multiple frailty and nutritional indexes on postoperative outcomes in critically ill patients undergoing lung transplantation. *Medicina, 60*. https://www.semanticscholar.org/paper/2a3eb4f1a75ef0dc4bdb4182a7209f4a0ab596e0 (accessed on 30th June 2025).
32. Maani, P. A. (2005). Pulmonary retransplant for a patient with bronchiolitis obliterans syndrome and hepatitis C viremia: An ethical case analysis. https://core.ac.uk/download/301286801.pdf (accessed on 30th June 2025).
33. Marinze, S., Marinze, S., Olawade, D. B., Olawade, D. B., et al. (2025). The impact of artificial intelligence and machine learning in organ retrieval and transplantation: A comprehensive review. https://core.ac.uk/download/637001221.pdf (accessed on 30th June 2025).
34. McQuiston, A., Emtiazjoo, A. M., Angel, P., Machuca, T., Christie, J., & Atkinson, C. (2021). Set up for failure: Pre-existing autoantibodies in lung transplant. *Frontiers in Immunology, 12*. https://www.semanticscholar.org/paper/490342be0b66d73793a5e2e3b4acfcb6d83685f1 (accessed on 30th June 2025).
35. Nguyen, E., Bayanati, H., Hurrell, C., Aitken, M., Cheung, E. M., Gupta, A., Harris, S., et al. (2022). Canadian Association of Radiologists/Canadian Association for Interventional Radiology/Canadian Society of Thoracic Radiology guidelines on thoracic interventions. *Canadian Association of Radiologists Journal, 74*, 272–287. https://www.semanticscholar.org/paper/ecfbc146211138e82ecbdb8809fe0df92e929776 (accessed on 30th June 2025).
36. Nourié, N., Boueri, C., Tran Minh, H., Divard, G., Lefaucheur, C., Salmona, M., Gressens, S. B., et al. (2024). BK polyomavirus infection in kidney transplantation: A comprehensive review

of current challenges and future directions. *International Journal of Molecular Sciences, 25.* https://www.semanticscholar.org/paper/0d33213d16c0511e391ed199b2b346a18bd501bd (accessed on 30th June 2025).

37. Palleschi, A., Mattioni, G., LoMauro, A., Privitera, E., Musso, V., Morlacchi, L., Vergari, M., et al. (2024). Diaphragm and lung transplantation. *Transplant International, 37.* https://www.semanticscholar.org/paper/381b4a04c7d797d2299f11112bbcfafa7ac3986a (accessed on 30th June 2025).

38. Ramineni, A., Faateh, M., Mehdizadeh-Shrifi, A., Hayes, D., & Morales, D. L. S. (2024). Outcomes of concomitant cardiac surgical procedures performed during pediatric lung transplantation in the United States. *Lung.* https://www.semanticscholar.org/paper/cb0a9d8de87e87fe919d772789f9a702356a919c (accessed on 30th June 2025).

39. Renaud-Picard, B., Koutsokera, A., Cabanero, M., & Martinu, T. (2021). Acute rejection in the modern lung transplant era. *Seminars in Respiratory and Critical Care Medicine, 42*, 411–427. https://www.semanticscholar.org/paper/ae27ad079b14d51205d3902558511235553179 71 (accessed on 30th June 2025).

40. Righi, I., Barone, I., Rosso, L., Morlacchi, L., Rossetti, V., Caffarena, G., Limanaqi, F., et al. (2024). Immunopathology of lung transplantation: From infection to rejection and vice versa. *Frontiers in Immunology, 15.* https://www.semanticscholar.org/paper/0cbb351f5f75bd19e2c50ecc672de9a17deaa812 (accessed on 30th June 2025).

41. Russell, C., & Keshavamurthy, S. (2022). Acute massive and submissive pulmonary embolism: Historical considerations, surgical techniques of pulmonary embolectomy, and novel applications in donor lungs with pulmonary emboli. *The International Journal of Angiology, 31*(3), 188–193. https://www.semanticscholar.org/paper/f152b705f091b3dfd626e54c57a1fd25c0b98223 (accessed on 30th June 2025).

42. Sarangi, A. K., Salem, M. A., Younus, M. D., El-Haroun, H., Mahal, A., Tripathy, L., Mishra, R., et al. (2024). Advanced biomaterials for regenerative medicine and their possible therapeutic significance in treating COVID-19: A critical overview. *International Journal of Surgery (London, England), 110*, 7508–7527. https://www.semanticscholar.org/paper/bb8e008647b6ec9928250463c7f982bddcedd38b (accessed on 30th June 2025).

43. Simanovski, J., & Ralph, J. (2022). A scoping review of the literature on sleep quality in adult lung transplant recipients. *Progress in Transplantation, 32*, 88–100. https://www.semanticscholar.org/paper/0350cc8673cb9c7a07af0b8832f2f3b0e65da3db (accessed on 30th June 2025).

44. Taghdiri, A. (2023). Exploring long-term outcomes in COPD patients: A comprehensive narrative review of bilateral and single lung transplantation. *The Cardiothoracic Surgeon, 31.* https://www.semanticscholar.org/paper/09b75b45737063c5e254328c86f4d1333afe97e4 (accessed on 30th June 2025).

45. Thaiparambil, J., Yin, Z., & El-Zein, R. (2023). Abstract 1948: Novel insights into lung cancer & chronic obstructive pulmonary disease racial disparities. *Cancer Research.* https://www.semanticscholar.org/paper/af2716ad5b2a735cefd5f351f663c95e62ee4b59 (accessed on 30th June 2025).

46. Tissot, A., Durand, E., Goronflot, T., Coiffard, B., Renaud-Picard, B., Roux, A., Demant, X., et al. (2024). Blood MMP-9 measured at 2 years after lung transplantation as a prognostic biomarker

of chronic lung allograft dysfunction. *Respiratory Research, 25.* https://www.semanticscholar.org/paper/e4c39cccda756ef2d9e4b6eb0bccc057b9da43b7 (accessed on 30th June 2025).

47. Upadhyay, B., Anstead, M. I., Keshavamurthy, S., & Gurley, J. (2024). Management of superior vena cava syndrome during lung transplantation for a patient with cystic fibrosis. *BMJ Case Reports, 17.* https://www.semanticscholar.org/paper/47dafb21bd71d3db89ce731cef92d521c547c656 (accessed on 30th June 2025).

48. Verleden, G., & Gottlieb, J. (2023). Lung transplantation for COPD/pulmonary emphysema. *European Respiratory Review, 32.* https://www.semanticscholar.org/paper/3f5c26166eaeaa47441afe4789727334d3d5c079 (accessed on 30th June 2025).

49. Vispo, N. S. (2025). Pioneering the future of organ transplantation: Lessons from the Spanish model. *Bionatura Journal.* https://www.semanticscholar.org/paper/6a515c12d7bd263d4c704b7fda3e2020ec7ac2d0 (accessed on 30th June 2025).

50. Wong, H. P. N., Selvakumar, S. V., Loh, P. Y., Liau, J. Y. J., Liau, M. Y. Q., & Shelat, V. G. (2024). Ethical frontiers in liver transplantation. *World Journal of Transplantation, 14.* https://www.semanticscholar.org/paper/f583aa5c55f09e90852571364b738560c85cfaae (accessed on 30th June 2025).

51. Yang, J., Xie, X., Li, J., Li, Y., Li, B., Wang, C., & Jiang, P. (2024). Which strategy is better for lung transplantation: Cardiopulmonary bypass or extracorporeal membrane oxygenation? *Perfusion.* https://www.semanticscholar.org/paper/c9b77baf1451c897293c0bded998578180d92dc0 (accessed on 30th June 2025).

52. Zarif, H. (2015). Distributive injustice and organ transplant waitlists. https://core.ac.uk/download/641025544.pdf (accessed on 30th June 2025).

CRITICAL CARE IN PULMONARY MEDICINE

12

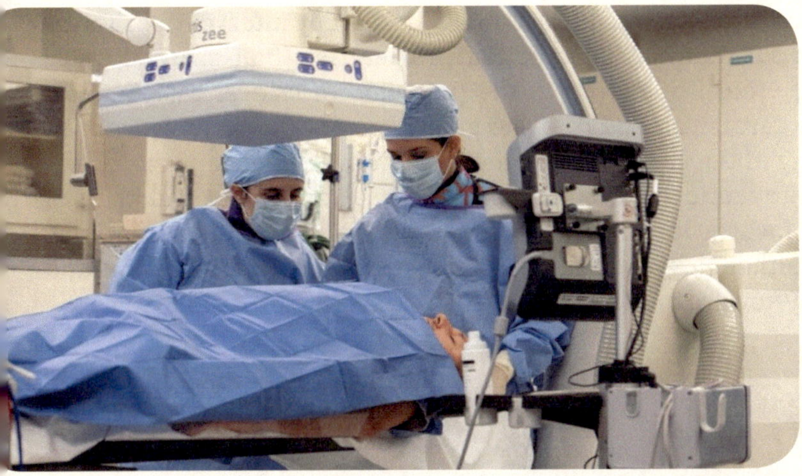

LEARNING OBJECTIVES

After studying this chapter, you will be able to:

1. Describe common pulmonary conditions in critical care;
2. List the diagnostic tools in pulmonary critical care;
3. Identify the management strategies for pulmonary patients;
4. Define the role of multidisciplinary teams;
5. Focus on the ethical considerations in pulmonary critical care;
6. Understand the advances in pulmonary medicine.

Introduction

The significance of critical care in pulmonary medicine has gained considerable attention in recent years due to rising cases of respiratory ailments and the need for advanced management of critically ill patients. The complicated lung conditions like acute respiratory distress syndrome (ARDS), chronic obstructive pulmonary disease (COPD), and pneumonia necessitate a multidisciplinary approach entailing novel interventions and evidence-guided guidelines. Awareness of the complexities present in such conditions is paramount to improving patient outcomes. Furthermore, the incorporation of personalized models of care and newer treatment modalities is becoming an increasingly targeted area in modern pulmonary medicine. Such a background opens the way for an in-depth examination of critical care practice with a view to tackling such concerns in a professional manner, looking at the importance of being attached to individualized therapeutic approaches as a way of enhancing the quality of care to be offered to critical patients. It requires both clinical competence and an effective system for decision-making and treatment delivery to handle pulmonary patients in the context of critical care. Recent studies indicate the potential to significantly enhance physician-patient communication in complicated care decisions through use of time-limited trials (TLTs) (Chang et al., 2019). The trials encourage healthy discussion and establish expectations, which can potentially abate the burden of futile therapies that might not be helpful to a patient with advanced pulmonary disease. Besides, the implementation of certain protocols for conditions such as acute heart failure (AHF) shows the value of evidence-based management protocols for emergency medical services (EMS) (Chang et al., 2019). These developments demonstrate the ongoing development of pulmonary medicine where protocolized care can expedite processes and improve health outcomes with the patient as the focal point of decision-making. As the critical care culture of pulmonary medicine evolves, the effect on healthcare systems, providers, and patients is profound. The integration of advanced diagnostics such as point-of-care testing and ultrasound with therapy interventions forms a culture of anticipatory care that can substantially alter patient trajectories (Banaszewski et al., 2020). Furthermore, the resolution of ethical dilemmas in the provision of critical care, namely in invasive procedures and end-of-life care, is essential to the guarantor of a humane practice of medicine. By virtue of an understanding of the complexity of these challenges, clinicians can better manage the subtleties of care, with therapeutic activity in accordance with the values and goals of patients and their families. Lastly, the focus given to critical care in pulmonary medicine not only reflects progress in technology and methodology but also highlights the role of compassion and mutual decision-making in the journey towards outstanding patient care (Figure 12.1).

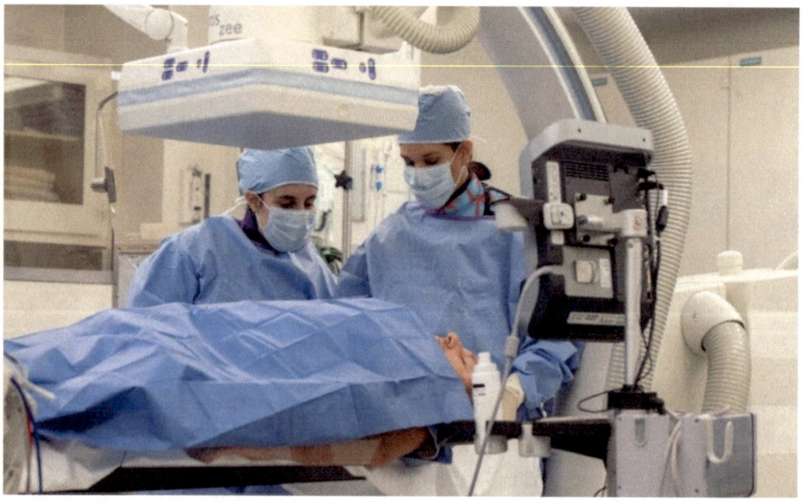

Figure 12.1. Critical care in pulmonary medicine.

Source: https://www.massgeneral.org/assets/mgh/images/medicine/pulmonary/pulmonary-137_1000x600.jpg.

Definition of Critical Care in Pulmonary Medicine

Critical care, in pulmonary medicine, refers to specialized medical care provided to patients with acute respiratory failure or distress. Critical care is characterized by a multidisciplinary strategy that incorporates essential aspects of patient management, such as the provision of advanced therapeutic modalities, monitoring, and support measures. This critical care aims to stabilize the patients by correcting the acute physiological derangements associated with severe lung diseases, like ARDS or COPD exacerbations. While working through complex clinical cases, adherence to set standards, including those published by the European Society of Cardiology, is important in order to achieve maximum patient outcomes (Kirchhof et al., 2016). The definition of critical care goes far beyond instant life support; it comprises continuous assessment of the patient, individualized treatment plans, and preventative intervention benefiting global respiratory function. Care teams, typically consisting of pulmonologists, intensivists, nurses, and respiratory therapists, rotate to observe the patient's vital signs, oxygenation level, and reaction to therapies. This integrative approach provides for each patient's own physiological status to be taken into account, thereby initiating person-specific therapeutic plans. Furthermore, the use of evidence-based practice ensures that clinicians are able to manage the dynamic nature of pulmonary medicine and ensure that interventions align with the latest in scientific knowledge while being respectful to the individual patient's rights and wishes (Kirchhof et al., 2016). Finally, the ethic of critical care of pulmonary medicine underscores the requirement to provide timely and effective intervention in preventing morbidity and mortality associated with acute respiratory illnesses. By targeting acute management and longer-term recovery strategies, pulmonary critical care aims not just to stabilize the patient but to optimize lung function and quality of life. A commitment to continuing education and adherence to changing evidence increases the capacity of health professionals to address changing needs of life-threatening pulmonary illnesses. Thus, the definition of critical care is not static but evolves with advances in medical science and technology, highlighting the need to keep oneself updated in this critical care specialty.

Importance of Pulmonary Health in Critical Care Settings

In critical care settings, the importance of pulmonary health cannot be overstressed as respiratory failure continues to be a leading cause of morbidity and mortality in patients. Care of pulmonary complications is extremely crucial, particularly in vulnerable populations such as those with comorbidities or states of immunocompromised conditions. Management of ARDS or COPD exacerbations involves timely and optimal clinical intervention to achieve normalization of oxygenation and ventilation. As physicians navigate the complexities of these conditions, they must be alert to the meticulous and watchful treatment of the etiologies for pulmonary distress. The integration of aggressive pulmonary health interventions in critical care not only enhances patient outcomes but also minimizes the occurrence of chronic respiratory handicaps, emphasizing the complementary nature of pulmonary care as part of the general framework of critical care medicine. The management of pulmonary health also involves the consideration of global challenges such as drug-resistant infections, which can complicate respiratory disease and treatment plans. The re-emergence of diseases like multidrug-resistant tuberculosis (MDR-TB) is a tremendous obstacle to effective pulmonary care. Particular recent research has put into context the horrifying tendency that defines MDR-TB, which is difficult to manage in critical care environments, particularly for those with high HIV prevalence. In such conditions, drug-resistant infections can create disturbing complications that raise alarm, and health care providers are compelled to develop invasive preventive and management strategies in an effort to avoid disruptions in pulmonary health programs. It is important to equip health care systems to combat such essential problems in an attempt to mitigate the impact of such diseases on the already compromised pulmonary environment in critical care units (Karim et al., 2010). In addition to managing infections, therapies such as inhaled nitric oxide (iNO) are also important components of pulmonary hypertension management, particularly in pediatric critical care. There were varied practices in initiating iNO among very preterm infants with pulmonary hypertension when their clinicians were surveyed, reflecting the complex decision-making of critical care. The varied reactions to iNO reflect not only individual practitioner outcomes but also the conflict between evidence-based and patient-centered care. As critical care professionals weigh the safety and efficacy of interventions, they must balance clinical recommendations with the complexities of patient needs, highlighting the prominent role of pulmonary health in achieving optimal results within critical care environments (Dukhovny et al., 2019). Finally, the development of pulmonary care within critical settings is at the heart of total patient health and well-being, setting the stage for complete recovery and ultimate wellness (Figure 12.2).

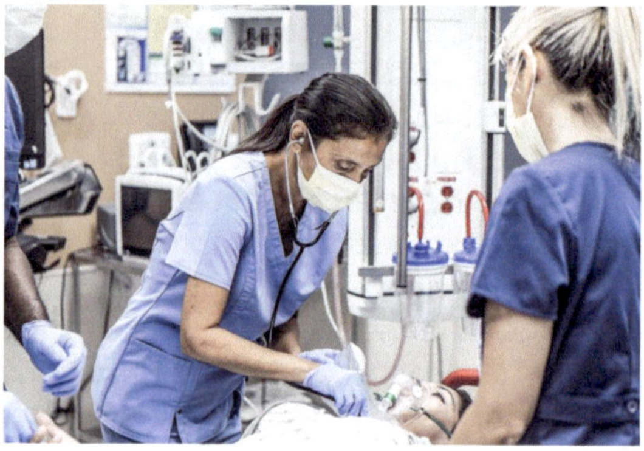

Figure 12.2. Pulmonary health in critical care settings.

Source: https://www.ngmcgme.org/wp-content/uploads/2025/02/GME-Pulm-Crit-Blog-1-1-1024x683.jpeg.

12.1. Common Pulmonary Conditions in Critical Care

Learning Outcome

1. Acute Respiratory Distress Syndrome (ARDS);
2. Chronic Obstructive Pulmonary Disease (COPD) exacerbations;
3. Pneumonia and complications.

The critical care environment of pulmonary medicine is often dominated by common but complex conditions that exert a staggering impact on outcomes. One such condition is idiopathic pulmonary fibrosis (IPF), which is characterized by progressive decline in lung function and high morbidity. IPF predominantly affects older patients, with a median survival of 3-5 years after the diagnosis, thereby ranking among the most fatal presentations of idiopathic interstitial pneumonia. The challenge inherent in managing IPF is its unpredictable course and the necessity of implementing an individualized treatment approach. Anti-fibrotic therapy has lately been approved to limit pulmonary function loss, a significant advancement. Yet, IPF management is not limited to the lung alone but also involves a global evaluation of comorbid conditions that affect the global well-being of the patient, according to critical care principles emphasizing global patient management (Collard et al., 2017). Comorbidities of pulmonary disorders in critical care need to be known to design successful treatment modalities. IPF patients commonly present with several comorbidities that add to the complexity of their clinical picture. Cardiovascular complications such as pulmonary hypertension and coronary disease frequently aggravate respiratory symptoms and complicate management regimens. Gastrointestinal complications, such as gastroesophageal reflux, are also common and should be considered in the management regimen, despite the debatable therapeutic benefit for such conditions. Besides, the presence of metabolic disorders like diabetes mellitus also poses other risks, as they have the potential to compromise immune and general health. This complexity further highlights the need for an integral and multidisciplinary approach within critical care settings to effectively address such intertwined health conditions and thereby improve patient outcomes and quality of life (Amaducci et al., 2018). Effective critical care of pulmonary diseases also requires accuracy in diagnosis. Accurate diagnosis not only guides therapeutic interventions but also allows disease progression and complications to be predicted. For instance, detection of associated comorbidities is important in the formulation of patient-specific care plans. For IPF, advanced diagnostic tools and disease-specific techniques have been developed to appreciate individual health profiles better. Clinicians must be highly sensitive in monitoring pulmonary function, assessing the impact of comorbidities, and altering treatment plans accordingly. Further, incorporation of routine screening for venous thromboembolism and obstructive sleep apnea can have a significant bearing on management outcomes. With the advancement of the discipline, the use of emerging diagnostic and therapeutic modalities will be central in treating prevalent pulmonary diseases in critical care, aiming to offer patients optimal and complete treatment (Collard et al., 2017).

12.1.1. Acute Respiratory Distress Syndrome (ARDS)

ARDS is a critical challenge in pulmonary critical care medicine, characterized by an abrupt onset of secondary respiratory failure due to increased alveolar-capillary membrane permeability. The pathologic change encourages the formation of non-cardiogenic pulmonary edema, which leads to critical hypoxemia and compromised respiratory mechanics. The etiologic heterogeneity of ARDS, ranging from pneumonia to sepsis, makes it essential to have a specially adapted management strategy. The universality of ARDS in critically ill patients necessitates profound knowledge of the disease since it drastically influences patients quality of life and survival. Literature shows that the combination of ventilatory and non-ventilatory interventions is significant, with a focus on clinical strategies that emphasize patient-specific preferences and intervention timing (Battalian et al., 2025). Ventilatory support strategies in ARDS have evolved, leading to many approaches aimed at maximizing oxygenation and minimizing lung injury. Conventional mechanical ventilation (CMV), high-flow nasal cannula therapy, and non-invasive ventilation are a few of the most prevalent treatments applied for the management of ARDS patients. Evidence indicates that the appropriate application of these practices has a strong influence on clinical outcomes. Notably, the proper use of such interventions is highly dependent on the severity of ARDS, along with each patient's reaction. A meta-analysis across a wide range of ventilatory approaches identified a clear majority of studies to emphasize the importance of tailoring these techniques to enhance patient survival rates (Battalian et al., 2025). Moreover, a discussion of the timing and order of interventions remains a significant issue to be explored in future research on efficient ARDS management. A recent controversy regarding the use of neuromuscular blocking agents (NMBAs) in ARDS treatment highlights a fascinating phenomenon of critical care medicine. NMBAs were hypothesized to optimize mechanical ventilation by reducing patient-ventilator asynchrony and improving hemodynamics in acute respiratory distress. However, the clinical application of NMBAs remains controversial. While they are deemed beneficial in reducing the work of breathing and enhancing oxygenation, apprehension of resulting adverse effects, such as neuromuscular weakness and thrombosis, has precluded their widespread application in managing ARDS. Thus, clinicians must strike a delicate balance between benefits and risks of applying NMBAs. A patient-centered model will allow an informed decision-making process regarding the application of these agents, again reflecting the subtleties of critical care for ARDS patients (Figure 12.3).

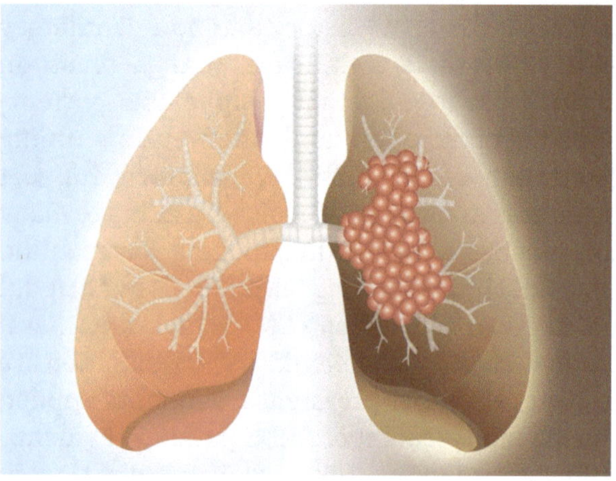

Figure 12.3. Acute respiratory distress syndrome (ARDS).

Source: https://external-content.duckduckgo.com/iu/?u=https%3A%2F%2Fwww.10faq.com%2Fassets%2Fimg%2Fwhat-is-acute-respiratory-distress-syndrome-06.jpg&f=1&nofb=1&ipt=a39d971378f1981ad057d4041a1790c466e8e1ffe5a22cf09054db79f275a33a.

12.1.2. Chronic Obstructive Pulmonary Disease (COPD) Exacerbations

COPD exacerbations represent acute episodes of precipitous worsening of respiratory symptoms, and they can require the use of additional therapeutic interventions. These exacerbations are brought about by numerous different causes that range from respiratory infections to environmental pollutants and even medication non-compliance. Understanding the underlying pathophysiological processes of exacerbations is relevant because these are associated with accelerated disease course and increased healthcare resource utilization. Existing evidence suggests that exacerbations have heterogeneous inflammatory profiles, with neutrophilic inflammation most prevalent. However, a significant subgroup of patients experiences type 2 inflammation, with other immune mechanisms implicated. The ability to identify these profiles can aid in the personalization of interventions. The awareness of the weight of such exacerbations heightens the need for continued monitoring and management interventions geared towards enhancing the quality of life in patients who have COPD (Singh et al., 2024). The management of COPD exacerbation is a complex intervention encompassing pharmacologic and non-pharmacologic management. Pharmacologically, the patients may receive bronchodilators, corticosteroids, and antibiotics, particularly where there is a suspicion of secondary infections. The effectiveness of the treatments, on the other hand, could vary, and hence, an individualized strategy for treatment is required. As well, emerging treatments specifically targeting certain inflammatory mechanisms, such as those of type 2 inflammation, propose a shift towards a more advanced perspective of therapy. As reviewed in the literature, integrating understanding of individual patient profiles with clinical strategies can lead to improved outcomes during exacerbation (Rabe et al., 2023). In addition, symptom identification and self-management education is important, allowing patients to promptly present themselves to the medical team. This intervention can reduce the severity of the exacerbation and its consequent complications. In critical care, treatment of COPD exacerbations frequently requires escalation to hospitalization, especially in severe or complicated cases. Acute respiratory failure patients may require advanced interventions such as invasive or non-invasive ventilation, and thus, the value of pulmonary specialists in the acute setting is emphasized. Furthermore, exacerbation-comorbidity interaction, which is common among the COPD population, complicates treatment and requires multidisciplinary care. Coordination between the healthcare providers is essential to address these complexities. Studies have further supported the concept that early diagnosis and intervention in exacerbations can reduce hospital admissions and improve patient outcomes. Finally, innovation in critical care practice in pulmonary medicine requires a focus on appreciating the nuances of COPD exacerbations and how they influence patient care and quality of life (Singh et al., 2024) (Figure 12.4).

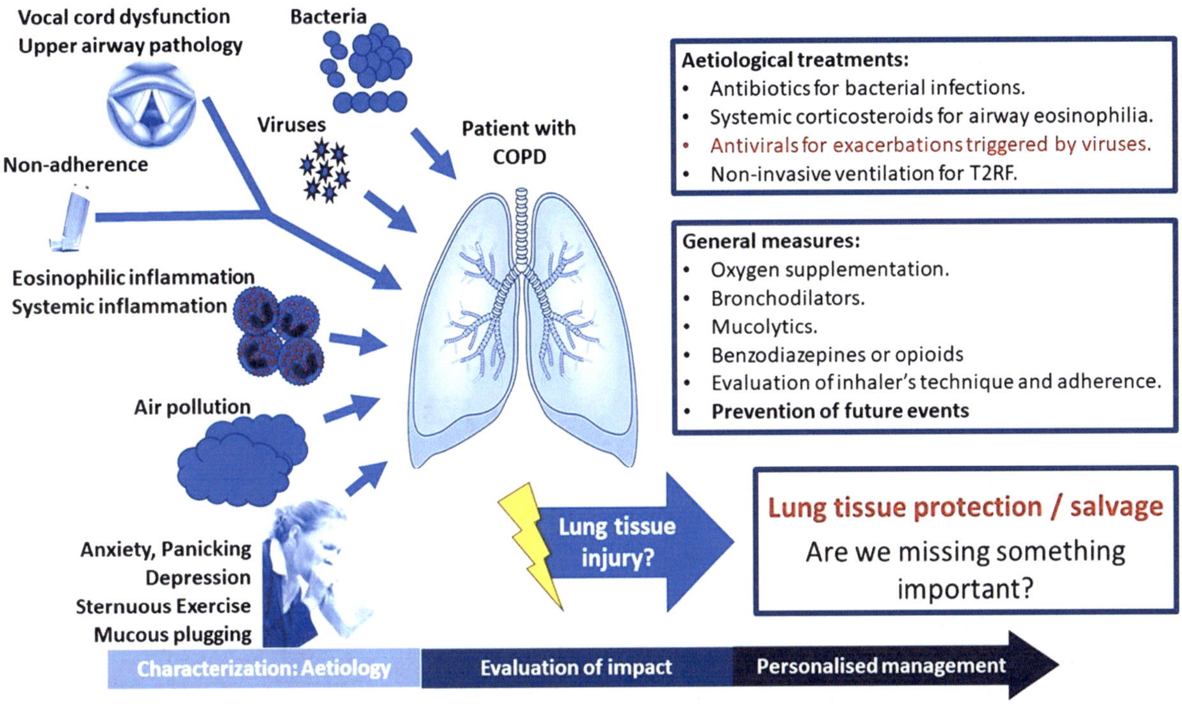

Figure 12.4. Acute exacerbations of chronic obstructive pulmonary disease (COPD).

Source: https://external-content.duckduckgo.com/iu/?u=https%3A%2F%2Fthorax.bmj.com%2Fcontent%2Fthoraxjnl%2Fearly%2F2020%2F03%2F26%2Fthoraxjnl-2019-214484%2FF1.large.jpg%3Fwidth%3D800%26height%3D600%26carousel%3D1&f=1&nofb=1&ipt=25b9522b1bebee7d160215527a10692e2db97735efe9f88104414f5ed3692068.

12.1.3. Pneumonia and Its Complications

Pneumonia is a critical challenge in intensive care, and the reason for this is predominantly due to its multiaspect presentation and the array of complications that can be encountered. The infectious process involving inflammation of the lung parenchyma can be severe and advance very quickly, leading to severe respiratory distress and necessitating intensive care. Pneumonia in pulmonary medicine is likely to occur in patients who are already compromised either by age or existing illness, thus complicating the success of its treatment. The interaction between pneumonia and underlying medical conditions may complicate the presentation, hence leading to more extended hospital stays and death. Therefore, an understanding of the pathophysiology of pneumonia and potential complications is a must for clinicians who practice pulmonary medicine and critical care. The association of pneumonia with serious complications such as ARDS is particularly concerning in intensive care units (ICUs). ARDS can occur as a direct response to the inflammatory process of pneumonia and lead to significant gas exchange derangements and mechanical ventilation requirements. Secondary infections, such as pleural effusion or empyema, can be precipitated by pneumonia, complicating the underlying infection and worsening pulmonary function. The challenge lies in detecting and treating these complications early on. Successful treatment regimens are usually multidisciplinary in scope, involving infectious disease specialists, pulmonary units, and critical care teams, all of whom contribute their knowledge in concert to achieve the best possible patient outcomes without the risk of pneumonia and its complications. In the grand scheme of pulmonary medicine, it is necessary to consider not only the infectious etiology of pneumonia but also the impact of noninfectious complications in critically ill patients. Postoperative patients with diseases such as obstructive sleep apnea are also more likely to develop pneumonia and other complications from procedures involving sedation and anesthesia (Doghramji et al., 2012). Patients who receive hematopoietic stem cell transplants most often have noninfectious pulmonary complications that can be a result of pneumonia, which can further be complicated by graft-versus-host disease and other immune responses (Baloglu et al., 2014). This highlights the importance of identifying patients at high risk preoperatively so that effective perioperative management measures can be taken to reduce both infectious and noninfectious complications of pneumonia. Preventive intervention in the intensive care setting is essential for improving patient outcomes in the context of this multilateral clinical situation (Figure 12.5).

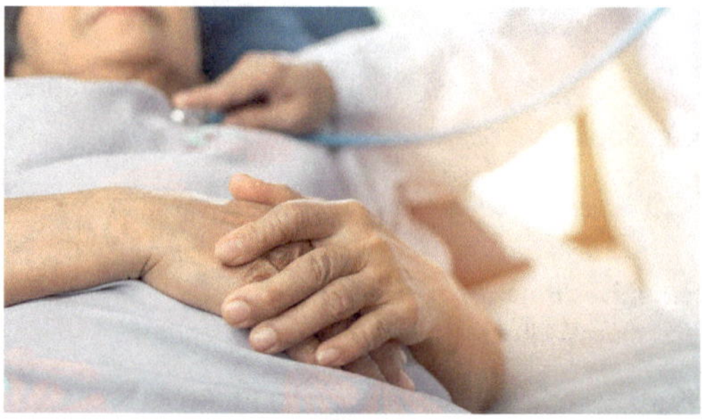

Figure 12.5. Pneumonia and its complications.

Source: https://external-content.duckduckgo.com/iu/?u=https%3A%2F%2Fs.yimg.com%2Fuu%2Fapi%2Fres%2F1.2%2FXdhUD6._p42yDhs1cq2dAA--~B%2FaD02NzQ7dz0xMTk5O3NtPTE7YXBwaWQ9eXRhY2h5b24-%2Fhttps%3A%2F%2Fmedia.zenfs.com%2Fen%2Fconsumer_reports_689%2F63d12f92e45c1693df1e92bb02e3ec90&f=1&nofb=1&ipt=33896de4408fabeb3a006c51fdb3c9d4e686ffd81275d0b320a75ec627925b59.

Test Your Knowledge

1. What is acute respiratory distress syndrome (ARDS)?
2. What is pneumonia and its complications?

12.2. Diagnostic Tools in Pulmonary Critical Care

Learning Outcome

1. Imaging methods: X-rays and CT scans;
2. Pulmonary function tests;
3. Blood gas analysis.

In pulmonary critical care, accurate and prompt diagnosis is very important for effective management and patient outcomes. Diagnostic tools must be robust, capable of handling a broad spectrum of conditions, such as pneumonia, ARDS, and tuberculosis. Among the various tools used, imaging modalities like chest X-rays and CT scans play a significant role in visualizing pulmonary pathology. Enhanced imaging technology has enabled more precise detection of lung infiltrates, consolidations, and other abnormalities, thus hastening diagnosis and early treatment. But their very limitations, including radiation exposure and availability, require ongoing innovation in the diagnostic process to keep pace with the evolving requirements presented by critically ill patients in the pulmonary setting. The treatment of diseases like tuberculosis presents unique challenges requiring certain consistent emphasis on dependably diagnosed tools in pulmonary critical care. The traditional diagnostic methods, while accurate, are likely to result in delay since confirmation by culture and sensitivity testing is needed in the laboratory. According to Harari et al. (2012), gold-standard tests for TB are more typically laboratory-based, involving multiple investigations over several weeks, and therefore likely to deter early intervention. Novel diagnostic devices, such as molecular diagnostics detecting Mycobacterium tuberculosis, have been introduced to rapidly diagnose but face enormous barriers to their widespread use. Moreover, breakdowns in point-of-care devices remind us of the ongoing need for new solutions that not only hasten diagnosis and enhance accuracy but also address tuberculosis transmission and drug adherence issues that are at the top of public health priorities. Besides, other critical conditions, such as AHF, also highlight the complexity of pulmonary critical care diagnostic instruments. A multinational survey indicated that the incidence rate is high among emergency medical services (EMS) regions in terms of setting guidelines for diagnosing AHF, but point-of-care testing and ultrasound remain in the stages of incomplete implementation, as mentioned in Banaszewski et al. (2020).

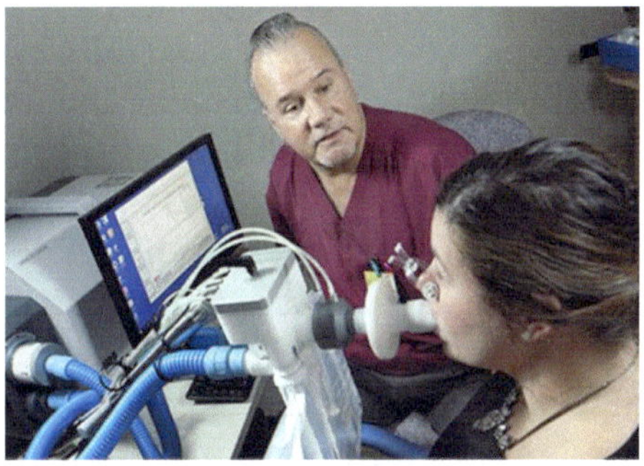

Figure 12.6. Diagnostic tools in pulmonary critical care.

Source: https://external-content.duckduckgo.com/iu/?u=https%3A%2F%2Ftse1.mm.bing.net%2Fth%3Fid%3DOIP.NmiOG9V3jRBn1lFhW_eKtQAAAA%26pid%3DApi&f=1&ipt=e201e9d94d4eb9281660db43b735324669fb143a7aab073c34085d82af34abbd.

The inaccessibility of full diagnostic arsenals may complicate pre-hospital management of patients presenting with respiratory distress. Secondly, the perceived difficulty in the diagnosis of AHF compared to other conditions reflects the challenge presented by health professionals to diagnose it in indeterminate emergency settings. This limitation suggests the necessity for ongoing training and procedural upgrades to improve the accuracy and efficiency of diagnosis for EMS practitioners in critical care situations. Enhancing these diagnostic skills is vital to enhance patient outcomes in pulmonary critical care as well as to enable timely interventions (Figure 12.6).

12.2.1. Imaging Techniques: X-rays and Computed Tomography (CT) Scans

The practice of pulmonary medicine is heavily dependent on advanced imaging techniques such as X-rays and CT scans for the diagnosis and treatment of lung conditions. X-rays are a very useful diagnostic tool, giving quick images of chest structures, including lungs, heart, and vessels. X-rays will reveal abnormalities, such as pneumonia, pleural effusions, and certain lung cancers. However, while the information provided by X-rays is important, their inability to provide the required level of detail often necessitates further investigation using more sophisticated methods like CT scans. CT scanning, by its cross-sectional images, provides accurate assessment of lung parenchyma as well as contiguous structures, in effect optimizing clinicians ability to interpret complex pulmonary conditions. Arguably, one of the most significant advances in pulmonary imaging is the application of High-Resolution Computed Tomography (HRCT) in the assessment of COPD and emphysema. New technical advancements in imaging analysis techniques have enabled the automatic measurement of emphysema regions from HRCT scans, eliminating the need for manually annotated scans for training. The auto-measurement relies on textural features from Gaussian filter banks and co-occurrence matrices to characterize lung tissue, a paradigm shift for the diagnostic field. Research indicates that classifiers like miSVM are superior to traditional methods in correlating imaging findings with pulmonary function tests (PFTs), highlighting the value of advanced imaging techniques in providing elusive diagnostic clues. Such advances hold significance in supporting patient care in intensive care settings. The use of X-rays along with CT scanning in pulmonary medicine enhances not only the reliability of diagnosis but also aids clinicians in following the progression of the disease and treatment effects. The ability to classify various severities of pulmonary disease, such as emphysema, using sophisticated imaging analytics has broad implications for personalized patient care. Recent studies have demonstrated that employing classifiers derived from imaging information can significantly improve the correlation between radiological and clinical findings, thereby minimizing inter-observer variability. This is extremely important in critical care, where precise and timely diagnosis can influence therapeutic maneuvers. With ongoing technological advances in imaging, the applications of X-rays and CT scans will extend further, eventually leading to better treatment options for patients with serious pulmonary conditions (N/A, 1992; Carl et al., 2018) (Figure 12.7).

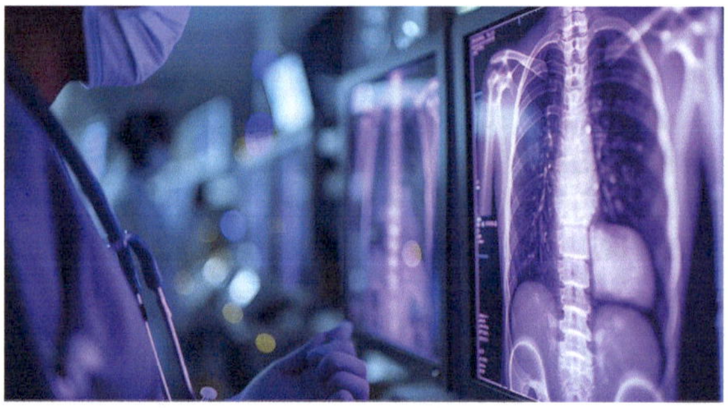

Figure 12.7. Imaging techniques.

Source: https://external-content.duckduckgo.com/iu/?u=https%3A%2F%2Fimg.freepik.com%2Fpremium-photo%2Funderstanding-different-medical-imaging-techniques-xrays-ct-scans-digital-radiography-concept-xrays-ct-scans-digital-radiography-medical-imaging-techniques-radiology_918839-120452.jpg%3Fw%3D826&f=1&nofb=1&ipt=7ea21a612785f6f3269c4cd7811bbdbdc16932dc9bd7e16f876a195d549a3456.

12.2.2. Pulmonary Function Tests (PFTs)

In pulmonary critical care, PFTs are essential diagnostic studies that measure the respiratory system's function. They quantify various regions of lung function, including airflow, lung volumes, and the effectiveness of gas exchange, providing clinicians with information to diagnose and manage pulmonary disease. Significantly, conditions like COPD and asthma rely heavily on PFTs in the assessment of severity, monitoring progression, and guiding suitable treatment interventions. Test results pinpoint the inherent pathophysiology of pulmonary disease, enabling clinicians to make evidence-based decisions that optimize patient outcomes and ensure efficient delivery of critical care. Traditionally, PFTs applied race-specific prediction equations in assessing lung function for diverse populations. However, more recent guidelines issued by the American Thoracic Society promote a race-neutral approach to minimize the risks of biases introduced by using race as an input variable in spirometry prediction equations. This change reflects practitioners' heightened awareness of the complexity of race and its intersection with physiology. As demonstrated in a study on the views of academic pulmonary practitioners, there is controversy on using race in PFT predictions and, consequently, an urgent need for continuous discussion within the profession (Banerjee et al., 2024). The discussions are crucial since they will influence the application of new guidelines and impact the standardization of care across various populations. Besides, the inclusion of body composition indices in pulmonary function tests has emerged as a significant field of study in the management of COPD patients. It is confirmed by evidence as having identified an association between body composition metrics—fat-free mass index (FFMI) and phase angle (PhA)—and exercise tolerance and promoting their role in nutritional and overall health status assessment in patients with chronic respiratory diseases (CRD) (Yang et al., 2024). As such, incorporation of these indices into routine PFTs may provide an enhanced understanding of the patient's status and enable risk stratification and tailoring of treatment regimens. This multi-faceted approach has the potential to the effectiveness of critical care provided in pulmonary medicine, resulting in better patient outcomes and a deeper understanding of the complexity of lung function and systemic health (Figure 12.8).

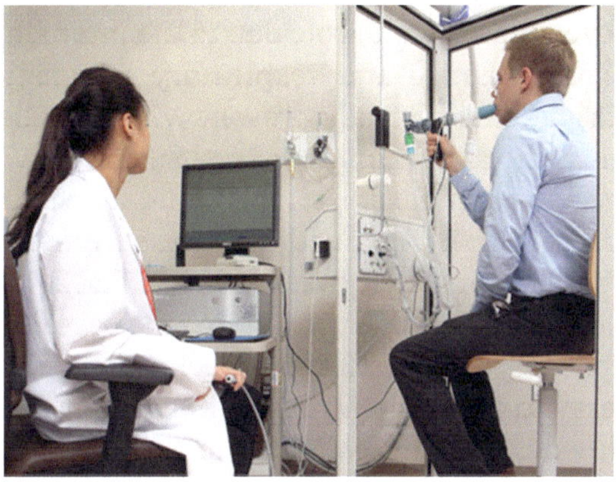

Figure 12.8. Pulmonary function tests (PFTs).

Source: https://external-content.duckduckgo.com/iu/?u=https%3A%2F%2Fmontgomerypulmonary.com%2Fwp-content%2Fuploads%2F2021%2F02%2FPulmonary-function-test.jpg&f=1&nofb=1&ipt=2b604385d5176744ac98bee76bae12515d52bac4762064dbc0b63cbb2cf3ee08.

12.2.3. Blood Gas Analysis

Blood gas analysis is a fundamental diagnostic tool in critical care, particularly in pulmonary medicine. The analysis provides essential information about a patient's respiratory status through measurements of values like arterial oxygen (PaO2) and carbon dioxide (PaCO2) levels, as well as pH. These measurements are important in assessing the efficiency of pulmonary gas exchange, enabling practitioners to identify respiratory failure and acid-base derangements early. Proper blood gas interpretation enables healthcare providers to prioritize management and follow up on treatment responses effectively. In acute illnesses, such as those of AHF syndromes, data that may be ascertained by blood gas analysis has an important function in altering respiratory support therapies so that patient outcomes within intensive care settings are improved, reflecting its function in managing conditions of respiratory distress and impaired oxygenation (Bueno et al., 2017). In ARDS and acute lung injury (ALI), blood gas analysis plays an even more pivotal role due to the interaction of gas exchange and respiratory mechanics. Such patients typically present with attendant non-cardiogenic pulmonary edema and varying degrees of hypoxemia from mild to severe, and early arterial blood gas measurement is essential. Parametric evaluation like PaO2/FiO2 ratio can be utilized in stratifying the severity of respiratory failure, thus influencing therapeutic interventions directly. Study findings indicate that worse prognoses follow lower PaO2/FiO2 ratios, thus guiding interventions like High Frequency Oscillation Ventilation (HFOV) and Nitric Oxide therapy (Chimbira et al., 2001). The quantitative results from blood gas analysis also assist in monitoring the response to treatment, which is essential for reducing the severe mortality and morbidity of the respiratory conditions. Moreover, the integration of blood gas analysis into critical care protocols enables ongoing evaluation of treatment effectiveness and stabilization of the patient. For instance, in acutely respiratory-failing non-invasive ventilated patients, the ability to observe real-time alterations in gas exchange parameters can lead to timely adjustment of therapeutic strategies. Effective use of blood gas data informs clinicians about respiratory mechanics, including the development of mechanical ventilation or oxygen therapy modalities. In addition, interpreting acid-base balance through blood gas testing aids in controlling comorbidities that complicate respiratory conditions. Therefore, rational understanding of this tool is important in the achievement of maximum patient outcomes, especially in patients with complex pulmonary pathologies within the critical care setting (Bueno et al., 2017) (Figure 12.9).

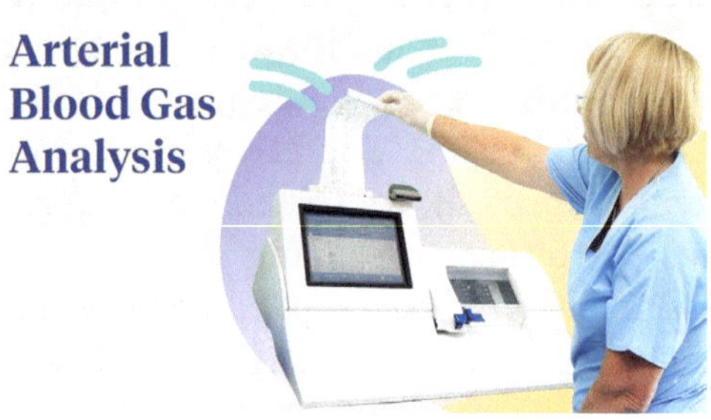

Figure 12.9. Blood gas analysis.

Source: https://external-content.duckduckgo.com/iu/?u=https%3A%2F%2Fi.ytimg.com%2Fvi%2F2wHP--s6-hA%2Fmaxresdefault.jpg&f=1&nofb=1&ipt=0ae4ed5a8a349e71d6671bebf6021a72ac8af4aa38c972c256f3efd9aefe3ac3.

Test Your Knowledge

1. What are the pulmonary function tests?
2. What is blood gas analysis?

12.3. Management Strategies for Pulmonary Patients

Learning Outcome

1. Mechanical ventilation techniques;
2. Pharmacological management;
3. Non-invasive ventilation strategies.

Effective pulmonary patient management strategies in critical care require a comprehensive approach that includes pre-operative and post-operative management. The critical period before lung transplantation is of utmost priority, as critical evaluation comes with the highest priority while checking the suitability of the patient. This evaluation typically includes a set of pulmonary function tests, sophisticated imaging, and assessment for comorbidities, all of which inform clinical decision-making. Pre-transplant therapy can substantially enhance patient outcomes by identifying possible complications and designing further therapy accordingly. Moreover, the findings also suggest that a multidisciplinary approach—which brings together professionals from various disciplines such as cardiology, respiratory therapy, and nutrition—is critical to creating a robust pre-operative strategy that caters to the physiological needs of the patient along with psychosocial elements that can affect recovery (Georgakopoulou, 2025). Once lung transplantation is done, post-operative care comes to the fore, in the sense that it plays a crucial role in preventing the complications of primary graft dysfunction and chronic lung allograft dysfunction (CLAD). Tailored immunosuppression protocols are critical in optimizing so that the risk of organ rejection is minimized while graft function is optimized. Active management through frequent follow-ups, the development of diagnostic modalities, and potential interventions like EVLP is becoming increasingly relevant. Having a dynamic and adaptive perspective for managing in the post-transplant setting allows for rapid alteration of therapeutic strategies, which directly impacts quality of life and patient survival after pulmonary disease. In the end, applying a complete framework in both the pre- and post-transplant phases can significantly increase the effectiveness of critical care interventions for patients with severe pulmonary disease (Georgakopoulou, 2025). Efficient communication is a central approach in end-of-life care for pulmonary patients in the ICU. Evidence indicates that poor communication tends to exacerbate the distress of patients and families under such circumstances. Therefore, emphasizing palliative training among Pulmonary and Critical Care Medicine (PCCM) fellowship programs is crucial to increase fellows' confidence in managing such complex conversations. There is evidence that active contributors to end-of-life care discussions—particularly those who utilize mentoring—are more self-assured about their skills. Incorporating successful communication instruction into fellowship programs ensures that future clinicians will have the ability to provide compassionate, patient-centered care. This emphasis on integral management not only improves the quality of care for patients but also reduces the emotional burden on families facing difficult treatment decisions in severe pulmonary cases (Figure 12.10).

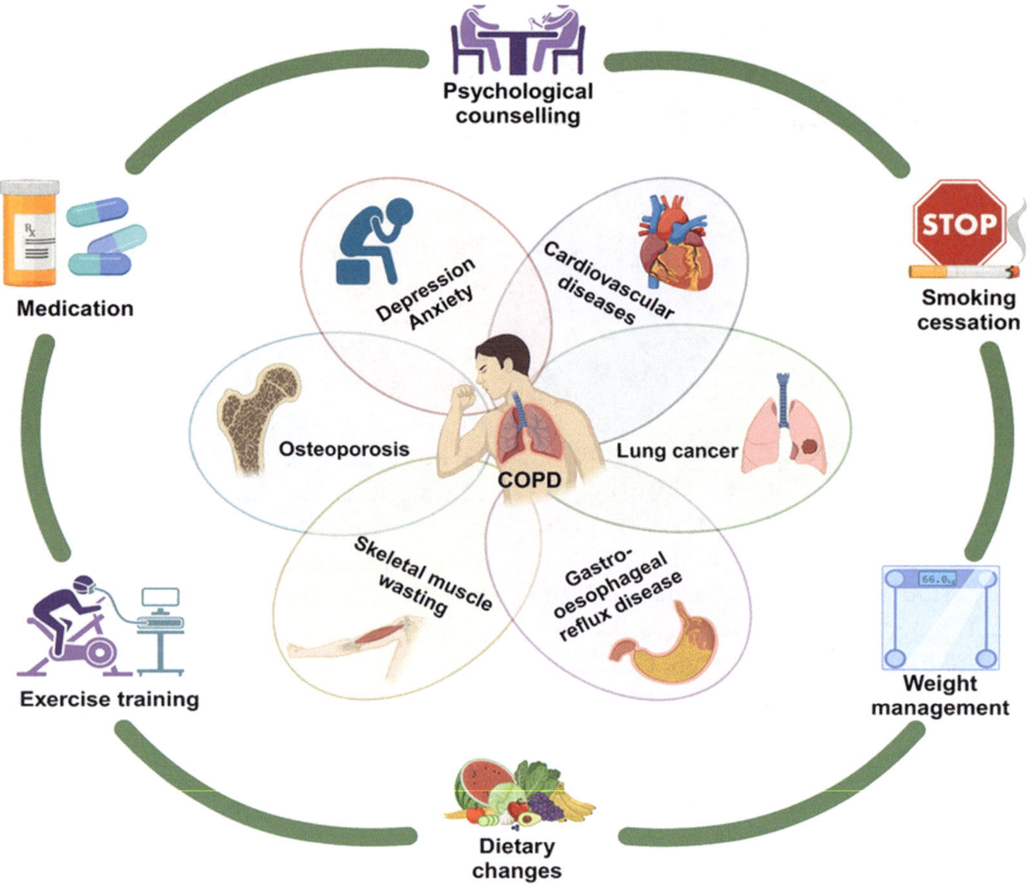

Figure 12.10. Management strategies for pulmonary patients.

Source: https://www.researchgate.net/publication/383950316/figure/fig2/AS:11431281277552128@1726107338369/Chronic-obstructive-pulmonary-disease-COPD-and-multimorbidity-and-the-management.png.

12.3.1. Mechanical Ventilation Techniques

Mechanical ventilation techniques are invaluable instruments in the management of critically ill patients, especially those suffering from respiratory failure. Among the various methods employed, CMV has been the established standard for the provision of ventilatory support. It is only now that it is increasingly recognized that there are significant benefits conferred by NPPV in certain groups, such as patients with AECOPD. Unlike CMV, which requires sedation and risks intubation-related complications, NPPV allows for less support, potentially preserving patient comfort and secretion clearance with reduced difficulty. This is particularly pertinent in those circumstances where less than optimal clearance of secretions might potentially contribute to worse outcomes, thus emphasizing the requirement for the most optimal available technique in each instance to be selected on a patient-specific basis. For patients on mechanical ventilation, bronchial hygiene therapy (BHT) is a critical component in enhancing respiratory function in the intensive care setting.

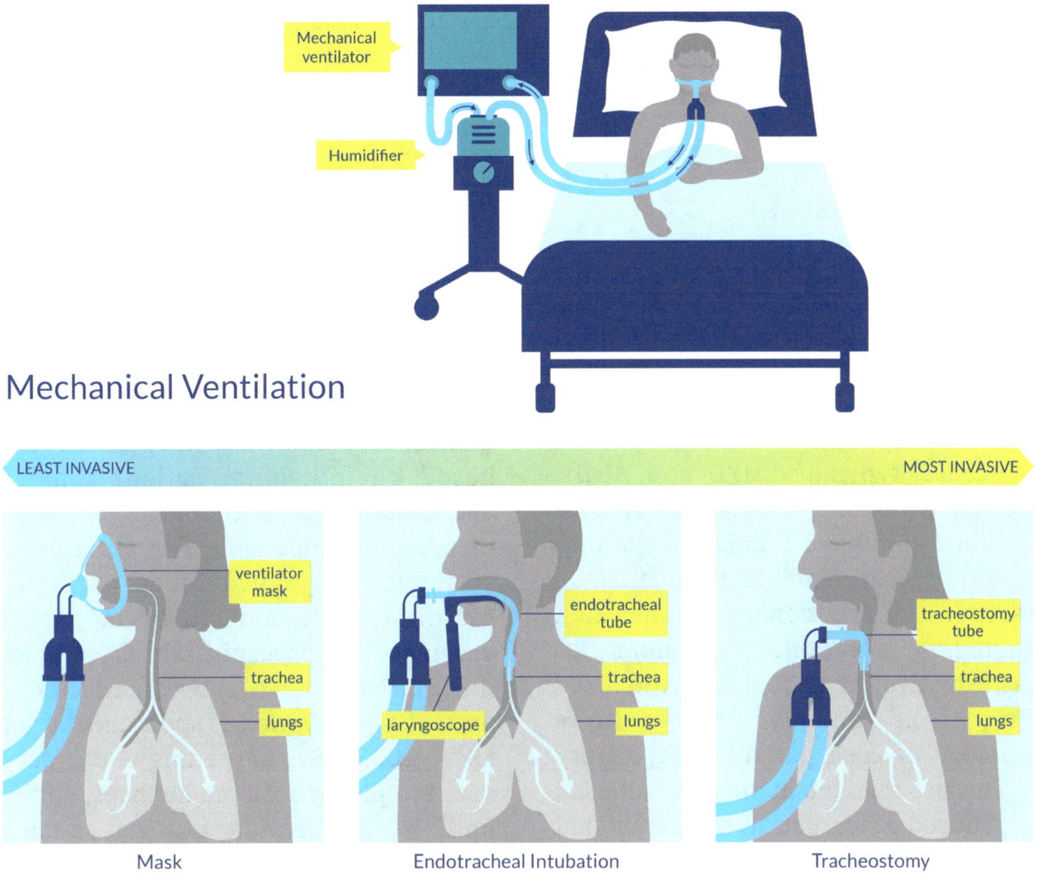

Figure 12.11. Mechanical ventilation techniques for pulmonary patients.

Source: https://scireproject.com/wp-content/uploads/2023/10/MechVent.png.

Techniques like chest physiotherapy, suction, and postural drainage try to improve secretion clearance and overall respiratory mechanics. Routine use of BHT has been shown to produce significant improvements in a variety of clinical outcomes. For example, research identified a significant increase in oxygen saturation levels after BHT interventions, as well as in the Horowitz index (PaO2/FiO2 ratio) and arterial oxygen saturation (SaO2) measures.

These increases are important because they are associated with improved pulmonary function as well as reduced ICU lengths of stay, underlining the complementary role of BHT to CMV approaches (Kushwaha et al., 2025). The second region to consider in mechanical ventilation approaches is the efficiency of NPPV combined with noninvasive assessments of the removal of respiratory secretions. Evidence indicated that this approach might be superior to CMV, particularly in hypercapnic encephalopathy and AECOPD patients. In a cohort study, evidence revealed that patients receiving NPPV evidenced better arterial blood gas adjustment, decreased complication rates, and shorter mechanical ventilation length. In addition, the reduced need for invasive equipment supports the potential of NPPV as an ideal first-line therapy in specific patient populations, thereby contributing to improved clinical outcomes. Based on these assumptions, the application of a variety of ventilation approaches that are based on patient profiles remains a cornerstone of effective critical care in pulmonary medicine (Wang et al., 2017) (Figure 12.11).

12.3.2. Pharmacological Interventions

In pulmonary critical care medicine, pharmacologic treatment is a cornerstone in the management of acute and chronic lung disease. The use of bronchodilators, corticosteroids, and antimicrobials is important in the management of such diseases, typically COPD and ARDS. Emerging evidence highlights the role of targeted therapy through combined inhalation therapy, achieving maximal bronchodilation with minimal systemic side effects. Additionally, the inclusion of new biologics in treatment regimens has been transformative, providing individualized approaches that address the unique pathophysiology of each patient's respiratory condition. This has resulted in improved clinical outcomes, reduced exacerbation frequency, and enhanced quality of life for chronic lung patients (Martins et al., 2025). The current research into pharmacologic developments underscores the dynamic character of pulmonary medicine and its applicability to critical care. Sedation and control of pain represent a significant area of pharmacologic intervention in critical care units. Invasive therapies used in critically ill patients with severe respiratory disease induce discomfort, which can lead to increased oxygen demand and stress response. Therefore, the application of analgesia and sedation protocols specifically to patients with respiratory disorders is important (N/A, 2023). The existing guidelines emphasize the evaluation and management of patient pain before the administration of continuous sedatives because this can lead to better outcomes in patients. In addition, combining pharmacological therapy with non-pharmacologic interventions such as early mobilization and rehabilitation can be beneficial in averting the undesirable effects of over-sedation. This integrative approach provides a more stable and comfortable environment for respiratory patients with critical illnesses, resulting in better patterns of recovery. The pharmacokinetic characteristics of medications used in ventilation and sedation introduce challenges when managing patients with respiratory failure, especially those undergoing extracorporeal membrane oxygenation (ECMO). Variability in drug absorption, distribution, metabolism, and excretion can significantly influence the therapeutic action and safety profile. Critical care clinicians need to titrate dosages based on individual patient considerations and disease states to adhere to the principles of precision medicine. For example, sedation strategies may need to be adjusted during recruitment maneuvers or in patients with varying levels of respiratory drive, where a fine line must be drawn between effective sedation and the preservation of spontaneous ventilation (N/A, 2023). By sharpening our understanding of these pharmacologic nuances, clinicians can optimize intervention strategies so that patients receive the optimal level of care tailored to their unique clinical environments (Figure 12.12).

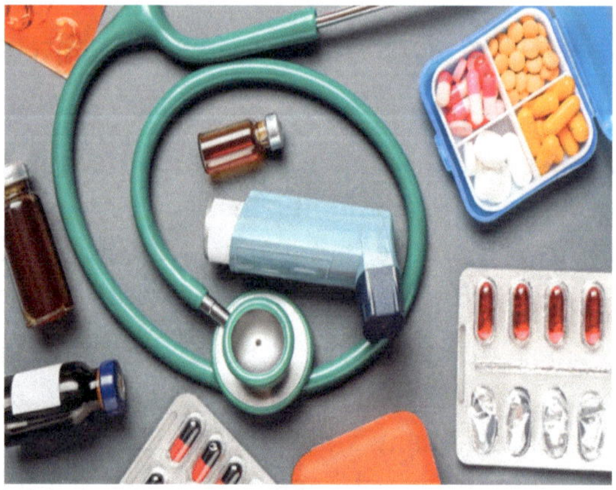

Figure 12.12. Pharmacological interventions for pulmonary patients.

Source: https://drkumo.com/wp-content/uploads/2023/01/copd-inhaler-with-medications-and-stethoscope.webp.

12.3.3. Non-invasive Ventilation (NIV) Options

NIV is now a standard part of critical care in pulmonary medicine and serves as a primary alternative to invasive mechanical ventilation. This approach utilizes several modalities, such as continuous positive airway pressure (CPAP) and bilevel positive airway pressure (BiPAP), to provide respiratory therapy without the need for intubation. These noninvasive therapies are particularly beneficial for the management of conditions such as ARDS and COPD, in which patient comfort and reduced risk of complications are paramount. The flexibility of NIV allows for tailored treatment protocols, which can significantly improve patient satisfaction and outcomes in critical care. Appropriate application of NIV not only contributes to proper oxygenation and ventilation but also decreases ICU stay duration, which proves its importance in current pulmonary therapy guidelines (Pan et al., 2023). Current clinical evidence has validated the effectiveness of NIV for high-risk patients, i.e., obese patients after extubation. Data indicate that the use of NIV with high-flow nasal oxygen significantly lowers rates of reintubation and mortality among such patients. Notably, the intermittent use of NIV during post-extubation intervals has been shown to provide the necessary respiratory support, leading to improved overall recovery trends. This is especially important in patients with extubation failure risk, who tend to be susceptible to adverse outcomes due to suboptimal respiratory management. Second, it is suggested that the use of NIV as part of a comprehensive, tailored strategy for treatment will enhance the therapeutic efficacy of treatment modalities within the intensive care setting. This form of evidence highlights the need for ongoing skills in applying these non-invasive techniques among healthcare professionals to improve patient prognosis (N/A, 2023). Similar to any therapy type, the application of non-invasive ventilation must consider patient-specific characteristics. Fatigue, compromised consciousness, or upper airway obstruction may require more tailored control of NIV. In addition, the use of sedation must be stringently managed because too much sedation can interfere with the efficacy of NIV therapy. Up-to-date evidence-based suggestions favor the optimal adjustment of NIV settings through enhanced patient assessment and dynamic monitoring, resulting in fewer complications. Application of many strategies, such as pharmacological and non-pharmacological methods, can significantly enhance comfort of patients during administration of NIV therapy. Given the heterogeneous pathophysiologic traits in severe respiratory diseases, tailoring ventilation measures to the needs of patients can mean improved clinical outcomes and a reduction of load on healthcare resources, thus underlining the pivotal role of NIV in critical care pulmonary medicine practice (Pan et al., 2023) (Figure 12.13).

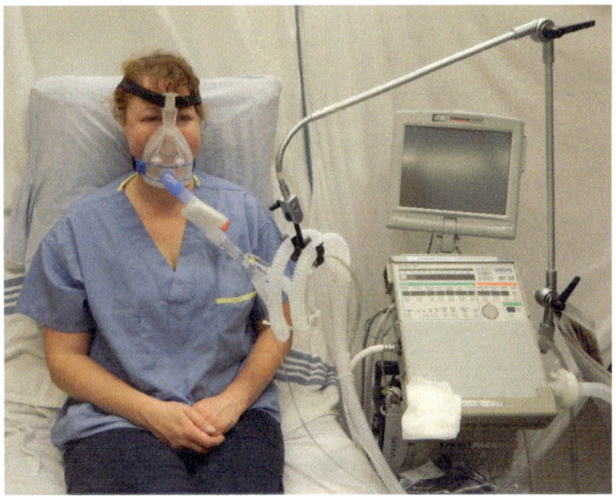

Figure 12.13. Non-invasive ventilation (NIV).

Source: https://upload.wikimedia.org/wikipedia/commons/0/04/BIPAP.JPG.

12.4. Role of Multidisciplinary Teams (MDTs)

Learning Outcome

1. Multidisciplinary collaboration between critical care and pulmonology specialists;
2. Role of nursing staff in pulmonary therapy;
3. Involvement of respiratory therapists.

The complexity of pulmonary critical care demands the involvement of MDTs to optimize patient outcomes and enhance the quality of care provision. These teams are most frequently made up of diverse healthcare professionals, such as intensivists, pulmonologists, respiratory therapists, nurses, physical therapists, and social workers, who collaborate to address the multifaceted issues presented by critically ill patients. This team of specialists allows for comprehensive patient assessments that involve medical, psychological, and rehabilitative elements. Such an additive approach is particularly urgent in ARDS and similar severe pulmonary diseases, where multimodal treatment can guide recovery pathways accordingly. Moreover, research emphasizes the role of such teams in implementing guidelines that enhance ventilation strategies for patients, thereby reducing mechanical ventilation time and enabling earlier weaning, ultimately resulting in an improved quality of life for survivors with severe respiratory disease (Yu et al., 2020).

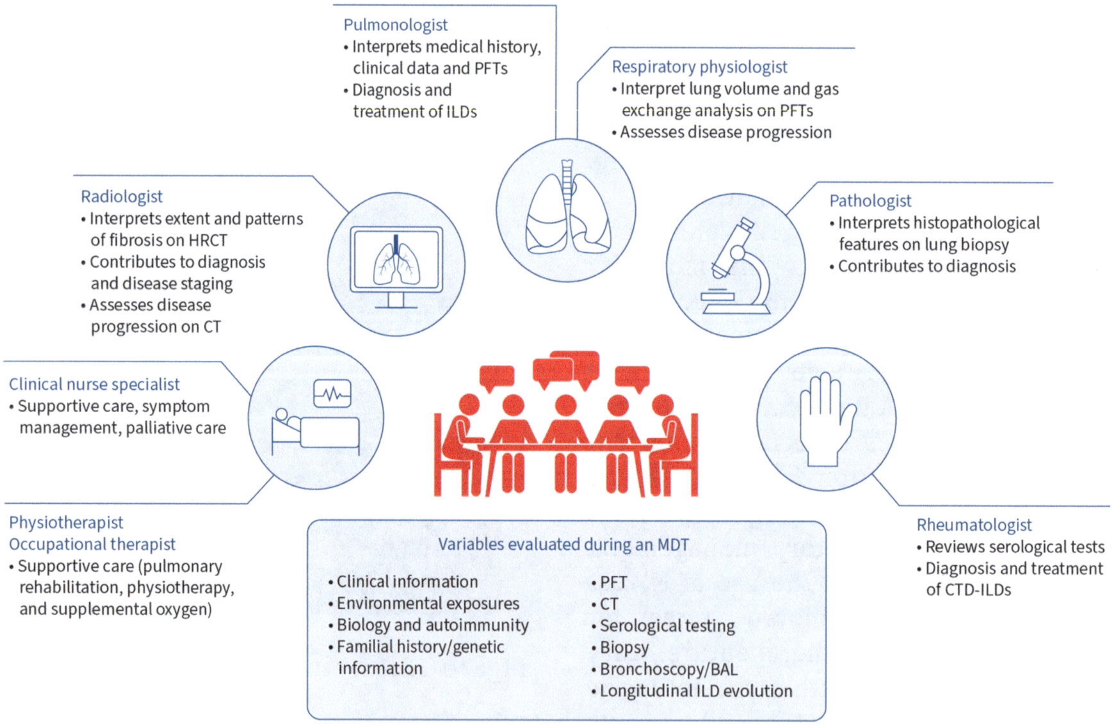

Figure 12.14. Role of multidisciplinary teams (MDTs).

Source: https://www.researchgate.net/publication/363379453/figure/fig1/AS:11431281083583290@1662661500426/Example-of-roles-in-an-multidisciplinary-team-MDT-for-diagnosis-and-management-BAL.png.

The role of the MDTs appears particularly pertinent about emerging health concerns, such as COVID-19, which has stretched healthcare systems globally. With hospitals filled with a growing number of critically ill patients, there is a necessity for effective coordination of multiple specialties to manage resources and deliver timely intervention. For instance, integration of professional competency among infectious disease specialists and respiratory therapists has a significant role to play in the creation of treatment guidelines for patients presenting with complex presentations of the virus. The COVID-19 pandemic witnessed hospital responses supported by geographic cohorting of patients and interprofessional collaboration, which enabled the management of the unique challenges of this epidemic, aimed at reducing infection levels and optimizing patient outcomes (Chopra et al., 2020). Consequently, the flexibility and comprehensive nature of MDTs are essential to enhancing healthcare delivery in times of crisis.

Furthermore, multidisciplinary team-led early rehabilitation intervention has emerged as a critical component in the management of pulmonary patients under intensive care. Early intervention is signaled to mitigate the adverse impacts commonly associated with prolonged mechanical ventilation and bed rest. MDTs supplement the rehabilitation process by ensuring that respiratory, physical, and psychological requirements are addressed holistically. Interventions such as positioning management, mobilization, and respiratory therapies have been observed to promote functional outcomes and shorten hospital stays for critically ill patients. These initiatives further attest to the necessity of interaction among various healthcare providers to create and implement personalized rehabilitation programs that facilitate recovery and overall patient prognosis in pulmonary medicine (Yu et al., 2020). Moving forward in this field, the necessity of multidisciplinary collaboration remains a fundamental pillar in best-practice critical care interventions and patient-focused care approaches (Figure 12.14).

12.4.1. Collaboration Between Pulmonologists and Critical Care Specialists

Interaction between critical care specialists and pulmonologists is critical in the treatment of serious pulmonary disorders that require intense medical intervention. Pulmonologists with their in-depth understanding of respiratory ailments often get to work with patients who have CRD that are likely to trigger critical health crises. As stated in existing literature, the optimal approach in such a case involves teleconsultation, which bridges the gap in access to medical services and allows timely intervention by critical care specialists. The collaboration, besides enhancing the quality of care, alleviates the CRD burden, particularly in the periphery where specialized units may be scarce (Fairhurst et al., 2021). Through cooperation, both specialties can devise more comprehensive treatment plans that address both the pulmonary and systemic effects of such illnesses. Ultimately, the merger is advantageous to patient care. Successful cooperation among pulmonologists and critical care physicians hinges on mutual communication and shared goal. Such nuances in patient management from each specialty must lead to improved diagnostic and therapeutic maneuvers. For instance, in pulmonary arterial hypertension, differing views from rheumatologists, pulmonologists, and cardiologists can inform therapy to address the complexity of the condition specifically. Use of a Delphi process has indicated that interprofessional collaboration yields consensus of significant endpoints for critical care, facilitating streamlined patient management (Avouac et al., 2010). This synchronization not only guarantees treatment effectiveness but also enhances the total patient satisfaction, as specialists harmonize their actions towards achieving the best care pathways. Moreover, clinical practice harmonization among critical care specialists and pulmonologists offers solidarity in treatment approaches. Mutual coordination spurs the development of best practices and evidence-based guidelines that enhance the quality of patient care. For example, the selection of successful outcomes related to management of CRD can be significantly improved by cross-fertilization of expertise from the two specialties. Periodic interdisciplinary meetings can serve as mechanisms for sharing case reports, treatment guidelines, and information regarding novel treatments. Lastly, an atmosphere of teamwork fosters professional relationships that can assist in encouraging innovation in treatment strategies, resulting in groundbreaking improvements in critical care and pulmonary medicine. Such cooperation is an essential step toward integrated patient care so that every aspect of respiratory well-being is brought into focus holistically.

12.4.2. Importance of Nursing Staff in Pulmonary Care

Nurses have an important role in pulmonary care, particularly intensive and critical care departments, where life-threatening respiratory disorders need enhanced vigilance and skills in their treatment. Nurses are typically the first medical professionals to assess and monitor patients' respiratory status, implementing measures that can prevent complications like atelectasis or pneumonia from happening. Their ability to promptly comprehend clinical data, coordinate initial intervention, and collaborate with multidisciplinary teams all have direct effects on patient outcomes. This central aspect of nursing practice not only enhances the quality of care but also emotionally consoles patients and families, thereby building a healing-conducive environment. Consequently, the intrinsic worth of nursing teams reinforces the necessity of their existence in pulmonary medicine within critical care scenarios, emphasizing their indispensable role in maintaining patient safety and well-being. In addition to direct clinical responsibilities, nurses in pulmonary care have a crucial role in establishing healthy communication patterns in the interprofessional care team. Their observations and direct experience equip them to represent patients, so that their treatment-related concerns are conveyed effectively to physicians and other specialists. This crucial role in communication is the counterpart to the overall effectiveness of the IPC process. Evidence proves that enhancing IPC in critical care environments leads to improved patient safety and satisfaction, as demonstrated by better management of complex cases that often require intricate interventions (Ghattas et al., 2025).

In this manner, the work of the nursing team transcends clinical practice; they also help shape the team model needed to deliver outstanding pulmonary care in critical care. In addition, ongoing education and in-service education of the nursing staff are key to responding to evolving pulmonary medicine challenges. Refresher information keeps nurses abreast of advances in respiratory therapy, technology, and best evidence-based practice. Nursing Education Reading List. The level of sophistication in caring for patients with respiratory distress syndromes, COPD, and other pulmonary conditions necessitates that nurses possess a profound grasp of theoretical foundations and technical skills. Such a competence is necessary in terms of using interventions that ensure not only patient recovery but end-of-life care as well, something critical in critical care settings (Joyce et al., 2025). The continuous development of nursing education and practice not only enhances the nursing staff but also sees to it that patients receive the quality care possible, emphasizing the need to invest in nursing staff in the field of pulmonary medicine (Figure 12.15).

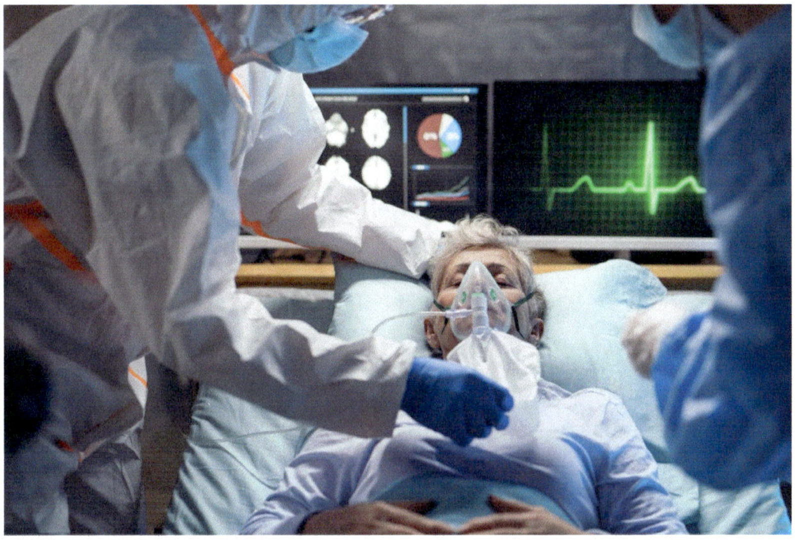

Figure 12.15. Nursing staff in pulmonary care.

Source: https://www.news-medical.net/images/Article_Images/ImageForArticle_10801_16623492556818693.jpg.

12.4.3. Involvement of Respiratory Therapists (RTs)

The role of RTs is a vital component of the multidisciplinary team working with patients in critical care, particularly in pulmonary medicine. Through their professional expertise, they can assess, diagnose, and facilitate interventions in patients with pulmonary disease and complications. RTs play an essential role in intubation procedures, especially in emergencies where immediate action is required to secure the airway of patients with cardiac or respiratory arrest. They utilize their high-level skills to verify correct endotracheal tube placement with the fewest possible complications, such as esophageal intubation, which occurs in approximately 3-17% of emergent cases (Elbaih et al., 2020). This high-level interaction emphasizes the role of respiratory therapists in effectively managing acute respiratory diseases and reinforces their value in producing positive patient outcomes. Additionally, integration of respiratory therapists within critical care teams enhances evidence-based guidelines and therapy application, particularly pulmonary rehabilitation. Research indicates that significant barriers such as poor interdisciplinary communication and low levels of awareness of RT roles can hinder adherence to these guidelines (Jia et al., 2025). Through active involvement in patient evaluation and educating patients and other health workers, RTs facilitate closure of such gaps. Their ability to conduct thorough assessments and deliver tailored treatment interventions provokes adherence to best practices, making them central advocates for respiratory well-being in the critical care setting. Perhaps most importantly, by doing away with these challenges, respiratory therapists make treatment not just compliant with available protocols, but also enhance the overall quality of offered healthcare services. In addition to their role in care and rehabilitation, respiratory therapists also play a central role in informing patients and families about respiratory ailments and management interventions. This is an important function in long-term care and prevention, which are critical in pulmonary medicine. RTs assist patients in understanding how vital medication, breathing technique, and lifestyle modification are in keeping chronic pulmonary disease under control. Apart from this, they provide continuity between acute and home care, where ongoing management and supervision are critical. In this sense, the respiratory therapist's role transcends direct clinical care to encompass ongoing support and advice, to equip patients and caregivers with the necessary tools to manage their respiratory condition effectively and independently in the long term (Figure 12.16).

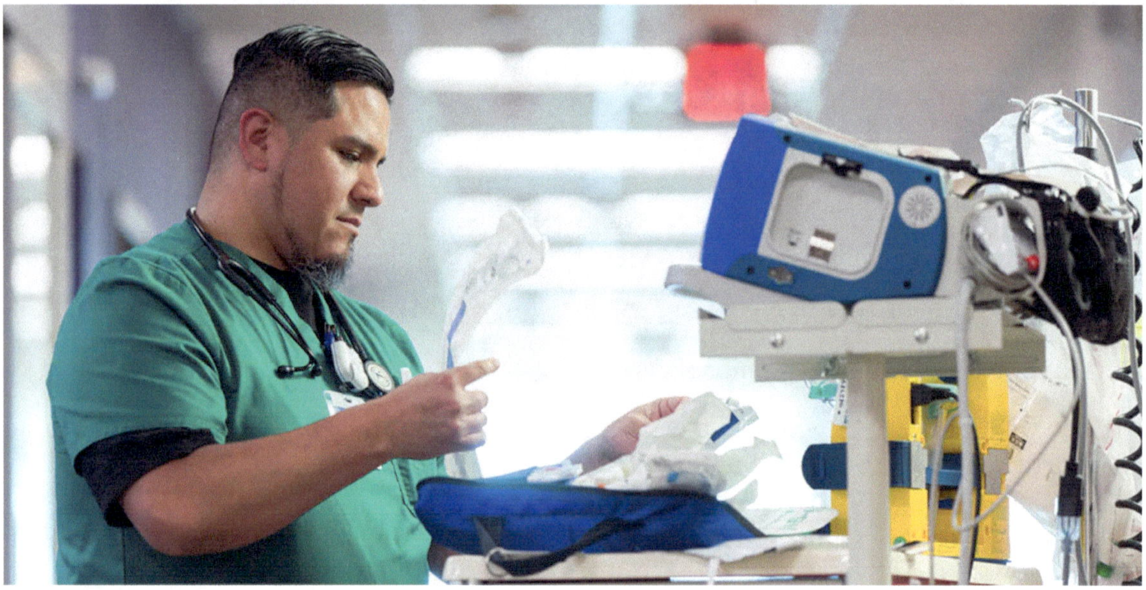

Figure 12.16. Respiratory therapist (RT).

Source: https://college.mayo.edu/media/mccms/content-assets/academics/explore-health-care-careers/mccms-respiratory-therapist-1024x512-WF2522104_0049.jpg.

Test Your Knowledge

1. Discourse the collaboration between pulmonologists and critical care physicians.
2. Role of nursing staff in pulmonary therapy?

12.5. Ethical Considerations in Pulmonary Critical Care

Learning Outcome

1. End-of-life decision-making;
2. Patient autonomy and informed consent;
3. Allocation of resources in critical care.

Ethical considerations in pulmonary critical care are of prime concern, particularly regarding patient autonomy and informed consent. ICUs challenge the independence of decisions made by patients due to their condition. As such, in such circumstances, healthcare providers must draw a tough line ethically so that patient rights remain protected. The informed consent process becomes even more crucial in scenarios such as lung transplantation, where risks, benefits, and potential outcomes must be weighed and disclosed freely with patients. This ethical duty extends to examining situations where patients might not have decisional capacity, and surrogate decision-makers are tasked with expressing the patients' wishes and values to ensure ethical integrity in treatment choices (Rodemund et al., 2023). Ultimately, a commitment to respecting patient autonomy in critical care settings not only facilitates ethical practice but also enhances the therapeutic relationship between providers and patients. Other than patient autonomy, confidentiality and data protection emerge as central ethical issues in pulmonary critical care. Given the sensitive nature of health information, especially in the presence of critical illness and potential transplantation, protecting patient data is critical. With the increased use of electronic health records and data sharing, healthcare professionals are confronted with challenges introduced by regulatory actions such as the GDPR. For instance, while databases like SICdb and AmsterdamUMCdb try to deidentify patients' data to comply with the law, the risk of reidentification persists (Rodemund et al., 2023). This requires a robust data handling practice that guarantees that ethical standards are upheld while maximizing the scientific value of disseminated data. Ethical stewardship in this area reiterates the highest importance of maintaining the trust of patients, as they must have confidence that their personal data is treated with the highest level of care and confidentiality. Finally, the ethical challenges of resource distribution and health inequities in pulmonary critical care cannot be overstated. Since healthcare networks strive to optimize results under the circumstances of limited resources available, the distribution of essential interventions of care can be contentious. Ethical models would anticipate that decisions regarding resource allocation be informed by equity and justice principles, ensuring all patients receive a fair opportunity at treatment, regardless of socio-economic status or demographic category. In lung transplant, for example, recipients may have complex eligibility criteria that may unwittingly discriminate against specific groups (Alrashdaa et al., 2023). Thus, policymakers and health administration leaders should continually reflect ethically and engage in dialogue with their communities, so that institutional practices promote fairness. Addressing ethical challenges to resource allocation could, at the same time, improve patient outcomes and increase trust in public action on health.

12.5.1. End-of-Life Decision-Making

In critical care, particularly pulmonary medicine, end-of-life decision-making is a complex and nuanced process at the heart of patient management. It is a period where the medical reality for the patient is generally balanced with their values and treatment choices. Health care workers must cope with various ethical concerns in respecting patients' autonomy, which tends to be complex in patients who are unable to express their will due to severe illness or mental disability. Added to these are the systemic determinants like healthcare policy and institutional procedure that do not necessarily facilitate withholding of life-sustaining treatment, for example, as reported in the case of Japan, where legal provisions guiding such decisions are unclear and do not facilitate universal acceptance of advanced care planning (Okada et al., 2021). These necessitate a collaborative approach by healthcare teams, patients, and families to offer respectful decisions that align with the patient-specific context. The work of skilled medical practitioners is most crucial in facilitating end-of-life discussions. Professional guidance from specialists, such as those practiced in critical care medicine, provides essential insight when deciding between aggressive continuing treatments and palliative options. Dr. Hassan Khouli, who has extensive experience dealing with patients who have complex critical diseases, identifies the necessity for training in collaborative communication and shared decision-making in such cases (Khouli et al., 2020). His experience highlights that the building of a foundation of trust and empathy is elemental to the discussion. Clinical practitioners with a thorough knowledge of medical, ethical, and emotional information can better support patients and families through the difficult process of end-of-life decisions, ensuring that the care received aligns with patients' values and preferred quality of life. Furthermore, the significance of advance care planning (ACP) for enhancing end-of-life decision-making is better understood. ACP allows patients to express their preferences for care and treatment before a crisis event, which can potentially take the burden off family members and healthcare providers during a crisis. ACCP models have evolved, reflecting changes in society and patient populations. The revised Japanese Society for Dialysis Therapy guidelines, for instance, recognize the importance of flexible decision-making and respect for patient autonomy, even in non-terminal illnesses (Okada et al., 2021). Through the incorporation of patient preference into care pathways, clinicians can engage in a participatory decision process that not only honors the patient's wishes but also optimizes overall quality of care and ultimately leads to more ethical and compassionate health care practice within critical care settings (Figure 12.17).

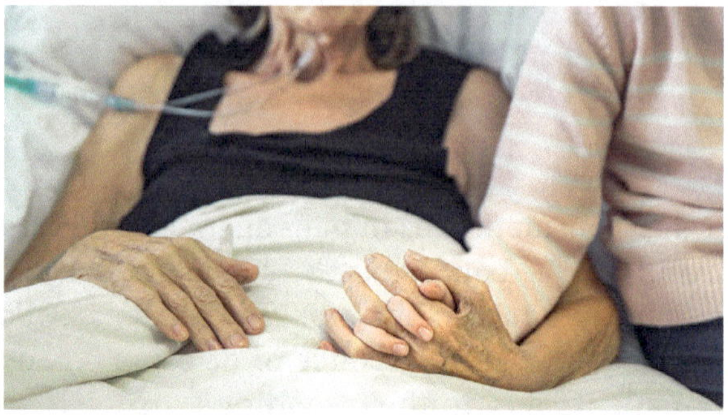

Figure 12.17. End-of-life decision-making.

Source: https://wp.technologyreview.com/wp-content/uploads/2024/08/GettyImages-1352063892.jpg.

12.5.2. Patient Autonomy and Informed Consent

In pulmonary medicine, patient autonomy and informed consent are pillars of ethics that guide practice. As patients are presented with make-or-break decisions regarding their care, particularly in the high-risk unit of intensive care, respect for an informed choice is paramount. Obtaining patients' comprehension of diagnosis, treatment options, and outcome is essential to establishing a climate of trust and respect. As doctors navigate through the complexities of severe pulmonary diseases, they must maintain open communication in order for patients to voice their wishes and fears. This form of communication not only upholds the value of autonomy but also promotes adherence to treatment guidelines, particularly crucial in intensive care where choices have long-term implications for the patient's well-being. Informed consent entails more than a signature on paper; it involves a comprehensive educational process about the benefits, risks, and possible alternatives to interventions that are recommended. Within the rubric of pulmonary medicine, where interventions may range from invasive therapy to complex pharmacologic regimens, patients must be fully informed about their choices. Discussing treatment options with patients can result in significant improvement in comprehension and satisfaction with care.

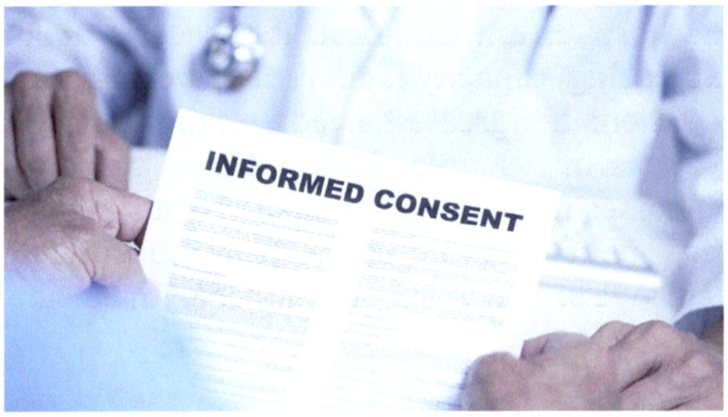

Figure 12.18. Patient autonomy and informed consent.

Source: https://www.aamc.org/sites/default/files/styles/scale_and_crop_1200_x_666/public/d/1/9-informed_consent_redboxxmain.jpg__992x558_q85_crop_subsampling-2_upscale.jpg?itok=GkA4exRo.

Moreover, a sensitivity to patients' diverse backgrounds and health literacy levels is key to this teaching process. Tailoring the presentation of information to the special needs of individuals can create a more inclusive method of consent, rather than risking the exclusion of the vulnerable. This ethical necessity eventually corresponds with one of its ends, that of facilitating value and preference-guided decision-making by patients. The combination of informed consent and patient autonomy in pulmonary critical care has difficulties. Conflicts can occur when clinicians' recommendations conflict with patients' desires and result in ethical problems for health professionals. The time pressure in critical care situations also reduces the time available for lengthy discourses on consent, risking ethical accountability. Acknowledging these challenges is necessary to improve the practice norms of pulmonary medicine. Educational courses that teach communication skills and ethical decision-making can equip clinicians to manage challenging consent cases effectively. Furthermore, organizational policies that encourage patients' participation in important decisions can develop a culture of respect for patient autonomy, ultimately translating into better patient outcomes and satisfaction in intensive care settings (Figure 12.18).

12.5.3. Resource Allocation in Critical Care

Resource distribution in critical care, especially in pulmonary medicine, is a significant concern due to the growing demand for healthcare delivery. As there is a rising burden of pulmonary diseases, including COPD and pneumonia, there is a demand for hospital facilities to ensure that the resources, such as ventilators, ICU beds, and well-qualified personnel, are distributed judiciously. Existing allocation methods have frequently left disparities, mostly between urban and rural health facilities. The unequal distribution of healthcare services has the possibility of bringing more morbidity and mortality to the vulnerable groups. Eliminating these disparities requires a thorough analysis of resource strengths, patient populations, and prevalence rates of diseases. By using systematic, data-driven processes, healthcare organizations can improve their capacity to divide limited resources efficiently and effectively, ultimately delivering better care to patients with life-threatening pulmonary diseases. A targeted strategy of resource allocation includes the rigorous analysis of spatial allocation within healthcare systems. Geographic information systems (GIS) techniques have been valuable tools for analyzing the provision of primary health care facilities, particularly in rural settings where health officers and institutions are minimal. Plotting the spatial distribution of general health resources like doctors, nurses, and beds provides policymakers with an idea of service deficits, as analyzed in Karur District by Umasankar et al. (2024). The application of spatial analysis not only identifies existing inequalities but also enables strategic planning of healthcare interventions to ensure that essential resources are directed to where they are most needed. Through targeted distribution, healthcare systems can maximize interventions aimed at managing pulmonary diseases and, consequently, overall patient care across different settings. Moreover, the deployment of personalized medicine in critical care requires an enhanced method of resource management, particularly in developing nations. The constraint of limited financial resources requires that healthcare professionals manage the allocation of resources effectively without sacrificing the quality of care for patients. The recent research highlights the importance of utilizing simulation-based models to estimate the allocation of beds in hospitals, aiming to identify inefficiencies and bottlenecks within the system (Kamal et al., 2024). By using predictive patient pathways and waiting time analysis, the hospital can make sensible choices about increasing capacity and redistributing staff to where the greatest need is. Such strategic reforms in resources lead not only to better outcomes for patients but also to a sustainable care model capable of meeting the growing demands of critical care in pulmonary medicine.

Test Your Knowledge

1. What is end-of-life decision-making?
2. What is patient autonomy?

12.6. Advances in Pulmonary Medicine

Learning Outcome

1. Innovations in therapeutic modalities;
2. Lung protective research;
3. Future directions of pulmonary critical care.

The foundation for pulmonary medicine has evolved at a dizzying speed, particularly with advances in metabolomics—a field of science concerned with the study of small molecule metabolites in biological systems. This frontier technique has penetrated the biochemical pathways of pulmonary disease, offering pulmonary medicine a whole new paradigm of understanding critical illnesses such as ARDS. Using advanced analytical methods, scientists can observe and quantify metabolic changes that correlate with disease states. The contribution of metabolomics goes beyond biomarker identification; they can provide enhancements to personalized medicine strategies in pulmonology. As outlined in recent reports, these advances aim to ultimately improve patient outcomes through tailor-made therapeutic strategies that correct specific metabolic derangements, thereby treating the causative factors of pulmonary dysfunction rather than merely managing symptoms (Simperson et al., 2024). Artificial intelligence (AI) has also hastened advances in pulmonary medicine by means of revolutionizing the manipulation of complex imaging data. Most notably in the diagnosis of pulmonary edema among ARDS patients, AI-driven automated lung segmentation enhances diagnostic accuracy and efficiency. In the past, techniques like single-indicator transpulmonary thermodilution (TPTD) have been essential in measuring extravascular lung water, but AI allows real-time assessment of chest CT scans. These developments have significantly reduced the time and skill required to achieve accurate assessments, enabling clinicians to make quicker, more informed decisions regarding patient care. While initial comparisons between TPTD and automatic segmentation reveal promising correlations, researchers note that additional validation is necessary to enhance accuracy in clinical use (Conrad et al., 2024).

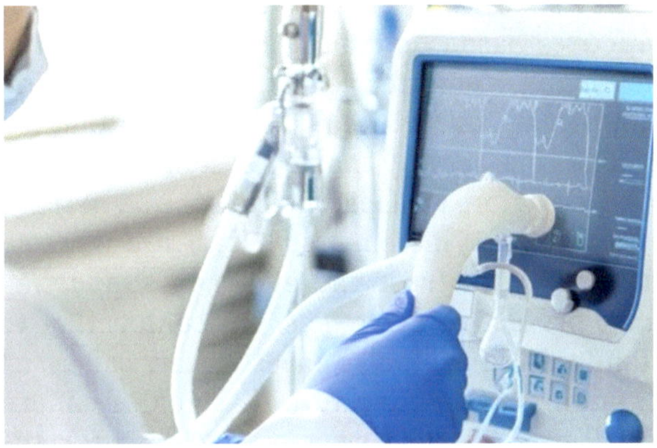

Figure 12.19. Advances in pulmonary medicine.

Source: https://drsomasaikiran.whitecoats.com/wp-content/uploads/sites/123/2025/03/Advanced-Pulmonary-Function-Testing-11.webp.

Furthermore, the therapeutic potential of progress in pulmonary medicine extends to the therapeutic domain, as new treatments and drugs continue to emerge. Targeted treatments and biologics have revolutionized treatment for CRD, such as asthma and COPD. Such medications, which typically work by modulating targeted pathways or molecules implicated in disease processes, are a divergence from mainstream broad-spectrum pharmacotherapies to more subtle interventions which consider the specificity of individual patient profiles. This is fueled by ongoing research activity working to deconstruct the intricacies of disease mechanisms and, hence, provide the platform for drug breakthroughs. The continuous quest for therapeutic solutions reflects both the intricate nature of lung diseases and the promising potential of personalized medicine, which optimizes hope for improved quality of life for patients with such disabling conditions (Simpson et al., 2024) (Figure 12.19).

12.6.1. Innovations in Treatment Modalities

In recent years, advancements in treatment strategies have revolutionized the approach to critical care in pulmonary medicine, particularly for longstanding diseases such as pulmonary arterial hypertension (PAH). Advances in telehealth services have gained strong momentum, allowing clinicians to observe patients' conditions remotely and make timely interventions. With the COVID-19 pandemic came the demand for minimizing physical contact, and it pushed the implementation of multiple telehealth modalities, which are being explored as viable options for patient assessment and treatment today. The continuous monitoring with telehealth facilitates better titration of therapy, and stronger validation is needed to ascertain that such developments are able to match traditional care standards in identifying minute changes in patients' status. As the technology continues to grow, it has the potential to propel patient activation and enhance compliance with the treatment regimen, ultimately leading to improved patient outcomes in patients with pulmonary disease in critical care (Milks et al., 2020). Furthermore, biometric and accelerometric devices have been identified as innovative technologies to treat pulmonary diseases. These technologies enable health care providers to quantify physical activity levels and monitor vital signs, illuminating patterns that may herald disease progression or decompensation. As an illustration, studies have shown that wearable devices can monitor parameters such as heart rate and oxygen saturation, providing valuable information about the patient's status between appointments. Ongoing monitoring of this nature is particularly crucial in PAH patients, whose condition can rapidly worsen without obvious symptoms. These technologies are being integrated into treatment modalities to allow practitioners to modulate care methods based on real-time information, perhaps decreasing the need for emergency interventions and allowing proactive management of chronic pulmonary disease (Davies et al., 2018). Furthermore, future treatment modalities are being designed through the development of telemonitoring and personalized medicine. The incorporation of machine learning programs can also potentially enhance decision-making by predicting outcomes from full patient details, including demographics, history, and presenting biometric values. This predictive capacity could potentially be harnessed to improve risk stratification aids so that treatment plans may be closer to each patient's individual needs. Future research will undoubtedly evaluate the role of remote health technologies in conjunction with existing modalities of treatment. As a result, the continuous progress of treatment methodologies in pulmonary medicine points toward the need for ongoing research and development, aimed at significantly improving patient quality of life as well as overall outcome in critical care (Milks et al., 2020).

12.6.2. Research on Lung Protective Strategies

In critical care, the significance of lung protective strategies has become a top agenda in pulmonary medicine. These strategies have been specifically designed to minimize ventilator-induced lung injury (VILI) in ARDS and other lung diseases. It has been found that employing lower tidal volumes during mechanical ventilation greatly reduces mortality in ARDS patients. The rationale behind this is the avoidance of alveolar over-distension and barotrauma. In addition, proper application of positive end-expiratory pressure (PEEP) will improve oxygenation and recruit atelectatic lung units. Such practice development reflects an in-depth understanding of the pathophysiological mechanisms involved, with an emphasis on the need for individualized ventilation strategies that provide protection for the lung without compromising patient safety. Critical evaluation of clinical guidelines for lung protective strategies is at the core of improving patient outcomes. Much effort has been put into synthesizing evidence through systematic reviews so that clinicians can apply best practices based on robust data. The Preferred Reporting Items for Systematic reviews and Meta-Analyses (PRISMA) statement plays a crucial role here by making systematic review reporting more transparent and consistent (Page et al., 2021). This ensures healthcare workers that they can trust the evidence supporting lung protective strategies. By conforming to standardized protocols, investigators can assist in adding to the literature that guides clinical application of such strategies. Thereafter, the integration of evidence-based recommendations into practice serves to clarify respiratory care for critically ill patients further. The COVID-19 pandemic has placed greater emphasis on lung protective interventions within the critical care setting, most importantly in patients requiring intensive care in the ICU. Research work has quickly advanced to manage the difficulties of Severe Acute Respiratory Syndrome Coronavirus 2 (SARS-CoV-2), and accordingly, specific guidelines have been formed for critically ill patients. The Surviving Sepsis Campaign COVID-19 panel of international experts has created a set of strong and weak recommendations on ventilatory support and lung protective strategies (Alhazzani et al.,

2020). These recommendations emphasize the need for personalized treatment in COVID-19-related hypoxemia and respiratory failure management. By critical review of new evidence and application of evidence-based practices, health practitioners are able to optimize treatment strategies in the context of challenges presented by this new disease and its impact on lung function in critically ill patients (Figure 12.20).

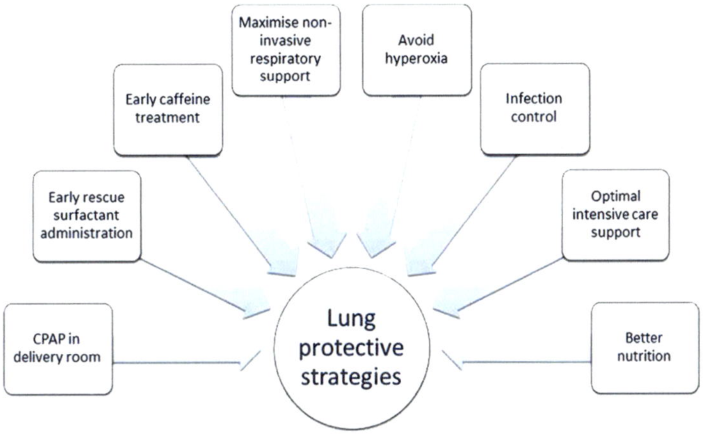

Figure 12.20. Lung protective strategies.

Source: https://www.researchgate.net/profile/Esra-Oezer-2/publication/338919991/figure/fig1/AS:853025941909507@1580388641497/Lung-protective-strategies-in-newborn-infants-with-respiratory-distress-syndrome.png.

12.6.3. Future Directions in Pulmonary Critical Care

With advancements in pulmonary critical care medicine, remarkable technological improvements in the shape of AI and machine learning are poised to play a key role in enhancing patient management. In a recent study, machine learning algorithms, namely those analyzing data from enormous databases like MIMIC-III, have been found to yield valuable insights into COPD severity classification. Using significant ICU parameters, like vital signs and blood gas data, such models are demonstrated to possess extremely high levels of accuracy. Such systems have the potential to enable clinicians to take quicker and more knowledgeable treatment protocol decisions, particularly in the acute setting. Future work should focus on validating such machine learning systems in large patient populations to determine their effectiveness and replicability, thereby demonstrating their value as highly useful decision-making tools in pulmonary medicine. Another area of immense potential in pulmonary critical care is the rapidly emerging field of metabolomics. As a branch of study focused on the global spectrum of metabolites in biological samples, it holds significant importance for promoting an understanding of pulmonary pathophysiology. Metabolomic investigations enable clinicians to identify certain biomarkers associated with various respiratory disorders, and in so doing, they can facilitate earlier diagnosis and personalized therapeutic strategy. For instance, through metabolomic analysis, researchers have started to characterize the metabolic changes associated with conditions like asthma and ARDS. As technology progresses over time, the integration of metabolomics in clinical applications can help individualize medicine, creating a more dynamic and responsive system of patient management in pulmonary critical care. Future directions will certainly require multidisciplinary collaborations to synthesize findings and bridge them to successful clinical applications. Lastly, developing an increased embedding of telemedicine in pulmonary critical care is an imperative direction for future development. Considering the recurring threat of respiratory diseases, with recent accelerated growth in telehealth use driven by world health emergencies, it is now more critical than ever to comprehend how virtual care can be used successfully to maximize patient outcomes. Telemedicine has the potential to allow for real-time monitoring of patients, timely interventions, and successful follow-up, especially in chronic disease management, such as in COPD. Moreover, as healthcare systems are more likely to adopt digital technologies, remote patient education, medication compliance support, and virtual consultation have the potential for much greater growth. Lastly, the successful application of telemedicine solutions in pulmonary critical care will depend on rigorous testing of their effectiveness and user acceptability to ensure they meet the complex needs of patients with respiratory diseases across various clinical settings.

Test Your Knowledge

1. What are the innovations in treatment modalities?
2. What is there to know about lung protective strategies?

Summary

The zenith of innovations in pulmonary critical care highlights the immediate need to overhaul the support mechanisms in healthcare systems. As per studies, burnout rates among healthcare professionals practicing in pulmonary, critical care, and sleep medicine are alarmingly high, with nearly 45% of clinicians expressing high levels of stress and exhaustion (Pamidi et al., 2025). This burnout not only endangers the well-being of healthcare workers but also harms the delivery of care to patients facing emergent scenarios. Organizations must embed interventions that foster a positive working environment, improve recovery, and address the roots of burnout. Precautionary strategies, as supported by clinicians, must place emphasis on the creation of an all-encompassing strategy that includes adequate rest and psychological safety among employees. Therefore, focusing on mental health in the organizational environment is crucial for enhancing both provider resilience and patient outcomes. The role of effective end-of-life care communication in the intensive care setting also cannot be overstated. The dynamics underlying critical illness necessitate empathetic and effective communication among healthcare clinicians, patients, and families. Results indicate that a considerable proportion of pulmonary and critical care fellows feel not confident enough to initiate end-of-life discussions, which is alarming given the emotional and ethical contexts (Yuan et al., 2025). The inadequacy of palliative care training in fellowship programs must be addressed as an urgent priority to support the competence and confidence of fellowship graduates. The combination of mentoring with workloads has been encouraging in solidifying fellows' ability to conduct these sensitive conversations. Complementing training in end-of-life communication offers two advantages: boosting provider confidence and ultimately improving the quality of care provided to patients and families at pivotal times. Lastly, resolution of the related problems of clinician burnout and effective end-of-life care communication is vital to the future of pulmonary medicine. By focusing on the emotional well-being of clinicians and on communication skill development, health centers can significantly improve the work climate for clinicians while increasing the level of patient care. Efforts to instill an effective work climate, implement robust mentorship initiatives, and provide high-quality training in palliative care should lead reform efforts. Ultimately, a balanced approach that considers both practitioner well-being and quality patient interaction will yield a more stable and more effective practice of pulmonary critical care. The achievement of these objectives can potentially benefit not only the health of providers but also more humane and effective care for patients who face dire health issues.

In pulmonary medicine, critical care treatments are an integral part of the successful management of severe respiratory diseases. One of the significant intervention methods that were discussed is the use of thoracic point-of-care ultrasound (T-POCUS). This minimally invasive medical imaging modality provides real-time lung visualization. T-POCUS allows for the identification of many pulmonary pathologies like pneumothorax, pleural effusion, pneumonia, and atelectasis, among others. Its ease and portability enable instant evaluation during emergencies, allowing medical professionals to make quick decisions. The importance of correct interpretation becomes evident when factors like scanning protocols and probe selection significantly influence diagnostic findings. However, additional studies would be required to establish standardized protocols and terminologies, as perceived within the ongoing controversies surrounding T-POCUSs application in veterinary medicine and human medicine too (Armenise, 2025). Secondly, the integration of Traditional Chinese Medicine

(TCM) therapies into the management of COPD has emerged as an intriguing part of the critical care debate. One bibliometric study revealed an increased number of studies dedicated to TCM, revealing a fascinating overlap between mainstream and complementary practices in respiratory management. China is the leading contributor to this growing body of work, predominantly from TCM universities. Primary interventions such as Tai Chi and acupuncture have similarly gained interest due to their therapeutic applications and implications in improving patients' lung function and quality of life. This new focus is an extension of the general appreciation for holistic therapies within medicine, signaling that subsequent research will continue to explore further the efficacy of combining ancient and modern therapeutic approaches (Yang et al., 2025). Incorporating these strategies highlights the evolving world of pulmonary critical care and confirms the relevance of ongoing research and inter-professional interaction. Specifically, the discussions identify that technical progress on diagnostics, i.e., T-POCUS, will continue to improve clinical practice through timely and precise diagnoses of respiratory disorders. Concurrently, the search for TCM as an adjunct treatment elicits reconsideration of how diverse treatment modalities can be harmoniously incorporated into patient care. In response to the sustained challenges posed by respiratory illnesses to healthcare systems worldwide, discussions on these major concerns will likely drive new ideas for treatment and improve patient outcomes in intensive care. This multilayered perspective emphasizes the importance of flexible strategies in addressing the multifaceted nature of pulmonary disease care.

KEY TERMS FROM THIS CHAPTER

Acute Respiratory Distress Syndrome
Airway management
Bronchospasm
Critical illness neuropathy
Extracorporeal membrane oxygenation
Hemodynamic monitoring
Hypercapnia
Hypoxemia
Lung-protective ventilation strategy
Mechanical ventilation
Non-invasive ventilation (NIV)
Oxygen therapy
Positive End-Expiratory Pressure (PEEP)
Pulmonary artery catheter
Pulmonary embolism
Tracheostomy
Ventilator-associated pneumonia (VAP)

Critical Thinking Questions

1. **What is the primary indication for endotracheal intubation in a patient with acute respiratory failure?**
    a. Mild hypoxemia
    b. Severe respiratory distress with inability to protect airway
    c. Fever and cough
    d. Chronic cough
2. **In acute respiratory distress syndrome (ARDS), what is the recommended tidal volume setting for mechanical ventilation?**
    a. 15 mL/kg ideal body weight
    b. 10 mL/kg ideal body weight
    c. 6 mL/kg ideal body weight
    d. 20 mL/kg ideal body weight
3. **Which of the following is the preferred oxygen delivery method for a patient with moderate hypoxemia?**
    a. Nasal cannula
    b. Non-rebreather mask
    c. Mechanical ventilation
    d. Room air
4. **What is the main complication to monitor for in patients receiving positive pressure ventilation?**
    a. Pulmonary embolism
    b. Barotrauma (pneumothorax)
    c. Pulmonary fibrosis
    d. Asthma exacerbation
5. **Which medication is commonly used as a first-line treatment for status asthmaticus in the ICU?**
    a. Intravenous corticosteroids
    b. Oral antihistamines
    c. Beta blockers
    d. Loop diuretics

Short Answer Questions

1. What are the indications for mechanical ventilation in patients with respiratory failure?
2. Describe the differences between hypoxemic and hypercapnic respiratory failure and their common causes.
3. What are the key ventilator settings to adjust when managing acute respiratory distress syndrome (ARDS)?
4. How is ventilator-associated pneumonia (VAP) diagnosed and prevented in the ICU?
5. What are the common causes and management strategies for acute exacerbations of chronic obstructive pulmonary disease (COPD) in critical care?

Answer to Critical Thinking Questions

1. (b); 2. (c); 3. (a); 4. (b); 5. (a)

References

1. Migliori, G. B., Dheda, K., Centis, R., Mwaba, P., Bates, M., O'Grady, J., Hoelscher, M., & Zumla, A. (2010). Review of multidrug-resistant and extensively drug-resistant TB: global perspectives with a focus on sub-Saharan Africa. *Tropical Medicine & International Health, 15*(9), 1052–1066. https://doi.org/10.1111/j.1365-3156.2010.02581.xAlhazzani, W., Møller, M. H., Arabi, Y. M., Loeb, M., Gong, M. N., Fan, E., Oczkowski, S., et al. (2020). Surviving Sepsis Campaign: Guidelines on the management of critically ill adults with Coronavirus Disease 2019 (COVID-19). *Intensive Care Medicine, 46*, 854–887. https://doi.org/10.1007/s00134-020-06022-5 (accessed on 30th June 2025).
2. Alrashdaa, S. N., Alanazi, S. N., Alanazi, M. M., Althobaiti, F. A., Khalf Alanazi, A. H., & Alinze, M. O. (2023). Lung transplant: Navigating challenges and advancements in pulmonary medicine. *International Journal of Engineering Applied Sciences and Technology*. https://www.semanticscholar.org/paper/0763090f68f74284c45b597036d548d22f9d5803 (accessed on 30th June 2025).
3. Amaducci, S., Bacci, E., Baldacci, S., Bartoli, L., et al. (2018). Inhalation therapy in the next decade: Determinants of adherence to treatment in asthma and COPD. https://core.ac.uk/download/152415584.pdf (accessed on 30th June 2025).
4. Armenise, A. (2025). Point-of-care lung ultrasound in small animal emergency and critical care medicine: A clinical review. *Animals: An Open Access Journal from MDPI, 15*. https://www.semanticscholar.org/paper/31d23dfd32491c3ab0d6d24a29d1c38bc4a5eb14 (accessed on 30th June 2025).
5. Avouac, J., Behrens, F., Denton, C. P., Distler, O., et al. (2010). Interactions between rheumatologists and cardio-/pulmonologists in the assessment and use of outcome measures in pulmonary arterial hypertension related to systemic sclerosis. https://core.ac.uk/download/604507164.pdf (accessed on 30th June 2025).
6. Baloglu, O., McArthur, J., & Rowan, C. (2014). Non-infectious pulmonary complications of hematopoietic stem cell transplantation. https://core.ac.uk/download/228066089.pdf (accessed on 30th June 2025).
7. Banaszewski, M., Bot, E., Braun, F., Celutkiene, J., et al. (2020). Pre-hospital management protocols and perceived difficulty in diagnosing acute heart failure. https://core.ac.uk/download/322829086.pdf (accessed on 30th June 2025).
8. Banerjee, D., Aijaz, S., Nassikas, N., Singh, P., Lakshman, S., Boyd, C., Brown, Q., et al. (2024). Perspectives on using race in pulmonary function testing: A national survey fellows and program directors. *Respiratory Care, 69*, 1371–1379. https://www.semanticscholar.org/paper/19429c2bd1532d7c109f7316f9ba99ae8867a1bc (accessed on 30th June 2025).
9. Battalian, T., Escudero Romero, R., & Barzaga Molina, A. (2025). Characteristics and temporality of the ventilatory techniques in the management of acute respiratory distress syndrome: A scoping review. *The Journal of Critical Care Medicine, 11*, 122–131. https://www.semanticscholar.org/paper/a414c24543da5b0470edeee0af2f18f259abb5a6 (accessed on 30th June 2025).
10. Bueno, H., Christ, M., Cowie, M., Cullen, L., et al. (2017). Indications and practical approach to non-invasive ventilation in acute heart failure. https://core.ac.uk/download/144473095.pdf (accessed on 30th June 2025).

11. Carl, J., Cheplygina, V., de Bruijne, M., Paschaloudi, S., et al. (2018). Automatic emphysema detection using weakly labeled HRCT lung images. https://core.ac.uk/download/161520273.pdf (accessed on 30th June 2025).

12. Chang, D., Kamangar, N., Lee, M., Liebler, J., et al. (2019). Time-limited trials among critically ill patients with advanced medical illnesses to reduce nonbeneficial intensive care unit treatments: Protocol for a multicenter quality improvement study. https://core.ac.uk/download/323082942.pdf (accessed on 30th June 2025).

13. Chimbira, W., Crawford, H., Gupta, S., Legg, J., et al. (2001). Acute lung injury in pediatric intensive care: Course and outcome. https://core.ac.uk/download/pdf/8715345.pdf (accessed on 30th June 2025).

14. Chinese Thoracic Society, Chinese Medical Association; Critical Care Medicine Group, Chinese Association of Chest Physician, Chinese Medical Doctor Association. (2023). [Expert consensus on management of pain, agitation and related issues in adult patients with critical respiratory diseases]. *Zhonghua Jie He He Hu Xi Za Zhi = Zhonghua Jiehe He Huxi Zazhi = Chinese Journal of Tuberculosis and Respiratory Diseases, 46*(12), 1162–1175. https://www.semanticscholar.org/paper/119452f6986d1bf3eee242f31957caf919db3151 (accessed on 30th June 2025).

15. Chopra, V., Toner, E., Waldhorn, R., & Washer, L. (2020). How should U.S. hospitals prepare for Coronavirus Disease 2019 (COVID-19)? *Annals of Internal Medicine, 172*, 621–622. https://doi.org/10.7326/m20-0907 (accessed on 30th June 2025).

16. Collard, H. R., & Oldham, J. M. (2017). Comorbid conditions in idiopathic pulmonary fibrosis: Recognition and management. https://core.ac.uk/download/323072212.pdf (accessed on 30th June 2025).

17. Conrad, A. M., Zimmermann, J., Mohr, D., Froelich, M., Hertel, A., Rathmann, N., Boesing, C., et al. (2024). Quantification of pulmonary edema using automated lung segmentation on computed tomography in mechanically ventilated patients with acute respiratory distress syndrome. *Intensive Care Medicine Experimental, 12*. https://www.semanticscholar.org/paper/1addccc3e6ab6679c222745589379e1f97ee9c68 (accessed on 30th June 2025).

18. Davies, M. J., D'Alessio, D. A., Fradkin, J., Kernan, W. N., Mathieu, C., Mingrone, G., Rossing, P., et al. (2018). Management of hyperglycemia in type 2 diabetes, 2018: A consensus report by the American Diabetes Association (ADA) and the European Association for the Study of Diabetes (EASD). *Diabetes Care, 41*, 2669–2701. https://doi.org/10.2337/dci18-0033 (accessed on 30th June 2025).

19. Doghramji, K., Grewal, R. G., Vasu, D., et al. (2012). Obstructive sleep apnea syndrome and perioperative complications: A systematic review of the literature. https://core.ac.uk/download/83049558.pdf (accessed on 30th June 2025).

20. Dukhovny, D., Guyatt, G., Jack, S., Kirpalani, H., et al. (2019). Factors influencing decision making in neonatology: Inhaled nitric oxide in preterm infants. https://core.ac.uk/download/323069963.pdf (accessed on 30th June 2025).

21. Elbaih, A., & Mousa, M. A. (2020). Teaching review on approach of esophageal intubation as complications in emergency airway management. https://www.semanticscholar.org/paper/e34aed638c2247a8e938bd3b48873d95f084905e (accessed on 30th June 2025).

22. Fairhurst, K., Juvekar, S., McKinstry, B., Patil, R., et al. (2021). Specialist to non-specialist teleconsultations in chronic respiratory disease management: A systematic review. https://

core.ac.uk/download/475141525.pdf (accessed on 30th June 2025).

23. Georgakopoulou, V. (2025). Optimizing patient outcomes in interstitial lung disease through pre- and post-transplant management strategies. *World Journal of Transplantation*. https://www.semanticscholar.org/paper/74d796ce4e10c18b673a1a8aa1a7e0fab37d130e (accessed on 30th June 2025).

24. Ghattas, A. H. S., & Abdou, H. A. A. (2025). Challenges and best practices for moving forward in interprofessional collaboration in critical care units: Nurses' perspectives. *BMC Nursing, 24*. https://www.semanticscholar.org/paper/55aa717c4753ec9a7e6ffd3803af6c8d05b5c6f2 (accessed on 30th June 2025).

25. Harari, A., Zumla, A., Armand, M., Axelsson-Robertson, R., Banada, P., Marais, B., Betsou, F., et al. (2012). Tuberculosis diagnostics and biomarkers: Needs, challenges, recent advances, and opportunities. https://core.ac.uk/download/9839032.pdf (accessed on 30th June 2025).

26. Iavarone, I. G., Al-Husinat, L., Vélez-Páez, J., Robba, C., Silva, P. L., Rocco, P., & Battaglini, D. (2024). Management of neuromuscular blocking agents in critically ill patients with lung diseases. *Journal of Clinical Medicine, 13*. https://www.semanticscholar.org/paper/b61694948466426ac13702e66e30ec13e34f1d55 (accessed on 30th June 2025).

27. Jia, Y., Cheng, G., Wang, H., Ma, B., Cai, Y., Ren, X., Guo, Y., et al. (2025). Barriers and facilitators to implementing pulmonary rehabilitation guidelines in China: A qualitative study using implementation science frameworks. *Health Research Policy and Systems, 23*. https://www.semanticscholar.org/paper/6c808604dec09cd4feb6460be0b04a93a7917312 (accessed on 30th June 2025).

28. Joyce, E., Guerin, S., Synman, L., & Ryberg, M. (2025). Exploring perspectives of supporting the process of dying, death and bereavement among critical care staff: A multidisciplinary, qualitative approach. *Journal of the Intensive Care Society, 26*, 21–28. https://www.semanticscholar.org/paper/aa5f9757e3fdaf7d118b28cbc37670390d312efb (accessed on 30th June 2025).

29. Kamal, M., Nagy, M., & Hassanain, O. (2024). Improving resource allocation in the precision medicine era: A simulation-based approach using R. *Personalized Medicine, 21*(3), 151–161. https://www.semanticscholar.org/paper/5da5b37042d4ed55e7952803b82f5c36679cc801 (accessed on 30th June 2025).

30. Khouli, H., & Nigam, A. (2020). Ten minutes with Hassan Khouli, chair of Department of Critical Care Medicine, Respiratory Institute, Cleveland Clinic. *BMJ Leader, 4*, 162–164. https://www.semanticscholar.org/paper/4e43f35cd0d69d5e02923481052170b481cabe16 (accessed on 30th June 2025).

31. Kirchhof, P., Benussi, S., Kotecha, D., Ahlsson, A., Atar, D., Casadei, B., Castellá, M., et al. (2016). 2016 ESC guidelines for the management of atrial fibrillation developed in collaboration with EACTS. *European Heart Journal, 37*, 2893–2962. https://doi.org/10.1093/eurheartj/ehw210 (accessed on 30th June 2025).

32. Kushwaha, N., Attry, S., Gugnani, A., & Saharan, A. (2025). Bronchial hygiene in critical care: Enhancing pulmonary function in mechanically ventilated patients. *European Journal of Molecular and Clinical Medicine*. https://www.semanticscholar.org/paper/faec94e79c6c96ab7f046949c81464adc232fda8 (accessed on 30th June 2025).

33. Lyon, A. R., López-Fernández, T., Couch, L. S., Asteggiano, R., Aznar, M. C., Bergler-Klein, J.,

Boriani, G., et al. (2022). 2022 ESC guidelines on cardio-oncology developed in collaboration with the European Hematology Association (EHA), the European Society for Therapeutic Radiology and Oncology (ESTRO) and the International Cardio-Oncology Society (IC-OS). *European Heart Journal, 43*, 4229–4361. https://doi.org/10.1093/eurheartj/ehac244 (accessed on 30th June 2025).

34. Martins, I. T., Golgher, S. A., Biagi, J., da Silva, U., Victor, G., & Freire, R. (2025). Advances in the management of chronic obstructive pulmonary disease. *Asclepius International Journal of Scientific Health Science*. https://www.semanticscholar.org/paper/edea14b439efca18c85037e6e05747b3334dab38 (accessed on 30th June 2025).

35. Milks, M. W., Sahay, S., Benza, R. L., & Farber, H. W. (2020). Risk assessment in patients with pulmonary arterial hypertension in the era of COVID-19 pandemic and the telehealth revolution: State of the art review. *The Journal of Heart and Lung Transplantation, 40*, 172–182. https://doi.org/10.1016/j.healun.2020.12.005 (accessed on 30th June 2025).

36. Okada, K., Tsuchiya, K., Sakai, K., Kuragano, T., Uchida, A., Tsuruya, K., Tomo, T., et al. (2021). Shared decision making for the initiation and continuation of dialysis: A proposal from the Japanese Society for Dialysis Therapy. *Renal Replacement Therapy, 7*, 1–23. https://www.semanticscholar.org/paper/36dbbd6e2437edaf4c10c6058d223e74c727c934 (accessed on 30th June 2025).

37. Page, M. J., Moher, D., Bossuyt, P. M., Boutron, I., Hoffmann, T., Mulrow, C. D., Shamseer, L., et al. (2021). PRISMA 2020 explanation and elaboration: Updated guidance and exemplars for reporting systematic reviews. *BMJ*. https://doi.org/10.1136/bmj.n160 (accessed on 30th June 2025).

38. Pamidi, S., Mehra, R., Gurubhagavatula, I., & Teodorescu, M. (2025). Initial self-reported data on sleep and burnout in pulmonary, critical care and sleep medicine: An initiative from the Assembly on Sleep and Respiratory Neurobiology of the American Thoracic Society. *Respiratory Research, 26*. https://www.semanticscholar.org/paper/80fbd4f01b2c994bdcd6a4d025e2439a6029ce7c (accessed on 30th June 2025).

39. Pan, P., & Xie, L. (2023). [Clinical update in critical care of pulmonary medicine 2022]. *Zhonghua Jie He He Hu Xi Za Zhi = Zhonghua Jiehe He Huxi Zazhi = Chinese Journal of Tuberculosis and Respiratory Diseases, 46*(1), 72–76. https://www.semanticscholar.org/paper/2ac3665a8901cf8587961eb12dfecca87159a9ca (accessed on 30th June 2025).

40. Rabe, K., Rennard, S., Martinez, F. J., Celli, B., Singh, D., Papi, A., Bafadhel, M., et al. (2023). Targeting type 2 inflammation and epithelial alarmins in chronic obstructive pulmonary disease: A biologics outlook. *American Journal of Respiratory and Critical Care Medicine*. https://www.semanticscholar.org/paper/7dd12fdacbbdd402ec7b3d02f84bbc5e58ca3439 (accessed on 30th June 2025).

41. Rodemund, N., Wernly, B., Jung, C., Cozowicz, C., & Koköfer, A. (2023). Striking the balance: Privacy protection and data accessibility in critical care research. *Intensive Care Medicine, 49*, 1029–1030. https://www.semanticscholar.org/paper/3aed6976a8d39144125861e06bb9b242acef5724 (accessed on 30th June 2025).

42. Shojaei, A., & Delrobaei, M. (2025). Severity classification of chronic obstructive pulmonary disease in intensive care units: A semi-supervised approach using MIMIC-III dataset. https://www.semanticscholar.org/paper/9091862b8f7ea915adcbb9e5471920e2b2c3826f (accessed on 30th June 2025).

43. Simpson, C., Ledford, J., & Liu, G. (2024). Application of metabolomics across the spectrum of pulmonary and critical care medicine. *American Journal of Respiratory Cell and Molecular Biology*. https://www.semanticscholar.org/paper/e7a23af69f8c45815260dd11f1a23dfbc71a5829 (accessed on 30th June 2025).

44. Singh, D., Han, M. K., Bhatt, S. P., Miravitlles, M., Compton, C., Kolterer, S., Mohan, T., et al. (2024). Is disease stability an attainable COPD treatment goal? *American Journal of Respiratory and Critical Care Medicine*. https://www.semanticscholar.org/paper/1a63287c992f29dcc697e34502f45ffe5c2a3b94 (accessed on 30th June 2025).

45. Umasankar, R., & Saravanabavan, V. (2024). Geospatial analysis of health care resource allocation in Karur district: Insights from GIS. *ShodhKosh: Journal of Visual and Performing Arts*. https://www.semanticscholar.org/paper/c689d6a7ab24d7e551a3fb39f73f506b25884d27 (accessed on 30th June 2025).

46. Wang, J., Cui, Z., Liu, S., Gao, X., Gao, P., Shi, Y., Guo, S., et al. (2017). Early use of noninvasive techniques for clearing respiratory secretions during noninvasive positive-pressure ventilation in patients with acute exacerbation of chronic obstructive pulmonary disease and hypercapnic encephalopathy. *Medicine, 96*. https://www.semanticscholar.org/paper/7b07d84d4d37da6db3e2d6916c24faf111d3a021 (accessed on 30th June 2025).

47. Yang, C., He, Q., Huang, L., Tian, H., Luo, Q., Xu, G., Sun, M., et al. (2025). Research trends of traditional Chinese medicine therapies on chronic obstructive pulmonary disease: A bibliometric analysis. *Complementary Medicine Research, 32*, 67–83. https://www.semanticscholar.org/paper/a28bb0a1bad513a1afdd3359b5059bab17928eef (accessed on 30th June 2025).

48. Yang, T., Qumu, M. S. W., Li, X. P., Wang, S. Y., He, J. Z., & Yang, T. (2024). [Correlation of body composition indicators with exercise capacity and nutritional status in male patients with chronic obstructive pulmonary disease]. *Zhonghua Yi Xue Za Zhi, 104*(36), 3402–3408. https://www.semanticscholar.org/paper/8e08a6c0bd4712429126ab8daaf935193336be34 (accessed on 30th June 2025).

49. Yu, P., Wei, Q., & He, C. (2020). Early rehabilitation for critically ill patients with COVID-19: More benefits than risks. *American Journal of Physical Medicine & Rehabilitation, 99*, 468–469. https://doi.org/10.1097/phm.0000000000001445 (accessed on 30th June 2025).

50. Yuan, L., Chaudhari, V., Rabin, S., McClintic, M., Desai, P., Beck, T., Chen, E., et al. (2025). Discussing end-of-life in the intensive care unit: Education practices in pulmonary and critical care medicine fellowship programs. *The American Journal of Hospice & Palliative Care*. https://www.semanticscholar.org/paper/9f41e419e026d3addd6cd3f612591a51fb531cdf (accessed on 30th June 2025).

51. Zeppenfeld, K., Tfelt-Hansen, J., Riva, M., Winkel, B. G., Behr, E. R., Blom, N. A., Charron, P., et al. (2022). 2022 ESC guidelines for the management of patients with ventricular arrhythmias and the prevention of sudden cardiac death. *European Heart Journal, 43*, 3997–4126. https://doi.org/10.1093/eurheartj/ehac262 (accessed on 30th June 2025).

INDEX

D

E

J

L

M

R

S